D1568422

The Pathology of
Congenital Heart Disease

A Personal Experience With More Than
6,300 Congenitally Malformed Hearts

Volume 2

by

Saroja Bharati, MD

and

Maurice Lev, BS, MD, MA (Phil.)

On the cover

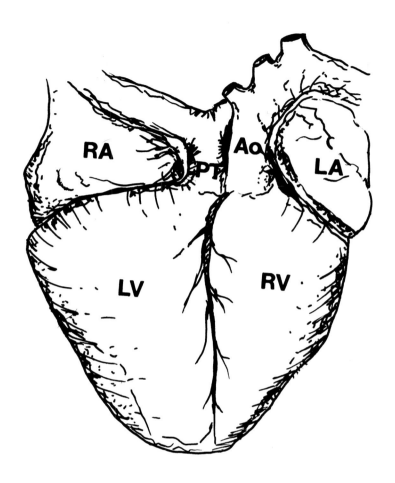

Mixed levocardia (atria in normal position, ventricles inverted) with complete inverted transposition (corrected transposition; external view of the heart. RA = morphological right atrium; LV = morphological left ventricle; PT = pulmonary trunk situated right and posterior and emerging from the morphological left ventricle; LA = morphological left atrium; RV = morphological right ventricle; Ao = aorta situated left and anterior and emerging from the morphological right ventricle. Note: The anterior descending coronary artery is situated to the right side of the aorta.

The Pathology of
Congenital Heart Disease

A Personal Experience With More Than 6,300 Congenitally Malformed Hearts

by

Saroja Bharati, MD

Director
Congenital Heart and Conduction System Center
The Heart Institute for Children of
Christ Hospital and Medical Center
Oak Lawn, Illinois;
Advocate Health Care
Professor of Pathology
Rush Medical College, Rush University
Rush-Presbyterian–St. Lukes Medical Center
Chicago, Illinois;
Clinical Professor of Pathology
Finch University of Health Sciences
Chicago Medical School
North Chicago, Illinois

and

Maurice Lev, BS, MD, MA (Phil.)[†]

Associate Director
Congenital Heart and Conduction System Center,
The Heart Institute for Children of
Christ Hospital and Medical Center
Oak Lawn, Illinois;
Advocate Health Care,
Distinguished Professor of Pathology
Medicine and Pediatrics
Rush Medical College, Rush University,
Rush-Presbyterian–St. Lukes Medical Center
Chicago, Illinois

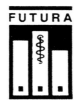

FUTURA

Futura Publishing Company, Inc.
Armonk, NY

[†]deceased

Library of Congress Cataloging-in-Publication Data

Bharati, Saroja, Lev, Maurice.
    The pathology of congenital heart disease : a personal experience
with more than 6,300 congenitally malformed hearts / by Saroja
Bharati and Maurice Lev.
        p.   cm.
    Includes bibliographical references and index.
    ISBN 0-87993-556-1 (2 v. set)
    1. Congenital heart disease.
II. Title.
    [DNLM: 1. Heart Defects, Congenital—pathology.   WG 220 B575p
1996]
RC687.B48   1996
616.1′2043—dc20
DNLM/DLC
for Library of Congress   95-24407
                                                       CIP

Copyright 1996
Futura Publishing Company, Inc.

Published by
Futura Publishing Company, Inc.
135 Bedford Road
Armonk, NY 10504-0418

LC #: 95-24407
ISBN#: 0-87993-556-1

Every effort has been made to ensure that the information in this book is as up to date and as accurate as possible at the time of publication. However, due to the constant developments in medicine, neither the authors or the publisher can accept any legal or any other responsibility for any errors or omissions that may occur.

Printed in the United States of America on acid-free paper.

*This book is dedicated
to the memory of my
beloved parents
Mr. and Mrs. L.R. Bharati*

Acknowledgments

We are indebted to the more than 6,300 infants, children, and adults whose congenitally malformed hearts made it possible for this newer knowledge to be created. We are also grateful to those people who took care of these sick people. This group of medical, surgical, nursing, and paramedical people constitutes those who practice in the profession and give their time to benefit mankind. This group also includes the families of the sick ones whom we professional people try to help in their misery and discomfort.

We thank the pediatric cardiologists, cardiologists, cardiac surgeons, pathologists, and medical examiners not only in Chicago and New Jersey but also all over the country and elsewhere in world for enriching us and constantly updating the knowledge in this field without which this book would not be possible. There are literally innumerable physicians involved in educating us, and we do not want to omit even one who contributed to our knowledge, but compiling such a list would include the entire cardiology community and we therefore say thank you to all our colleagues, co-workers, and friends who taught us and expanded our thinking. A list of the entire cardiology community all over the globe and those who donated the hearts to our Center would form a monograph by itself.

Our very special thanks to all the secretaries who helped us in many ways. Although many were involved, there are four who helped more than others. They are Edie Webster, Vicki Crump, Joyce Conti, and, last but not least, my secretary Kay Pinson, who worked with me enthusiastically and made it all possible. Had it not been for her help and understanding, this project would not be completed. I sincerely thank my artist, Marilyn Uhl, who has stood by me ever since I entered this field and did most of the art work in this project.

We want to thank all our dear and near ones, which includes our families, friends, and our well wishers who understood our quest for knowledge. To the dear and near ones who we know always felt that we did not spend much time with them, we wish to tell them that we were not away from them intentionally. To do our best, a book of this nature takes a certain amount of time and energy in a given period of time to accomplish this task.

And finally, had it not been for the good will, good wishes, and prayers of my sisters and brothers, Babs, An, Chin, Vardu, Sarasa, Viji, and their families, this work would not have been accomplished.

My very special thanks to my publishers, Steven Korn and Jacques Strauss, for their constant encouragement over the last many years. Words cannot express my gratitude to Linda Shaw, Senior Editor at Futura, who worked not only on this book but also on our previous two books, *The Cardiac Conduction System in Unexplained Sudden Death* in 1990, and *Cardiac Surgery and the Conduction System* in 1992. She worked tirelessly and enthusiastically, making this task a great joy.

Saroja Bharati, MD
Maurice Lev, MD

Preface

I am humbly presenting to you the cumulative knowledge in pathology of congenital heart disease as seen by Dr. Maurice Lev and myself. This includes 6,307 congenitally malformed hearts out of almost 7,000 congenitally malformed hearts that we had the privilege to study in detail. A systematic study of pathological examination of congenitally malformed hearts was initiated by Dr. Lev nearly 60 years ago to which is added my experience in this field for the last 25 years. Since 1970 I have had the good fortune of working with Dr. Lev until February of 1994. This, therefore, includes the experience in this field starting from where the great Maude Abbott left off (pathology of 1,000 congenitally malformed hearts originally published in 1932 and later republished in her Atlas in 1936) until now.

Thus, this may be considered the 20th century's accumulated knowledge in pathology of congenital heart disease. However, I emphasize that this by no means is complete or perfect, and that is not the intention of this presentation. No knowledge is complete, and congenital heart disease is not an exception. The sole purpose of this presentation is to share with you all the knowledge that we accumulated in this field in this century. We hope that our book will help the clinicians and surgeons in making the diagnosis of congenital heart disease and correcting the lesions, nonsurgically or surgically, as best they can. We also hope that our book will stimulate the basic scientists, particularly in the field of genetics, immunology, and molecular biology. Finally, we also hope the epidemiologists, statisticians, and computer experts will find this book useful.

Again, the main purpose of this book is to share our experience in the pathology of congenital heart disease with those who are interested in this subject. I sincerely hope that the knowledge presented in this book will revitalize this field and stimulate newer thinking in the creation of newer concepts in the care of the patient with a congenitally malformed heart.

Saroja Bharati, MD

Contents

x • *THE PATHOLOGY OF CONGENITAL HEART DISEASE*

Abbreviations Used in This Book

AA = aortic arch or ascending aorta
AAL = aorta anterior and left
AAR = aorta anterior and right
AI = aortic insufficiency
AL = anterior leaflet
AO = aorta
APM = anterior papillary muscle
AS = aortic stenosis
ASD = atrial septal defect
AV = atrioventricular
AV valve = atrioventricular valve

Bi = bicuspid
Bicuspid AV = bicuspid aortic valve

CAVO = common atrioventricular orifice
CFB = central fibrous body
CS = coronary sinus
CT = complete transposition

D = defect
DOLV = double outlet left ventricle
DORV = double outlet right ventricle

FC = fetal (preductal) coarctation
FOD = fossa ovalis defect

LA = left atrium
LAP = left atrial appendage
LAV = left atrioventricular valve
LLPV = lower left pulmonary vein
LPV = left pulmonary vein
LSVC = left superior vena cava
LSVC → CS = left superior vena cava entering coronary
  sinus
Lt = left
LUPV = left upper pulmonary vein
LV = left ventricle

MC = main chamber
MI = mitral insufficiency
MS = mitral stenosis

MV = mitral valve
MVC = main ventricular chamber

PA = pulmonary atresia
PAPVD = partial anomalous pulmonary venous
  drainage
PB = parietal band
PDA = patent ductus arteriosus
PFO = patent foramen ovale
PPL = pulmonary posterior and left
PPM = posterior papillary muscle
PPR = pulmonary posterior and right
PM = papillary muscle
Pvein = pulmonary vein
PS = pulmonary stenosis
PT = pulmonary trunk
PV = pulmonary valve

RA = right atrium
RAA = right aortic arch
RAP = right atrial appendage
RAV = right atrioventricular valve
RSVC = right superior vena cava
Rt = right
RV = right ventricle

SA = sinoatrial
SAN = sinoatrial node
SB = septal band
SBE = infective endocarditis
SOC = small outlet chamber
SVC = superior vena cava

TAPVD = total anomalous pulmonary venous drainage
TI = tricuspid insufficiency
TS = tricuspid stenosis
TV = tricuspid valve

VF = ventricular fibrillation
VSD = ventricular septal defect

51

Ventricular Septal Defect with Pulmonary Stenosis

In this entity, the defect may be situated anywhere in the ventricular septum, and the pulmonary stenosis is usually infundibular associated with valvular stenosis. There is either a fossa ovalis defect or a patent foramen ovale accompanying the lesion. There is hypertrophy and enlargement of the right atrium with hypertrophy of the right ventricle.

Analysis of Our Material

There was a total of six cases: four males, one female, and one unknown. The youngest was 19 weeks of age and the oldest 12 years, with a mean of 5 years.

The Complex

The right atrium was either hypertrophied and enlarged or hypertrophied. The right ventricle was usually hypertrophied or hypertrophied and enlarged. The left side of the heart was either normal or atrophied and rarely hypertrophied and enlarged.

The Valves

The tricuspid orifice size had a tendency to be smaller than normal and the pulmonic orifice size was usually smaller than normal, and in one it was very small. The mitral and the aortic orifices were either normal or smaller than normal, and in one they were enlarged. The tricuspid valve was normally formed in three with distinctly increased hemodynamic change. In two, the valve revealed considerable thickening or space between the anterior and septal leaflets with thickening close to the region of the defect. In one case, the valve was an Ebstein-like malformation with re-

dundant, thickened leaflets and a poorly developed anterolateral papillary muscle. The pulmonic valve was bicuspid in three, and was markedly thickened or dome-shaped. In one, there was poststenotic dilatation of the main pulmonary trunk. The mitral valve was normally formed in all except one, where the anterolateral papillary muscle proceeded to the base of the valve. The aortic valve was normally formed in four, markedly thickened in one, and was bicuspid and thickened in another. The complex associated with each heart is as follows:

1. Right aortic arch, usual VSD, pulmonary valvular and infundibular stenosis, large bronchial artery going to the right lung with a patent foramen ovale.

2. Pulmonary valvular and infundibular stenosis with VSD and surgical closure of the defect resulting in heart block. This was accompanied by a left superior vena cava entering the coronary sinus.

3. Infundibular and pulmonary valvular stenosis with spontaneously closed VSD (Figs. 1, 2). This was associated with a high origin of the right coronary ostium and an oblique patent foramen ovale.

4. Stenosis of the pulmonary veins with infundibular and valvular pulmonary stenosis and surgical closure of VSD and ASD.

5. Pulmonary valvular and infundibular stenosis with tricuspid stenosis and insufficiency, muscular VSD, fossa ovalis ASD, anomalous chordal connections in the left ventricle, common brachiocephalic trunk, and left subclavian artery away from it.

6. Double VSD, infundibular pulmonary stenosis, infective endocarditis (Figs. 3, 4), and fossa ovalis defect extending proximally.

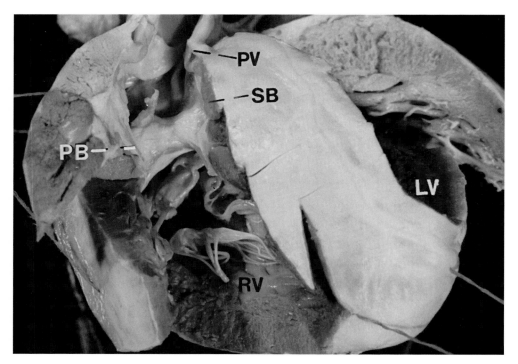

Figure 1: Anomalous parietal band in the outflow tract of the right ventricle producing infundibular pulmonary stenosis. RV = right ventricle; LV = left ventricle; PV = small pulmonary valve with stenosis; SB = abbreviated hypertrophied septal band; PB = anomalous parietal band criss-crossing the outflow tract of the right ventricle causing infundibular pulmonary stenosis.

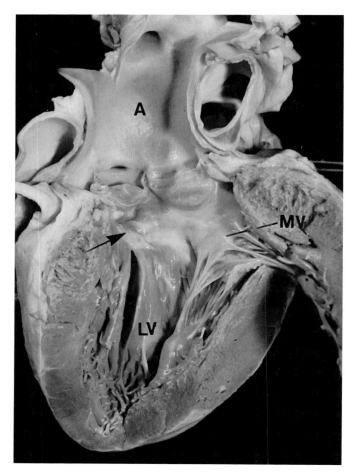

Figure 2: Left ventricular view of Figure 1 demonstrating the spontaneously closed ventricular septal defect by means of a small aneurysm. A = aorta; MV = mitral valve; LV = left ventricle. Arrow points to the small aneurysm of the membranous septum. Note the high origin of the right coronary ostium.

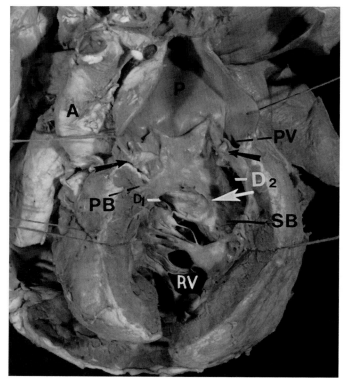

Figure 3: Outflow tract of the right ventricle demonstrating infundibular pulmonary stenosis, marked right ventricular hypertrophy, with infective endocarditis of the pulmonary valve and the infundibular region. A = aorta; P = pulmonary trunk showing poststenotic dilatation; PV = pulmonary valve; RV = right ventricle; SB = septal band; PB = markedly abbreviated deviated parietal band; D_1 = defect beneath the junction of the anterior and septal leaflets of the tricuspid valve; D_2 = second ventricular septal defect in an oblique angle beneath the pulmonary valve in the conus area. Arrows point to infective endocarditis.

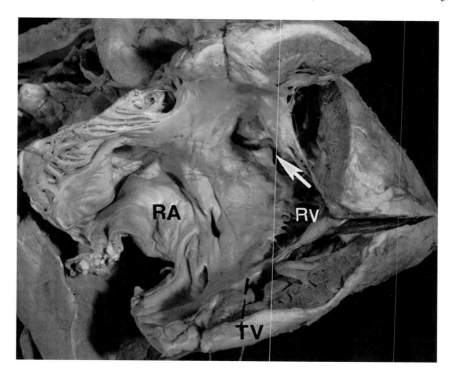

Figure 4: Right atrial, right ventricular view of Figure 3. RA = right atrium; TV = tricuspid valve; RV = right ventricle. Note the tremendous hypertrophy of the right ventricle, hypertrophy and enlargement of the right atrium, and diffusely thickened tricuspid valve, with considerable thickening at the junction of the anterior and septal leaflets. Arrow points to the thickened tricuspid valve near the VSD.

Comment

The one common denominator that emerges from all of the six cases is that there is always infundibular pulmonary stenosis, and the ventricular septal defect can be situated anywhere in the septum. However, the defect is not a tetralogy of Fallot type with U-shaped deficiency in the ventricular septum. Thus, we are dealing with a distinct anatomic abnormality where the architecture of the right ventricle presents abnormal orientation of the septal and parietal band muscles to a varying extent beneath the pulmonic valve with, in general, a small pulmonary orifice and thickened valvular tissue. It is of interest that the defect had closed spontaneously in one case.

If attempts are made to close the defect and open the valve by nonsurgical methods, the infundibular anatomy and the relationship of the tricuspid valve should be well delineated. It is also of interest that the atrial septum presents a defect or there may be an oblique patent foramen ovale.

52

Aortic Stenosis

There are three types of aortic stenosis: (1) valvular (Fig. 1), (2) subvalvular (Fig. 2), and (3) supravalvular (Fig. 3).

The Complex (Fig. 4)

There is pressure hypertrophy of the left ventricle to a varying extent and often of the left atrium and hemodynamic changes of the mitral valve, in some cases with stenosis and/or insufficiency of the valve. In the subaortic and supravalvular types, the aortic valve is always thickened and usually with a smaller than normal anulus. This may be either a hemodynamic effect or a structural part of the malformation. Poststenotic dilatation of the ascending aorta may or may not be present.

Valvular Aortic Stenosis

This must be distinguished as to the age group in which it is found. Below the age of about 2 years, such stenosis is both anular and valvular. The valve consists of a unicuspid, bicuspid (Fig. 1), or tricuspid but abnormally formed valve. The valvular tissue is irregularly thickened and nodular. The term now used to describe this valve is *dysplastic*. This lesion in most cases in this group is associated with fibroelastosis of the left ventricle and/or preductal (fetal) coarctation of the aorta (Fig. 1). In addition, the mitral valve may present abnormalities such as arcade and/or parachute-like malformations that may give rise to mitral stenosis and/or insufficiency.

There is some left ventricular hypertrophy with a normal or enlarged left ventricle. In extreme cases, this type of lesion may simulate a hypoplastic left heart syndrome. The myocardium of the left ventricle most frequently shows fibrotic and necrotic changes. The left atrium is also hypertrophied. In children and teenagers, the stenosis is usually more valvular than anular, but an anular element remains. In adulthood, the stenosis is usually valvular and related to the hemodynamic vicissitudes of a bicuspid valve. In middle and old age, bicuspid aortic valve with calcific stenosis is the usual eventuality. In some there may be some insufficiency of the valve as well (Fig. 5). A bicuspid valve may show no stenosis and be an incidental finding at autopsy in old age.

Subaortic Stenosis

Subaortic stenosis has a protean picture. It may be produced by a shelf or membrane, a plaque, or a ridge of fibroelastic tissue extending from the anterior part of the ventricular septum to the anterior leaflet of the mitral valve (Fig. 2). This lies a varying distance from the aortic valve starting from the base of the aortic valve itself and may extend up to ½ to 1 cm beneath the valve, producing a variously sized subaortic pocket or narrowed area, which may be in the form of a tunnel or a shelf or a platform.

Subaortic stenosis may be produced by a protuberance of muscle from the septum narrowing the outflow tract. This protuberance may be in the upper, middle, or lower third of the chamber (Fig. 6). Pressure hypertrophy of the left atrium and ventricle ensues. The main characteristic of this disease is the relatively greater hypertrophy of the septum as compared to the parietal wall of the left ventricle with distinct ventricular septal bulge. There may also be various developmental or hemodynamic changes in the mitral valve producing insufficiency. This involves the aortic leaflet of the mitral valve especially. In some, the posterior leaflet may be redundant or segmented with profuse elongated chordae. The protuberance of the muscle producing subaortic stenosis hemodynamically today is referred to as hypertrophic cardiomyopathy and this is

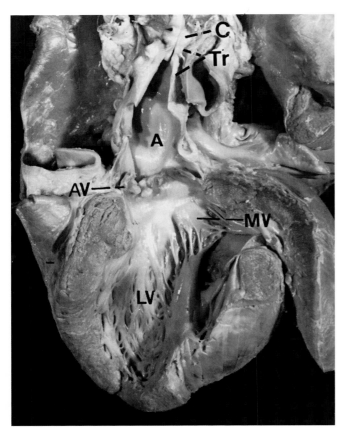

Figure 1: Bicuspid dysplastic aortic valve with stenosis. AV = bicuspid dysplastic thickened aortic valve; A = aorta; LV = left ventricle; MV = mitral valve; C = coarctation; Tr = transverse arch.

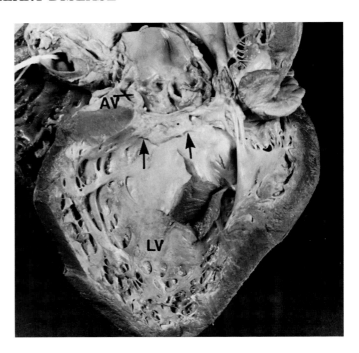

Figure 2: Subaortic stenosis of fibroelastic type; left ventricular view with aortic stenosis and insufficiency. Note the enlarged left ventricle. AV = markedly thickened deformed aortic valve with small anulus; LV = left ventricle. Arrows point to the irregular fibroelastic ridge beneath the aortic valve. Note the diffuse fibroelastosis of the left ventricle. (Used with permission from Lev M. See Figure 3.)

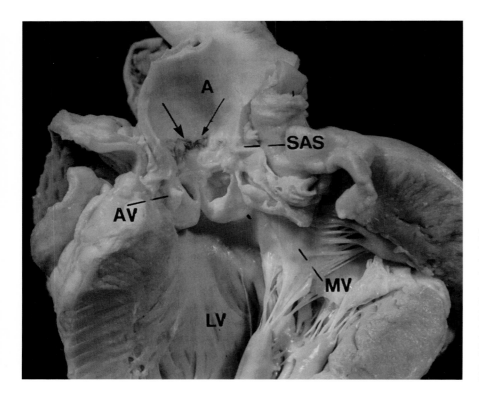

Figure 3: Supravalvular aortic stenosis with infective endarteritis. LV = left ventricle; MV = mitral valve; AV = thickened with mild aneurysm of the sinus of Valsalva of the aortic valve; SAS = supravalvular aortic stenosis; A = mild poststenotic dilatation of the ascending aorta. Arrows point to the infective endarteritis. (Used with permission from Lev M: *Autopsy Diagnosis of Congenitally Malformed Hearts.* Charles C. Thomas, Springfield, Illinois, 1953.)

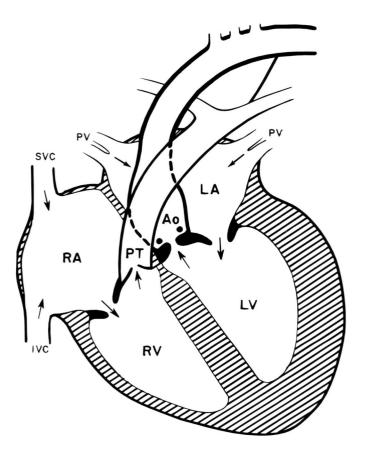

Figure 4: Schematic diagram of aortic stenosis complex. SVC = superior vena cava; IVC = inferior vena cava; RA = right atrium; RV = right ventricle; LA = left atrium; LV = left ventricle; PV = pulmonary vein; Ao = aorta; PT = pulmonary trunk.

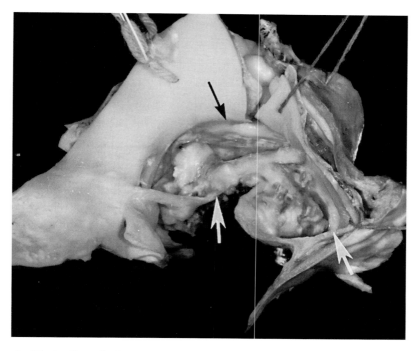

Figure 5: Markedly calcified bicuspid aortic valve with aortic stenosis and insufficiency, a close-up view of the calcified valve. Arrows point to the irregular calcification of the aortic valve.

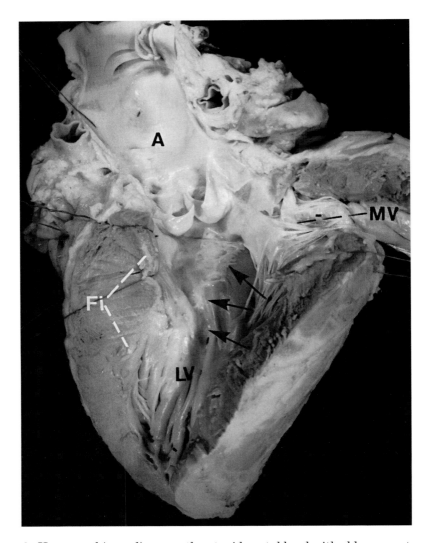

Figure 6: Hypertrophic cardiomyopathy at mid-septal level with old myomectomy and residual subaortic stenosis and sudden death. A = ascending aorta; LV = left ventricle; MV = mitral valve; Fi = fibroelastosis of the left ventricle. Arrows point to residual subaortic stenosis.

related to abnormal genes located on chromosome 14q, 15, 11, 7, 1, and probably many more. Sudden death may be the first manifestation of this disease.

Supravalvular Aortic Stenosis

Supravalvular aortic stenosis is of two types. There may be an accentuation of the supravalvular ridge, producing a narrowing at the upper margins of the sinus of Valsalva (Fig. 3). The aortic valve edge is thickened, the commissures are widened, and the mouths of the sinuses of Valsalva narrowed. In the other type, there is a narrowing about 1 cm above the sinuses of Valsalva produced by a ledge of thickening protruding into the aorta. In either case, there is again pressure hypertrophy of the left ventricle and atrium.

This entity may occur as an isolated lesion or may be associated with peripheral pulmonary stenosis, abnormal calcium metabolism, and abnormal-looking infant (atypical facies).

Although aortic stenosis may be classified into the above three distinct categories, it is emphasized that the stenosis frequently is at multiple levels in the left side of the heart and not an isolated obstructive phenomenon at one particular area related to the valve. This is especially true when there is subaortic obstruction.

Analysis of Our Material

In order to understand this lesion in its entirety, the material was classified as follows:

I Aortic stenosis below the age
   of 3 months   46–28%
II Aortic stenosis above the age
   of 3 months and below the   } 39%
   age of 2 years   18–11%
III Aortic stenosis above the age
    of 2 years   101–61%
                          Total   ‾‾165‾‾

I. Aortic Stenosis Below the Age of 3 Months

Analysis of Our Material

There was a total of 46 cases; 30 (65%) were male subjects and 16 (35%) were female subjects. The youngest was a 23.8-weeks' gestation fetus, and the oldest 2 months and 13 days, with a mean of 15.43 days.

The Complex

The heart was hypertrophied and enlarged in all with the apex formed by the left ventricle in 16 (35%), the right ventricle in 15 (32.5%), and by both ventricles in 15 (32.5%). The right atrium was hypertrophied and enlarged in 36 (78%) (Fig. 7), was hypertrophied in four

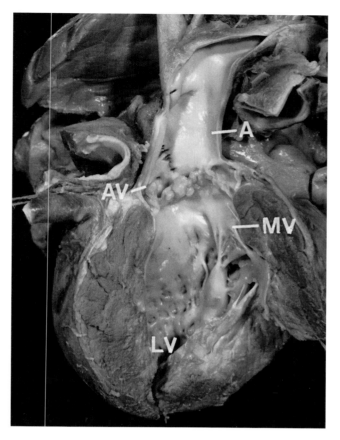

Figure 8: Unicuspid aortic valve with stenosis and marked left ventricular hypertrophy. AV = dysplastic unicuspid aortic valve; LV = small left ventricle with thick wall and hypertrophy; A = ascending aorta; MV = mitral valve.

(9%), enlarged in three (6.5%), and normal in size in three (6.5%). The right ventricle was hypertrophied and enlarged in 38 (83%) (Fig. 7), was hypertrophied in five (11%), normal in two (4%) and was enlarged in one (2%). The left atrium was hypertrophied and enlarged in 26 (57%), hypertrophied in 14 (30%), enlarged in three (6.5%), and was of normal size in three (6.5%). The left ventricle was hypertrophied and small with thick wall and fibroelastosis in 22 (48%) (Fig. 8), hypertrophied and enlarged in 18 (39%), enlarged in three (7%), minute chamber with thick wall and fibroelastosis in one (2%), atrophied in one (2%), small with thin wall in one (2%).

The Valves

The tricuspid orifice was enlarged in 21 (46%) (Fig. 7), was normal in size in 20 (43%), and was smaller than normal in five (11%). The pulmonic orifice was enlarged in 26 (57%), was normal in size in 16 (34%), and was smaller than normal in four (9%). The mitral orifice was smaller than normal in 28 (61%), was normal in size in 16 (35%), and was enlarged in two (4%). The

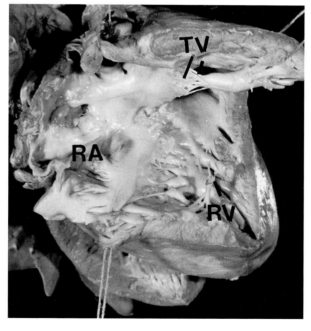

Figure 7: Hypertrophy and enlargement of the right atrium and right ventricle with closed foramen ovale in an infant less than 2 months of age. RA = right atrium; RV = right ventricle; TV = tricuspid valve. Note the intact atrial septum.

aortic orifice size was distinctly smaller than normal in 40 (87%), was normal in size in five (11%), and was minute in one (2%).

The tricuspid valve, although normally formed in the majority of cases (37–80%) (Fig. 7), was abnormal in nine (20%). There was considerable redundancy and thickening, especially of the anterior leaflet in three (6.5%). In one, the anterolateral papillary muscle was quite large and proceeded to the base of the valve. In another, the anterolateral papillary muscle was poorly developed. In two cases where the valve was markedly redundant and nodose, there were blood cysts. One was a case of mild Ebstein-like malformation. In one the anterolateral papillary muscle revealed infarction. The pulmonic valve was normally formed and presented increased hemodynamic change in all except three (6.5%). In one it was a markedly dysplastic bicuspid pulmonic valve, and in two others, the valve was considerably thickened and irregular.

The Mitral Valve

In one the mitral valve formed an Ebstein-like malformation. There was arcade-like malformation of the mitral valve with no chordae between the papil-

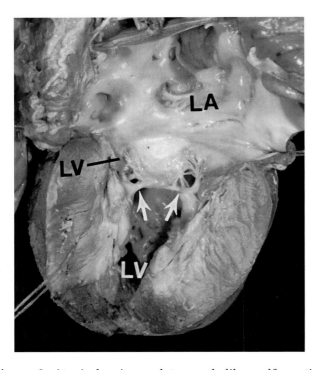

Figure 9: Atypical or incomplete arcade-like malformation of the mitral valve with mitral stenosis. LA = hypertrophied and enlarged left atrium; LV = left ventricle; MV = mitral valve. Arrows point to the arcade-like malformation of the mitral valve. Note the fusion of the anterior and posterior papillary muscles to the edge of the leaflet with markedly abbreviated chordae.

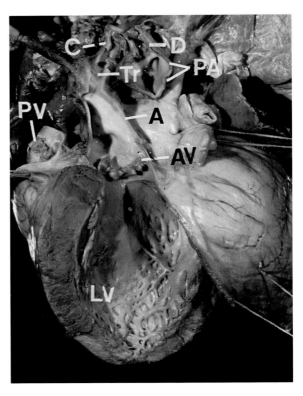

Figure 10: Unicuspid aortic valve with stenosis and insufficiency with preductal coarctation of the aorta. A = ascending aorta; AV = dysplastic unicuspid aortic valve; LV = hypertrophied and enlarged left ventricle with diffuse fibroelastosis; Tr = transverse arch; C = coarctation; D = ductus arteriosus; PV = pulmonary valve; PA = two pulmonary arteries.

lary muscles and the edge of the leaflet with redundant leaflet structure or sheet of tissue in six (13%). The valve was irregularly thickened with bizarre connections in 10 (22%). There were markedly abbreviated chordae with atypical arcade-like malformation in nine (20%) (Fig. 9). In one the papillary muscles were absent, in another it was a parachute type of a valve. The papillary muscles were extremely small in one, and markedly fibrotic in one. Significant mitral stenosis was present in 17 (37%), mitral stenosis and insufficiency in four (9%), mitral insufficiency in four (9%).

The Aortic Valve

The aortic valve was unicuspid in 25 (54%) (Fig. 10), bicuspid in 15 (33%) (Fig. 1), tricuspid in six (13%). The bicuspidality was formed by either the noncoronary with the right or the left with the noncoronary cusp. The valve was markedly redundant, nodose and irregularly thickened.

Classification

Aortic valvular stenosis—41 (89.1%)
Hypertrophic cardiomyopathy—3 (6.5%)
Supravalvular aortic stenosis—2 (4.4%)

The major left-sided associated cardiac anomalies are a part of the spectrum of this entity. Hence, the above broad classification is subdivided into the following subtypes of aortic stenosis:

The Types of Aortic Stenosis Seen Below the Age of 3 Months

Aortic stenosis and fibroelastosis of the left ventricle—7 (15%)
Aortic valvular stenosis, mitral stenosis, and fibroelastosis of the left ventricle—8 (17%)
Aortic stenosis, preductal coarctation, and fibroelastosis of the left ventricle—5 (11%) (Figs. 10, 11)
Aortic stenosis, mitral stenosis, mitral insufficiency and fibroelastosis of the left ventricle—4 (9%)
Isolated valvular aortic stenosis—3 (6.5%)

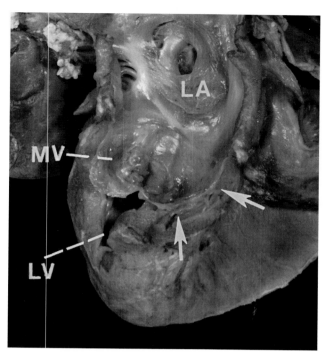

Figure 12: Aortic stenosis and Ebstein's malformation of the mitral valve with stenosis in a 1-day-old infant. LA = left atrium; LV = left ventricle; MV = mitral valve. Arrows point to the downward displacement of the posterior leaflet.

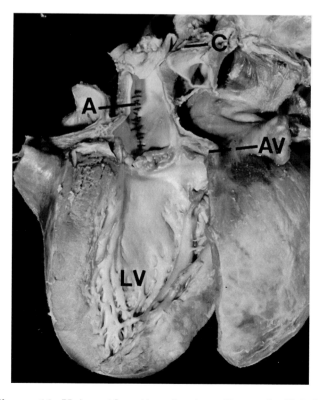

Figure 11: Unicuspid aortic valve in a 1½-month-old baby with aortic stenosis and insufficiency, diffuse fibroelastosis of the left ventricle, and surgical intervention. LV = hypertrophied and enlarged left ventricle with diffuse fibroelastosis; AV = dysplastic unicuspid aortic valve; A = ascending aorta; C = coarctation.

Aortic stenosis, mitral stenosis, paraductal coarctation, and fibroelastosis of the left ventricle—2 (4%)
Aortic stenosis, mitral insufficiency, paraductal coarctation, and fibroelastosis of the left ventricle—1
Aortic stenosis and preductal coarctation—1
Aortic stenosis, preductal coarctation, and mitral stenosis—2 (4%)
Aortic stenosis, mitral stenosis, preductal coarctation, and fibroelastosis of the left ventricle—2 (4%)
Aortic stenosis and mitral stenosis—1
Aortic stenosis, Ebstein-like malformation of the mitral valve, with mitral stenosis and double VSD—1 (Figs. 12–14)
Aortic stenosis and mitral insufficiency—1
Aortic stenosis, mitral insufficiency, and preductal coarctation—1
Aortic stenosis, mitral insufficiency, and fibroelastosis—2 (4%)
Supravalvular aortic stenosis with fibroelastosis of the left ventricle—1
Supravalvular and valvular aortic stenosis and fibroelastosis of the left ventricle—1
Hypertrophic cardiomyopathy with mitral stenosis—1
Hypertrophic cardiomyopathy (1 with subpulmonary stenosis)—2 (4%)

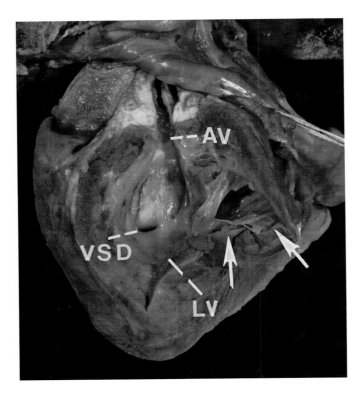

Figure 13: Left ventricular outflow tract showing the ventricular septal defect and aortic stenosis. LV = left ventricle; VSD = muscular ventricular septal defect—1; AV = aortic valve. The second defect is close to the base of the mitral valve and cannot be seen. Arrows point to displaced posterior mitral leaflet.

Atrial Septal Morphology

Atrial septal defect, fossa ovalis type—19 (41%)
Large atrial septal defect, fossa ovalis type—9 (20%)
Small aneurysm of fossa ovalis—2 (4%)
Premature closure of foramen ovale (1-day-old, 30-weeks' gestation fetus)—1
Aneurysm of space of His—3 (6.5%)
Left superior vena cava entering coronary sinus—2 (4%)
Chiari network—1
Cor triatriatum dexter, incomplete—1
In addition to the above, the following were noted:
Foramen ovale closed in an 8-day-old infant—1 (2%)
Oblique foramen ovale in infants (1–3 days old)—3 (6.5%)
Oblique foramen ovale from 3 days to 20 days—5 (11%)
Oblique foramen ovale from 5 weeks to 2 months—5 (11%)
Closed foramen ovale in 2 month old—2 (4%) (Fig. 7)

Other Associated Cardiac Anomalies on the Left Side

Fibroelastosis of the left ventricle—30 (65%) (Fig. 15)
Aneurysm formation of interventricular septum—2 (4%)
Aneurysm of sinus of Valsalva, right aortic cusp—1 (2%)
Aortic insufficiency—1 (2%)

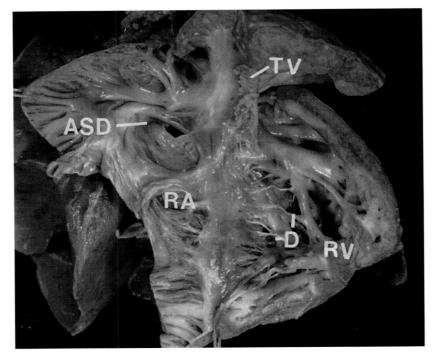

Figure 14: Right atrial, right ventricular view showing anomalous muscle bands in the inlet and ventricular septal defects. RA = right atrium; RV = right ventricle; ASD = atrial septal defect; TV = tricuspid valve; D = defects 1 and 2.

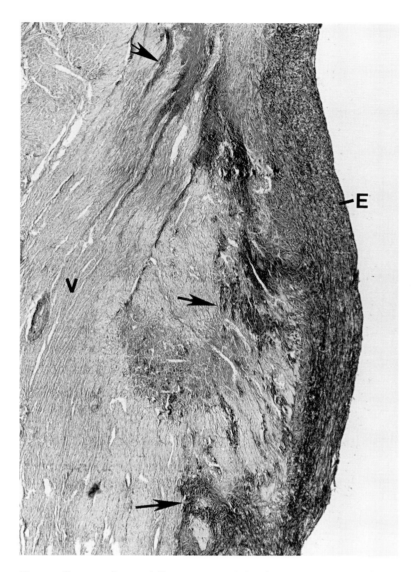

Figure 15: Photomicrograph showing diffuse fibroelastosis of the left ventricle. Weigert-van Geison stain, ×45. E = endocardial fibroelastosis; V = ventricular myocardium. Arrows point to fibroelastosis.

Forme fruste of overriding aorta—1 (2%)
Single left coronary ostium—1 (2%)
High origin of coronary ostia—1 (2%)
High origin of right coronary ostium—3 (6.5%)
High origin of left coronary ostium—1 (2%)
Prominent coronary artery circulation (enlarged or tortuous)—1 (2%)
Ascending aorta, small—12 (26%)
Ascending aorta, minute—1 (2%)
Poststenotic dilatation of the ascending aorta—4 (9%)
Outpouching of the aorta—10 (22%)
Transverse arch smaller than normal—8 (17%)
Right subclavian from descending aorta—1 (2%)

Other Cardiac Anomalies

Spontaneous closure of muscular VSD—1 (2%)
Double VSD—1 (2%)
Pulmonary artery smaller than normal—1 (2%)
Pulmonary hypertension—2 (4%)

Diverticulum of right ventricle—1 (2%)
Congenital polyvalvular disease—1 (2%)
Tricuspid stenosis—1

The Status of Ductus Arteriosus

Huge ductus arteriosus—7 (15%)
Circuitous, either elongated or wide patent ductus arteriosus—5 (11%)

Microscopic Examination

Histologic examination of the myocardium and the aortic valve was done in eight cases of aortic stenosis in infancy.

Aortic Valve

There was disorganization of the cusp layers, hypoelastification, and an increase in mucopolysaccharides (Fig. 16).

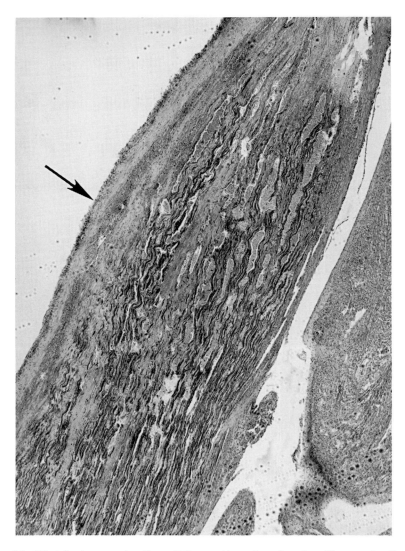

Figure 16: Histologic examination of the aortic valve showing disorganization of the cusp layers, hypoelastification, and an increase in mucopolysaccharides. Weigert-van Geison stain, ×45. Arrow points to aortic valve.

Myocardium

There was necrosis with proliferation of young and old connective tissue and perivascular increase in connective tissue. These changes were maximally seen subendocardially (Fig. 17). The above findings were present even in a case of a 1-day-old infant. The right ventricle revealed an increase in connective tissue.

Myocardial changes in aortic stenosis in infancy are of great interest. These changes present mostly subendocardially, consisted of necrosis, and the presence of young and old connective tissue and a perivascular increase in connective tissue. These findings were present even in a 1-day-old child, indicating that the changes in the myocardium of the left ventricle had been going on during fetal life. These were present in the absence of changes in the large coronary arteries.

II. Aortic Stenosis Above the Age of 3 Months and Below the Age of 2 Years

Analysis of Our Material

There was a total of 18 cases, 11 (61%) were males and six (39%) were female subjects. The youngest was 3½ months of age, and the oldest 19 months, with a mean age of 9 months, and 21.5 days.

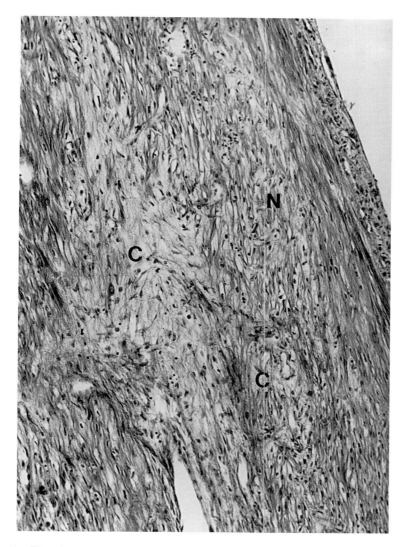

Figure 17: Histology of myocardium showing necrosis with proliferation of young and old connective tissue. Weigert-van Geison stain, ×150. N = necrosis; C = young and old connective tissue; N = necrosis.

The Complex

The heart was hypertrophied and enlarged in all. The apex was formed by the left ventricle (94%) in all but one where the apex was formed by both ventricles. The right atrium was hypertrophied and enlarged in 15 (83%), hypertrophied in two (11%), and was of normal size in one (6%). The right ventricle was hypertrophied and enlarged in 14 (78%) and was hypertrophied in four (22%). The left atrium was hypertrophied and enlarged in 17 (94%) (Fig. 18), and hypertrophied in one. The left ventricle was hypertrophied and enlarged in 12 (67%) and was markedly hypertrophied alone in six (33%) (Fig. 19).

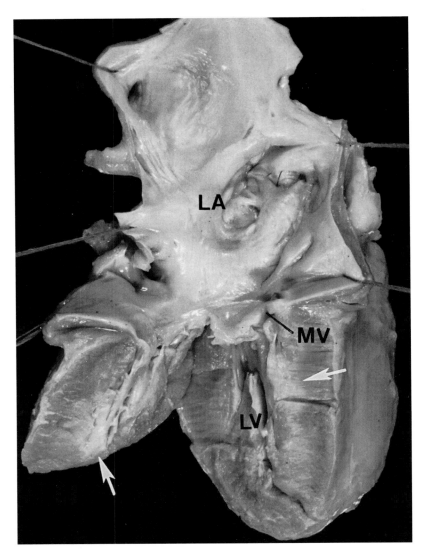

Figure 18: Markedly abbreviated chordae and fusion of papillary muscles and fibrosis of the left ventricle, with mitral stenosis and insufficiency. Note the left atrial hypertrophy and enlargement. LA = huge left atrium; LV = hypertrophied left ventricle with scars; MV = considerably thickened and short, thick chordae for the mitral valve. Arrows point to fibrosis of the left ventricle.

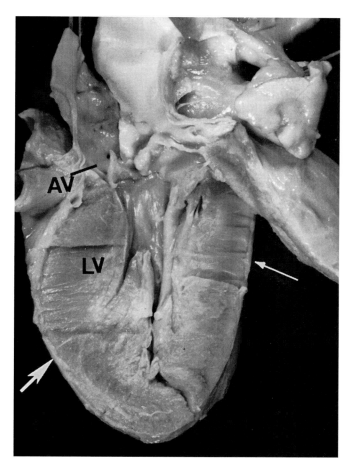

Figure 19: Left ventricular hypertrophy in unicuspid dysplastic aortic valve with stenosis. AV = dysplastic aortic valve; LV = small left ventricle with marked hypertrophy and fibroelastosis. Arrows point to the marked thickening of the posterior and anterior walls of the left ventricle.

The Valves

The tricuspid orifice was enlarged in 10 (56%) and was normal in size in eight (44%). It was normally formed in 15 (83%) but presented increased hemodynamic change. In two others (11%), the anterolateral leaflet was quite large with two papillary muscles proceeding to the base of the valve, and the valvular tissue was quite redundant. In one (6%) the posterior and medial leaflets were joined together.

The pulmonic orifice was enlarged in 10 (56%), was normal in size in six (33%), and smaller than normal in two (11%). The valve, in general, presented distinctly increased hemodynamic change. In one (6%) there was distinct narrowing at the bifurcation, the right smaller than the left, with marked thickening of the pulmonary tree and its branches. In one (6%), multiple stenosis of the peripheral pulmonary arteries with thickening was noted. In three (17%) the pulmonary trunk was quite thickened. The mitral orifice was distinctly smaller than normal in seven (39%). The orifice was enlarged in three (17%). In the remaining eight (44%) it was normal in size. In two (11%) it was smaller than normal; in four (22%) of the normal-sized orifices and in two (11%) enlarged valves the chordae were abbreviated and thickened and the valve itself presented increased nodularity and thickening from the line of closure to the edge (Fig. 18). The valve formed a complete arcade-like malformation with markedly thickening papillary muscles fusing with the edge of the leaflet in two (11%) and in another two (11%) it formed an incomplete arcade-like malformation. In two (11%) others the entire valvular structure was connected to a short stubby posterior papillary muscle in a parachute type of malformation. Thus, 12 (67%) cases, including those with normal sized, enlarged, or smaller than normal valves, presented some type of an abnormality of the mitral valve.

The Aortic Valve

The aortic orifice size was smaller than normal in 14 (78%), was normal in size in two (11%), and was enlarged in two (11%). The valve was bicuspid in six (33%), unicuspid in five (28%) (Fig. 19), and was a tricuspid valve in seven (39%). The valve was irregularly thickened, nodose, and was not subdivided into two cusps in two (11%), and there was a low raphé and thickened commissures, resulting in an incompletely formed bicuspid valve in two (11%). The subaortic area immediately adjacent to or beneath the base of the aortic valve was distinctly smaller than normal in all.

The major left-sided associated cardiac anomalies constituted a part of the spectrum of aortic stenosis in this age group. Hence, aortic stenosis in this group may be further subdivided.

The types of aortic stenosis in this group were:

Aortic valvular stenosis with diffuse fibroelastosis of the left ventricle—5 (28%)

Aortic stenosis, mitral stenosis, and coarctation—2 (11%)

Aortic stenosis and mitral insufficiency—2 (11%)

Aortic stenosis, mitral stenosis, and insufficiency—1 (6%) (Fig. 18, 19)

Aortic stenosis, subaortic stenosis, and mitral stenosis—1 (6%)

Aortic stenosis, subaortic stenosis, mitral stenosis, and coarctation—1 (6%)

Supravalvular aortic stenosis with peripheral pulmonary stenosis—3 (17%)

Supravalvular aortic stenosis and pulmonary stenosis—1 (6%)

Aortic stenosis, subaortic stenosis, supravalvular aortic stenosis, mitral stenosis, closing VSD, overriding aorta, and coarctation of the aorta—1 (6%)

Hypertrophic cardiomyopathy—muscular subaortic stenosis with subpulmonary stenosis produced by the ventricular septal bulge—1 (6%)

The Other Major Associated Cardiac Abnormalities on the Left Side

Fibroelastosis of the left ventricle—10 (56%) (Fig. 19)
Infarct of the left ventricle—1 (6%)
Fibrosis of the myocardium—1 (6%)
Marked atherosclerosis of aortic mitral anulus and base of the aortic valve—1 (6%)
Abnormal chordal extensions in the left ventricle—1 (6%)
High origin of coronary ostia—1 (6%)
Small ascending aorta—2 (11%)
Poststenotic dilatation and residual coarctation—1 (6%)

The Other Major Associated Cardiac Abnormalities on the Right Side

Atrial septal defect, fossa ovalis type, or patent foramen ovale—2 (11%)
Probe patent foramen ovale—3 (17%)
Spatio intersepto valvulare—1
Aneurysm of space of His—1
Intermediate chamber with pouch formation in the septum primum—1
Tricuspid stenosis—1
Diverticulum of right ventricle—1
Infundibular pulmonary stenosis—1

Aortic Stenosis Above 2 Years of Age
Analysis of Our Material

There was a total of 101 cases; 71 (77%) were male subjects, 22 (23%) were female subjects, two were unidentified, and six were dogs. The oldest was 81 years of age and the youngest was 2 years, 3 months, and the mean age was 27.68 years.

The Complex

The heart was hypertrophied and enlarged in all. The apex was formed by the left ventricle in 91 (90%) cases, by both ventricles in seven (7%), and by the right ventricle in three (3%). The right atrium was hypertrophied and enlarged in 61 (60%), hypertrophied in 21 (21%), and was normal in size in 19 (19%). The right ventricle was hypertrophied and enlarged in 75 (74%), hypertrophied in 18 (18%), and was normal in size in eight (8%). The left atrium was hypertrophied and enlarged in 73 (72%) (Fig. 20), hypertrophied in 24 (24%), and was normal in size in four (4%). The left ventricle was hypertrophied and enlarged in 77 (76%), and hypertrophied in 24 (24%). Although the left ventricle was hypertrophied, only rarely was it smaller than normal in size.

The Valves

The tricuspid orifice was normal in size in 67 (66%), enlarged in 33 (33%), and was smaller than normal in one (1%). The pulmonic orifice was enlarged in

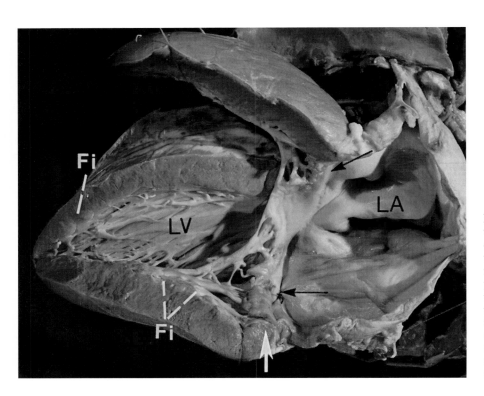

Figure 20: Left atrial, left ventricular view demonstrating the markedly thickened posterior leaflet of the mitral valve with insufficiency in a 2-year, 10-month-old child. LA = left atrium, hypertrophied and enlarged; LV = left ventricle; Fi = fibroelastosis of the left ventricle. Arrows point to irregular thickening of the posterior leaflet of the mitral valve. Note the thickened chordae and fibrotic papillary muscles proceeding directly to the edge or the undersurface of the valve.

49 (48.5%), normal in size in 47 (46.5%), and was smaller than normal in five (5%). The mitral orifice was normal in 50 (50%), enlarged in 33 (33%), and was smaller than normal in 18 (17%). The aortic orifice was smaller than normal in 68 (67%), normal in size in 26 (26%), and was enlarged in seven (7%).

The Tricuspid Valve

Although, in general, the tricuspid valve was normally formed in 72 (71%), it was abnormally formed in 29 (29%) cases. The majority of the normally formed valves presented increased hemodynamic change. The most common abnormalities were a poorly developed inferior leaflet giving rise to the mitralization of leaflets, and the division of medial and anterior leaflets into several components with accessory connections of the leaflets to the papillary muscles. In two there were large accessory openings, and in five the valve was redundant and was segmented into several components. In others the valve presented considerably increased thickening, and the anterolateral papillary muscle was poorly developed in three.

The pulmonary valve, although, in general, was normally formed, was quadricuspid in one, it was

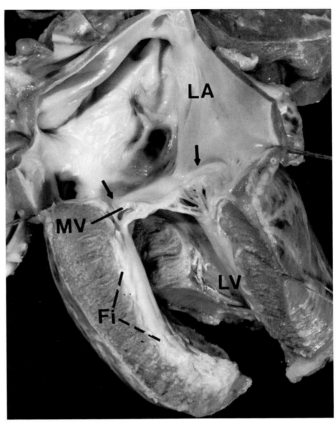

Figure 22: Supravalvular aortic stenosis with thickening of the mitral valve, short chordae with anular mitral stenosis, and fibroelastosis of the left ventricle. LA = left atrium; MV = thickened mitral valve with short chordae and anular stenosis; LV = left ventricle; Fi = fibroelastosis of the left ventricle. Arrows point to ridge formation in the mitral anulus.

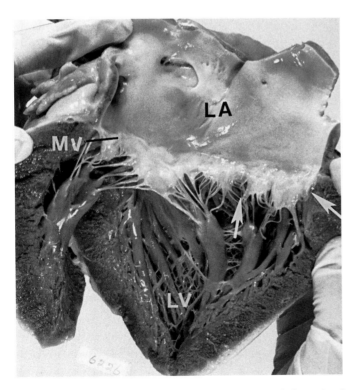

Figure 21: Segmented large posterior leaflet of the mitral valve and elongated chordae in hypertrophic cardiomyopathy. LA = hypertrophied and enlarged left atrium; LV = hypertrophied left ventricle; MV = mitral valve. Arrows point to segmented posterior leaflet.

thickened with widening of the commissure in two, the valve was bicuspid and thickened in two and it was fenestrated in one. Thus, the valve was abnormal in six (6%).

The Mitral Valve

The mitral valve was abnormally formed in 43 (42.5%) cases. The abnormalities included a markedly thickened mitral valve (Fig. 20), redundant leaflets, a large posterior leaflet divided into several segments (Fig. 21), elongated or markedly abbreviated chordae, anular ridges (Fig. 22), markedly hypertrophied and/or fibrotic papillary muscles (Fig. 20), arcade-like malformation, and extension of the anterolateral papillary muscle to the aortic valve base in five. Rarely, an accessory opening was seen. The valve was calcific in five. *The types and frequency of mitral valve anomalies in various types of aortic stenosis were as follows:*

(MI = mitral insufficiency; MS = mitral stenosis; AI = aortic insufficiency; AS = aortic stenosis.)

Hypertrophic cardiomyopathy—14 (MI2) (Fig. 21)

Subaortic stenosis of fibroelastic ridge formation type—9 (MI1, MS1)

Subaortic stenosis of both muscular and endocardial ridge thickening—3

Aortic stenosis and subaortic stenosis—1

Bicuspid aortic valve with calcification and with or without infective endocarditis—7 (AI4, MS2)

Markedly irregularly thickened mitral valve and bicuspid aortic valve with stenosis—3 (MS, MI, and/or AI3) (Fig. 20)

Accessory mitral orifice with insufficiency (1 with VSD)—2

Bicuspid aortic valve with stenosis and subaortic stenosis with infective endocarditis of the mitral valve—1

Aortic valvular stenosis and irregular thickening of the mitral valve and mitral insufficiency—1

Coarctation of the aorta with aortic stenosis and irregular thickening of the mitral valve—1 (MS)

Supravalvular aortic stenosis with irregularly thickened mitral valve—1 (MI) (Fig. 22)

The above changes produced either mitral stenosis or insufficiency or both to a varying extent.

The Aortic Valve

The valve was abnormally formed in 44 (43.5%)

The aortic valve was bicuspid with irregular thickening—37 (37%) (Figs. 5, 23)

Unicuspid valve—4 (4%)

Quadricuspid valve—1

Incompletely divided tricuspid with a low raphé—2

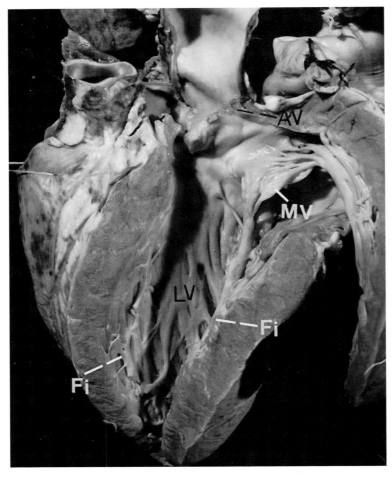

Figure 23: Calcific bicuspid aortic valve with aortic stenosis and mitral insufficiency; left ventricular view. LV = left ventricle; AV = bicuspid calcified with irregular thickening of the aortic valve; MV = markedly thickened mitral valve; Fi = fibroelastosis of the left ventricle.

The Aortic Valve in Various Types of Aortic Stenosis

A bicuspid aortic valve was present in the following:

Valvular aortic stenosis—31 (22 calcific) (Figs. 5, 23)
Subaortic, fibroelastic type—1
Subaortic, fibroelastic muscular type—1
Valvular, fibroelastic subvalvular aortic stenosis—2
Valvular, subvalvular, and supravalvular stenosis—1
Familial hypertrophic cardiomyopathy—1
Unicuspid aortic valve was seen with aortic valvular stenosis—4 (1 with calcification, 1 with infective endocarditis)
Almost quadricuspid aortic valve was seen with aortic stenosis and infective endocarditis—1

Classification of Aortic Stenosis Beyond the Age of 2 Years

Aortic valvular stenosis—20 (20%)
Calcific valvular aortic stenosis—25 (25%)
Subaortic stenosis—45 (45%)
    Hypertrophic cardiomyopathy—19 (out of 45—42%) (out of 101—19%)
    Fibroelastic ridge—13 (13%)
    Muscular and fibroelastic ridge—3 (3%)
    Membranous subaortic stenosis—2 (2%)
    Valvular and subvalvular aortic stenosis
    Valvular and fibroelastic subvalvular stenosis—4 (4%)
    Valvular, muscular subaortic stenosis—2 (2%)
    Valvular, muscular, and fibroelastic subvalvular stenosis—1 (1%)
    Valvular, muscular, fibroelastic, and membranous subvalvular stenosis—1
Supravalvular aortic stenosis—8 (8%)
Aortic valvular and supravalvular aortic stenosis—1
Severe aortic stenosis, sub AS, coarctation and PDA repair (old)—1
Marked obesity, hypertrophic cardiomyopathy, hypertension and coronary artery disease, arrhythmias, and sudden death—1

Associated Cardiac Abnormalities in Bicuspid Aortic Valve

Calcific bicuspid aortic valve with stenosis and insufficiency with infective endocarditis of aortic and mitral valve—1
Bicuspid aortic valve with aortic stenosis and VSD—1
Bicuspid aortic valve with aortic stenosis and arrhythmias—1
Calcific bicuspid aortic valve with double mitral orifice—1

Bicuspid aortic valve with old infarct (posteroseptal and apical), old surgery—1
Bicuspid aortic valve with calcification, AS, and coronary artery disease with posteroseptal infarct—1
Bicuspid aortic valve with marked sclerosis and 2 right coronary ostia and calcification of the valve—1
Bicuspid aortic valve with calcific AS and subendocardial myocardial infarction—1
Bicuspid aortic valve with calcific AS and recent infarction of the myocardium—1
Bicuspid aortic valve with calcific stenosis AI following surgery—1
Bicuspid aortic valve with aortic and mitral stenosis and mild pulmonary stenosis and tricuspid stenosis—1
Bicuspid aortic valve calcific, with coronary artery disease—1
Bicuspid aortic valve with calcification and origin of both coronaries from anterior cusp—1
Bicuspid aortic valve calcific, marked coronary artery disease, old infarct aneurysm formation, mitral insufficiency, and thrombosis in the left ventricle—1
Calcific bicuspid aortic valve with aortic stenosis and insufficiency with huge left superior vena cava entering coronary sinus and thrombosis in right atrium—1
Bicuspid aortic valve, severe 3-vessel disease, extensive infarction, huge aneurysm and rupture, dominant left coronary artery, and small right coronary—1 (Figs. 24, 25)
Bicuspid aortic valve calcification and left superior vena cava entering coronary sinus with moderate 3-vessel disease—1
Bicuspid aortic valve calcification and aortic valve replacement with aortic insufficiency, fibrosis and anomalous muscle in the left ventricle, left superior vena cava entering coronary sinus, accessory tricuspid orifice—1
Bicuspid calcific aortic stenosis and insufficiency, viral myocarditis, 3-vessel disease and aneurysm of the lower third of the ventricular septum—1
Bicuspid aortic valve, huge aneurysm of ascending aorta and rupture with dominant left coronary artery and two small right coronaries—1 (Figs. 26—28)
Unicuspid aortic valve, infective endocarditis, aortic insufficiency—1 (Fig. 29)
Unicuspid aortic valve with AS and AI, old surgery, myocardial infarction, and pulmonary hypertension—1
Quadricuspid aortic valve with subacute bacterial endocarditis (SBE) rupture and fistulas track formation and AI—1
Incomplete division of 3 cusps (low raphé) with marked fatty infiltration of the right ventricle and both coronaries from the right cusp and high origin—1

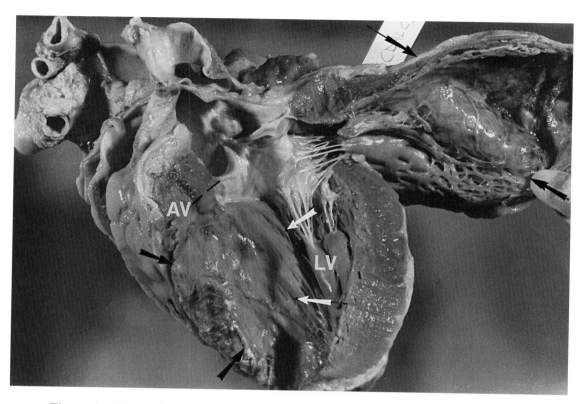

Figure 24: Bicuspid aortic valve with coronary artery disease with old aneurysm of the anteroseptal wall with recent myocardial infarction and rupture of the anterolateral wall; left ventricular view. AV = bicuspid aortic valve; LV = left ventricle. Arrows point to the huge anteroseptal and lateral wall aneurysm with rupture.

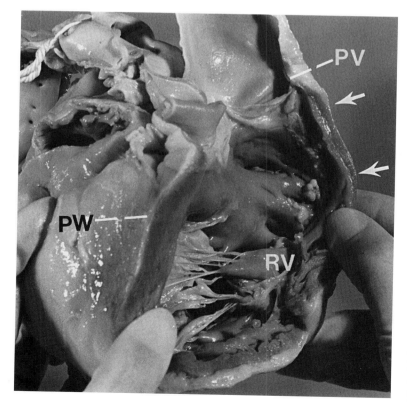

Figure 25: Right ventricular outflow tract view demonstrating the extension of the myocardial infarction into the right ventricular aspect of the septum. RV = right ventricle; PV = pulmonary valve; PW = hypertrophied parietal wall. Arrows point to the extension of the infarct. Note in contrast to the anteroseptal wall the parietal wall of the right ventricle is markedly hypertrophied.

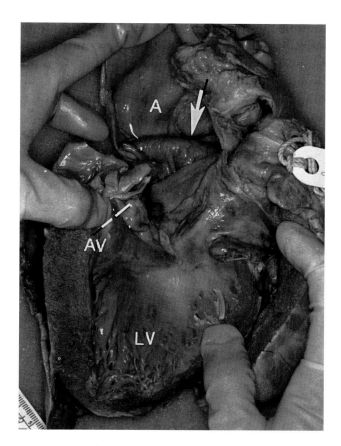

Figure 26: Bicuspid aortic valve with aortic insufficiency and aneurysmal dilatation of the ascending aorta with rupture; left ventricular view demonstrating the enlarged left ventricle and the aneurysm of the ascending aorta with rupture. AV = bicuspid aortic valve; LV = left ventricle; A = ascending aorta aneurysm. Arrow points to the rupture.

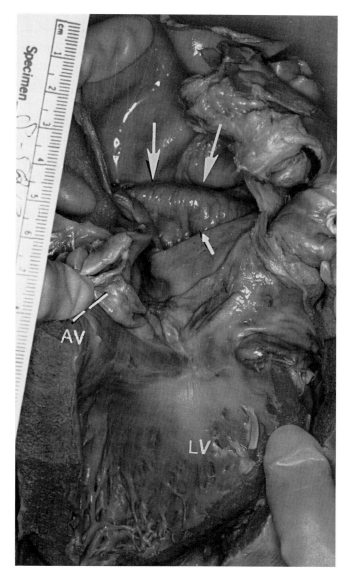

Figure 27: Markedly dilated anulus of the bicuspid aortic valve with rupture of the ascending aorta; close-up view. LV = left ventricle; AV = aortic valve, bicuspid. Arrows point to the rupture in the ascending aorta.

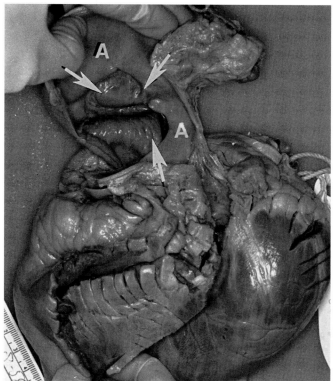

Figure 28: External view of the heart demonstrating the aneurysmal dilatation of the ascending aorta with rupture. A = ascending aorta. Arrows point to the rupture.

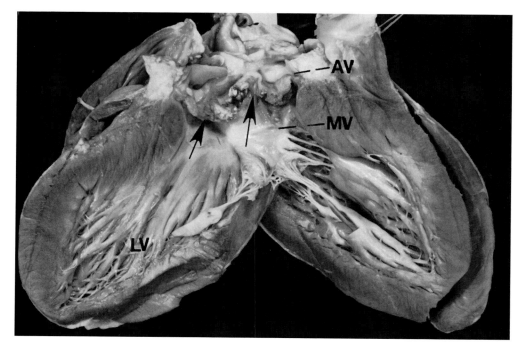

Figure 29: Unicuspid or incompletely divided tricuspid aortic valve with infective endocarditis and aortic insufficiency. LV = left ventricle; MV = mitral valve; AV = markedly deformed aortic valve with infective endocarditis. Arrows point to the valve. Note the enlargement of the left ventricle with fibroelastosis.

Subaortic Stenosis–Fibroelastic Ridge, Membranous, Shelf, and Other Discrete Types

In subaortic stenosis, in general, irregular bands of thickened endocardial tissue or a fibroelastic ridge formed a constricting band of tissue which proceeded in a circumferential manner from the anterior part of the muscular ventricular septum up to the aortic mitral anulus (Figs. 30—32). These ridges usually extended up the base of the aortic valve with a small aortic valve anulus. In six of them, there was associated muscular hypertrophy, thus adding the muscular element to the powerful endocardial ridge of tissue (Fig. 33). In others, either a membranous shelf was present beneath the aortic valve (Figs. 34—36) or the subaortic area was narrowed and formed a tunnel with a fibroelastic ridge (Fig. 37). The aortic valve was thickened and the sinuses of Valsalva formed a thickened pouch with the small anulus of varying degree. The mitral valve likewise was thickened to a varying degree (Fig. 38). The subaortic obstruction in some was quite prominent, similar to hypertrophic cardiomyopathy, producing marked bulges beneath the tricuspid and pulmonic valves (Figs. 39, 40).

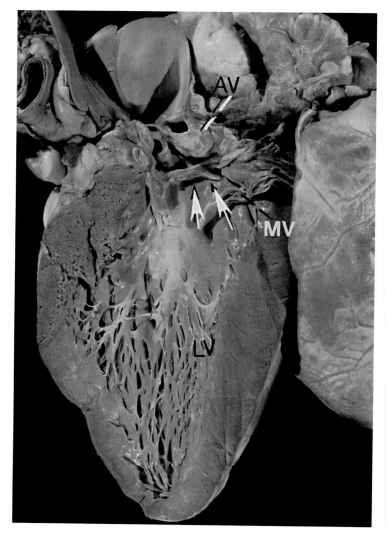

Figure 30: Subaortic stenosis of fibroelastic ridge beneath the aortic valve; left ventricular view. LV = left ventricle; MV = thickened mitral valve; AV = note the small aortic valve with markedly thickened cusps. Arrows point to the fibroelastic ridge beneath the aortic valve.

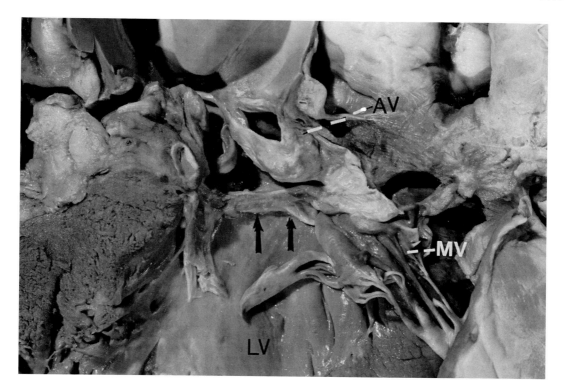

Figure 31: Close-up view of Figure 30. AV = markedly thickened aortic valve; MV = mitral valve; LV = left ventricle. Arrows point to the fibroelastic ridge beneath the aortic valve.

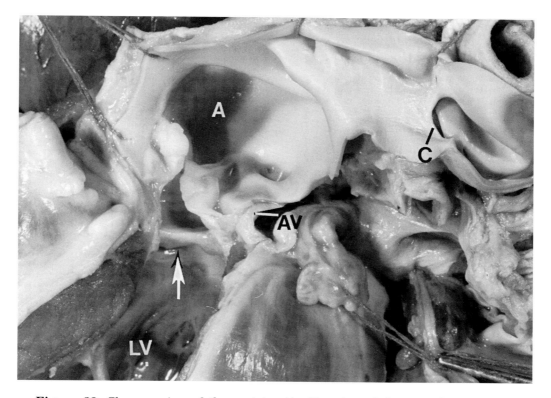

Figure 32: Close-up view of the poststenotic dilatation of the ascending aorta in subaortic stenosis with coarctation of the aorta. LV = left ventricle; A = poststenotic dilatation of the ascending aorta; AV = aortic valve markedly thickened; C = coarctation. Arrow points to the fibromuscular subaortic stenosis.

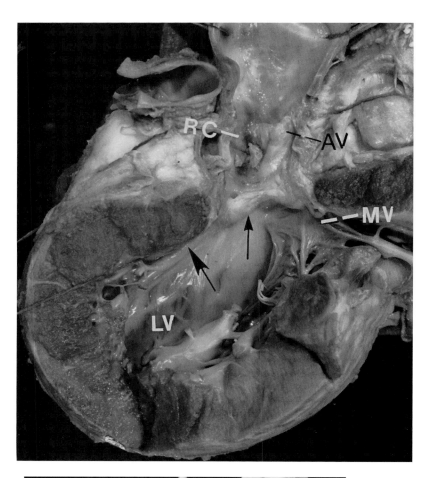

Figure 33: Aortic stenosis and subaortic stenosis (fibromuscular type) with surgical correction and narrowing of right coronary artery; left ventricular view. LV = hypertrophied left ventricle; MV = mitral valve; AV = remnant of the dysplastic aortic valve; RC = occluded right coronary artery. Arrows point to the subaortic fibromuscular ridge.

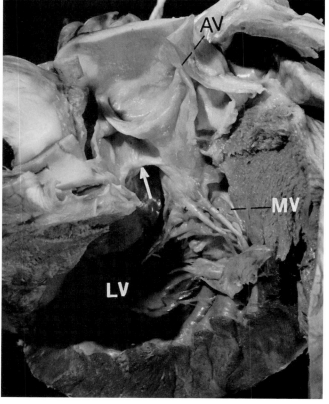

Figure 34: Subaortic stenosis, a membranous or a shelf-like formation beneath the aortic valve. AV = aortic valve; MV = mitral valve; LV = left ventricle. Arrow points to the subaortic shelf or membrane.

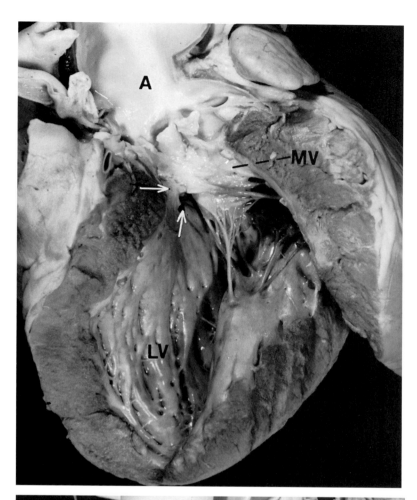

Figure 35: Aortic valvular stenosis and subaortic stenosis. LV = left ventricle; MV = mitral valve; A = aorta. Arrows point to the fibroelastic thickening and narrowing of the subaortic area. Note the markedly deformed thickened aortic valve.

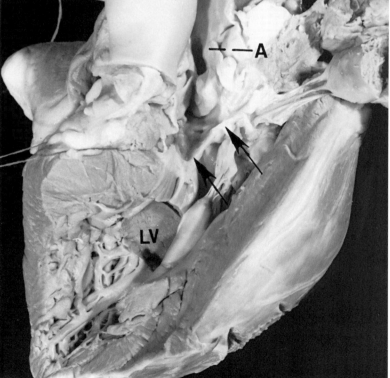

Figure 36: Subaortic stenosis of fibroelastic ridge extending from the base of the aortic mitral anulus to the summit of the ventricular septum in an oblique manner producing subaortic stenosis. LV = left ventricle; A = aorta. Arrows indicate the oblique extension of the fibroelastic ridge causing marked narrowing beneath the aortic valve. (Used with permission from Gasul BM, Arcilla RA, Lev M: *Heart Disease in Children: Diagnosis and Treatment*. JB Lippincott Co, Philadelphia, PA, 1966.

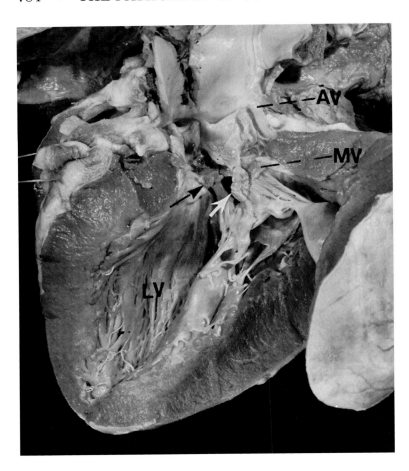

Figure 37: Aortic stenosis and tunnel type of subaortic stenosis with irregular fibroelastic ridge. LV = left ventricle; MV = mitral valve; AV = aortic valve. Arrows point to the irregular fibroelastic ridge immediately beneath the deformed aortic valve and tunnel type of narrowing.

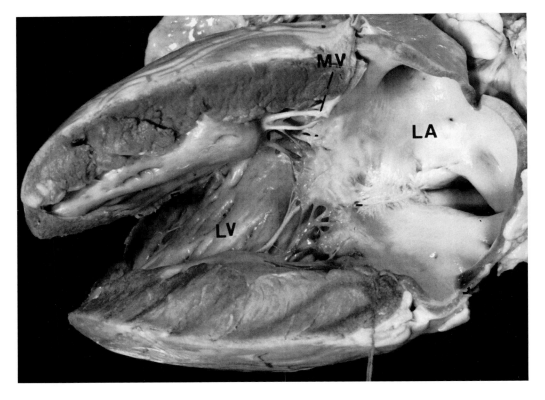

Figure 38: Left atrial, left ventricular view showing the thickening of the mitral valve and hypertrophy of the left atrium. LA = left atrium; LV = left ventricle; MV = thickened mitral valve.

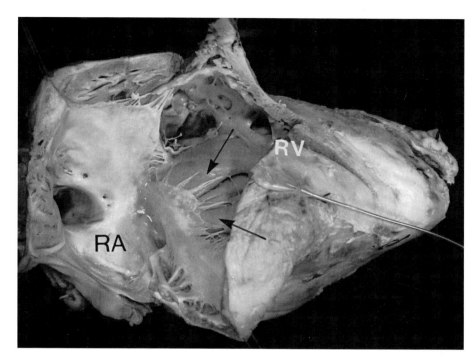

Figure 39: Right atrial, right ventricular view demonstrating the tremendous ventricular septal hypertrophy bulging into the right ventricle beneath the septal leaflet of the tricuspid valve. RA = right atrium; RV = right ventricle. Arrows point to the right ventricular septal bulge.

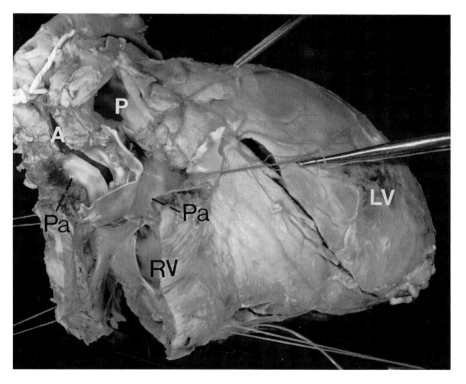

Figure 40: Right ventricular outflow tract in aortic and subaortic stenosis (operated several times) with recent Konno procedure. Note the enormously hypertrophied and enlarged heart with residual infundibular stenosis. LV = left ventricle; RV = right ventricle; P = pulmonary trunk; A = aorta; Pa = patch enlargement of the outflow tract of the right ventricle following the Konno procedure.

Associated Abnormalities in Subaortic Stenosis (Fibroelastic Ridge and Muscular Type)

Quadricuspid pulmonary valve—1

Bicuspid aortic valve with infective endocarditis, mycotic aneurysm of mitral valve, aorta, and atrial septum—1

Necrosis of the myocardium and rupture—1

Probe patent foramen ovale—1

Mitral insufficiency, anomalous muscle bands in RV, tricuspid stenosis, and high origin of coronary ostia—1 (Figs. 41—43)

Bicuspid aortic valve with calcification with thickened tricuspid valve—1

Irregularly thickened tricuspid valve, complete AV block following aortic valve replacement—1

Systemic hypertension—1

Narrowing and occlusion of right main coronary following surgery in the aortic valve—1

Paraductal coarctation, single coronary artery, anomalous muscle bundle in left ventricle, mitral stenosis—1 (Fig. 44)

Previous commissurotomies and false aneurysm of the ascending aorta, calcific aortitis, high origin of both coronary ostia—1

Aortic valvotomy and resection of subaortic muscle, replacement of aortic valve and Konno procedure—1

Pulmonary valvular and probably infundibular stenosis—1

Valvular, subvalvular, and muscular subaortic stenosis, several surgeries and Konno procedure, and high origin of right coronary with fibrosis of the papillary muscles of both the right and left ventricles—1 (Figs. 39, 40, 45, 46).

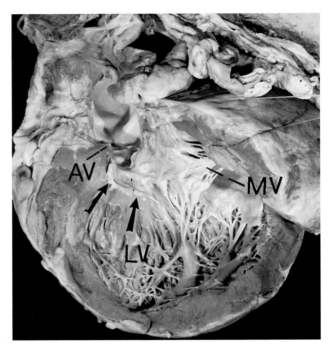

Figure 41: Subaortic stenosis with huge mitral valve, redundant chordal connections, and mitral insufficiency, left ventricular outflow tract view. LV = huge left ventricle; MV = markedly enlarged mitral valve with numerous chordal connections; AV = aortic valve. Arrows point to the irregular fibroelastic ridge beneath the aortic valve.

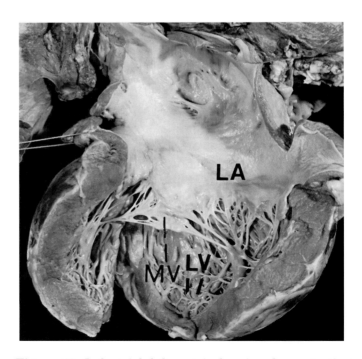

Figure 42: Left atrial, left ventricular view demonstrating the abnormally formed mitral valve with mitral insufficiency. LA = huge left atrium; MV = abnormally formed mitral valve; LV = left ventricle.

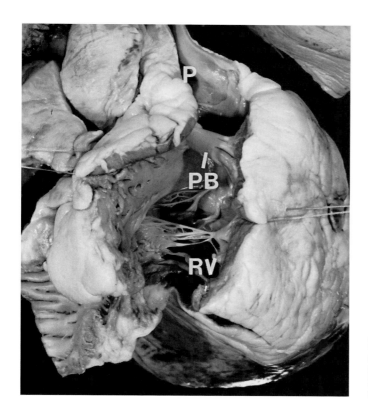

Figure 43: Right ventricular outflow tract view demonstrating an anomalous parietal band criss-crossing the outflow tract of the right ventricle beneath the pulmonary trunk. RV = right ventricle; PB = anomalous parietal band beneath the pulmonary trunk; P = pulmonary trunk.

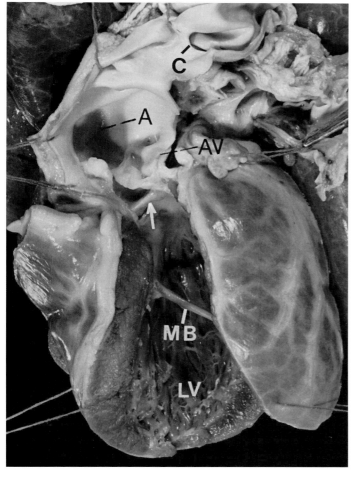

Figure 44: Subaortic stenosis of fibromuscular type with coarctation of the aorta, poststenotic dilatation of the ascending aorta; left ventricular view. LV = left ventricle; A = poststenotic dilatation of the ascending aorta; AV = aortic valve; mb = anomalous muscle band stretching across the outflow tract of the left ventricle; C = coarctation. Arrow points to the subaortic ridge.

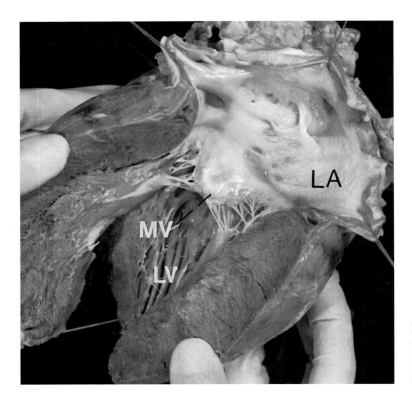

Figure 45: Left atrial, left ventricular view demonstrating the marked hypertrophy of the left-sided chambers thickened mitral valve. LA = left atrium; LV = left ventricle; MV = markedly thickened mitral valve.

Hypertrophic Cardiomyopathy

In this entity the muscular hypertrophy of the septum varied considerably. In some the hypertrophy extended from the base to the apex both anteriorly and posteriorly (Figs. 47, 48). In some there was hypertrophy at the mid-part (Fig. 6) or lower third of the septum. In some there was no significant hypertrophy at the gross level but there was hemodynamically significant left ventricular outflow tract obstruction.

There was fibrosis in the ventricular septum along the course of the anterior leaflet of the mitral valve with associated mitral valve abnormalities (Figs. 49, 50). This was in the form of calcification in two, and the posterior leaflet was quite large and segmented into several components in five (Fig. 21). There was a mild cleft-like malformation in two, in one the valve was distinctly floppy in nature, in the remainder the chordae were profuse with marked thickening of the mitral valve, especially from the line of closure to the edge (Fig. 51), and there was fibrosis of the papillary muscle in two. There were two cases of

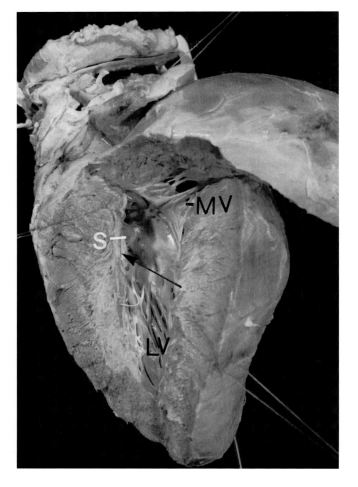

Figure 46: Left ventricular outflow tract demonstrating the marked left ventricular hypertrophy with fibroelastosis. Note the thickened endocardium and small cavity and residual subaortic obstruction. S = residual subaortic stenosis; LV = left ventricle; MV = mitral valve. Arrow points to the muscular subaortic bulge.

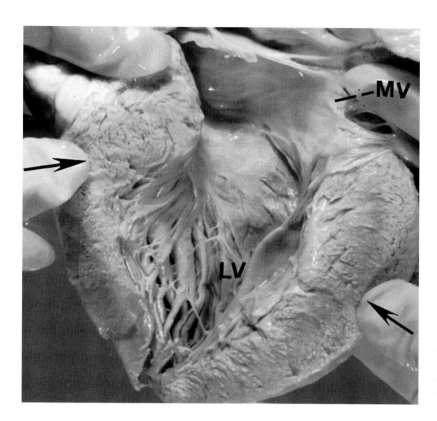

Figure 47: Left ventricular outflow view in a child with hypertrophic cardiomyopathy and sudden death. Note the hypertrophy extending from the base to the apex anteriorly and posteriorly. LV = left ventricle; MV = mitral valve. Arrows point to the left ventricular wall thickness.

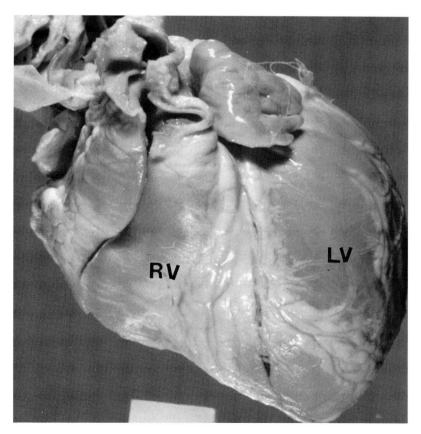

Figure 48: External view of the heart demonstrating the marked left ventricular hypertrophy. LV = left ventricle; RV = right ventricle.

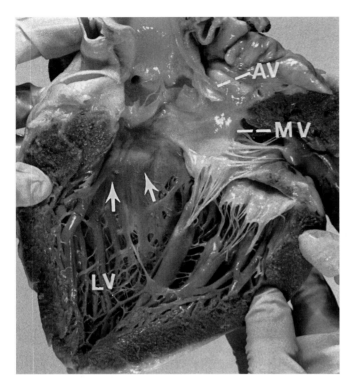

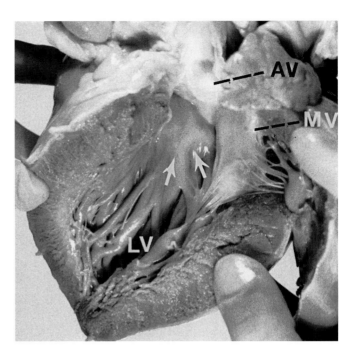

Figure 49: Left ventricular hypertrophy and enlargement with fibroelastosis on the summit of the septum along the course to the anterior leaflet of the mitral valve. LV = left ventricle; MV = mitral valve; AV = aortic valve. Arrows point to the fibrosis.

Figure 50: Marked trabeculations of the left ventricle and uniform hypertrophy of the ventricular septum from base to apex. LV = left ventricle; MV = mitral valve; AV = aortic valve. Arrows point to the fibroelastosis on the summit of the septum.

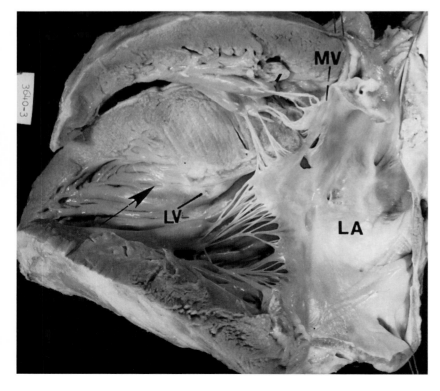

Figure 51: Left atrial, left ventricular view of thickened mitral valve with profuse chordae. LA = left atrium; MV = mitral valve; LV = left ventricle. Arrow points to hypertrophic cardiomyopathy.

Figure 52: Hypertrophic cardiomyopathy with clinically demonstrated subaortic obstruction but anatomically not a classic hypertrophy. AV = aortic valve; RAC = subluxated right aortic cusp; LV = left ventricle. Arrows point to the oblique hypertrophy of the septum.

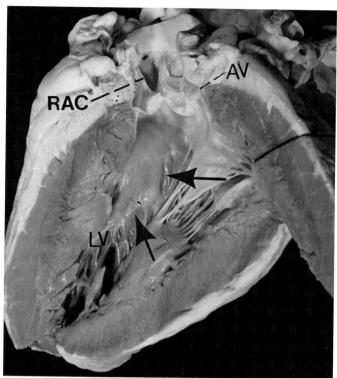

familial hypertrophic cardiomyopathy and both died suddenly. There was one case of subluxation of right aortic valve cusp, small right coronary artery arrhythmias, and sudden death (Fig. 52). The ventricular septal hypertrophy, when marked, resulted in bulging of the septum on the right side beneath the tricuspid and pulmonic valves (Figs. 53, 54).

Histologically, there was myocardial fiber disarray with fibrosis to a varying degree with or without mononuclear cells. Similar findings were also noted in the various parts of the conduction system, especially disrupting the fibers of the left bundle branch.

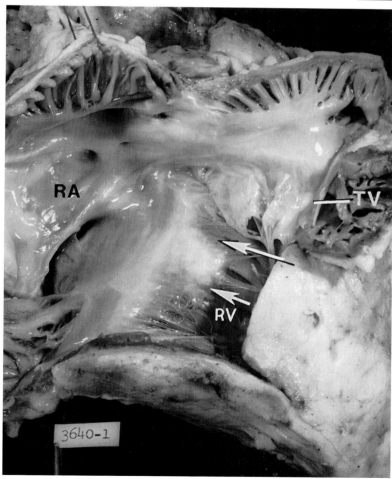

Figure 53: Right atrial, right ventricular view demonstrating the ventricular septal bulge beneath the septal leaflet of the tricuspid valve. RA = right atrium; RV = right ventricle; TV = tricuspid valve. Arrows point to the ventricular septal bulge.

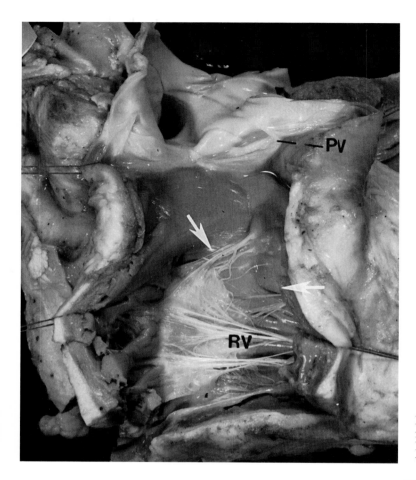

Figure 54: Outflow tract of the right ventricle showing the ventricular septal bulge. RV = right ventricle; PV = pulmonary valve. Arrows point to the bulge in the outflow tract of the right ventricle.

Supravalvular Aortic Stenosis

In supravalvular aortic stenosis, three had peripheral pulmonary stenosis as well. The walls of the main pulmonary trunk and the pulmonary arteries were quite thick (Figs. 55—59). This was associated with a prominent supravalvular ridge that produced pocket-like sinuses of Valsalva. The coronary arteries were also markedly thickened. The mitral valve was also thickened. The left ventricle was markedly hypertrophied in all.

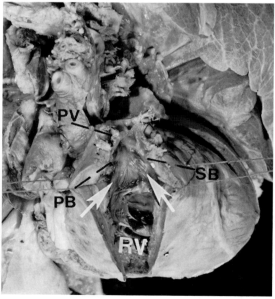

Figure 55: Supravalvular aortic stenosis, pulmonary valvular, infundibular and peripheral arterial stenosis. External view demonstrating the hypertrophied heart with infundibular pulmonary stenosis. RV = right ventricle; PV = thickened pulmonic valve; SB = septal band; PB = parietal band. Note the small pulmonic valve. Arrows point to infundibular pulmonary stenosis.

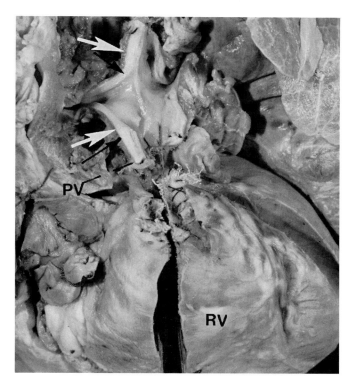

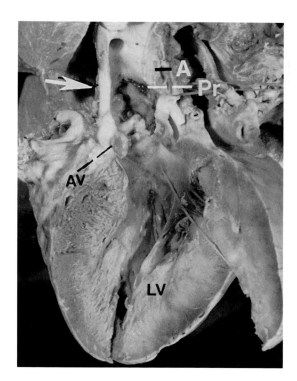

Figure 56: Close-up view of the pulmonary arteries demonstrating marked thickening of the pulmonary arterial walls. RV = right ventricle; PV = pulmonary valve. Arrows point to thickening of the walls of the pulmonary arteries.

Figure 57: Supravalvular aortic stenosis with peripheral pulmonary stenosis and surgery. LV = hypertrophied left ventricle and fibroelastosis; A = ascending aorta; Pr = enlargement of the ascending aorta with prosthesis; AV = thickened aortic valve. Arrow points to the thickened aortic wall.

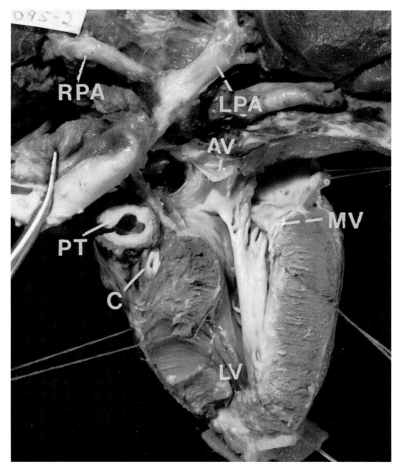

Figure 58: Supravalvular aortic stenosis with peripheral pulmonary stenosis and thickening and narrowing of the pulmonary arteries. LV = left ventricle, hypertrophied with small chamber; RPA = small thickened right pulmonary artery; LPA = small thickened left pulmonary artery; AV = aortic valve; MV = thickened mitral valve; C = thickened coronary artery; PT = thickened main pulmonary trunk.

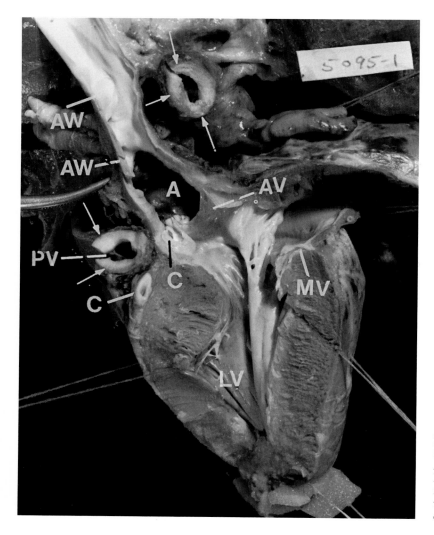

Figure 59: Supravalvular aortic stenosis and peripheral pulmonary stenosis. LV = left ventricle; AW = aortic wall; A = aorta; AV = aortic valve; MV = mitral valve; C = thickened coronary artery; PV = pulmonary valve. Arrows point to thickened pulmonary trunk. Note the thickening of the aortic wall close to the aortic valve.

Fibroelastosis of the Left Ventricle

In 35 (35%) (Fig. 60), there was fibroelastosis of all the chambers and fibroelastosis was diffuse in nature in the left ventricle.

Other Major Associated Cardiac Abnormalities in All Types of Aortic Stenosis

Patent foramen ovale—5
Divided right ventricle—1 (Fig. 61)
Residual pulmonic or subpulmonary stenosis—2
Pulmonary hypertension—5
Mitral stenosis—4
Mitral insufficiency—7
Floppy mitral valve—2
Residual subaortic stenosis—11
Aortic stenosis with valve replacement—AI and development of sub-AS—1
Aortic insufficiency—12 (Fig. 62)
Poststenotic dilatation of the ascending aorta—23
Origin of both coronaries from left sinus of Valsalva and anomalous right subclavian artery—1

Aortic stenosis—surgery—AI—prosthesis—1
Aortic stenosis with VSD, anomalous muscle bundles in the left ventricle and surgical replacement of the aortic valve—1
Calcific aortic stenosis with patent ductus with old surgery and aortic valve replacement—1
Aortic stenosis with prosthetic valve replacement—supravalvular aortic stenosis and coronary artery disease—1
Irregularly thickened 3 cusps with fenestrations, dominant right circulation, hypoplastic left and mild atherosclerosis in a 29-year-old—1
Marked irregular thickening of aortic valve, mitral valve, pulmonary valve, and aortic stenosis with replacement of aortic valve—1
Aortic stenosis valvotomy, old residual AS and insufficiency and mitral insufficiency with valve replacement, old, with pulmonary hypertension—1
Single coronary ostium—2
High origin of both coronary ostia—4
High origin of left coronary ostium—1
Origin of both coronaries from left sinus of Valsalva—1

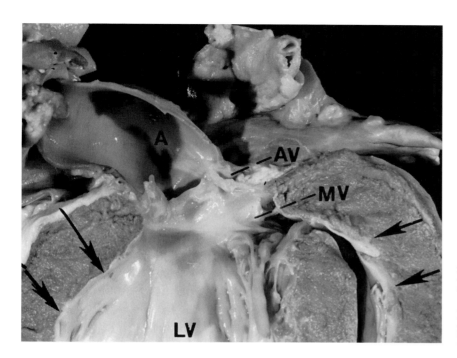

Figure 60: Aortic stenosis with fibroelastosis of the left ventricle. A = ascending aorta; AV = markedly thickened bicuspid aortic valve; MV = mitral valve; LV = left ventricle. Arrows point to the diffuse fibroelastosis of the left ventricle.

Small right coronary ostium—1
High origin of right coronary artery—1
Coronary ostia emerging from anterior cusps—1
Rupture of aortic valve with fistulous tract—1
Fatty infiltration of the right ventricle—2
Fibrosis of the left ventricle and anomalous muscle bands in the left ventricle—1
Left superior vena cava entering coronary sinus—1

Accessory tricuspid orifice with tricuspid insufficiency—1
Cholesterolemia left ear—1
Posterobasal aneurysm—1
Aneurysm of the lower third of the ventricular septum—1

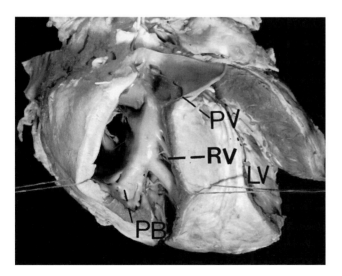

Figure 61: Divided right ventricle in a case of valvular aortic stenosis; right ventricular view. LV = left ventricle; PV = pulmonary valve; RV = right ventricle; PB = markedly hypertrophied parietal band dividing the right ventricle into an inlet and an outlet.

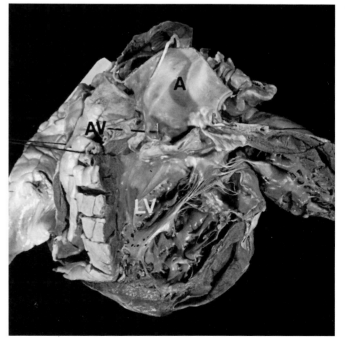

Figure 62: Bicuspid aortic valve with calcification and aortic insufficiency with enlarged left ventricle. A = aorta; AV = markedly irregularly thickened calcified aortic valve with aortic insufficiency; LV = enlarged left ventricle.

Comment

As seen from our material, aortic stenosis in infancy may be broadly grouped into three categories:

Group 1: Small left ventricle, thick wall, and fibroelastosis.

Group 2: Large left ventricle, thick wall, and diffuse fibroelastosis.

Group 3: Hypertrophied left ventricle with mild to moderate fibroelastosis.

In all of the above, the mitral valve may or may not be smaller than normal with an arcade-like malformation with significant mitral stenosis and/or insufficiency. Likewise, there may or may not be hypoplasia of the transverse arch to a varying degree with or without coarctation of the aorta.

The major anatomic problems in aortic stenosis in infancy (below the age of 3 months) are: (1) dysplastic unicuspid or bicuspid aortic valve with small anulus (Fig. 63) (2) small left ventricle, (3) mitral stenosis and/or insufficiency, (4) fibroelastosis of the left ventricle, with or without enlargement of the chamber, (5) hypoplasia of the transverse arch with or without coarctation of the aorta, and the necrotic changes in the myocardium.

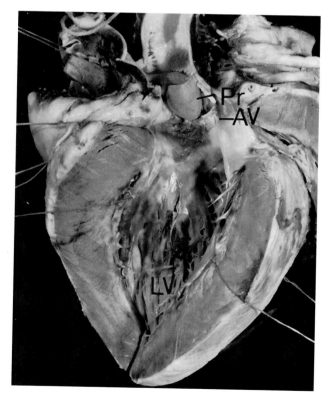

Figure 63: Aortic stenosis with surgical correction (several times) (infancy and childhood); left ventricular view. LV = left ventricle; AV = aortic valve; Pr = prosthesis. Note the markedly deformed aortic valve with tremendous fibroelastosis of the summit of the ventricular septum.

The anatomic findings suggest that aortic stenosis in this age group is a complicated disease. In addition to the altered hemodynamic factors in intrauterine life during the later stages of pregnancy at the atrial level in the developing heart, there probably is an abnormality in the development and formation of the distal bulbar cushions. The presence of fibroelastosis of the left ventricle in 66% suggests intrauterine viral or other infections that might have played a role in the development of this entity, especially when this entity is seen in the newborn.

It is obvious that in a selected few, a balloon dilatation may be helpful. Likewise, the repair of coarctation may be feasible in those with a reasonable-sized left ventricle and a normal-sized or near-normal-sized mitral valve.

It is of significance that in 15 (33%) the atrial septal defect was not present but an oblique small foramen ovale was seen. In one there was a premature closure of the foramen ovale. In this group one may hypothesize that the abnormal formation of the atrial septum might have altered the hemodynamics at the atrial level at a critical stage in the developing heart, resulting in diminished flow to the left side and resulting in critical aortic stenosis. This also suggests the possibility that the abnormal hemodynamics at the atrial level in intrauterine life might have resulted and/or promoted the formation of fibroelastosis of the left ventricle in some. The fibroelastosis of the left ventricle extending to the papillary muscles of the mitral valve may impede the function of the mitral valve, resulting in significant mitral insufficiency and/or stenosis, thereby raising the left atrial pressure and further closing the atrial shunt hemodynamically. Thus, a vicious cycle may be produced.

The development of distal bulbar cushions and the genetic tendency for a specific viral infection to affect the left side of the heart at a critical stage of pregnancy are the areas to be explored further.

The myocardial changes in this group also suggest the possibility that at least in some there might have been a primary myocardial problem at a genetic level. The myocardial changes, per se, to critical aortic stenosis in infancy deserve further research.

Aortic stenosis above the age of 3 months is frequently associated again with fibroelastosis of the left ventricle and mitral valve anomalies. The next in frequency is coarctation of the aorta with or without subaortic stenosis of the discrete type. The left ventricle is hypertrophied and enlarged in the majority. Therefore, in a selected few, balloon dilatation may be attempted in a more or less normally formed aortic valve and occasionally a bicuspid (a less dysplastic) valve may be amenable for such a treatment. Here again the sizes of the left ventricle, the mitral valve anomalies, and fibroelastosis of the left ventricle have to be evaluated thoroughly before any type of management.

The dysplastic aortic valve seen in aortic stenosis is reflected in the disorganization, hypoelastification, and increase in mucopolysaccharides. This is seen whether the valve is uni-, bi-, or tricuspid. This type of valve is similar to congenital polyvalvular disease. The dysplastic nature of the valve suggests that those infants who survive surgery may develop restenosis or insufficiency as they grow older, requiring second surgery at a later date. The myocardial fibrosis seen in infancy raises more doubts as to the success of surgery in the long run. The fibrosis may not only impair the contractibility of the myocardium but may form a nidus for reentry phenomenon resulting in an arrhythmogenic ventricle, and sudden death.

When aortic stenosis is seen beyond the age of 2 years, it is usually an irregular thickened bicuspid valve. There is a greater tendency for a bicuspid valve to get calcific with aging. Likewise, there is a tendency for infective endocarditis to develop in a malformed valve. The calcification is usually in the form of an irregular mass affecting all the valve cusps.

The function of a bicuspid aortic valve with calcification in asymptomatic individuals at various age groups should be compared with a normally formed tricuspid aortic valve. This might shed a light as to the development of calcification with aging in a bicuspid valve versus a normally formed tricuspid aortic valve. An isolated bicuspid aortic valve is probably the most common congenital cardiac anomaly that remains asymptomatic for a long period of time. Unless a specific genetic marker system is identified, this entity probably may remain a challenge for a long time to come.

The association of coronary artery disease, myocardial infarction, and aneurysm formation in the left ventricle in older individuals in this entity is not an unexpected finding. However, a ductus arteriosus, coarctation of the aorta, and/or ventricular septal defect was seen rarely (Figs. 64—66) in the older age group.

When there is subaortic stenosis of the fibroelastic ridge or shelf, recurrence of the lesion is seen frequently following surgery. It is likely that the subaortic area is abnormally developed and hence the susceptibility for recurrence of subaortic obstruction following

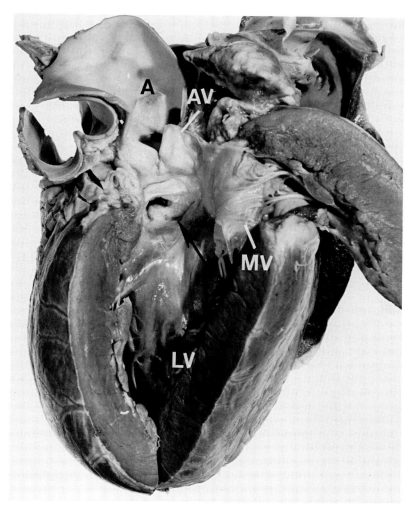

Figure 64: Aortic stenosis with VSD and accessory tricuspid and mitral orifices with insufficiency. AV = aortic valve; A = aorta; MV = mitral valve; LV = left ventricle. Arrow points to the endocardial ridges beneath the aortic valve and along the rim of the VSD.

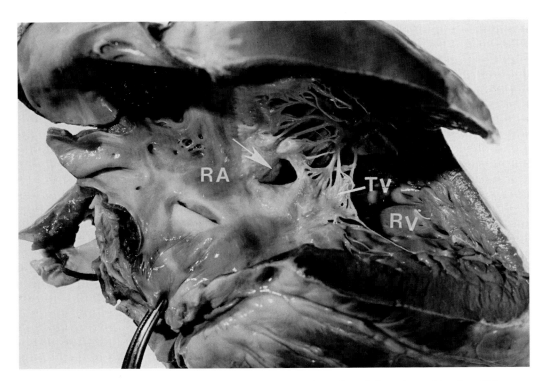

Figure 65: Accessory tricuspid orifice in the septal leaflet of the tricuspid valve. RA = right atrium; TV = tricuspid valve; RV = right ventricle. Arrow points to the accessory orifice.

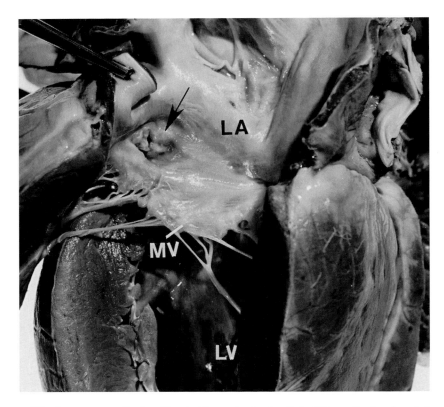

Figure 66: Accessory mitral orifice in the anterior leaflet of the mitral valve. LA = left atrium; LV = left ventricle; MV = mitral valve. Arrow points to the accessory orifice.

surgical intervention. The abnormal development of the subaortic area in turn may be related to a specific genetic marker system that might have been altered during normal embryogenesis. On the other hand, the abnormal formation of the aortic valve may be related to the abnormal formation of distal bulbar cushions. In some there may be an alteration in both the distal and proximal bulbar cushions that might have produced aortic valvular and subaortic obstructive phenomena. The frequent association of a smallness of the valve with a small anulus (Figs. 27—34) and thickening of the aortic valve in subaortic stenosis favors the above theory.

Although hypertrophic cardiomyopathy is an autosomal dominant pattern of inherited genetic disease, it is emphasized that the disease may manifest in very many variations both at the genetic and the clinical level. Today the genetic abnormalities are noted on chromosomes 15, 14q, 11, 7, and 1. With time, many more abnormal genes will be discovered and there may be several subgroups to this entity that may manifest at different age groups with various symptoms. It is again stressed that different genes will be affected differently at different levels.

In summary, aortic stenosis of any type when seen in infancy is definitely a complicated disease. The complications, as discussed previously, include (1) dysplastic aortic valve with a small anulus, (2) anomalies in the mitral valve—stenosis or insufficiency, (3) subaortic stenosis, (4) small left ventricle and fibroelastosis, (5) uncommonly large left ventricle with fibroelastosis, (6) coarctation of the aorta and hypoplasia of transverse arch, and (7) the myocardial changes.

The above findings suggest that in some there may be abnormal hemodynamics in intrauterine life with or without a genetic tendency for abnormal formation of the proximal and distal bulbar cushions. In addition, there may be an infective element or a tendency for a viral infection to occur at the vulnerable stages of development of the heart. Thus, it appears that there probably are several etiologic factors responsible for the development of various types of aortic stenosis.

The marked left ventricular hypertrophy and fibroelastosis are obvious impediments for the contractility of the chamber postoperatively. It appears that the chamber mass attains a critical stage of hypertrophy and is unable to contract any further.

It would be worthwhile to explore a noninvasive method of relieving the stenotic calcific aortic valve by focusing on a special kind of laser beam to affect only the aortic valvular area. Since symptomatic aortic stenosis is seen at various age groups, new innovative methods of treating this disease have to be developed starting at the molecular and genetic levels as well as to refine some of the interventional methodologies that are being used today. Certainly treating aortic stenosis by surgical replacement of the aortic valve in the older age group may remain the method of choice in the immediate future. The fact that an ideal prosthetic valve has not been developed thus far strongly indicates that noninvasive methods of treating this disease by means of pharmacological or other means have to be developed in the future.

One cannot forget the innumerable variations in the aortic valvular and subacute areas that produce aortic and subaortic obstruction that may or may not manifest significant hemodynamic obstruction clinically. The concept of treating the anatomic obstruction without hemodynamic evidence of subaortic and valvular stenosis of varying types, that is, in the so-called "silent types," by means of innovative methods have to be entertained. This may be considered a form of prophylaxis against the development of hypertrophy of the muscle mass.

The tendency for aortic valvular and the entire spectrum of left-sided anomalies to occur in males more so than in females deserves further research.

53

Idiopathic Hypertrophy with Fibroelastosis

In the dilated type, the heart is hypertrophied and enlarged (Fig. 1) without known cause and the endocardium showed fibroelastosis (Fig. 2). The apex is formed by the left ventricle, occasionally by both ventricles. The hypertrophy and enlargement involves all chambers, although in a few cases only the left side is involved. The fibroelastosis involves the left ventricle (Fig. 2) and left atrium maximally and diffusely, while the right atrium and ventricle are, in most cases, more focally involved, occasionally diffusely. The mitral valve is thickened in most cases. It is not known whether this is purely a hemodynamic change or whether it is an extension of the fibroelastic process on the valve. The aortic valve is less frequently involved than the mitral valve. The pulmonary trunk is, in most cases, larger than the aorta, and in a smaller number of cases, equal to the aorta.

In some cases of the contracted type of fibroelastosis, the right side of the heart is dominant (Fig. 3), while the left side is either normal or slightly hypertrophied. Here, marked mitral stenosis is present, with markedly thickened and amorphous valvular tissue (Figs. 4, 5). Here, the apex is formed by the right ventricle (Fig. 6).

Analysis of Our Material

There were 81 cases in our series: 45 males and 36 females. The age ranged from 1 hour to 47 years. The average age was 3 years, 3 months, and 4 days. Nine cases were of the contracted type and in one, fibroelastosis was present in both the right and the left ventricle (Figs. 7, 8). The remainder were of the dilated type.

The Complex

The apex was formed by both ventricles in 12, by the right ventricle in five, and by the left ventricle in 64. In the dilated type, there were hypertrophy and enlargement in all chambers. The tricuspid valve was normal in size in 33 cases and small in two. In the remaining it was enlarged. The pulmonic orifice was normal in size in 34, enlarged in 45, and small in two. The mitral orifice was normal in size in 33, enlarged in 38, and small in 10. The aortic orifice was normal in 46 cases, enlarged in 20, and small in eight. In seven cases, the size of the orifices was not stated.

In the dilated type, all chambers were enlarged. In the contracted type, the left chambers were small or sometimes enlarged (Fig. 9), while there was marked hypertrophy of the right chambers. In one contracted type, there was mild Ebstein-like malformation of the tricuspid valve with redundancy of the valve and insufficiency. In one, the fibroelastosis affected both ventricles. All hearts showed diffuse thickening and whitening of the left ventricle.

The Valves
Tricuspid Valve

The tricuspid valve was in general normally formed and showed the usual or sometimes increased hemodynamic change. The valve leaflets were at times attached to the aberrant papillary muscles. In some cases, the papillary muscles proceeded to the base of the valve rather than to the edge. Occasionally, blood cysts were present on the tricuspid valve. In one, there was a mild Ebstein-like malformation with a nodose, thickened valve which was insufficient.

801

Idiopathic Hypertrophy
with fibroelastosis

DEFINITION

As in title.

HEMODYNAMICS

LV endiastolic pressure elevated; LA, RA & RV pressures elevated.

· No shunts.

· Normal flows.

· Normal cardiac output at rest, decreased with exercise.

PATHOLOGIC COMPLEX

LV & LA hypertrophied and dilated; RA & RV usually hypertrophied, fibroelastosis of LV and sometimes other chambers.

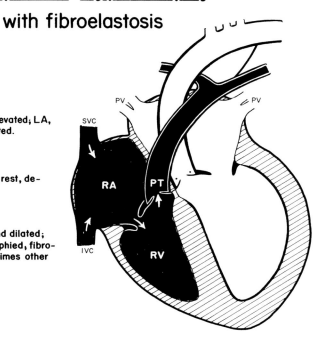

Figure 1: The hemodynamics of idiopathic hypertrophy with fibroelastosis is shown schematically in the diagram. SVC = superior vena cava; IVC = inferior vena cava; RA = right atrium; RV = right ventricle; PT = pulmonary trunk; PV = pulmonary vein.

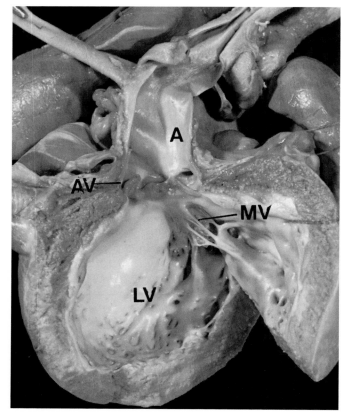

Figure 2: Left ventricular view showing the diffuse fibroelastosis. A = aorta; AV = aortic valve; LV = left ventricle; MV = mitral valve. (Used with permission from Hastreiter AR, Oshima M, Miller RA, Lev M, Paul MH: Congenital aortic stenosis syndrome in infancy. *Circulation* 1963, 28: 1084—1095.)

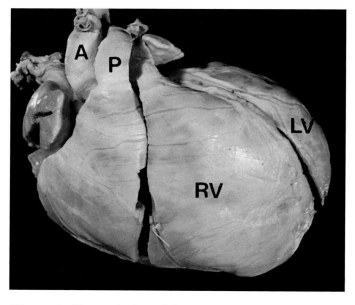

Figure 3: External view of the contracted type of fibroelastosis showing that the apex of the heart is formed by the right ventricle. A = aorta; P = pulmonary trunk; RV = right ventricle; LV = left ventricle.

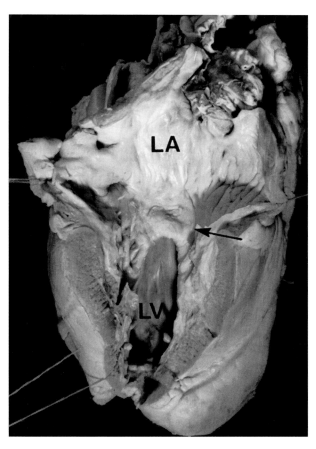

Figure 4: Left atrial view of the contracted type of fibroelastosis showing the markedly thickened mitral valve with marked mitral stenosis and large left atrium. LA = left atrium; LV = left ventricle. Arrow points to the arcade-like malformation of the thickened stenotic mitral valve. (Used with permission from Fixler DA, Cole RB, Paul MH, Lev M, Girod DA: Familial occurrence of the contracted form of endocardial fibroelastosis. *Am J Cardiol* 26:208—213, 1970).

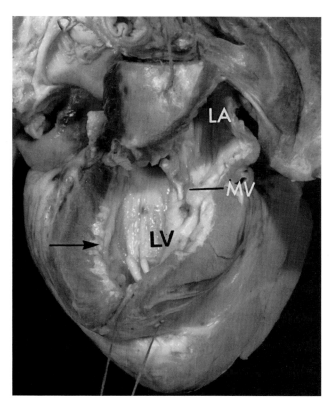

Figure 5: Left atrial-left ventricular view of a case of contracted type of fibroelastosis showing small, thickened mitral valve. LA = left atrium; MV = mitral valve; LV = left ventricle. Arrow points to the diffuse fibroelastosis of the left ventricle.

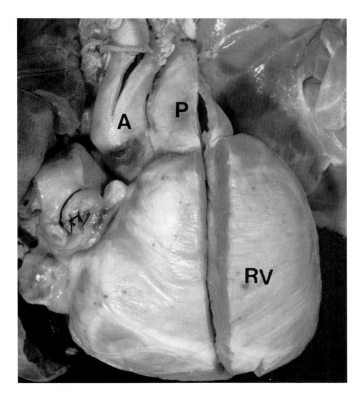

Figure 6: An example of contracted type of fibroelastosis; external view showing the apex formed by the right ventricle. A = smaller aorta; P = larger pulmonary trunk; RV = right ventricle.

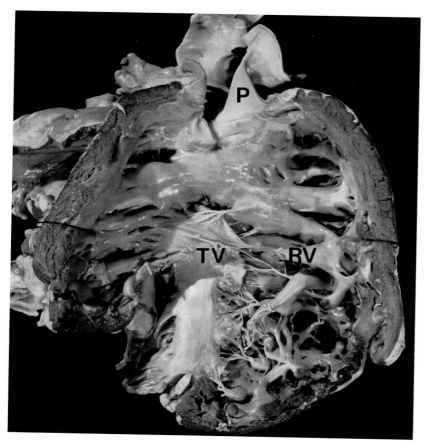

Figure 7: Right ventricular view from a case of contracted type of fibroelastosis with fibroelastosis of the right and left ventricle. P = pulmonary trunk; TV = tricuspid valve; RV = right ventricle.

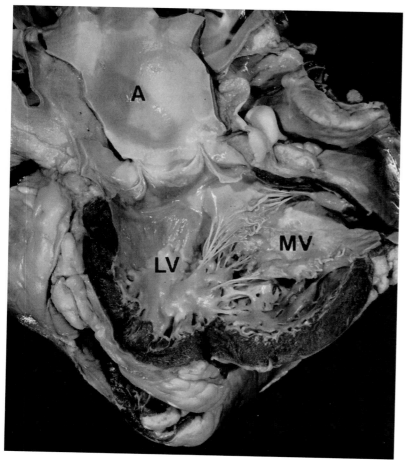

Figure 8: Left ventricular view from a case of contracted type of fibroelastosis with fibroelastosis of both right and left ventricles. Left ventricular view of Figure 7. A = aorta; LV = left ventricle; MV = mitral valve.

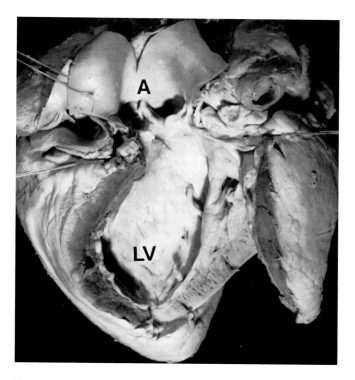

Figure 9: Left ventricular view from a case of contracted type of fibroelastosis showing large left ventricle. A = aorta; LV = left ventricle. (Used with permission from Fixler DA, et al. See Figure 4.)

Pulmonic Valve

The pulmonic valve was almost always normally formed and showed either the usual or increased hemodynamic change. In one, there was dilatation of the sinuses of Valsalva, and in another, widening of the commissures.

Mitral Valve

In 19, the chordae were abbreviated and thick. In two, there were blood cysts. In some, the chordae were shrunken, nodose, and fibrotic. In the majority, however, they were normally formed but showed increased hemodynamic change (Fig. 10). Where the size of the left ventricle was large, the papillary muscles were situated more towards the base of the heart. In addition, papillary muscles were flattened and fibrosed in many (Fig. 11).

Aortic Valve

Most of the valves were markedly thickened with increased hemodynamic change. Four were bicuspid. In one, the right and posterior sinuses of Valsalva were aneurysmally dilated.

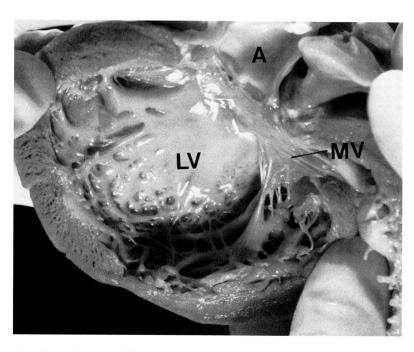

Figure 10: Dilated type of fibroelastosis showing normally formed mitral valve. A = aorta; LV = left ventricle; MV = mitral valve showing increased hemodynamic change.

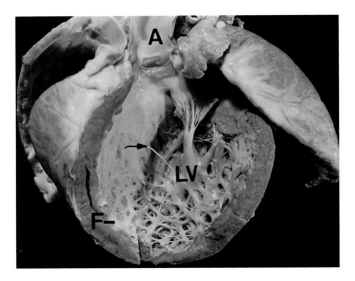

Figure 11: Left ventricular view of a dilated type of fibroelastosis showing fibrosis of the posterior papillary muscle. LV = left ventricle; A = aorta; F = fibroelastosis. Arrow points to the accessory chordae.

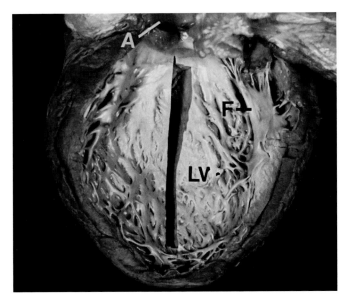

Figure 12: Left ventricular view of a dilated type of fibroelastosis showing fibrotic scars and accessory chordae and muscle bands. A = aorta; LV = left ventricle; F = fibrotic scar. Arrow points to the fibrotic papillary muscle.

The Endocardium

The endocardium of all chambers was thickened and whitened, especially that of the left ventricle. In some, distinct fibrotic scars were present with accessory chordal or muscle bands in the left ventricle (Fig. 12).

Microscopic Examination

This showed marked thickening of the endocardium, consisting of a mixture of collagen connective tissue with elastic tissue (Fig. 13). There was no evidence of myocarditis in the cases studied.

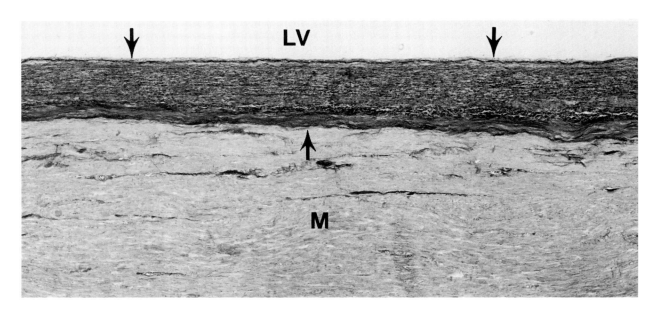

Figure 13: Microscopic examination of the left ventricle demonstrating the fibroelastosis. LV = left ventricular cavity; M = myocardium. Arrows point to the marked endocardial fibroelastosis of the left ventricle.

Comment

The associated cardiac abnormalities are given in Tables 1 and 2.

Table 1

Associated Cardiac Abnormalities

In general, they were not seen. Occasionally, they were seen.

Patent foramen ovale	13
Fossa ovalis defect	4
Abnormal architecture of the atrial septum	1
Aneurysm of fossa ovalis	2
Entry of coronary sinus into both atria	1
Tricuspid insufficiency with diverticulum of right ventricle	1
Abnormal architecture of the right ventricle	4
Abnormal ridge in left atrium	1
Mitral stenosis	1
Absent chordae in the left ventricle	2
Division of left ventricle into two parts	1
Aortic stenosis and mitral stenosis of a mild nature	1
Abnormal mitral valve	1
Anatomic adult coarctation	1
Fetal coarctation	1
High origin of right coronary ostium	1
High origin of left coronary ostium	3
Large left coronary artery with small right coronary artery	1
Cirsoid wide patent ductus arteriosus	1 (1 day old)
Sudden death	1 (21 months)
Congenital AV block	1 (2 days)
Wolff-Parkinson-White syndrome	1 (1 yr)

Table 2

Contracted Type of Fibroelastosis of the Left Ventricle

With fibroelastosis of the right ventricle	1
With mitral stenosis and ASD	1
With mitral stenosis	4
With deformed arcade mitral valve, mitral stenosis and insufficiency, and marked pulmonary hypertension	1
Familial congestive cardiomyopathy and ventricular tachycardia with mild Ebstein's anomaly with redundant tricuspid valve with tricuspid insufficiency; aneurysm of membranous septum and pulmonary hypertension	1
With normal mitral valve	1

Etiogenesis of Fibroelastosis

It is not known whether this is a primary phenomenon due to altered changes in the synthesis of collagen connective tissue, with or without alteration in the formation of elastic tissue. Some believe the fibroelastosis is the end result of previous myocarditis or endocarditis in intrauterine life. Whether it is primary or secondary in nature, we also have to entertain the fact that in at least some cases this may be related to abnormal (obstructive) lymphatic drainage of the heart.

In still others, this may represent a primary genetic abnormality or may be the end result of an antigen, antibody reaction due to varying types of allergic states at the molecular genetic level.

54

Origin of One or Both Coronary Arteries from the Pulmonary Arterial Tree

Origin of the Left Coronary Artery from the Pulmonary Trunk

In this anomaly, the left coronary artery arises from the left posterior sinuses of Valsalva of the pulmonary trunk (Fig. 1). The right coronary artery emerges normally (Fig. 2) and is a large and tortuous vessel. Dominance of the right coronary artery is of great importance in the longevity of the patient.

The heart is greatly enlarged. The apex is formed by the left ventricle. The anterior descending coronary artery courses in its usual position and is shifted somewhat to the right. In some cases this vessel characteristically rides over the hump of the left ventricle.

The basic internal pathology lies in the left ventricle (Fig. 2). This chamber is markedly dilated with a wall of average thickness, or somewhat thickened wall, or focal or generalized thinness of the myocardium. There may be an associated infarct of the myocardium which in some cases may be extensive. The endocardium shows diffuse fibroelastosis. The left atrium is hypertrophied and enlarged. The infarction of the left ventricle may extend to the posterior and anterior groups of papillary muscles, resulting in mitral insufficiency, clinically. We are dealing with poor perfusion of the myocardium of the left ventricle and anterior part of the septum with deoxygenated blood under low pressure in the early stages of the disease. As the right coronary artery takes over the circulation, there results a runoff of blood into the left coronary artery and into the pulmonary trunk. The extent of this runoff is variable (Fig. 3).

Analysis of Our Material

There were 23 cases in our series; 11 were males and 12 were females. The youngest patient was 2 days old and the oldest was 20 years, 11 months, 11 days. The average age was 2 years, 2 months, 14 days. Eight were white and eight were black patients. The race of the remainder is unknown.

The Complex

The apex was formed by the left ventricle in all except one case. The anterior descending coronary artery was pushed to the right side. In the exceptional case, the apex was formed by both ventricles. There was hypertrophy and enlargement of all chambers, especially the left atrium and ventricle. The wall of the left ventricle was often thin.

The tricuspid orifice was normal in size in 11, enlarged in 10, and smaller than normal in two. The pulmonic orifice was normal in 11, enlarged in 10, questionably small in one, and not stated in one. The mitral orifice was normal in size in nine, enlarged in 12, and not stated in two. The aortic orifice was normal in size in 11, enlarged in nine, small in one, and not stated in one. The tricuspid valve, in general, was normally formed and showed either normal or increased hemodynamic change and occasional blood cysts. The medial leaflet was ballooned out in one case, and in another there was tricuspid stenosis. The medial leaflet was connected to an irregularly formed septal band in one. In one the valvular material was considerably thick, ir-

809

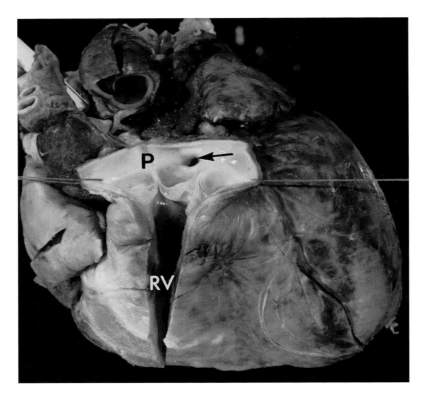

Figure 1: Origin of left coronary artery from the pulmonary trunk. Right ventricular view. P = pulmonary trunk; RV = right ventricle. Arrow points to the left coronary artery emerging from the left posterior pulmonic cusp.

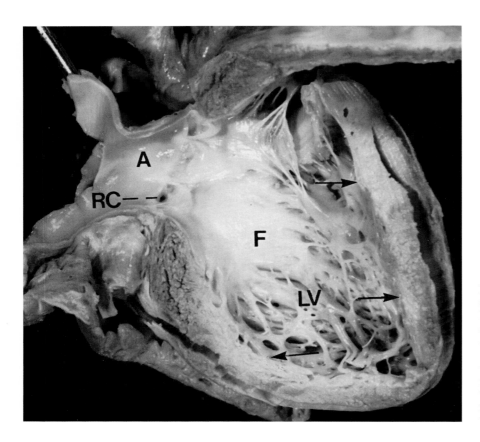

Figure 2: Origin of left coronary artery from the pulmonary artery. Left ventricular view showing the normal origin of right coronary artery from the aorta, and enlarged left ventricle with fibroelastosis and infarct in the anterior and inferior walls. A = aorta; LV = left ventricle; RC = right coronary artery; F = fibroelastosis of the left ventricle. Arrows point to the infarct in the anteroseptal and inferior walls.

<u>L</u>eft <u>C</u>oronary from <u>P</u>ulmonary

DEFINITION

As in title.

HEMODYNAMICS

- **Pressures normal in all heart chambers, low in left coronary artery.**
- **Small L→R shunt at pulmonary level.**
- **Slightly increased pulmonary flow.**
- **Blood flows from right coronary artery through left coronary artery into PA.**

PATHOLOGIC COMPLEX

LA & LV hypertrophied and dilated; endocardial fibroelastosis of LV; myocardial infarct may be present.

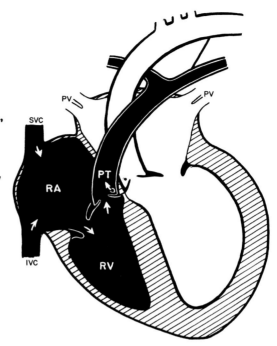

Figure 3: The hemodynamics of this anomaly is depicted schematically in the diagram. SVC = superior vena cava; IVC = inferior vena cava; RA = right atrium; RV = right ventricle; PV = pulmonary vein; PT = pulmonary trunk.

regular, and nodose. The pulmonic valve in all cases was normally formed and showed increased hemodynamic change.

The mitral valve was normally formed and showed considerably increased hemodynamic change in all but five. In one it was a sheet of valvular tissue plastered onto the ventricular septum and connected to a single papillary muscle in the posterior wall. In another case it was ballooned out. In three cases the chordae were short with a papillary muscle lying close to the valve, and the line of closure was thick and nodose.

The aortic valve was normally formed in all but one case where it was bicuspid. It usually showed increased hemodynamic change.

The endocardium showed focal thickening and whitening in the right atrium and right ventricle, and diffuse thickening and whitening and fibroelastosis in the left atrium and left ventricle. The fibroelastosis extended to the anterior and posterior groups of papillary muscles.

In four cases there was marked fibrosis of the myocardium and subendocardium. Infarction of the left ventricle occurred in six cases. Marked mitral insufficiency was present in four. In one case there was massive infarction of the ventricular septum, which created a bulge into the right ventricle with obstruction of the mouth of the pulmonary artery with secondary tricuspid stenosis. In three cases both papillary muscles were fibrotic and flattened and displaced proximally. Associated cardiac abnormalities were scarce. There was one common brachiocephalic trunk, one patent ductus arteriosus, two foramen ovale defects, one rete Chiari, and one case of coarctation.

Comment

The marked fibrosis of the ventricular myocardium present in some cases points to the necessity of early operative intervention.

In one unique 2-day-old infant, there was an oblique patent foramen ovale, closing ductus arteriosus, and infarct of the left ventricle. The left coronary artery was larger than the right coronary artery. This infant died suddenly. This was the youngest in our series. The presence of an oblique patent foramen ovale suggests that the transition from fetal circulation to the adult type of circulatory pattern might have occurred immediately after birth rather than in a gradual manner within the 48 hours after birth. In addition, the ductus arteriosus was closed or closing functionally. Thus, in the presence of an adult type of circulation immediately after birth, the pressure in the pulmonary artery could have dropped rapidly resulting in a steal-like phenomenon. Histologically, the myocardium revealed fresh infarction of the left ventricle. This unique case suggests that significant clinical problems can occur in the neonatal period, which may result in sudden death in cases of origin of the left coronary artery from the pulmonary arterial tree with a dominant left coronary circulation and a small right coronary artery.

Location of the Coronary Ostium and its Surgical Significance

In general, the left coronary artery either emerged from the left or the right posterior pulmonic cusp. It may be easier for the surgeon to relocate the left coronary artery when it emerges from the left pulmonic cusp than when it emerges from the right posterior pulmonic cusp. In the latter as well as when the coronary artery emerges from the right pulmonary artery, there may be technical problems associated with relocation that may in the long run produce kinking and narrowing.

The left coronary ostium either emerged from the base of the sinuses of Valsalva, or at the higher level up to the level of the supravalvular ridge, or above the sinuses of Valsalva. This is an important anatomic detail for the surgeon to tailor the appropriate kind of surgical technique in each case.

Depending on the location of the coronary ostium, the size of the pulmonary flap would vary from small to large during the surgical relocation of the coronary ostium to the left aortic sinus of Valsalva. In these cir-cumstances, graft enlargement of the pulmonary trunk may be required. At the same time, a kink at the anastomotic site in the aortic sinus region and/or close to the right coronary ostium should be prevented. A supravalvular relocation of the left coronary ostium close to the right coronary ostium may result in the left coronary artery coursing between the aorta and the pulmonary trunk with the future possibility of coronary ischemia and sudden death.

On the other hand, in some selected cases with extensive myocardial infarction (septal, anterolateral, and inferior walls) of the left ventricle and fibrosis of the papillary muscles of the mitral valve, cardiac transplantation may be entertained.

Origin of the Right Coronary Artery from the Pulmonary Trunk

This permits survival to adult life, but the patient may die suddenly with an infarct in the posterior wall of the left ventricle. The right ventricle may or may not show ischemic changes. No case of this anomaly was present in this series.

Origin of the Left Coronary Artery from the Right Pulmonary Artery

This is rare and, of course, produces the same effect as origin from the pulmonary trunk. There were two cases of origin of the left coronary artery from the beginning of the right pulmonary artery in our series (Fig. 4). One was 3½ months old and the other was 3

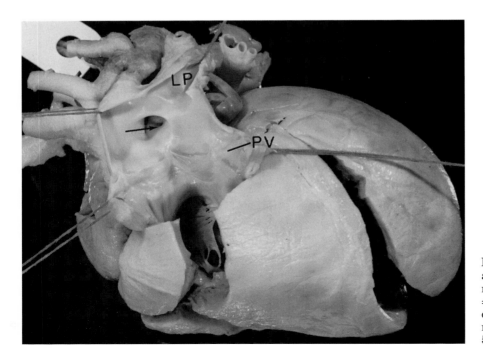

Figure 4: Origin of the left coronary artery from the beginning of the right pulmonary artery. PV = pulmonary valve; LP = left pulmonary artery. Arrow points to origin of the left coronary. (Used with permission from Bharati S, et al. See Figure 5.)

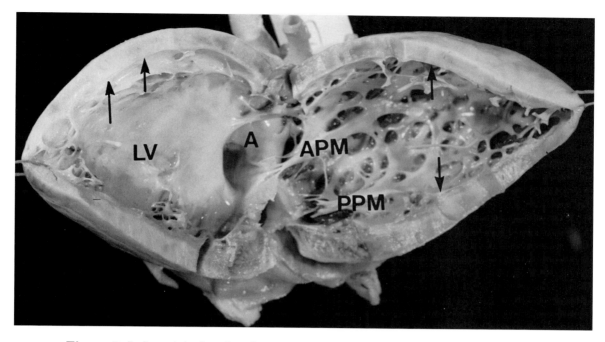

Figure 5: Left ventricular view demonstrating the large left ventricle with infarction of the anterolateral and inferior walls of the septum. Also note the fibrosed anterior (APM) and posterior (PPM) papillary muscles situated more proximally than normal. LV = left ventricle; A = aorta. Arrows point to the fibrosed areas in the anterolateral and inferior walls. (Used with permission from Bharati S, Chandra N, Stephenson L, et al: Origin of left coronary artery from the right pulmonary artery. *J Am Coll Cardiol* 3:1565—1569, 1984.)

months old. Both were male and white. One was associated with coarctation of the aorta. The electrocardiogram was compatible with infarction of anterolateral and inferior left ventricular walls. There was extensive fibrosis of the septum and free walls with fibrotic papillary muscles (Fig. 5). The other case was associated with a dysplastic tricuspid valve that was considerably enlarged with tricuspid insufficiency. In addition, this was a case of sequestrated right lung with abnormal distribution of right pulmonary artery branch and an anomalous celiac artery branch to part of the right lung. There was a spontaneously closed ventricular septal defect in one case.

Origin of Both Coronary Arteries from the Pulmonary Trunk

This again is very rare and is seen in neonates. There was one case in our series (Fig. 6). This was a 3-day-old white female infant. It was associated with hypoplasia of the aortic tract complex (Fig. 7). Also present were marked mitral stenosis (Fig. 8) with an aneurysm of the fossa ovalis and a dysplastic tricuspid orifice with tricuspid insufficiency, coarctation, patent ductus arteriosus, and a small muscular ventricular septal defect.

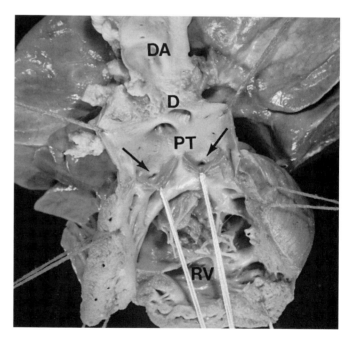

Figure 6: Origin of both coronaries from the pulmonary trunk. Right ventricular outflow tract view showing the origin of both coronary arteries from the posterior sinus of Valsalva. D = ductus arteriosus; DA = descending aorta; PT = pulmonary trunk; RV = right ventricle. Note the two strings that open up the sinuses of Valsalva and the arrows pointing to the coronary ostia. (Used with permission from Bharati S, et al. See Figure 8.)

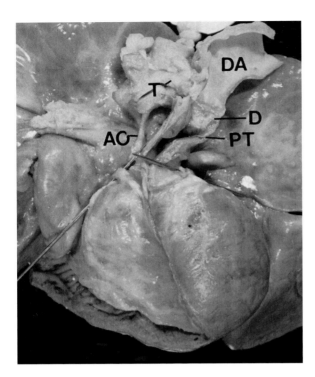

Figure 7: External view of the heart of Fig. 6 showing the hypoplasia of the ascending aorta. AO = aorta; D = ductus arteriosus; DA = descending aorta; PT = pulmonary trunk; T = transverse arch. Note the minute ascending aorta that widens out to form the transverse arch and the ductus forming the descending aorta. Note also two probes lifting the right and left coronary arteries as they form a sling around the base of the pulmonary trunk. (Used with permission from Bharati S, et al. See Figure 8.)

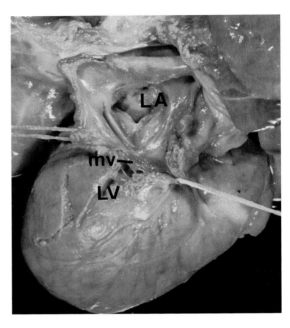

Figure 8: Left atrial view of Figures 6 and 7 showing the small mitral valve and small left ventricle. LA = left atrium; LV = left ventricle; MV = mitral valve. (Used with permission from Bharati S, Szarnicki RJ, Popper R, Fryer A, Lev M: Origin of both coronary arteries from the pulmonary trunk associated with hypoplasia of aortic tract complex: A new entity. *J Am Coll Cardiol* 3:437—441, 1984.)

Ebstein's Anomaly

In Ebstein's anomaly, there is downward displacement of part or all of the effective ring of the tricuspid valve, with associated abnormality of the valvular apparatus and hence, of the architecture of the right ventricle (Fig. 1). The downward displacement and the associated valvular abnormality vary considerably in each heart resulting from a marked Ebstein-like malformation in a moderate to mild form. It is self-evident that when it is markedly malformed, the hemodynamics of Ebstein's anomaly is severe, and if mild to moderate, the hemodynamics are mild to moderate and permit survival to older age. This disease may be classified as follows:

1. Simple Ebstein's anomaly
2. Complicated
   a. with pulmonary stenosis or atresia
   b. with VSD
   c. with mitral stenosis, with or without VSD
   d. with tetralogy of Fallot or double outlet right ventricle or overriding of the aorta
   e. with mixed levocardia or mesocardia (corrected transposition).

Simple Ebstein's Anomaly

The ring or base (anulus) of the anterior leaflet is usually completely anchored on the original right AV orifice. In a few cases, the lateral portion of the ring is deviated and in occasional instances, the entire ring is gradually deviated downward into the right ventricle, but remains anchored on the pars membranacea. The anterior leaflet is large, often converted into a large sail-like sheet in which are embedded one or more anterolateral papillary muscles. Occasionally, this leaflet is perforated, producing one or several openings into the conus (Fig. 2). The ring of the medial leaflet is gradually deviated a varying distance downward into the right ventricle. It is a relatively small leaflet, often im-

mobile and sometimes deficient or absent. The ring of the inferior leaflet is displaced downward into the right ventricle. It is connected in most cases, to aberrant, inferior papillary muscles (Fig. 2). It is often deficient and, in some cases, completely absent. In an occasional case, the tricuspid valve ring may not be displaced, but the proximal part of the valve is adherent to the wall of the right ventricle so that the effective ring is displaced.

The original AV orifice is in all cases greatly enlarged. The effective orifice or orifices present at the distal portion of the valve funnel is usually normal in size, but in some cases, distinctly smaller than normal, producing stenosis (Fig. 3). Insufficiency of the valve is present in many cases due to deficiency or absence of the medial and inferior leaflets.

Thus, the right ventricle is divided into proximal and distal chambers. The proximal chamber is equal to, smaller than, or larger than the distal chamber, dependent on the degree of tricuspid ring displacement. The proximal chamber is usually thin-walled, often with a markedly thickened endocardium. It may be aneurysmally dilated and paper-thin (Figs. 4, 5). The distal chamber consists of a conus in all cases, apical recess in almost all cases, and a portion of sinus in most cases. On the septum, the demarcation between proximal and distal chambers may be in the form of a ridge of fibrous tissue and muscle. The size of the distal chamber, in most cases, is less than that of the definitive right ventricle in a normal person of the same age, weight, and height. The wall of the chamber is of average thickness for the given age or thinner than normal. There is a tendency for the arch produced by the junction of the septal and parietal bands to be shallower than normal. The muscle of Lancisi, thus, is implanted high in the conus and in some it is enlarged (Fig. 5).

The right atrium is markedly hypertrophied and enlarged in all cases. The eustachian valve has a ten-

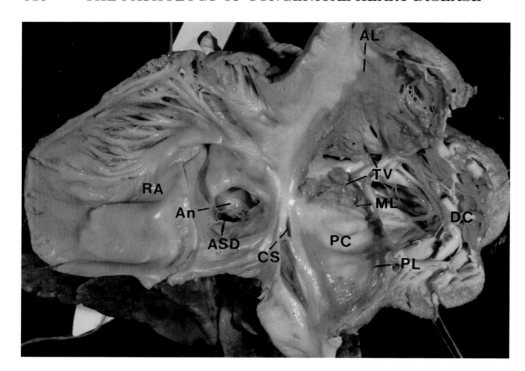

Figure 1: Ebstein's anomaly depicting the downward displacement of the medial and posterior leaflets of the tricuspid valve into the sinus of the right ventricle dividing the ventricle into a proximal and a distal chamber. CS = coronary sinus; RA = right atrium; An = aneurysm of fossa ovalis; ASD = atrial septal defect, fossa ovalis type; PC = proximal chamber; TV = tricuspid valve; PL = posterior leaflet; ML = medial leaflet; AL = anterior leaflet; DC = distal chamber.

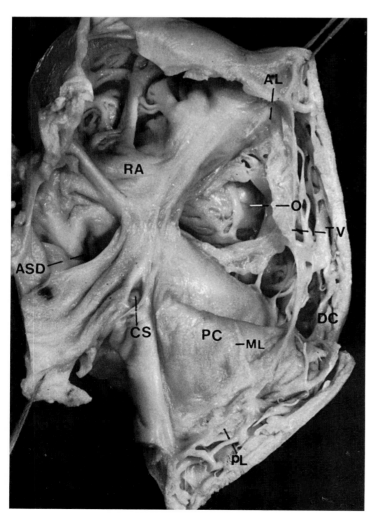

Figure 2: Ebstein's anomaly showing large opening in the anterior leaflet. RA = right atrium; PC = proximal chamber; DC = distal chamber; CS = coronary sinus; ASD = atrial septal defect; TV = tricuspid valve; ML = medial leaflet; PL = posterior leaflet; O = opening in the anterior leaflet; AL = anterior leaflet.

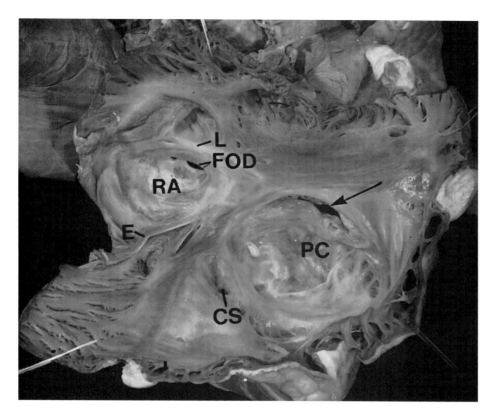

Figure 3: Marked Ebstein malformation with tricuspid stenosis. Right atrial, right ventricular view. RA = right atrium; L = limbus fossa ovalis; FOD = fossa ovalis defect; E = eustachian valve; CS = coronary sinus; PC = proximal chamber, with displaced septal and inferior leaflets. Arrow points to the marked stenosis of the effective tricuspid orifice with stenosis.

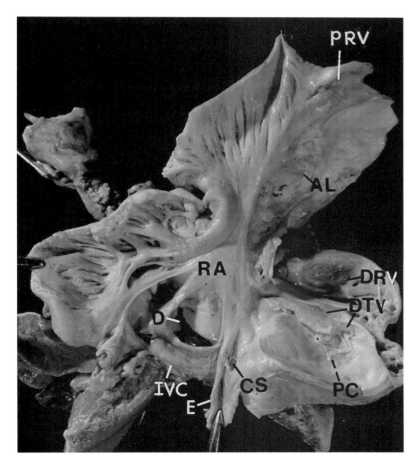

Figure 4: Aneurysmally dilated and paper-thin right ventricle in a case of Ebstein's anomaly with marked pulmonary stenosis. Right atrial, right ventricular view. RA = right atrium; D = atrial septal defect; IVC = inferior vena cava; E = eustachian valve; CS = coronary sinus; PC = proximal chamber; DTV = displaced tricuspid valve; DRV = distal right ventricular chamber; AL = anterior leaflet; PRV = paper thin right ventricle. (Used with permission from Lev M, et al. See Figure 42.)

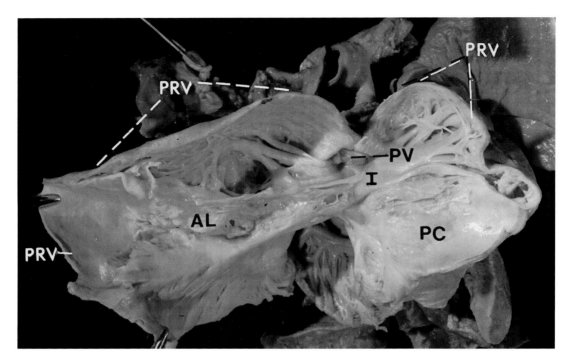

Figure 5: Outflow tract of right ventricle depicting the paper-thin right ventricle in a case of Ebstein's anomaly with marked pulmonary stenosis. PRV = paper-thin right ventricle; AL = anterior leaflet; PC = proximal chamber; I = infundibulum; PV = pulmonary valve. (Used with permission from Lev M, et al. See Figure 42.)

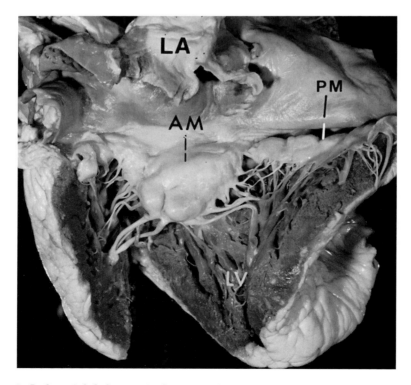

Figure 6: Left atrial, left ventricular view showing the redundant mitral valve. LA = left atrium; AM = anterior mitral leaflet; PM = posterior mitral leaflet. Note the marked redundancy of both the leaflets with elongated and thickened chordae (floppy mitral valve).

Ebstein's Complex

DEFINITION

Downward displacement of tricuspid orifice.

HEMODYNAMICS

- RA pressure elevated; RV, PA, LA & LV pressures normal, (or decreased).
- R→L shunt at atrial level if ASD present.
- Decreased pulmonary flow.
- Cyanosis if ASD present.

PATHOLOGIC COMPLEX

RA hypertrophied and dilated; proximal and distal RV chambers; small pulmonary artery; ASD usually; LA & LV normal.

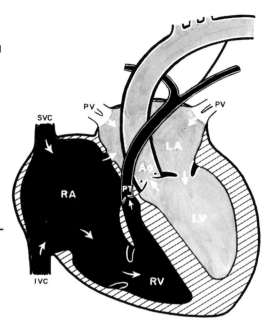

Figure 7: The hemodynamics of this entity is depicted schematically in the diagram. SVC = superior vena cava; IVC = inferior vena cava; RA = right atrium; RV = right ventricle; PA = pulmonary artery; PT = pulmonary trunk; PV = pulmonary veins; LA = left atrium; LV = left ventricle; Ao = aorta; R→L = right to left; ASD = atrial septal defect.

dency to be prominent. An atrial septal defect of the fossa ovalis type or a patent foramen ovale is most often seen, and a patent ductus is frequently present. The pulmonary orifice and trunk are either normal in size or smaller than normal and the pulmonic valve is normal. The size of the left side of the heart varies according to the amount of pulmonary flow and the presence of an atrial septal defect. The mitral valve is often greatly thickened. This may be a hemodynamic alteration produced by the deviation of the septum to the left. In some, the mitral valve is redundant and floppy and may be either stenotic or insufficient hemodynamically (Fig. 6). The aortic orifice and valve are usually normal.

The fundamental hemodynamic alteration in Ebstein's anomaly may be considered to lie in the atrialized right ventricle (proximal chamber) (Fig. 7). Since this portion contracts at the same time as the distal chamber, it thus forces blood into the right atrium. In cases with true tricuspid insufficiency, the above effects are exacerbated. If there is tricuspid stenosis, the filling of the distal chamber may be impaired. The altered hemodynamics causes a peculiar left ventricular septal bulge.

Complicated Types of Ebstein's Anomaly

With Pulmonary Stenosis or Atresia

The pulmonic valve may be abnormally formed, or diaphragm-like with enlargement of the proximal and distal chambers, or there may be pulmonary atresia.

With Ventricular Septal Defect

If the defect enters the proximal chamber, there may be exacerbation of the usual findings. If it enters the distal chamber, there may be pulmonary hypertension.

With Mitral Stenosis, with or without Ventricular Septal Defect

The thickening of the mitral valve alluded to above may be associated with a small mitral orifice producing stenosis (Figs. 8, 9).

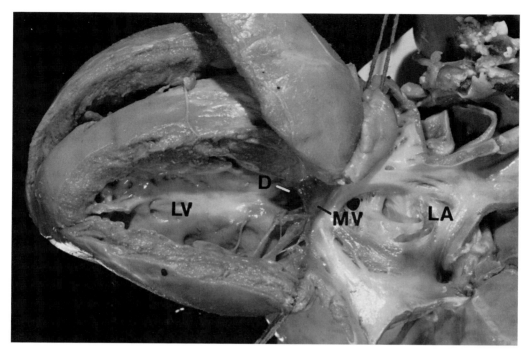

Figure 8: Small mitral orifice with mitral stenosis in a case of Ebstein's anomaly and ventricular septal defect. Left atrial, left ventricular view showing the small mitral valve. LA = left atrium; LV = left ventricle; MV = mitral valve; D = ventricular septal defect. Note that the anterior and posterior leaflets are not well demarcated into two distinct components with poorly developed papillary muscles. (Used with permission from Lev M, et al. See Figure 42.)

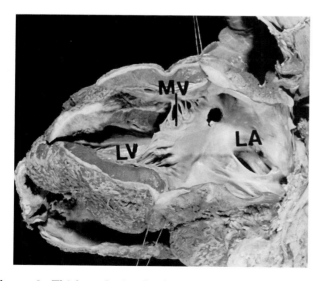

Figure 9: Thickened mitral valve with small mitral and mitral stenosis in a case of Ebstein's anomaly without ventricular septal defect. Left atrial, left ventricular view. LA = left atrium; LV = left ventricle; MV = mitral valve.

With Tetralogy of Fallot or Double Outlet Right Ventricle

These are rarities (Figs. 10, 11).

With Mixed Levocardia or Mesocardia

In these anomalies, the left-sided AV orifice is the seat of the abnormality. Hence, it is the left atrium that is markedly hypertrophied and enlarged, accompanied by hypertrophy and enlargement of the distal chamber of the morphological right (left-sided) ventricle and the morphological left ventricle (right-sided). This will be discussed further in the chapter on mixed levocardia (corrected transposition).

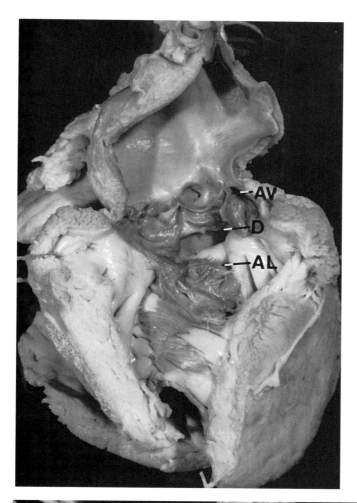

Figure 10: Overriding aorta and pulmonary atresia with ventricular septal defect or tetralogy of Fallot with pulmonary atresia in a case of Ebstein's malformation. Right ventricular outflow tract view depicting the aorta emerging in an overriding manner. AV = aortic valve; D = defect; AL = attachment of the anterior leaflet of the tricuspid close to the base of the VSD. (Used with permission from Lev M, et al. See Figure 42.)

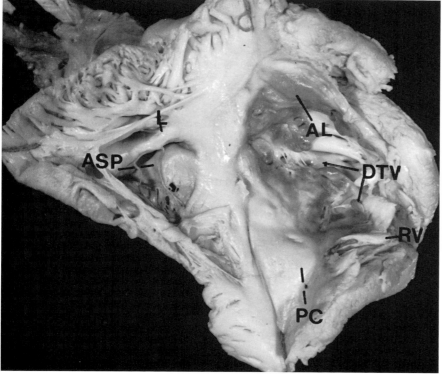

Figure 11: Ebstein's malformation of the tricuspid valve from the case shown in Figure 10. Right atrial, right ventricular view. ASP = aneurysm of the septum primum with a small atrial septal defect; PC = proximal chamber; RV = distal right ventricular chamber; AL = anterior leaflet of the tricuspid valve; DTV = displaced tricuspid valve. (Used with permission from Lev M, et al. See Figure 42.)

Figure 12: Ebstein's malformation from a case of a stillborn infant. Right atrial, right ventricular view. FOD = fossa ovalis defect; L = limbus fossa ovalis; CS = coronary sinus; PC = proximal chamber; DTV = displaced tricuspid valve; AL = anterior leaflet; RV = distal right ventricular chamber.

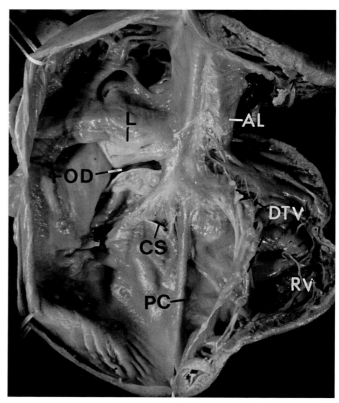

Analysis of Our Material

There were 67 cases in our series. Their age ranged from stillbirth (Fig. 12) to 84 years of age (Fig. 13). Forty-one were female and 26 were male. The median age was 9 years. Table I shows the occurrence of Ebstein's anomaly in various age groups. Approximately 62% were below the age of 6 months.

The heart was hypertrophied and enlarged in all (Fig. 14). The apex was formed by the right ventricle in 15 (Fig. 15), by the left ventricle in 26, by both ventricles in 24, and in one it was not determined. In one case, the apex was bifid.

The right atrium was markedly hypertrophied and enlarged in all cases. The eustachian valve had a tendency to be prominent (Fig. 16). In the majority of cases, there was an atrial septal defect of either medium or large size (Fig. 17). The status of the atrial

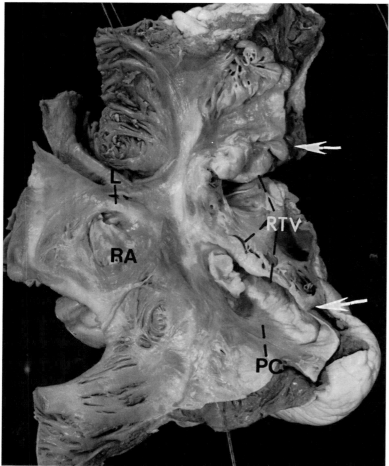

Figure 13: Ebstein's malformation from a case of an 84-year-old male. Right atrial, right ventricular view depicting the markedly redundant tricuspid valve leaflets with mild Ebstein-like malformation. RA = right atrium; RTV = redundant tricuspid valve leaflet; PC = proximal chamber; L = limbus. Arrows point to the redundant leaflets. (Used with permission from Lev M, et al. See Figure 42.)

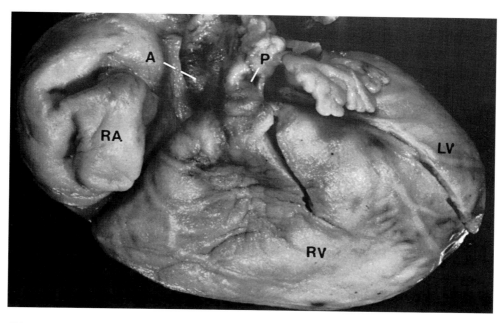

Figure 14: Enlarged heart, external view showing the apex formed by both ventricles. RA = right atrium; RV = right ventricle; LV = left ventricle; A = aorta; P = pulmonary trunk.

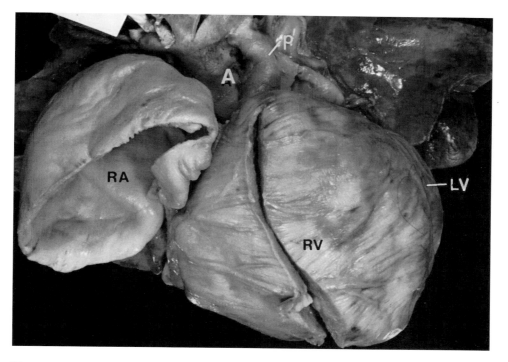

Figure 15: External view showing the apex formed by the right ventricle. RA = huge right atrium; RV = right ventricle; LV = left ventricle; A = aorta; P = pulmonary trunk.

Table 1

Number of Cases in Various Age Groups

Stillborn	3	(4.5%)	
Less than 1 month (32 weeks' gest.— 2)	29	(43%)	62.5%
1—6 months	10	(15%)	
6 months—1 year	1		
1—5 years	5		
5—10 years	5		
10—20 years	1		
20—30 years	5		
30—40 years	3		
40—50 years	1		
50—60 years	2		
60—70 years	1		
70—80 years	0		
80—90 years	1		

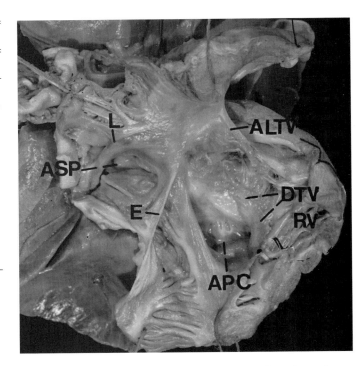

Figure 16: Markedly hypertrophied and enlarged eustachian valve in a case of Ebstein's anomaly. Right atrial, right ventricular view. ASP = aneurysm of the septum primum; L = limbus fossa ovalis; E = enlarged eustachian valve; APC = atrialized proximal chamber; DTV = displaced tricuspid valve; ALTV = anterior leaflet of the tricuspid valve; RV = right ventricle.

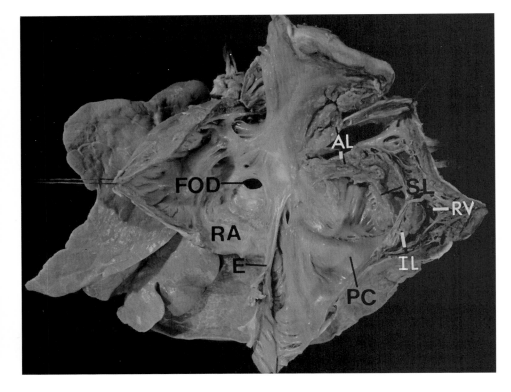

Figure 17: Ebstein's anomaly showing a good-sized atrial septal defect. Right atrial, right ventricular view. FOD = fossa ovalis defect; SL = septal (medial) leaflet; RA = right atrium; E = enlarged eustachian valve; PC = proximal chamber; IL = inferior leaflet of the tricuspid valve; AL = anterior leaflet of the tricuspid valve; RV = distal right ventricular chamber.

Table 2

Morphology of the Atrial Septum

ASD fossa ovalis type	35	(52%)
Huge ASD	11	(16%)
Patent foramen ovale	7	
Closed foramen ovale	6	
Surgically closed ASD	3	
Oblique PFO	2	
Common atrium	1	
Coronary sinus ASD small	1	
Proximal ASD with straddling right upper pulmonary veins	1	

Table 3

Morphology of the Ventricular Septal Defect

VSD in 11 cases (16%) and usually this entered the distal chamber. In two cases, the VSD entered the proximal changer.

Anterior large defect entered distal chamber	4
Moderate defect entered distal chamber	3
Anterior small defect entered distal chamber	1
Small defect entered distal chamber	1
Large defect entered proximal chamber	1
Small defect entered proximal chamber	1

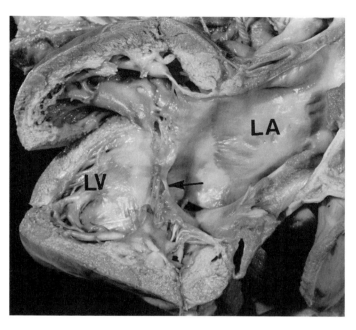

Figure 19: Same heart as shown in Figure 18. Left atrial side of the common atrium and left ventricular view. LA = left atrial side of the common atrium; LV = left ventricle. Arrow points to the incomplete cleft-like malformation of the anterior leaflet of the mitral valve.

septum is given in Table 2. An atypical primum defect was found in one with a common atrium (Figs. 18, 19).

There was a ventricular septal defect in 11 cases (16%). Usually, this entered the distal chamber (Figs. 20—22). In two cases, the VSD entered the proximal chamber (Figs. 23—25). The morphology of the defect is given in Table 3.

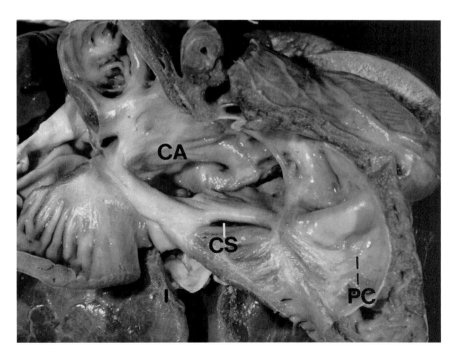

Figure 18: Common atrium with proximal atrialized chamber in a case of Ebstein's malformation. CA = common atrium; CS = coronary sinus; PC = proximal atrialized chamber.

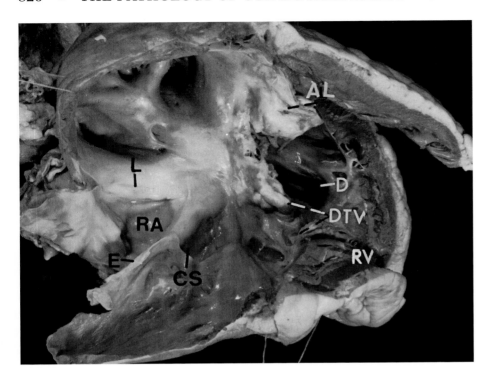

Figure 20: Ventricular septal defect in a case of Ebstein's malformation of a mild type where the defect is situated in the distal chamber. Right atrial, right ventricular view. RA = right atrium; L = limbus; E = eustachian valve; CS = coronary sinus; RV = distal right ventricle; DTV = mildly displaced septal and inferior leaflets of the tricuspid valve; D = defect; AL = anterior leaflet. (Used with permission from Lev M, et al. See Figure 42.)

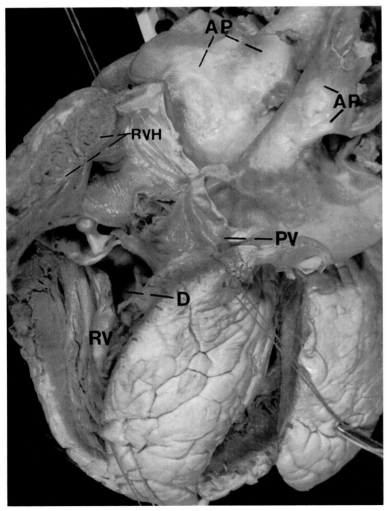

Figure 21: Outflow tract of the right ventricle in the same case as shown in Figure 20. D = defect; RVH = right ventricular hypertrophy; RV = right ventricle; PV = pulmonary valve; AP = atherosclerosis of the pulmonary trunk.

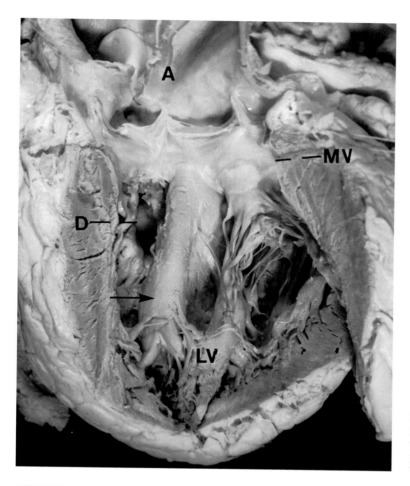

Figure 22: Same case as in Figures 20 and 21 showing the left ventricular view. A = aorta; LV = left ventricle; D = defect; MV = mitral valve. Arrow points to the anomalous muscle bundle in the left ventricle.

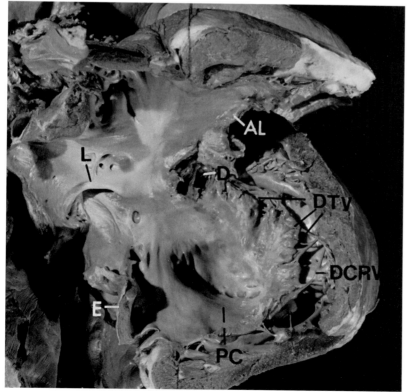

Figure 23: Ventricular septal defect in the proximal atrialized portion of Ebstein's anomaly. Right atrial, right ventricular view. L = limbus; E = eustachian valve; PC = proximal atrialized portion of the right ventricle; DCRV = distal chamber of the right ventricle; DTV = markedly displaced septal and inferior leaflets of the tricuspid valve; D = defect entering the proximal chamber; AL = anterior leaflet.

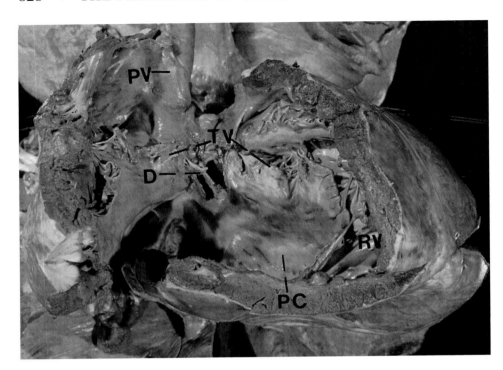

Figure 24: Outflow tract of the right ventricle depicting the defect entering the atrialized portion of the right ventricle. PV = pulmonary valve; TV = displaced tricuspid valve; D = defect; PC = proximal atrialized portion of the right ventricle; RV = distal right ventricle.

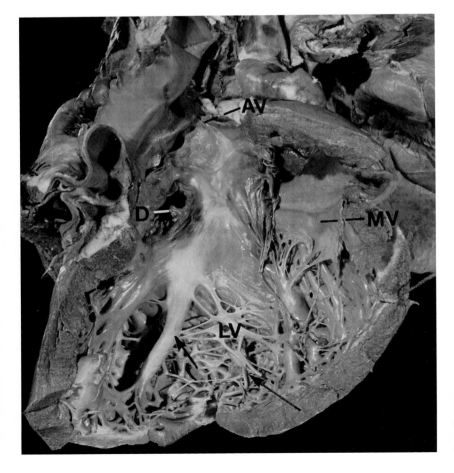

Figure 25: Left ventricular outflow tract showing the defect. LV = left ventricle; MV = mitral valve; AV = aortic valve; D = defect. Arrows point to the anomalous muscle bundles in the left ventricle

The Tricuspid Valve in Ebstein's Anomaly

The tricuspid orifice was small in nine cases and enlarged in 50 cases. It was normal in size in six cases. In two cases, there was tricuspid atresia (Fig. 26). This valve was insufficient in 21 cases (Fig. 27) and stenotic in four (Fig. 28). In general, the medial and inferior leaflets were displaced and plastered on the inferior septal wall. Uncommonly, the leaflets were absent in part or completely. There were nubbins of valvular material on the tricuspid, medial, and inferior leaflets (Fig. 29). Although the anulus was normal in all but two, the anterior leaflet was redundant, thick, and often formed an aneurysm and obstructed the outflow tract of the right ventricle. It was often converted into a large sail-like sheet (Fig. 30). In two cases, part of the anterior leaflet was displaced downward (Figs. 31, 32). The ring of the medial leaflet was gradually deviated a varying distance downward into the right ventricle from its anchor on the pars membranacea. This leaflet was usually connected by chordae to the septal band. It was a relatively small leaflet, often immobile and sometimes deficient or absent. The ring of the inferior leaflet was displaced downward into the right ventricle, but in a few cases, its actual position had a tendency to approach the original atrioventricular orifice. It was connected, in most cases, to an aberrant inferior papillary muscle. It was often displaced and, in some cases, completely absent. In an occasional case, the tricuspid valve ring was not displaced, but the proximal part of the valve was adherent to the wall of the right ventricle. The effective ring was thus displaced, and therefore, the heart belonged to the category of Ebstein's anomaly (Fig. 33). Occasionally, accessory orifices were present (Figs. 2, 34). Often the papillary muscles and the chordae were bizarre, hypoplastic, or even absent (Figs. 26—34).

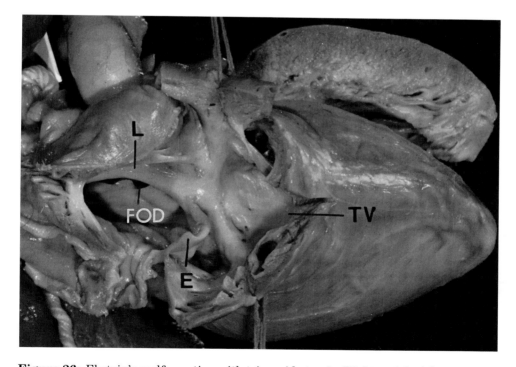

Figure 26: Ebstein's malformation with tricuspid atresia. Right atrial, right ventricular view. L = limbus fossa ovalis; FOD = fossa ovalis defect; E = eustachian valve; TV = tricuspid valve. Note that the entire tricuspid valvular apparatus is displaced into the right ventricle and the valvular tissue completely occluding the orifice. (Used with permission from Lev M, et al. See Figure 42.)

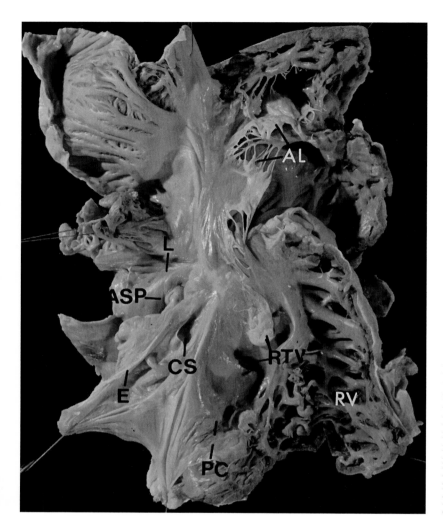

Figure 27: Marked enlargement of the tricuspid orifice with displacement of the septal and inferior leaflets and plastering of the valve into the inlet with marked tricuspid insufficiency. Right atrial, right ventricular view. L = limbus fossa ovalis; ASP = aneurysm of the septum primum; E = eustachian valve; CS = coronary sinus; AL = anterior leaflet of the tricuspid valve; RTV = redundant tricuspid valvular tissue mildly displaced into the right ventricle; PC = proximal chamber; RV = distal right ventricular chamber.

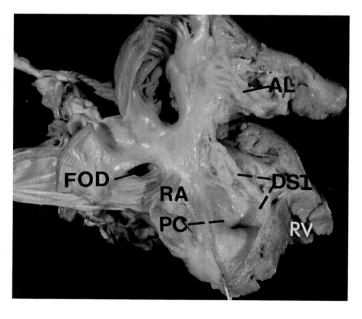

Figure 28: Ebstein's anomaly with stenosis of the tricuspid valve. Right atrial, right ventricular view. FOD = fossa ovalis defect; RA = right atrium; PC = proximal atrialized chamber; AL = anterior leaflet of the tricuspid valve; DSI = displaced septal and inferior leaflets of the tricuspid valve; RV = distal right ventricular chamber.

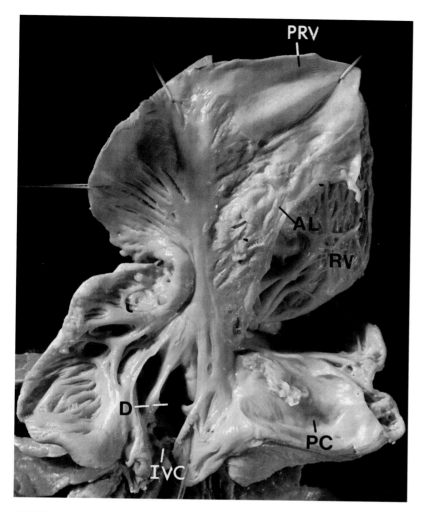

Figure 29: Nubbins of valvular tissue in the proximal atrialized chamber. D = atrial septal defect; IVC = inferior vena cava; PC = proximal chamber with tricuspid valve tissue; RV = distal right ventricle; AL = redundant anterior leaflet; PRV = paper thin right ventricle. (Used with permission from Lev M, et al. See Figure 42.)

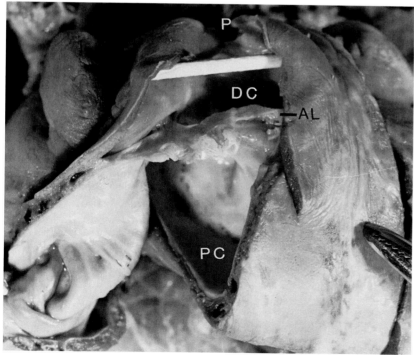

Figure 30: Large anterior leaflet of the tricuspid valve forming a sail-like sheet obstructing the outflow into the pulmonary trunk. P = pulmonary trunk; DC = markedly abbreviated distal chamber; PC = proximal chamber; AL = anterior leaflet of the tricuspid valve. (Used with permission from Lev M: See Figure 36.)

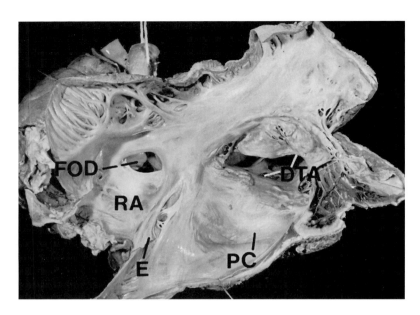

Figure 31: Displacement of all the leaflets into the right ventricle. FOD = fossa ovalis defect; RA = right atrium; E = eustachian valve; PC = proximal atrialized chamber; DTA = displaced tricuspid anterior leaflet.

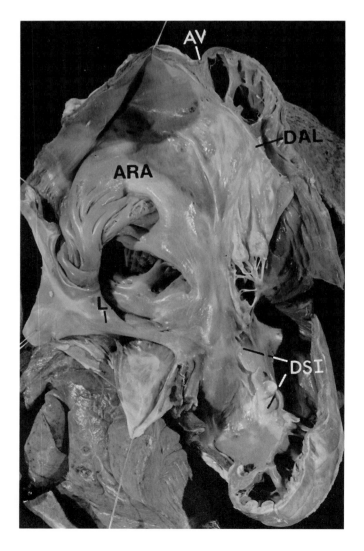

Figure 32: Mild to moderate displacement of all the three leaflets from another case of Ebstein's malformation. ARA = aneurysm of right atrium; L = limbus fossa ovalis; DSI = displaced septal and inferior leaflets of the tricuspid valve; DAL = displaced anterior leaflet; AV = atrioventricular sulcus.

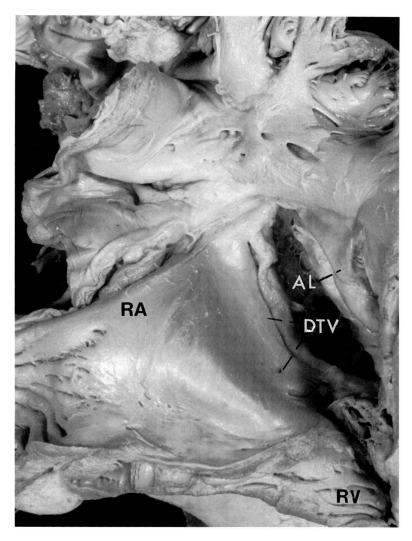

Figure 33: Plastered proximal part of the septal and inferior leaflets of the tricuspid valve with a displaced effective ring. RA = right atrium; RV = right ventricle; AL = anterior leaflet; DTV = plastered septal and inferior leaflets with displacement of the effective ring of the tricuspid valve.

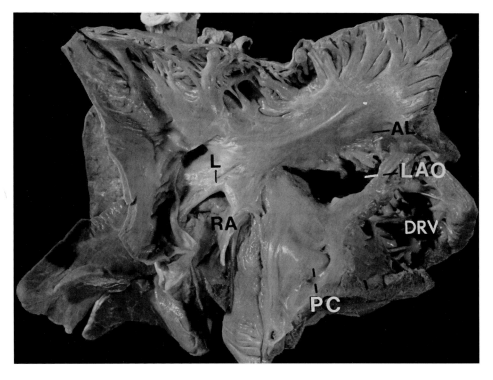

Figure 34: Huge accessory opening in the tricuspid valve. Right atrial, right ventricular view. RA = right atrium; L = limbus fossa ovalis; PC = proximal atrialized chamber of the right ventricle; AL = anterior leaflet of the tricuspid valve; LAO = large accessory opening; DRV = distal right ventricular chamber.

The Right Ventricle in Ebstein's Anomaly

The right ventricle was hypertrophied and enlarged in 46, enlarged in six, hypertrophied in 12, very small in two, and normal in size in one. The above includes both the sinus and the conus part of the right ventricle.

As discussed previously, the right ventricle was divided into proximal and distal chambers in most cases. The proximal chamber was equal to, smaller than, or larger than the distal chamber, dependent on the degree of the tricuspid ring displacement. The proximal chamber was usually thin-walled, often with a markedly thickened endocardium but the wall was thickened in some (Fig. 35). It was aneurysmally dilated and paper-thin in some. It was, to a variable extent, surrounded by the distal chamber on the lateral inferior and distal walls of the right ventricle. The distal chamber consisted of a conus in all cases, apical recess, and the portion of sinus in most cases which markedly encircled the tricuspid funnel (Fig. 36). On

the septum, the demarcation between the proximal and distal chambers was in the form of a ridge of fibrous tissue and muscle, or there was no demarcation between the two chambers in this area. In most cases, the size of the distal chamber was less than that of the definitive right ventricle in a normal person of the same age, weight, and height and its wall was of either average thickness or thinner than normal. The septal band was normal in most cases, but the parietal band (crista) showed abnormal orientation of its fibers with anomalous papillary muscles (Fig. 37), with a tendency for the arch produced by the junction of the septal and parietal bands to be shallower than normal (Figs. 37, 38). The muscle of Lancisi (conal band) thus was either situated high in the conus or was enlarged. The endocardium of the distal chamber was focally thickened. Where there was absence of medial and inferior leaflets of the tricuspid valve, the right ventricle was not subdivided into proximal and distal chambers. The valve was floppy and redundant in older age groups (Fig. 13). The amount of displacement of the tricuspid valve in the right ventricle varied considerably. In general, marked

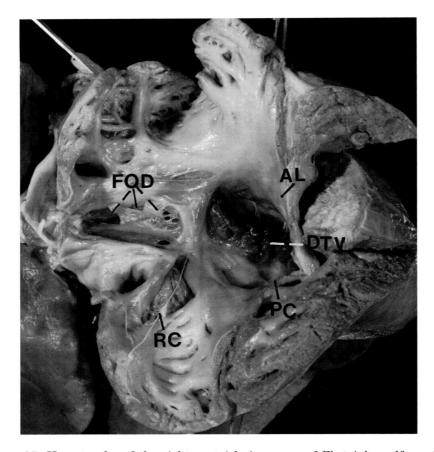

Figure 35: Hypertrophy of the right ventricle in a case of Ebstein's malformation. Right atrial, right ventricular view. FOD = fossa ovalis defect; RC = Rete Chiari network; PC = proximal chamber; DTV = displaced tricuspid valve; AL = anterior leaflet. Note the markedly hypertrophied right ventricular wall.

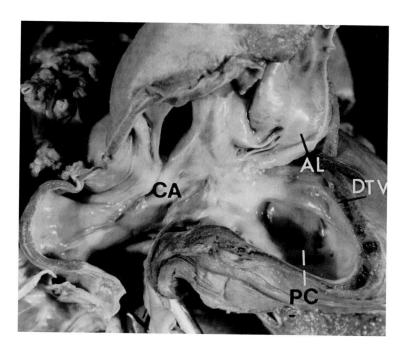

Figure 36: A case of Ebstein's malformation with common atrium showing the sinus encircling the entire tricuspid valve that is displaced. CA = common atrium; AL = anterior leaflet; PC = proximal atrialized chamber; DTV = displaced tricuspid valve. (Used with permission from Lev M: *Autopsy Diagnosis of Congenitally Malformed Hearts.* Charles C. Thomas, Springfield, Illinois, 1953.)

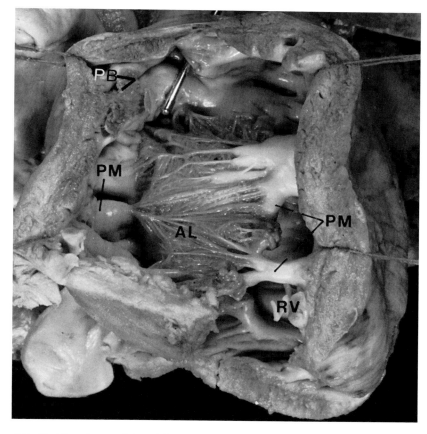

Figure 37: Outflow tract of the right ventricle showing the large anterior leaflet of the tricuspid valve connected to anomalous papillary muscles and deviated parietal band. PM = anomalous papillary muscles; RV = right ventricle; AL = anterior leaflet of the tricuspid valve; PB = parietal band. Note the probe passing through the stenotic pulmonary valve.

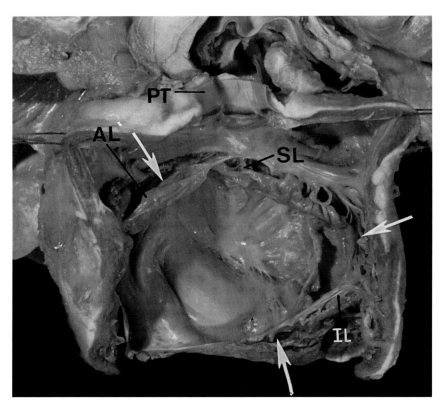

Figure 38: Abnormally formed outflow tract of the right ventricle in a case of a marked Ebstein malformation of the tricuspid valve. IL = displaced inferior leaflet; SL = septal leaflet; AL = anterior leaflet; PT = pulmonary trunk. Note the septal and parietal bands showing abnormal orientation. Also note the bicuspid pulmonary valves. The arrows point to the marked Ebstein-like malformation of the tricuspid valve.

displacement of the valve close to the apex of the right ventricle was usually seen in infancy, implying abnormal hemodynamics in the right side of the heart in intrauterine life. On the other hand, mild-to-moderate displacement was present in the older age group suggesting less severe hemodynamics to the right side of the heart.

The pulmonic orifice was enlarged in 16 cases, normal in size in 18, small in 21, very small in four, and atretic in eight (Fig. 39). Its valve was bicuspid in four (Fig. 40), calcified in one (Fig. 41), and fenestrated in two. The status of the ductus arteriosus is given in Table 4.

The size of the left side of the heart varied according to the amount of pulmonary flow and the presence or absence of an atrial septal defect. The left atrium was hypertrophied and enlarged in 33, normal in size in 20, hypertrophied in five, enlarged in eight, and atrophied in one. The mitral orifice, in the majority of cases, was enlarged (31) or normal in size (24) and was small in 12. The mitral valve was often redundant, thickened, and nodular, especially the posterior leaflet in 14 cases, and was distinctly floppy in five (Fig. 6).

There was distinct mitral stenosis in three (Figs. 8, 9) and mitral insufficiency in two. The changes in the mitral valve are probably due to the fact that there was a concomitant atrial septal defect, which probably caused considerable hemodynamic changes in the mitral valve, similar to that found in the atrial septal defect in older age group. It was not common to find the left ventricle bulging towards the outflow tract. This, we believe, is due to the altered hemodynamics of the right ventricle affecting the posterior ventricular septum. The chordae were abbreviated and not uncommonly, the papillary muscles proceeded to the base of the valve or the chordae were markedly thickened and irregular. The anterior leaflet was, in some cases, redundant, forming an aneurysm.

The left ventricle was hypertrophied and enlarged in 33, normal in 20, enlarged in eight, hypertrophied in five, and was atrophied in one.

In 10 cases, the left ventricular architecture was abnormal. There were many trabeculations and anomalous muscle bundles in this chamber (Figs. 22, 25). In addition, the ventricular septum bulged into the left ventricular cavity. Occasionally, the left ventricle

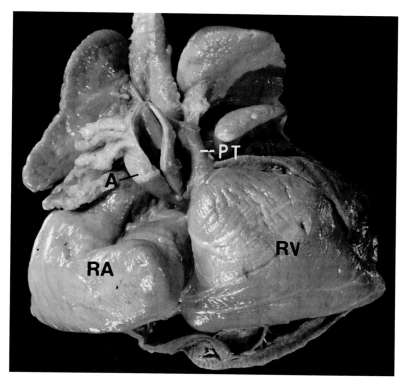

Figure 39: External view of the heart depicting pulmonary atresia in a case of Ebstein's anomaly. RA = right atrium; RV = right ventricle; A = aorta; PT = pulmonary trunk. Note the very small pulmonary trunk.

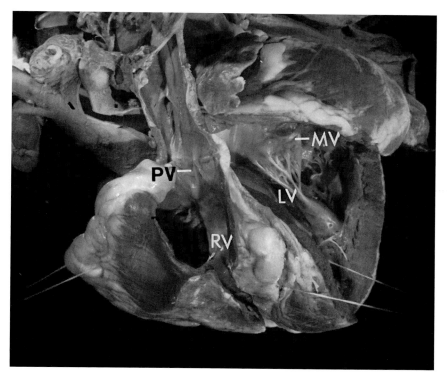

Figure 40: Ebstein's anomaly with pulmonary stenosis. PV = bicuspid pulmonary valve; RV = right ventricle; MV = mitral valve; LV = left ventricle.

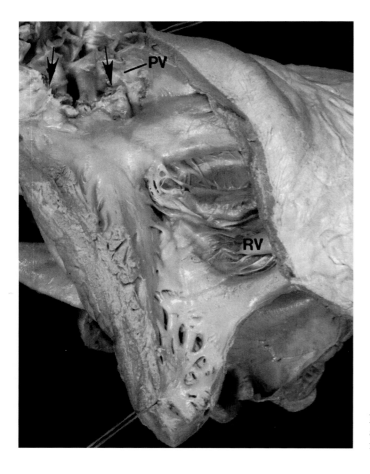

Figure 41: Calcific pulmonic valve in a case of Ebstein's anomaly. RV = right ventricle; PV = pulmonary valve. Arrows point to the markedly calcific irregular thickened valve.

was spongy. The aortic orifice, in general, was either normal (37) or enlarged in (21), and occasionally small (9). A bicuspid valve was seen in one (Fig. 42), fenestrations in one, calcification in one, and in one the noncoronary cusp was rotated to the right. The associated cardiac abnormalities are listed in Table 5.

Table 4

Status of Patent Ductus Arteriosus

Wide in a 3-month-old	1
Small or closing with pulmonary atresia (1 stillborn, 1 newborn)	2
Tortuous aneurysmally dilated (stillborn)	1
Elongated, tortuous, and closing (newborn)	2
Directly entering left lung	1
Intrauterine sudden death with tortuous, long and huge RSVC	1
Cirsoid in a 3-month-old	1

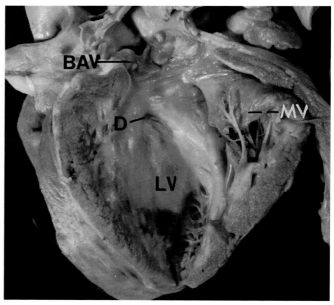

Figure 42: Left ventricular view demonstrating a bicuspid aortic valve in a case of Ebstein's anomaly with a small VSD. BAV = bicuspid aortic valve; D = small ventricular septal defect; LV = left ventricle; MV = mitral valve. Note the bulge of the ventricular septum. (Used with permission from Lev M, Liberthson RR, Joseph RH, Seten CE, Kunske RD, Eckner FAO, Miller RA: The pathologic anatomy of Ebstein's disease. *AMA Arch Pathol* 1970, 90:334—343.)

Table 5

Associated Cardiac Abnormalities

Fetal coarctation	2
Absent transverse arch with mitral stenosis	1
Tricuspid atresia with pulmonary atresia	2
Aneurysm of fossa ovalis	7
Aneurysm of space of His	5
Aneurysm of pars membranacea	2
Double right coronary ostium	1
High origin of left coronary	1
Coronary artery disease in a 52-year-old	1
Aortic stenosis with fibroelastosis	2
Subaortic stenosis	1
LSVC → CS	4
Enlargement of pulmonary venous segment of LA	1
Partially divided left atrium with diverticulum of proximal part of LA	1
Pulmonary atresia with VSD (overriding aorta)	2
Double mitral orifice	1
Trunco conal inversion with straddling conus with straddling PT and MS, FC and PDA	1
Fibroelastosis of the left ventricle (contracted type)	1
Pulmonary stenosis, marked	8
Pulmonary stenosis, mild	1
Pulmonary stenosis and pulmonary insufficiency	2
Pulmonary insufficiency	1
Small coronary sinus	2
Rete Chiari	2
Cor triatriatum dexter	1
Obstruction between sinus and conus	1
Partial Uhl's anomaly	1
Marked pulmonary hypertension	3
Right aortic arch	1
Sudden infant death	2
Fetal coarctation, elongated PDA with PSVT	2
Displaced coronary sinus close to TV	1
Cocaine-addicted mother with cardiomegaly	1
Common brachiocephalic trunk	2
Sudden death (1 intrauterine)	5
WPW—documented	3

Comment

As seen from our material, the majority of Ebstein's anomaly cases are seen below the age of 6 months. These hearts show marked displacement and varying abnormalities of the tricuspid valve apparatus associated with other cardiac abnormalities. The marked variations in the tricuspid valve and the right ventricular morphology suggest the possibility of genetic variability of this disease. This may be one of the reasons for the increase in mortality and morbidity following surgical repair in infancy.

The severe pulmonary stenosis or atresia in the presence of a marked Ebstein's anomaly with a huge heart in the neonatal period raises the issue as to the development of innovative methods of possibly correcting these anomalies by genetic and/or pharmacological means in intrauterine life.

Likewise, in the older age group, when operated, marked cardiomegaly as such may increase the mortality and/or the morbidity in some. In a few, the heart weighed close to or even reached 1,000 gm.

It is evident that the floppy mitral valve, or stenosis, the altered ventricular septum, and fenestrations in the aortic valve are equally important anatomical findings that may alter the surgical outcome in some.

Although we have included some cases of sudden death with mild Ebstein's malformation, this subject will be dealt with later in detail.

Briefly, there appears to be an increased tendency for sudden death in the relatively young and healthy with mild Ebstein-like malformation. The occurrence of preexcitation and paroxysmal supraventricular tachycardia was observed uncommonly. The above finding suggests that some of the sudden deaths may indeed be due to preexcitation with concealed conduction and/or due to the abnormal formation of the atrioventricular junction including the septal leaflet of the tricuspid valve, the central fibrous body, the membranous septum, and the coronary sinus region.

Is Ebstein's Anomaly a Connective Tissue Disorder or a Forme Fruste of a Connective Tissue Disorder?

Recently we encountered a unique heart that presented the characteristics of both the Ebstein's anomaly and a connective tissue disorder. This was a 46-year-old white male who died suddenly following rupture of the thoracic-aortic aneurysm at the inferior end of the old graft anastomotic site. He had surgical repair of coarctation of the aorta with a Dacron patch graft 13 years prior to death. In addition to the rupture of the aortic aneurysm there was Ebstein's anomaly of the tricuspid valve, aneurysm of the pulmonic sinuses of Valsalva, a floppy mitral valve, and a bicuspid aortic valve with aneurysm of the sinuses of Valsalva.

The involvement of all the four valves in the presence of the ruptured aortic aneurysm at the site of the previously repaired coarctation of the aorta, suggests the possibility that Ebstein's anomaly, at least in some, may indeed be a variant of a connective tissue disorder yet to be described. This may or may not be related to Marfan's or forme fruste Marfan's syndrome. The relationship of connective tissue disorders to Ebstein's anomaly needs further research at the molecular and genetic level. It is understood that the genetics of the simple Ebstein's anomaly as such should be explored in the future.

56

Vascular Rings

Vascular rings, unassociated with other anomalies, were uncommon in our material. The most common anomaly was right aortic arch with a left ductus arteriosus (Figs. 1, 2). Less common was double aortic arch (Fig. 3). When there was a double aortic arch, usually the right arch was larger (dominant) than the left.

Analysis of Our Material

There were a total of 21 cases. Seventeen were males, three were females, and one was an animal heart. The age ranged from stillborn to 12 years with a median age of 1 year and 8 months.

The Complex

The apex in the majority was formed by the left ventricle, less frequently by both ventricles, and rarely by the right ventricle. The right atrium and right ventricle were hypertrophied and enlarged in 50% of our cases. The remainder were either normal or hypertrophied. The left side of the heart was either normal or hypertrophied and enlarged. In general, the valves were mostly normal in size and normally formed. Less commonly, the valves were enlarged with accessory papillary muscles for the right or left ventricle. The mitral and aortic valves in most cases were normal. Fifteen were associated with a right aortic arch and a ductus arteriosus or ligamentum arteriosum. There were six cases of double aortic arch. The right aortic arch was larger than the left aortic arch in four cases (Figs. 4—8). The details of the aortic arch anomalies in each case are given in Table 1. The associated cardiac and extracardiac anomalies are given in Table 2.

Comment

One may hypothesize that the genes related to the aortic arch derivatives are probably abnormal to start with and/or altered by the abnormal hemodynamics during the early stages of the developing embryo resulting in various types of anomalies in the aortic arch system.

Regarding the treatment, it is self evident that when relieving the tracheal and/or the esophageal obstruction it is important that the function of these structures is maintained adequately many years following surgery. Likewise the associated cardiac anomalies such as the ASD, coarctation of the aorta, and pulmonary arterial anomalies deserve attention.

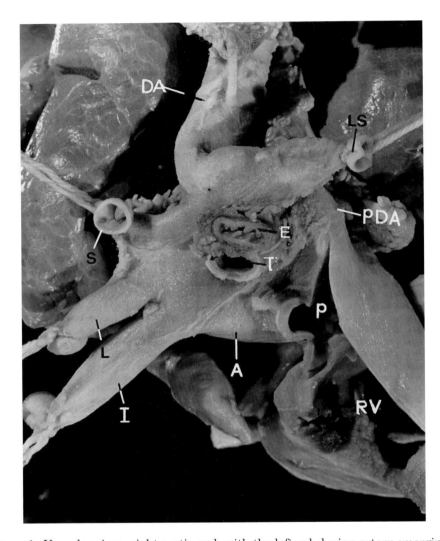

Figure 1: Vascular ring—right aortic arch with the left subclavian artery emerging at the junction of the ductus with the descending aorta, superior view. A = ascending aorta; I = innominate artery; L = left common carotid artery; S = right subclavian artery; DA = descending aorta; LS = left subclavian artery; PDA = patent ductus arteriosus; T = trachea; E = esophagus; P = pulmonary trunk; RV = right ventricle.

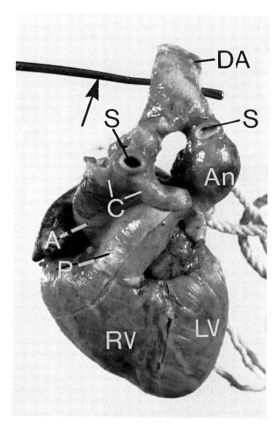

Figure 2: Right aortic arch with vascular ring formed by the aneurysmally dilated ductus arteriosus as it joins the descending aorta with the left subclavian artery emerging distal to the ductus (trachea and esophagus removed from the specimen). RV = right ventricle; LV = left ventricle; A = aorta; P = pulmonary trunk; An = aneurysmally dilated patent ductus arteriosus; C = carotid arteries; S = subclavian arteries (one from the right aortic arch and the other from the ductus arteriosus as it joins the descending aorta; DA = descending aorta. Arrow points to the probe behind the vascular ring.

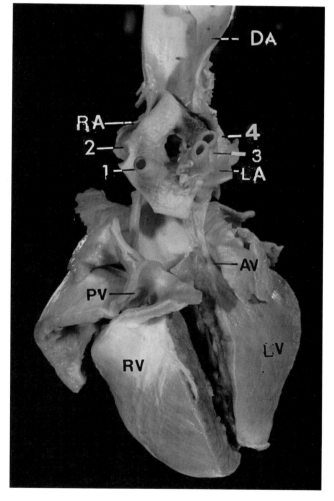

Figure 3: Double aortic arch, two vessels emerging from each arch (1, 2, 3 and 4)—both arches, of more or less equal size, joining together forming the descending aorta. RV = right ventricle; LV = left ventricle; PV = pulmonary valve; AV = aortic valve; RA = right aortic arch; LA = left aortic arch; DA = descending aorta. Numbers 1, 2, 3 and 4 depict the two vessels emerging from each side, joining together posteriorly to form the descending aorta.

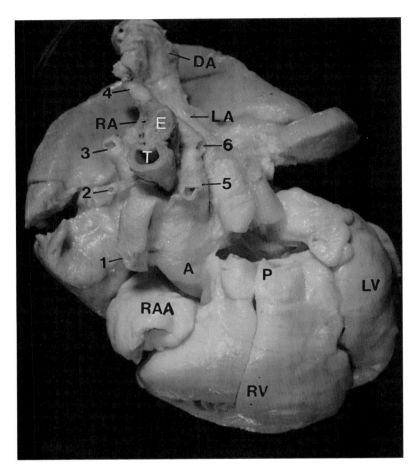

Figure 4: Double aortic arch with vascular ring, external view of the heart. RAA = right atrial appendage; RV = right ventricle; LV = left ventricle; RA = right aortic arch; LA = left aortic arch; P = pulmonary trunk; T = trachea; A = aorta; E = esophagus; DA = descending aorta. Numbers 1, 2, 3, and 4 depict the vessels emerging from the larger posterior segment of the right arch; 5 and 6 depict vessels emerging from the smaller left anterior segment of the arch. Note the larger right and the smaller left aortic arch joining together distally behind the trachea and esophagus.

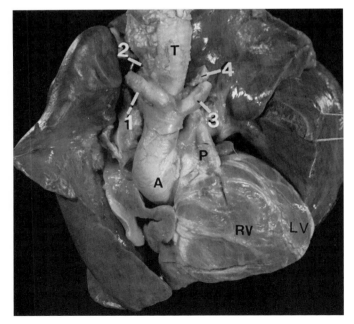

Figure 5: External view of the heart, depicting a case of double aortic arch, with dominant right arch. Numbers 1, 2, 3 and 4 depict the two vessels from each side of the arch winding around the trachea and esophagus to join or form the descending aorta. RV = right ventricle; LV = left ventricle; A = ascending aorta; P = pulmonary trunk; T = trachea.

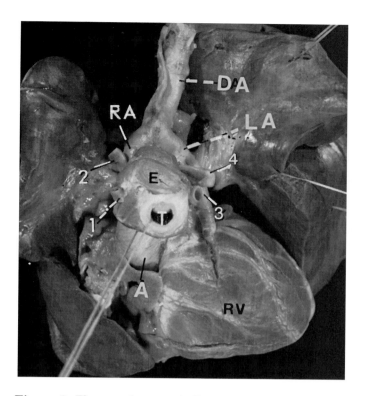

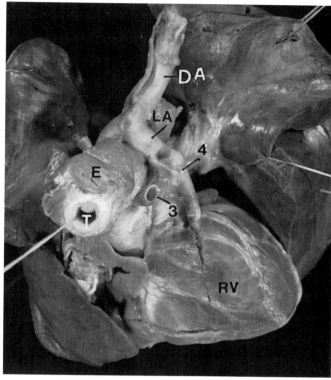

Figure 6: The same heart as in Figure 5 as seen from the superior view. Trachea and esophagus are pulled anteriorly or forward. T = trachea; E = esophagus. 1, 2, 3, and 4 represent the two brachiocephalic vessels from each side of the aortic arch (right and left) forming the sling around the trachea and esophagus to form the descending aorta. DA = descending aorta; A = ascending aorta; RA = right aortic arch; LA = left aortic arch; RV = right ventricle.

Figure 7: Same as in Figures 5 and 6. The trachea and esophagus are pulled towards the right showing the left-sided component of the aortic arch as it forms the descending aorta. The abbreviations and numbers are the same as in Figures 5 and 6.

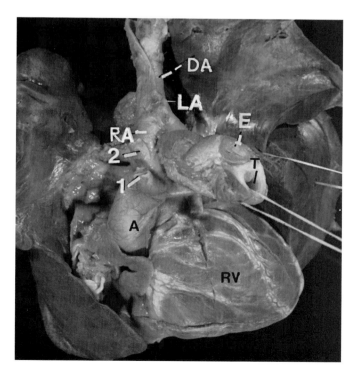

Figure 8: Same as in Figures 5, 6, and 7. The trachea and esophagus are pulled towards the left side to demonstrate the dominant right aortic arch. The abbreviations and numbers are the same as in Figures 5 and 6.

Table 1

The Anatomy of the Aortic Arch

	No. of Cases
Double aortic arch with dominant right and small left with right common carotid artery and right subclavian artery from right arch and left common carotid artery and left subclavian artery from left arch.	2
Double aortic arch with dominant right and minute left aortic arch with three vessels from the right arch and two vessels from the smaller arch.	1
Double aortic arch with two vessels from right and 2 from left.	1
Double aortic arch with two vessels from anterior arch and four from posterior arch, joined together posteriorly distal to patent ductus arteriosus.	1
Double aortic arch with large right posterior segment and small left anterior segment and two vessels from each segment.	1
Right aortic arch with left patent ductus arteriosus.	6
Right aortic arch with patent ductus arteriosus from left subclavian artery.	1
Right aortic arch with aneurysmally dilated ductus arteriosus with left subclavian artery at its junction with the descending aorta.	1
Right aortic arch with left subclavian artery from descending aorta at its junction with ligamentum arteriosum.	3
Right aortic arch with left subclavian artery from right descending aorta at its junction with the ligamentum arteriosum.	1
Right aortic arch with large patent ductus arteriosus and right descending aorta with right subclavian artery at its junction.	1
Right aortic arch with tortuous probe patent ductus arteriosus and right descending aorta giving rise to right subclavian artery.	1
Right aortic arch with a diverticulum-like structure giving off the left subclavian artery and tortuous ductus joining the junction of the left subclavian artery and the diverticulum.	1

Table 2

Associated Cardiac and Extracardiac Abnormalities

	No. of Cases
Atrial septal defect, fossa ovalis type	7
Patent foramen ovale	7
Aneurysm of fossa ovalis	1
Rete Chiari network	1
Patent foramen ovale in a stillborn	1
Aneurysm of space of His	2
Accessory tricuspid orifice with insufficiency	1
Large right pulmonary artery and small left pulmonary artery	1
Large usual VSD with fetal coarctation of the aorta and aortic stenosis	1
High origin of both coronary ostia	1
High origin of right coronary ostium	1
Double left atrium (mild form)	1
Abnormal architecture of right ventricle	1
Mild pulmonary stenosis	1
Dwarf	1
Leukemia with vegetations in the mitral valve	1

57

Abnormal Position of the Heart or Its Component Chambers– Mixed Levocardia

If the base-apex axis of the heart points to the left and downward, and this position is due to the inherent structure of the heart, then it is said to be in levocardia. If the base-apex axis points to the right and downward, and this position is due to the inherent structure of the heart, then the heart is said to be in dextrocardia. If the longitudinal axis of the heart points to the midline of the body and there is no apex, and this is due to the inherent structure of the heart, then the heart is said to be in mesocardia position. If the heart is basically in levocardia, or mesocardia, or dextrocardia in structure, but it is pushed laterally to an opposite position by extraneous pathology, then there is dextroposition, levoposition, or mesoposition. In all of these positions, if the atria and ventricles correspond, then they are said to be concordant. If not, they are discordant. In levocardia, mesocardia, or dextrocardia, if the atria and ventricles are discordant, we call this condition mixed or discordant dextrocardia, mesocardia, or levocardia. In mixed (discordant) levocardia, the atria may be in situs solitus (normal position) and the ventricles inverted. Or, the atria may be in situs inversus and the ventricles in normal position (Fig. 1).

In the chest, if the right lung has three lobes and the left has two, we call this condition situs solitus thoracis. If the converse is true, then we call this condition situs inversus thoracis. We accordingly have the same conditions in the abdomen: situs solitus abdominalis and situs inversus abdominalis.

If the spleen is normal in structure, the situs of the atria in almost all cases follows the situs of the abdominal organs. We do not speak of the situs of the ventri-

cles since their embryology is different from that of the atria. If there is polysplenia or asplenia, then any type of position of the heart, organs, or chambers of the heart may be present. Under these circumstances, there is a tendency for defective septation truncoconal abnormalities and abnormalities in the systemic and or pulmonic venous return.

From the standpoint of the relationship of the arterial trunks to the ventricles from which they arise, if their origin is normal, then we may use the term ventriculoarterial concordance. If they arise from the wrong ventricles, the term ventriculoarterial discordance may be used. We prefer to keep the term *transposition* where vessels arise from the wrong ventricles. The term *overriding* is retained where an arterial trunk arises from two ventricles.

If the chambers of the heart in dextrocardia are such as would be obtained if the heart were rotated in a horizontal position towards the right with the atria as a fulcrum, then the condition is called dextroversion (Fig. 1). In this condition, the right atrium is to the right or to the right and posterior. The left atrium is to the left or to the left and anterior. The right ventricle is to the right and posterior and the left ventricle is to the left and anterior. The other organs are in situs solitus.

In mirror-image dextrocardia, the chambers of the heart are in a mirror-image position of the normal (Fig. 1). That is, there is a disturbance in laterality but not in anteroposteriority. Thus, the right atrium and ventricle are anterior and to the left, and the left atrium and ventricle are posterior and to the right. The organs

LEVOCARDIA

Pure Levocardia;
Normal position of heart
with normal relationship
of chambers

Mixed Levocardia,
with Atrial Inversion

Mixed Levocardia
with Ventricular Inversion

Levoversion

MESOCARDIA

Mesoversion
Type I

Mixed Mesocardia
with Ventricular Inversion

Mixed Mesocardia
with Atrial Inversion

Mesoversion
Type II

DEXTROCARDIA

Mirror-image

Mixed Dextrocardia:
Atria in Mirror-image;
Ventricles in
Pivotal Position

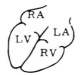

Mixed Dextrocardia:
Atria in Pivotal Position;
Ventricles in Mirror-image

Dextroversion

Figure 1: The position of the chambers in the various directions of the base apex of the heart. LA = left atrium; LV = left ventricle; RA = right atrium; RV = right ventricle. (Used with permission from Lev M, Bharati S. Abnormal position of the heart and its chambers. In *The Heart*, ed. by JE Edwards, et al. Baltimore, MD, The Williams and Wilkins Co, Chap. 16, 1974, pp. 327—331.)

are in situs inversus if the spleen is normal in structure.

If the basic structure of the heart is concordant levocardia, but the heart is pivoted around so that the longitudinal axis of the heart points to the midline of the body, then there is mesoversion. In this type of mesoversion, the atria are posterior, the right atrium is situated to the right side and the left atrium to the left side, and the ventricles are anterior, the right ventricle is situated to the right side and the left ventricle to the left side. If the basic structure of the heart is concordant mirror-image dextrocardia, if it is pivoted around to the left, then there is a second type of mesoversion. In this type, the atria are posterior, but the right atrium is to the left side and the left atrium is to the right side, and the ventricles are anterior, the right ventricle is to the left side and the left ventricle is to the right side. We have not seen any heart in this type of mesoversion.

Mixed Levocardia

As stated above, this is a condition in which the base-apex axis points to the left and down but the atria and ventricles do not correspond (discordance) (Fig. 1). There are three types of mixed levocardia (Figs. 1, 2).

I. With ventricular inversion
    a. With inverted transposition
    b. With complete transposition (noninverted)
II. With atrial inversion
III. 1. With relatively normally positioned chambers with *criss-cross atrioventricular connection*
    a. Noninverted transposition
    b. Inverted transposition
  2. With ventricular inversion and *normal atrioventricular connection in a criss-cross manner*
    a. Noninverted transposition
    b. Complete inverted transposition

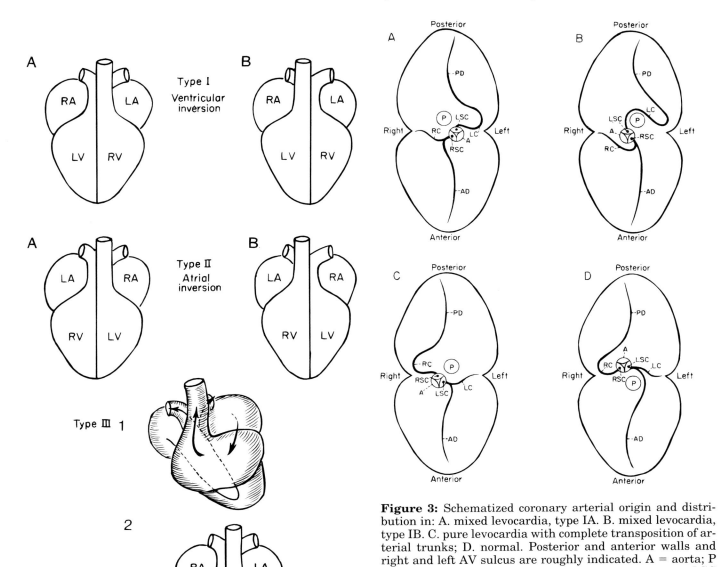

Figure 3: Schematized coronary arterial origin and distribution in: A. mixed levocardia, type IA. B. mixed levocardia, type IB. C. pure levocardia with complete transposition of arterial trunks; D. normal. Posterior and anterior walls and right and left AV sulcus are roughly indicated. A = aorta; P = pulmonary artery; RSC = right-sided coronary cusp; LSC = left-sided coronary cusp; LC = left circumflex coronary artery; AD = anterior descending coronary artery; RC = right circumflex coronary artery; PD = posterior descending coronary artery. (Used with permission from Lev M, Rowlatt UF. See Figure 95.)

Figure 2: Types of mixed levocardia: I.A. with ventricular inversion and complete inverted transposition of arterial trunks. I.B. with ventricular inversion and complete non-inverted transposition of the arterial trunks. II.A. with atrial inversion with normal position of the efferent vessels. IIB. with atrial inversion with complete transposition of arterial trunks. III.1. atria and ventricles in relatively normal position but abnormally connected. LA = left atrium; LV = left ventricle; RA = right atrium; RV = right ventricle. III.2. Mixed levocardia with ventricular inversion and normal atrioventricular connection in a criss-cross manner.

The flow of blood may or may not be corrected in a physiological sense. If it is so corrected, then the term *corrected transposition* may pertain. The term *inversion* means that the atria or ventricles are in opposite position vis-à-vis its fellow (accompanying chamber). The coronary artery and accompanying coronary venous drainage are shown schematically in the three types of mixed levocardia in the diagram (Figs. 3, 4).

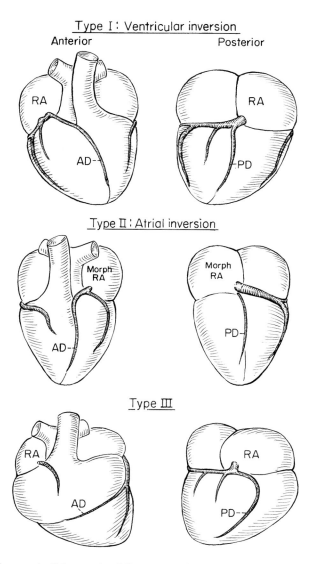

Figure 4: Schematized diagrams of coronary venous circulation in mixed levocardia. RA = right atrium; AD = anterior descending vein; PD = posterior descending vein. (Used with permission from Lev M, Rowlatt UF. See Figure 95.)

I. Mixed Levocardia with Ventricular Inversion

In these cases, the atria are in the normal position, but the ventricles are inverted. The mitral and tricuspid valves correspond to the ventricles. There are two types: (a) with inverted transposition and (b) with noninverted transposition.

(a) With Inverted Transposition

In these cases, the aorta is situated to the left and anterior while the pulmonary trunk is situated to the right and posterior (Fig. 5). The aorta emerges from the morphologically right ventricle which is present poste-

riorly and to the left, while the pulmonary trunk emerges from the morphologically left ventricle which is present anteriorly and to the right. All cases have an abnormal left atrioventricular (AV) valve. This valve may be markedly thickened, or irregular with bizarre connections. It is usually insufficient. There may, however, be left AV valve stenosis (tricuspid stenosis), or Ebstein's anomaly. The sinus of the morphologically right ventricle is accordingly abnormal architecturally, and may be markedly abbreviated. The septal and parietal bands are abnormal. The septal band is very sharply demarcated while the parietal band is flat. The right AV valve (mitral) is more often normal architecturally, but the anterior and posterior papillary muscles may be widely distributed. There are usually accessory muscle bands accompanying the posterior group of papillary muscles. The pars membranacea or the membranous part of the ventricular septum is usually large.

The coronary artery distribution is as follows (Fig. 3): The right-sided coronary artery comes from the right sinus of Valsalva and gives off the anterior descending coronary artery from the right side of the aorta, and all the other branches of the normal right coronary artery. The left-sided coronary artery comes from the posterior sinus of Valsalva and gives off the usual branches of the right coronary artery. The noncoronary or the posterior aortic cusp is rotated anteriorly.

The morphologically left (right-sided, pulmonary) ventricle under normal conditions would be thinner than the normal left ventricle, while the morphologically right (left-sided, aortic) ventricle under normal conditions is always thicker than normal. The complexes usually found are: (1) left AV valve insufficiency, (2) ventricular septal defect, (3) ventricular septal defect with pulmonary stenosis, (4) ventricular septal defect with pulmonary atresia, (5) coarctation of the aorta, and (6) other complex cardiac anomalies.

(b) With Complete Noninverted Transposition

In these hearts, the ventricles are inverted. The aorta, however, emerges from the left ventricle while the pulmonary trunk comes from the right ventricle. The aorta is anterior and to the right and the pulmonary trunk is posterior and to the left. In one case there was mitral-aortic continuity and in the other case there was not. Some of these hearts in the literature have been called isolated ventricular inversion. We do not believe this is a correct term, since this term does not take into the account the abnormal position of the vessels vis-à-vis each other. Furthermore, physiologically, these hearts are complete transpositions. It is for these reasons we have called these hearts complete

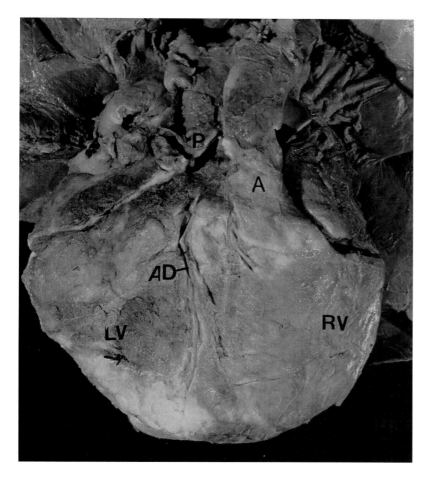

Figure 5: External view of corrected transposition. A = aorta to the left and anterior; P = pulmonary trunk to the right and posterior; LV = left ventricle; RV = right ventricle; AD = anterior descending on the right side of aorta. (Used with permission from Lev M, Rowlatt UF. See Figure 95.)

noninverted transpositions. In one case there was a ventricular septal defect and in the other there was not.

II. Mixed Levocardia with Atrial Inversion

Here the atria are in opposite position. The veins usually enter the correct morphological chamber, but on the wrong side positionally. When this is associated with complete noninverted transposition, then corrected transposition may be present physiologically. It may, however, be associated with overriding aorta (partial transposition), pulmonary stenosis, or pulmonary atresia. These cases are usually a type of isolated levocardia with or without asplenia.

III. With Relatively Normally Placed Chambers with Criss-Cross Connection of the AV Valves

These hearts today are called criss-cross or upstairs-downstairs hearts. In this entity, the chambers were in a relatively normal position, yet the connec-

tions of this chamber were abnormal. Thus, the right atrium present anteriorly was connected by way of a mitral orifice with the left ventricle present posteriorly. This orifice was inferiorly placed vis-à-vis its fellow (the tricuspid). The left atrium was connected with the right ventricle by way of a tricuspid orifice which was situated superiorly. There was a tendency for double outlet right ventricle of the Taussig-Bing type to occur frequently.

In the second rare type, the right atrium was connected with the right ventricle situated anterosuperiorly and to the left by means of a tricuspid orifice. The left atrium was connected with the morphologically left ventricle situated posteroinferiorly and to the right by means of a mitral valve. Thus, although the AV connections are criss-cross, there is no AV discordance. It is debatable whether this type of heart should be described along with mixed levocardia. We find it useful to include this in this discussion.

Analysis of Our Material

There was a total of 79 cases; the oldest was 39 years of age and the youngest a stillborn, with an average age of 7 years. There were 48 males, 28 females, one animal heart, and two unknowns.

Position of the Vessels

The aorta was anterior and to the left and the pulmonary trunk to the right and posterior in 77% of the cases (Fig. 5). In 15%, the aorta was anterior and to the right and the pulmonary trunk posterior and to the left. The aorta and the pulmonary trunk were anteroposterior in 5% and were side by side in 3%.

Composition of the Apex

The apex was formed by both ventricles in 47% (Fig. 5), by the morphologically left ventricle in 37% (Fig. 6), and by the morphologically right ventricle in 16%.

The Complex

The right atrium was hypertrophied and enlarged in 77%, was hypertrophied in 15%, was normal in size in 3%, and in 4% there was a common atrium that was hypertrophied and enlarged. In 1% there was a huge

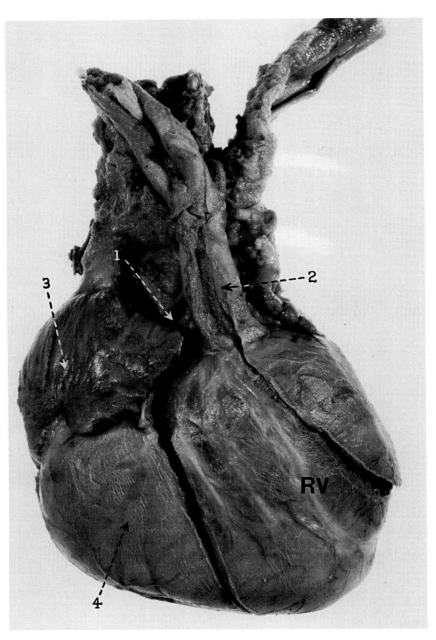

Figure 6: External view of mixed levocardia with ventricular inversion with the apex formed by the morphologically left ventricle. 1 = pulmonary trunk; 2 = aorta; 3 = right atrial appendage; 4 = left ventricle; RV = morphologically right ventricle.

aneurysm of the right atrium. The morphologically left ventricle was hypertrophied and enlarged in 63%, was only hypertrophied in 27%, was atrophied in 6%, and was normal in 4%. The morphologically left atrium was hypertrophied and enlarged in 74%, was only hypertrophied in 12%, was normal in size in 7%, and was aneurysmally dilated with thin walls in 5%, and was atrophied in 2%. The morphologically right ventricle was hypertrophied and enlarged in 51%, was only hypertrophied in 39%, was normal in only 1%, and in the remainder (9%), either it was aneurysmally dilated with thin walls or actually atrophied. There was a distinct tendency for both ventricular chambers to be abnormally formed. There were abnormal muscle bundles proceeding to the undersurface of the AV valves. The inlet or the sinus of the right ventricle was quite abbreviated with hypoplastic papillary muscles. The septal band in general was hypertrophied and the parietal band flattened and segmented into trabeculae carneae. Rarely there was a divided right ventricle.

Size of the Orifices

The morphologically mitral orifice was enlarged in 49%, was normal in size in 27%, was smaller than nor-

mal in 16%, was atrophied in 4%, was huge in 2%, and was very small in 2%. The aortic orifice was enlarged in 51%, normal in size in 23%, was smaller than normal in 22%, and was atretic in 4%. The tricuspid orifice was smaller than normal in 55%, enlarged in 31%, normal in size only in 11%, was huge in 3%, and one was associated with double tricuspid orifice. In this last case, one tricuspid orifice was larger and the other smaller than normal in size. The pulmonic orifice size was enlarged in 43%, was smaller than normal in 32%, very small in 4%, was atretic in 13%, and was normal in size in only 8%.

The Valves

The Left-Sided AV Valve–or the Morphologically Tricuspid Valve

Anatomically this valve was abnormally formed to a varying degree in *all* cases. In 35% there was moderate to marked Ebstein-like malformation of the valve (Figs. 7, 8). In many there was mild Ebstein-like malformation (Fig. 9). The septal and the posterior (inferior) leaflets were displaced to a varying extent and more or less plastered onto the posteroinferior wall of

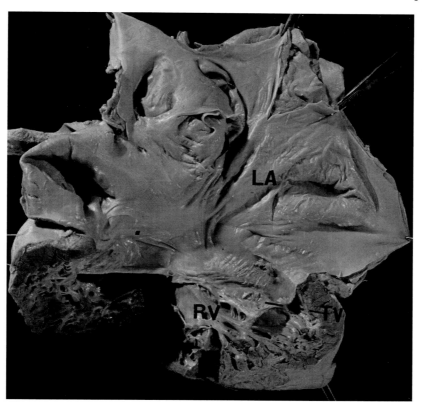

Figure 7: Ebstein's anomaly of the left AV valve in a case of corrected transposition with tremendous left AV valve insufficiency. LA = huge left atrium; TV = Ebstein's malformation of the tricuspid valve displaced and attached into the inlet of the right ventricle; RV = right ventricle. Note the practical absence of chordae and the papillary muscles. (Used with permission from Lev M, Rowlatt UF. See Figure 95.)

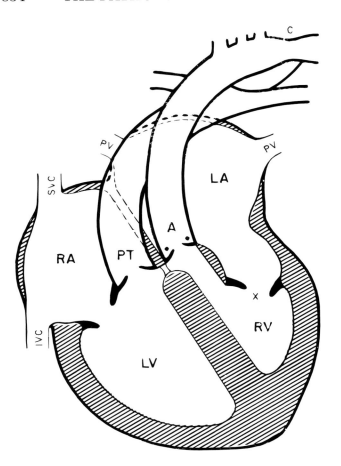

Figure 8: Diagrammatic sketch of heart seen in Figure 7. RA = right atrium; LV = left ventricle; IVC = inferior vena cava; SVC = superior vena cava; PV = pulmonary veins; C = coarctation; LA = left atrium; A = aorta; RV = right ventricle. X indicates Ebstein's anomaly of the left AV valve with insufficiency. (Used with permission from Lev M, Rowlatt UF. See Figure 95.)

the morphologically right ventricle with either absent chordae or markedly abbreviated chordae. Likewise, the papillary muscles were either hypoplastic or poorly developed or abnormally located anywhere in the inlet or the sinus of the right ventricle. In addition, the valvular tissue frequently showed considerable redundancy or irregular thickening and nodulation. The anterior leaflet was also abnormally formed. This was quite large and the junction of the anterior and septal or medial leaflets was frequently anchored onto the lower margin of the ventricular septal defect either covering the defect or in part covering the defect. In 18% of the cases the valve was markedly thickened and nodular with bizarre connections and was segmented into several components and was attached to the ventricular septum to a varying degree (Figs. 10, 11). Often, anomalous muscle bands proceeded to the undersurface or the base of the inferior leaflet. Where there was a defect, which occurred quite frequently in this entity, the valve either directly or by means of chordae was anchored onto the margins of the defect to a varying ex-

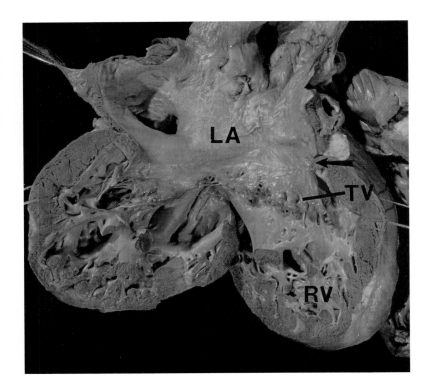

Figure 9: Mild Ebstein-like malformation of the tricuspid valve. LA = left atrium; RV = right ventricle; TV = tricuspid valve. Arrow points to the mild displacement of the septal and posterior leaflets into the morphologically right ventricle. Note the irregular thickening of the valvular tissue and abbreviated chordal connections. (Used with permission from Lev M, Rowlatt UF. See Figure 95.)

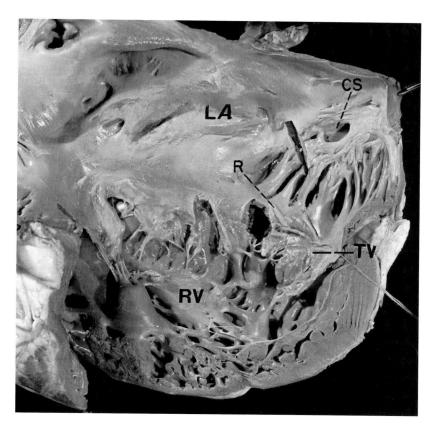

Figure 10: Corrected transposition with irregular thickening of the left AV valve (tricuspid) with marked insufficiency. LA = left atrium; TV = tricuspid valve, markedly thickened; R = irregular thickening of the tricuspid valve; RV = hypertrophied and enlarged right ventricle; CS = entry of coronary sinus into the left atrium. (Used with permission from Lev M, Rowlatt UF. See Figure 95.)

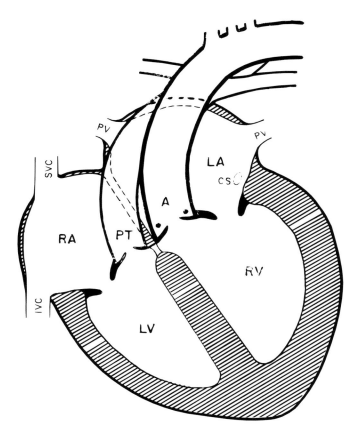

Figure 11: Diagrammatic sketch of heart seen in Figure 10. CS = coronary sinus entering left atrium; SVC = superior vena cava; IVC = inferior vena cava; RA = right atrium; RV = right ventricle; LA = left atrium; LV = left ventricle; PV = pulmonary vein; A = aorta; PT = pulmonary trunk. (Used with permission from Lev M, Rowlatt UF. See Figure 95.)

tent (Fig. 12). Although the valve was smaller than normal in many, physiological stenosis of the valve was uncommon (Figs. 13, 14):

In about 15% there was a distinct straddling tricuspid (the left AV valve) where a part or the entire valvular apparatus (the anulus, the leaflet, the chordae, and the peripheral connections) were in the morphologically left ventricle (Figs. 15, 16). Thus, there was a tendency for the valve to straddle the ventricular septum from a mild to a severe extent, resulting in either basilar or complete straddling tricuspid valve. In the remainder of the cases, the valve was either mildly displaced into the inlet or the sinus of the right ventricle and/or divided into several segments. The variations in the left AV valve were remarkable in that no two left AV valves looked identical in this entity. The

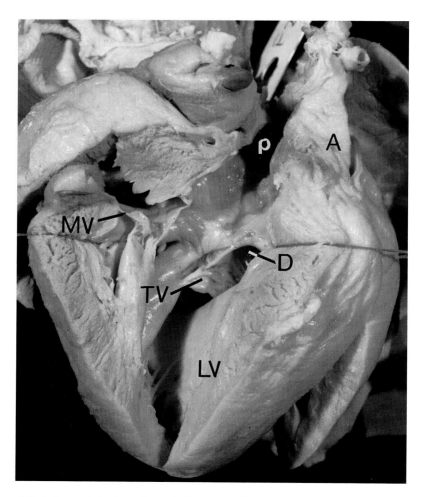

Figure 16: Left ventricular view of Figure 15 demonstrating a part of the tricuspid valve anulus, leaflet structure, and chordal extensions are connected to a large papillary muscle in the morphologically left ventricle. LV = left ventricle; MV = mitral valve; TV = straddling tricuspid valve; D = ventricular septal defect; P = pulmonary trunk; A = aorta.

Mitral Valve

This was normal in 64% (Fig. 17), in 10.5% there was a common AV orifice, the valve was atretic in 4.5%, the valve was straddling in 6%, in another 6% the valve presented a cleft-like malformation (Fig. 18), and in 9% the valve was divided off into several segments with irregular thickening with or without stenosis and/or insufficiency. The right AV valve thus was significantly insufficient in 16.5%. The papillary muscles had a tendency to be widely distributed or bizarre with accessory muscle bands to the base of the posterior or the anterior leaflet of the valve. Uncommonly, the papillary muscles of either the anterior or the posterior group were poorly developed with abbreviated chordae. Rarely, there was an accessory opening within the mitral valve.

Pulmonary Valve

This was normal in 57%, was bicuspid and stenotic in 25%, and the valve was atretic in 13%. In 1% the valve presented widened commissures, in 2% the valve cusps were unequal in size, in 1% with aneurysm of the sinuses and supravalvular stenosis. Rarely in longstanding cases of pulmonary hypertension was there atherosclerosis of the pulmonary trunk. The valve was dome-shaped in 1%.

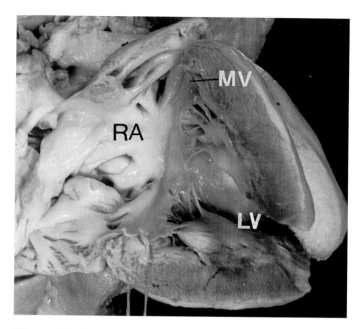

Figure 17: Right atrial, left ventricular view showing the more or less normally formed mitral valve. RA = right atrium; MV = mitral valve; LV = left ventricle.

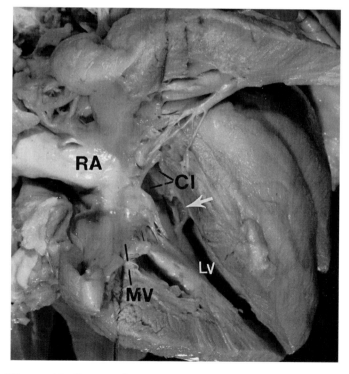

Figure 18: Corrected transposition with cleft in the anterior leaflet of the mitral valve. Right atrial, left ventricular view. RA = right atrium; MV = mitral valve; LV = left ventricle; Cl = cleft in the anterior leaflet of the mitral valve. Arrow points to the straddling tricuspid valve attached to the left ventricle.

I. Mixed Levocardia with Atria in Normal Position and Ventricles Inverted

Type I. Mixed Levocardia with Atria Normal, Ventricles Inverted

    1 (a). with inverted transposition
    1 (b). with complete transposition (noninverted).

Type I (a). The various complexes associated with this entity are:

(1) left AV valve insufficiency
(2) ventricular septal defect and abnormal left AV valve
(3) ventricular septal defect and Ebstein-like anomaly of the left AV valve
(4) ventricular septal defect with straddling left AV valve
(5) Ventricular septal defect with pulmonary stenosis and anomalous formation of the left AV valve
(6) ventricular septal defect and left AV valve stenosis
(7) ventricular septal defect with pulmonary stenosis and overriding aorta associated with left AV valve abnormality
(8) ventricular septal defect with pulmonary atresia and overriding aorta and left AV valve stenosis
(9) coarctation of the aorta with anatomic aortic stenosis and abnormal left AV valve
(10) hypoplasia of the transverse arch with coarctation of the aorta with Ebstein's anomaly of the left AV valve, or left AV valve abnormality
(11) double outlet right ventricle and subpulmonary ventricular septal defect and coarctation of the aorta
(12) double outlet right ventricle with subaortic or doubly committed or noncommitted type of ventricular septal defect
(13) common AV orifice
(14) right AV valve atresia
(15) aortic atresia with intact ventricular septum and atypical Ebstein's anomaly
(16) with intact ventricular septum
(17) with AV block and/or preexcitation

(1) *Left AV Valve Insufficiency.* A fundamental feature of this entity is the abnormal formation of the left AV valve and the hemodynamic alteration of the left AV valve with insufficiency and its hemodynamic effects on the myocardium and the endocardium (Figs. 10, 11).

(2) *Ventricular Septal Defect and Abnormal Left AV Valve*. When there was a defect, it was usually large and was situated at the base of the ventricular septum and was not confluent with the mouth of the pulmonic valve (Figs. 19, 20). It entered the morphologically right ventricle in the lower part of the conus or the infundibulum and in the upper part of the sinus or the inlet and it almost always impinged upon the tricuspid valve. The tricuspid valve was always abnormally formed and it was difficult to ascertain the physiological insufficiency the valve might have produced in the presence of the large ventricular septal defect. The complex was thus typical of ventricular septal defect with left-to-right shunt and pulmonary hypertension. Uncommonly, the defect was small or multiple (Figs. 21, 22). Often the tricuspid valve or endocardial tissue or aneurysm of the membranous septum protruded through the defect, and not only restricted the flow at the level of the defect (Figs. 23, 24), but produced subpulmonary obstruction. In some the defect was situated in an oblique angle with mild overriding of the pulmonary trunk (Fig. 25).

(3) *Ventricular Septal Defect and Ebstein-like Malformation of the Tricuspid Valve*. Here the Ebstein's malformation varied from a mild to a moderate degree and the valve was anchored to the defect to a varying extent. The defect, although usually large, was small in some.

(4) *Ventricular Septal Defect and Straddling Left AV valve*. This was a distinct entity. The morphologically tricuspid valve had a tendency to straddle the defect and enter the morphologically left ventricle and connected to well-developed papillary muscles in the left ventricle or connected to a varying degree along the rim of the ventricular septal defect (Fig. 26). Sometimes this resulted in subpulmonary obstruction.

(5) *Ventricular Septal Defect with Pulmonary Stenosis and Abnormal Formation of the Left AV Valve*. The defect was usually large in nature and the pulmonary stenosis was either mild or moderate. The com-

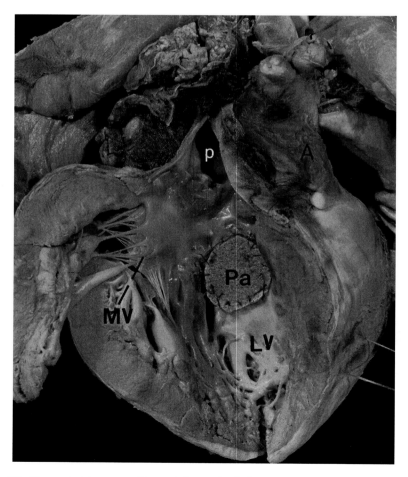

Figure 19: Corrected transposition with surgical closure of a large ventricular septal defect. MV = mitral valve; LV = left ventricle; A = aorta; P = pulmonary trunk; Pa = patch closure of the large defect. (Used with permission from Lev M, Rowlatt UF. See Figure 95.)

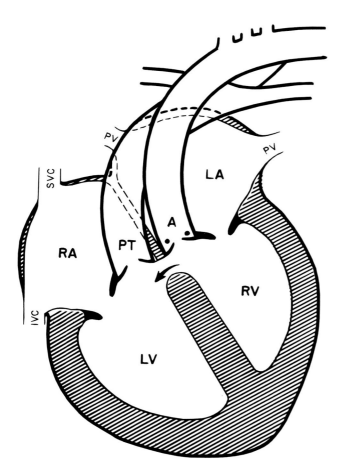

Figure 20: Diagrammatic sketch of heart seen in Fig. 19. Arrow points to the flow of blood at the ventricular septal defect level. SVC = superior vena cava; IVC = inferior vena cava; RA = right atrium; RV = right ventricle; LA = left atrium; LV = left ventricle; PV = pulmonary vein; A = aorta; PT = pulmonary trunk. (Used with permission from Lev M, Rowlatt UF. See Figure 95.)

plex is typical of that of left-to-right shunt at the VSD level with mild pulmonary stenosis (Figs. 27, 28).

(6) *Ventricular Septal Defect with Left AV Valve Stenosis.* The defect was present in the usual position and often the tricuspid valve covered the defect (Fig. 29). The left AV valve, however, showed marked abnormality with abnormal architecture of the inflow and outflow tracts of the right ventricle. The physiological results of these appear to be mild stenosis of the left AV valve. It is again emphasized that in the presence of a large ventricular septal defect, it would be almost difficult to evaluate the function of the stenotic left AV valve. Usually this complex is typical of left-to-right shunt at the ventricular level with mild AV valve (tricuspid) stenosis.

(7) *Ventricular Septal Defect, Pulmonary Stenosis, and Overriding Aorta and Left AV Valve Stenosis* (Figs. 30—32). In this type, the ventricular septal defect was so situated that the aorta distinctly overrode the septum. The pulmonic stenosis, coupled with the tricuspid stenosis, resulted in a right-to-left shunt at the ven-

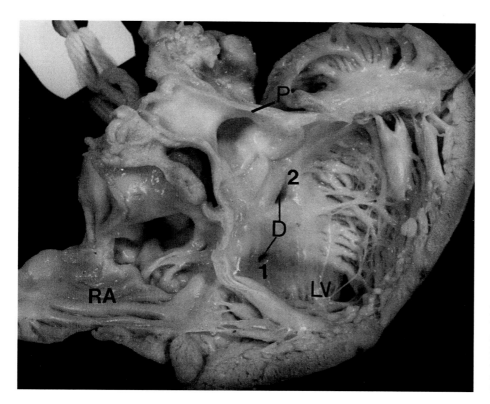

Figure 21: Mixed levocardia with ventricular inversion with double small ventricular septal defects. RA = right atrium; LV = morphologically left ventricle; D = ventricular septal defect, small, 1 and 2; P = pulmonary trunk.

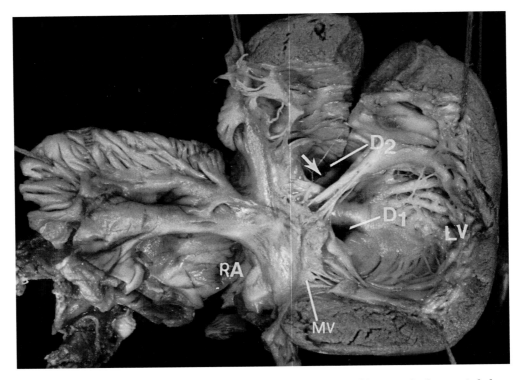

Figure 22: Right atrial, left ventricular view showing double ventricular septal defects. RA = right atrium; MV = mitral valve; LV = left ventricle; D$_1$ = common AV canal type of a somewhat posteriorly located defect; D$_2$ = anteriorly located defect with straddling conus. Arrow points to the straddling conus.

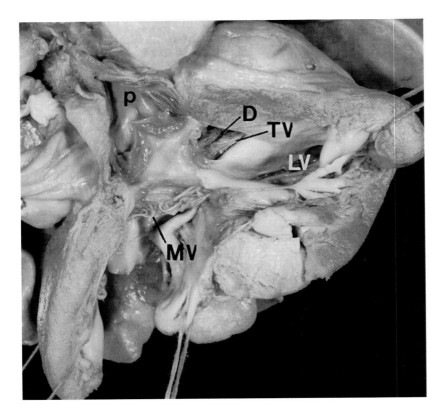

Figure 23: Morphologically left ventricle and the VSD with the tricuspid valve attached along the rim of the defect, restricting the defect. LV = left ventricle; MV = mitral valve; P = pulmonary trunk; D = defect; TV = attachment of the tricuspid valve along the margin of the defect.

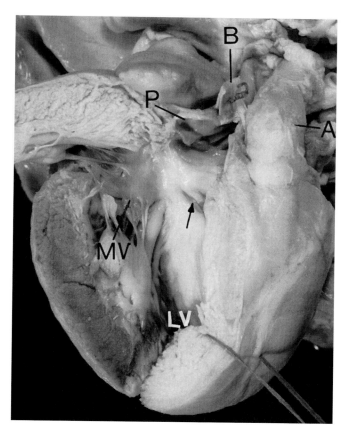

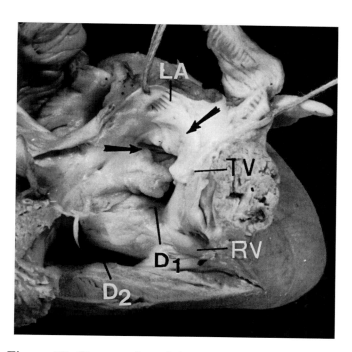

Figure 26: Close-up view of the straddling tricuspid valve through a large common AV canal type of VSD. LA = left atrium; RV = right ventricle; TV = tricuspid valve; D_1 = common AV canal type of a defect; D_2 more anteriorly located defect. Arrows point to the straddling tricuspid valve.

Figure 24: Left ventricular view of the VSD covered by the tricuspid valve. LV = left ventricle; MV = mitral valve; P = pulmonary trunk; B = banding of the pulmonary trunk; A = aorta. Arrow points to the defect situated in an oblique manner and covered by the tricuspid valve.

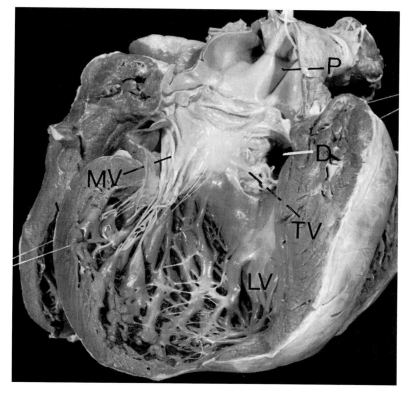

Figure 25: Morphologically left ventricular view demonstrating the overriding pulmonary trunk and the basilar straddling tricuspid valve through an oblique VSD. P = pulmonary valve; D = defect; TV = basilar straddling tricuspid valve along the rim of the defect; LV = left ventricle; MV = mitral valve. Note that the location of the VSD is oblique and although it involves the membranous septum to a minimal extent, it extends further anteriorly and confluent, in part, with the pulmonary valve.

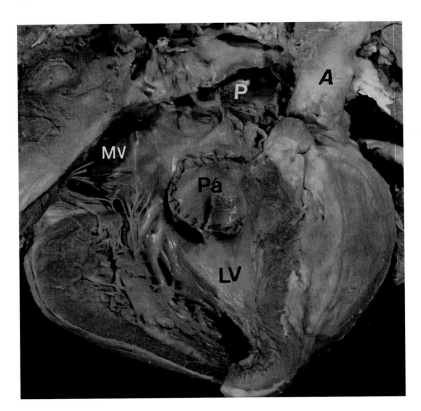

Figure 27: Corrected transposition with large ventricular septal defect and pulmonary stenosis with surgical repair. A = aorta situated to the left and anterior; P = pulmonary trunk to the right and posterior; MV = mitral valve; LV = left ventricle; Pa = patch closure of the large ventricular septal defect. Note the irregular, thickened bicuspid pulmonary valve. (Used with permission from Lev M, Rowlatt UF. See Figure 95.)

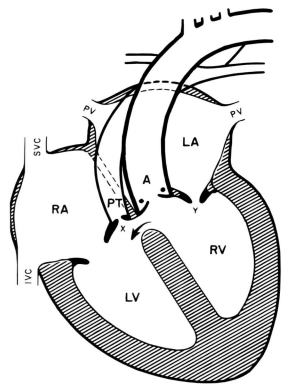

Figure 28: Diagrammatic sketch of heart seen in Figure 27. SVC = superior vena cava; IVC = inferior vena cava; RA = right atrium; RV = right ventricle; LA = left atrium; LV = left ventricle; PV = pulmonary vein; A = aorta; PT = pulmonary trunk; X = pulmonary stenosis; Y = left AV valve stenosis. (Used with permission from Lev M, Rowlatt UF. See Figure 95.)

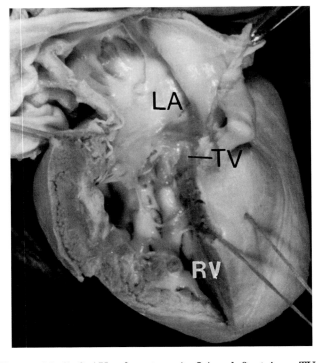

Figure 29: Left AV valve stenosis. LA = left atrium; TV = thickened, small tricuspid valve covering the ventricular septal defect; RV = right ventricle.

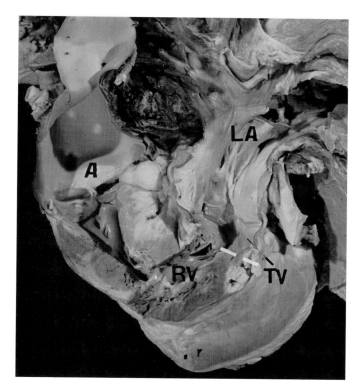

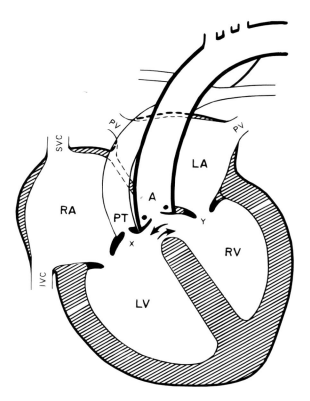

Figure 30: Corrected transposition with marked tricuspid stenosis and ventricular septal defect. LA = left atrium; A = aorta; RV = right ventricle; TV = small tricuspid with marked stenosis. Note the parietal wall of the right ventricle obstructing the view of the VSD.

Figure 32: Diagrammatic sketch of hearts shown in Fig. 30 and Fig. 31. Note the arrows at the ventricular septal defect indicating shunting of blood bidirectionally. X = pulmonary stenosis; Y = left AV valve stenosis; SVC = superior vena cava; IVC = inferior vena cava; RA = right atrium; RV = right ventricle; LA = left atrium; LV = left ventricle; PV = pulmonary vein; A = aorta; PT = pulmonary trunk. (Used with permission from Lev M, Rowlatt UF. See Figure 95.)

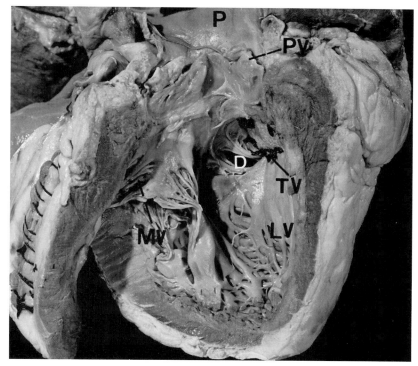

Figure 31: Morphologically left ventricle demonstrating the large ventricular septal defect with pulmonary infundibular stenosis and the anomalous attachment of the tricuspid valve to the lower margin of the defect and overriding aorta. MV = mitral valve; LV = left ventricle; D = large ventricular septal defect; PV = bicuspid pulmonary valve, thickened; P = pulmonary trunk; TV = attachment of the tricuspid valve to the lower margin of the defect. (Used with permission from Lev M, Rowlatt UF. See Figure 95.)

Figure 33: Mixed levocardia with pulmonary atresia. External view of the heart. LV = morphologically left ventricle; RV = morphologically right ventricle; A = aorta to the left and anterior; P = pulmonary trunk, very small, to the right and posterior; RPA = right pulmonary artery. (Used with permission from Lev M, Rowlatt UF. See Figure 95.)

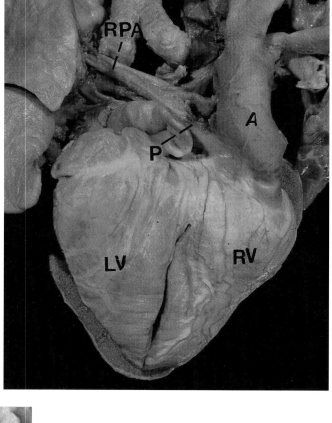

tricular level, giving a complex physiologically reminiscent of cyanotic tetralogy of Fallot. However, the morphology of the left AV valve (tricuspid) and the inflow tract of the morphologically right ventricle (left-sided) differed markedly from tetralogy. Likewise, the relationship of the arterial trunks was that of complete inverted transposition.

(8) *Mild Overriding Aorta and Pulmonary Atresia with Ventricular Septal Defect or Pseudotruncus.* This is a type of complete inverted transposition, although there is pulmonary atresia (Figs. 33—35). There were a total of seven cases: four with ventricular septal defect and three with common AV orifice. The VSD was either confluent with the aorta or located in an oblique manner close to the tricuspid valve (Figs. 36, 37). The details of this complex are given below:

Pulmonary atresia and PDA—1
Pulmonary atresia with large VSD and PDA—2
Pulmonary atresia with straddling parietal band, over-

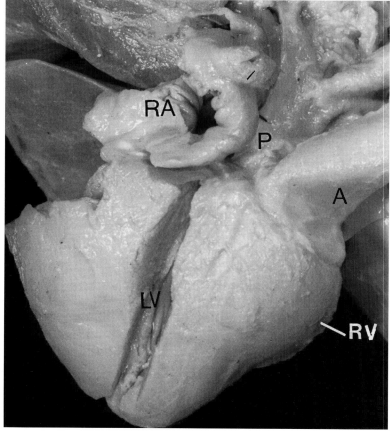

Figure 34: Mixed levocardia with ventricular inversion and pulmonary atresia, external view. A = aorta; P = small pulmonary trunk; RA = right atrium; RV -right ventricle; LV = left ventricle.

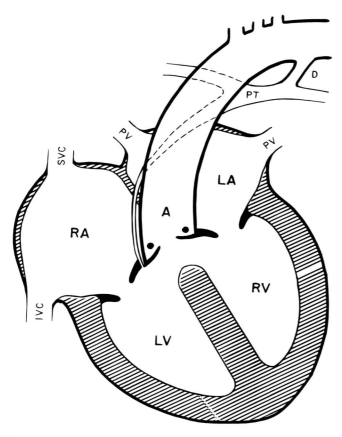

Figure 35: Diagrammatic sketch of hearts shown in Figures 33 and 34. Note the atretic main pulmonary trunk. D = patent ductus arteriosus; SVC = superior vena cava; IVC = inferior vena cava; RA = right atrium; RV = right ventricle; LA = left atrium; LV = left ventricle; PV = pulmonary vein; A = aorta; PT = pulmonary trunk. (Used with permission from Lev M, Rowlatt UF. See Figure 95.)

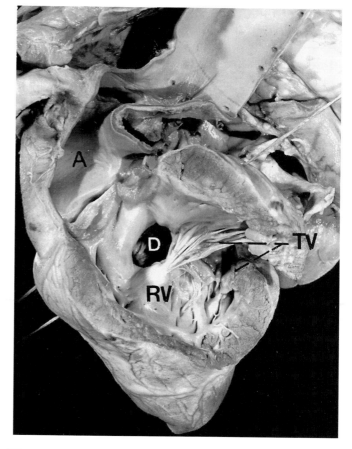

Figure 36: Right ventricular outflow tract in a case of a corrected transposition with a large ventricular septal defect and pulmonary atresia. TV = tricuspid valve; RV = right ventricle; D = large defect; A = aorta emerging from the right ventricle.

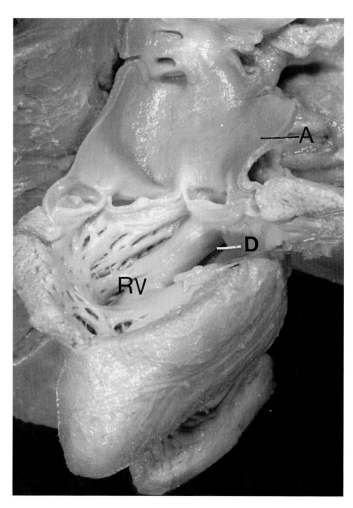

Figure 37: Outflow tract of the right ventricle depicting the aorta emerging from this chamber in an oblique manner, somewhat facing the defect. D = defect; RV = right ventricle; A = aorta.

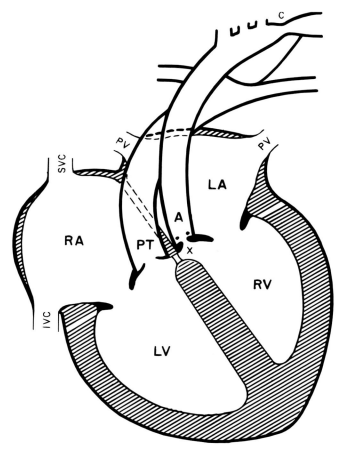

Figure 38: Diagrammatic sketch of coarctation of the aorta in mixed levocardia with ventricular inversion. C = coarctation of the aorta; X = aortic stenosis; SVC = superior vena cava; IVC = inferior vena cava; RA = right atrium; RV = right ventricle; LA = left atrium; LV = left ventricle; PV = pulmonary vein; A = aorta; PT = pulmonary trunk. (Used with permission from Lev M, Rowlatt UF. See Figure 95.)

riding aorta, marked tricuspid stenosis and insufficiency, small left pulmonary artery, large VSD, and both lungs bilobed—1

Pulmonary atresia with CAVO, fossa ovalis defect, left superior vena cava entering left atrium—1

Pulmonary atresia with CAVO, total anomalous pulmonary venous drainage, PDA and asplenia—1

Pulmonary atresia with CAVO, fossa ovalis defect, left superior vena cava entering the left atrium, right aortic arch, right PDA, and hepatic veins entering the left atrium and asplenia—1.

(9) *Coarctation of the Aorta with Anatomic Aortic Stenosis and Abnormal Left AV Valve.* When there was anatomic coarctation, it was difficult to evaluate the nature of the coarctation (Fig. 38).

(10) *Hypoplasia of Transverse Arch with Coarctation of the Aorta with Ebstein's Anomaly of the Left AV Valve, or Left AV Valve Abnormality.* The left AV valve presented features of either an atypical Ebstein-like malformation or was markedly thickened with irregular valvular tissue with hypoplastic papillary muscles and abbreviated chordae (Figs. 39, 40). This may be associated with an aneurysm in the foramen ovale (Figs. 40, 41). A VSD was seen frequently (Figs. 42—44). When there was severe hypoplasia of the transverse arch, there was an associated patent ductus arteriosus.

(11) *Double Outlet Right Ventricle with Subpulmonary Ventricular Septal Defect and Coarctation of the Aorta.* In this entity the defect was confluent to the pulmonary trunk (Fig. 45) and either there was hypoplasia of the transverse arch with interrupted aortic

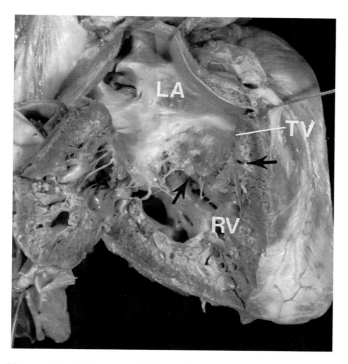

Figure 39: Mild case of Ebstein's anomaly of the tricuspid valve with tricuspid stenosis. Left atrial, right ventricular view. LA = left atrium; RV = right ventricle; TV = tricuspid valve. Arrows point to the mild displacement and plastering of the septal leaflet of the tricuspid valve with a small anulus.

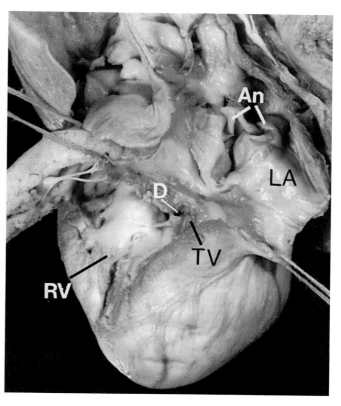

Figure 40: Mixed levocardia with tricuspid stenosis, ventricular septal defect, and coarctation of the aorta. Left atrial, right ventricular view demonstrating the aneurysm of the fossa ovalis and tricuspid stenosis. LA = left atrium; TV = tricuspid valve; An = aneurysm of the fossa ovalis; D = ventricular septal defect; RV = morphologically right ventricle. Note the attachment of the tricuspid valve along the margin of the defect.

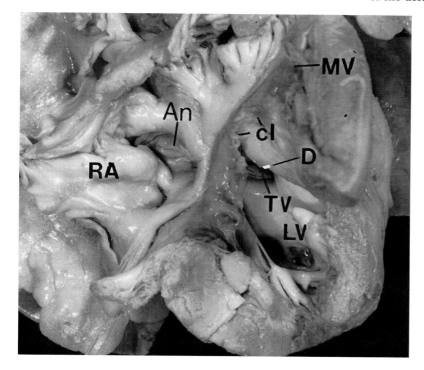

Figure 41: Right atrial, left ventricular view demonstrating the aneurysm of the fossa ovalis and the ventricular septal defect. RA = right atrium; An = aneurysm of the fossa ovalis; MV = mitral valve; cl = cleft in the mitral valve; D = ventricular septal defect; TV = tricuspid valve attachment along the crest of the defect; LV = left ventricle.

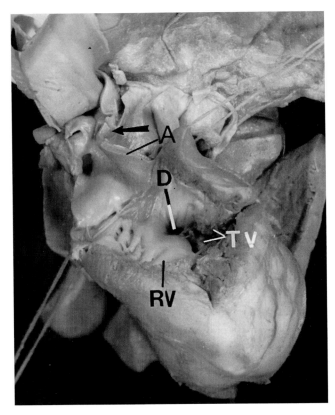

Figure 42: Morphologically right ventricle demonstrating the defect and coarctation of the aorta. RV = right ventricle; TV = tricuspid valve; D = defect; A = ascending aorta. Arrow points to coarctation.

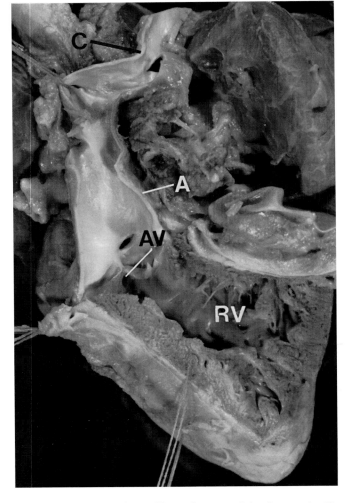

Figure 43: Morphologically right ventricle demonstrating the bicuspid aortic valve and coarctation of the aorta. RV = right ventricle; A = ascending aorta; C = coarctation of the aorta; AV = bicuspid aortic valve. Note the high origin of the right coronary ostium.

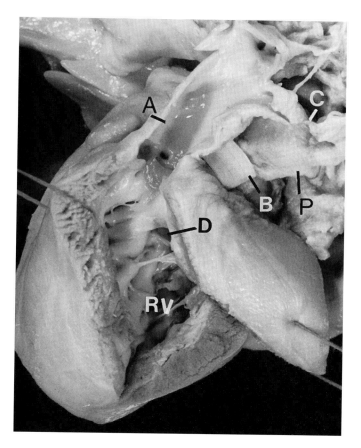

Figure 44: Mixed levocardia with ventricular inversion, hypoplasia of transverse arch, and coarctation of the aorta with overriding pulmonary trunk and recent banding procedure. RV = right ventricle; A = aorta; B = banding procedure; P = pulmonary trunk; C = coarctation; D = defect.

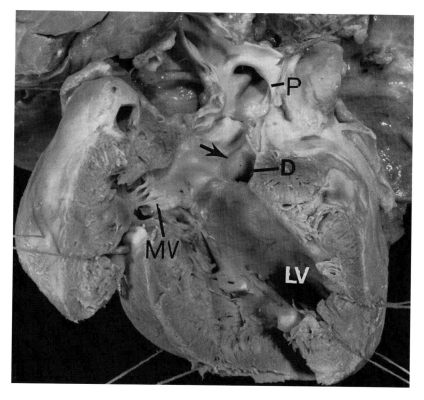

Figure 45: Left ventricular outflow tract demonstrating straddling conus and mild overriding of the pulmonary trunk. LV = left ventricle; MV = mitral valve; P = pulmonary trunk; D = defect. Arrow points to the straddling conus.

arch or marked coarctation. This heart may be considered similar to that of the Taussig-Bing group of hearts with AV concordance. The complexes are:

VSD, straddling conus with overriding pulmonary trunk and coarctation—1
Taussig-Bing complex with coarctation and PDA—1
Double outlet right ventricle with regular (noninverted type) with Taussig-Bing and absent transverse arch and VSD—1.

(12) *Double Outlet Right Ventricle with Subaortic or Doubly Committed or Noncommitted Type of Ventricular Septal Defect.* There was either pulmonary stenosis, fetal coarctation, and/or Ebstein's anomaly of the left AV valve and the great arteries were in the noninverted (regular) type of transposition. The complexes are as follows:

Double outlet right ventricle (noninverted) noncommitted VSD with pulmonary stenosis—1
Double outlet right ventricle (noninverted) doubly committed type VSD with common atrium—1

Double outlet right ventricle (regular type) with fetal coarctation, Ebstein's anomaly of the tricuspid valve with stenosis, VSD, PDA—1

(13) *Mixed Levocardia with Ventricular Inversion and Common AV Orifice.* There were four cases, three associated with infundibular and valvular pulmonary stenosis, and one with fetal coarctation. Total anomalous pulmonary venous drainage was usually present (Figs. 46—49). They are presented in detail as follows:

CAVO, TAPVD, right upper pulmonary vein to right superior vena cava and other veins to left superior vena cava to coronary sinus, pulmonary stenosis, and infundibular stenosis, and PDA.
CAVO, inverted DORV, small right-sided coronary ostium, right aortic arch, right descending aorta and right PDA, common atrium, noncommitted type of CAVO with pulmonary stenosis and infundibular stenosis, absent coronary sinus, both coronary ostia from posterior sinus.
CAVO, dominant RV type, TAPVD—mixed type, aneurysm of membranous septum producing subpulmonary stenosis, ASD.

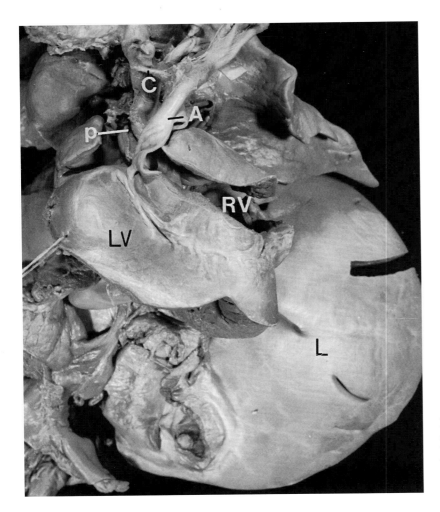

Figure 46: Mixed levocardia with common AV orifice and coarctation of the aorta. External view of the heart with the liver. RV = right ventricle; LV = left ventricle; A = aorta; P = pulmonary trunk; C = coarctation of the aorta; L = liver.

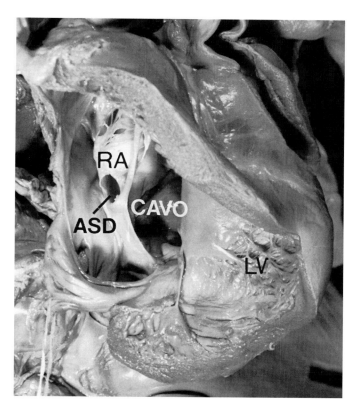

Figure 47: Right atrial, left ventricular view in common AV orifice of complete type. RA = right atrium; CAVO = common atrioventricular orifice, complete type; LV = left ventricle; ASD = atrial septal defect, fossa ovalis type.

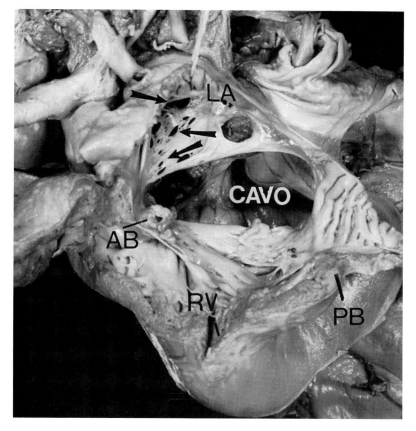

Figure 48: Left atrial, right ventricular view in a large common AV orifice. LA = left atrium; RV = right ventricle; CAVO = common atrioventricular orifice of complete type; PB = posterior bridging leaflet of the common AV valve; AB = anterior bridging leaflet of the common AV valve. Arrows point to the fenestrated opening in the septum primum and the atrial septal defect.

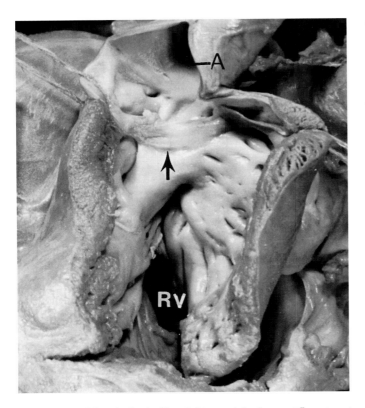

Figure 49: Morphologically right ventricular outflow tract demonstrating the aorta emerging from the right ventricle with a small bicuspid aortic valve. RV = right ventricle; A = aorta. Arrow points to the bicuspid aortic valve. Note also that the aorta emerges unrelated to the common AV orifice defect.

CAVO, TAPVD → RA, FC, AS, PDA, LSVC → LA, absent coronary sinus, asplenia, right lung 2 lobes, left lung 3 lobes, and accessory liver.

(14) *Mixed Levocardia with Right AV Valve Atresia.* There were three such cases, two of them with double ventricular septal defects and one with CAVO type of a ventricular septal defect associated with double outlet right ventricle or overriding aorta. The details of this entity are as follows:

Double VSD, DORV, Ebstein's with marked LV valve insufficiency, pulmonary stenosis, right aortic arch, large fossa ovalis defect, and probe PDA (Figs. 50—54).
Straddling tricuspid valve with CAVO-type VSD, DORV with pulmonary stenosis, left superior vena cava entering the coronary sinus (Figs. 55, 56).
Double small VSD (1 U-shaped, 1 below the first), small right coronary ostium, right aortic arch, right descending aorta, right PDA with abnormal architecture of the right ventricle.

(15) *Mixed Levocardia with Aortic Atresia or Marked Aortic Stenosis and Intact Ventricular Septum.* There were four such cases (three with aortic atresia and one with aortic stenosis), all associated with atypical Ebstein-like anomaly of the left AV valve with incomplete formation of the valvular tissue with a huge orifice and practical absence of valvular tissue resulting in tremendous left AV valve insufficiency in in-

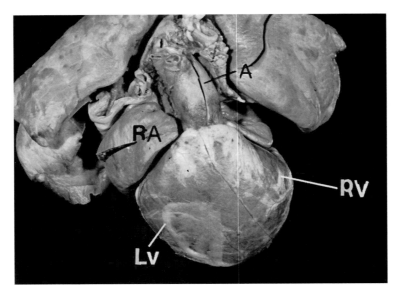

Figure 50: External view of the heart of mixed levocardia with right AV valve atresia. RA = right atrium; A = aorta; RV = right ventricle; LV = left ventricle.

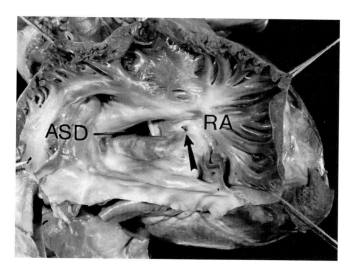

Figure 51: Mixed levocardia with ventricular inversion and right AV valve atresia, right atrial view. RA = right atrium; ASD = atrial septal defect, fossa ovalis type. Arrow points to the dimple where the right AV valve and orifice and valvular apparatus should be.

trauterine life. This had resulted in a paper-thin left atrium that was aneurysmally dilated, and a paper-thin huge right ventricle. Rarely, a marked Ebstein's anomaly was associated with marked aortic stenosis.

Aortic atresia with almost absence of tricuspid valve with marked tricuspid insufficiency, paper-thin right ventricle, and huge ASD.

Aortic atresia with atypical Ebstein's anomaly and almost absence of the tricuspid valve leaflet with left AV valve insufficiency, stenosis of the pulmonary vein, pulmonary artery and coronary sinus, atypical

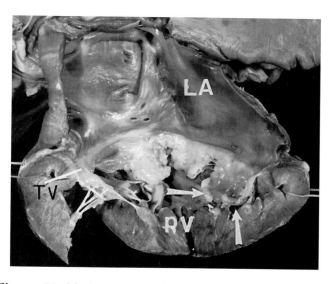

Figure 53: Markedly redundant tricuspid valve with Ebstein-like malformation and significant tricuspid insufficiency. Left atrial, right ventricular view. LA = left atrium; RV = right ventricle; TV = markedly redundant segmented tricuspid valve with Ebstein-like malformation. Arrows point to the Ebstein-like malformation.

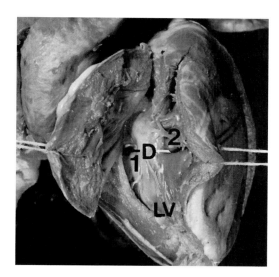

Figure 52: Left ventricular outflow tract depicting two ventricular septal defects. LV = left ventricle; D = defects 1 and 2. Note that no vessel emerges from this chamber.

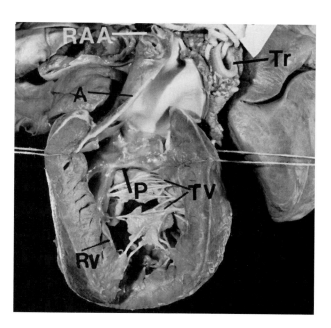

Figure 54: Right ventricular outflow tract depicting double outlet right ventricle with marked pulmonary stenosis and right aortic arch. RV = right ventricle; TV = tricuspid valve; A = aorta; P = pulmonary trunk emerging also from the right ventricle with markedly narrowed opening; RAA = right aortic arch; Tr = trachea.

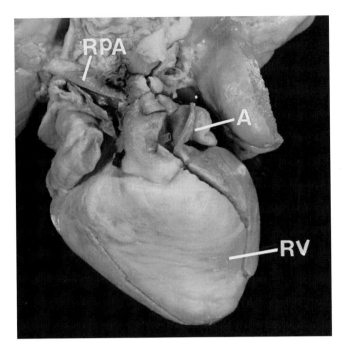

Figure 55: External view of mixed levocardia with ventricular inversion and right AV valve atresia with double outlet right ventricle and pulmonary stenosis. RV = right ventricle; A = aorta; RPA = right pulmonary artery.

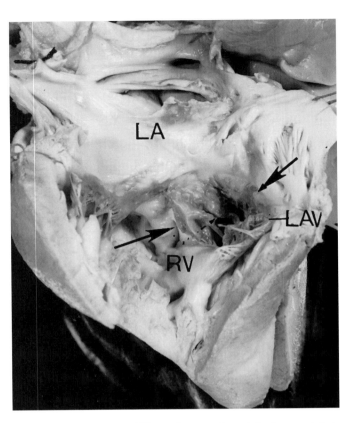

Figure 56: Common AV canal type of ventricular septal defect with straddling tricuspid valve. LA = left atrium; RV = right ventricle; LAV = left AV valve — tricuspid valve. Note that it is quite large and redundant and straddles through the defect to the opposite chamber. Arrows point to the straddling left AV valve.

large proximal and fossa ovalis defect, abnormal architecture of the right ventricle (Figs. 57—60).

Aortic atresia with almost absent tricuspid valve with tricuspid insufficiency and obstruction to outflow tract of the right ventricle with abnormal architecture of the right ventricle (Figs. 61—65).

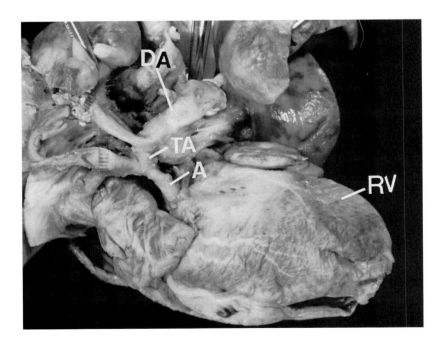

Figure 57: External view of mixed levocardia with aortic atresia and absent tricuspid valve with huge right ventricle. RV = right ventricle; A = ascending aorta comes to the base of the heart without entering the heart—aortic atresia; TA = transverse arch; DA = descending aorta.

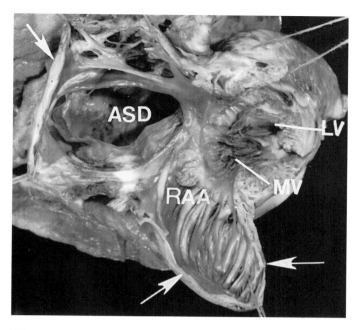

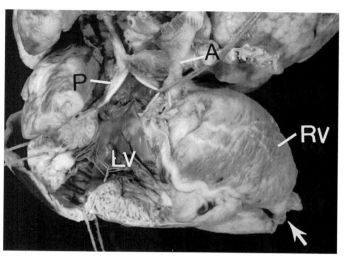

Figure 59: Outflow tract of the left ventricle. LV = left ventricle; P = pulmonary trunk; A = ascending aorta, very small; RV = morphologically right ventricle. Arrow points to the thin wall, right ventricle. Note also the ventricular septal bulge into the morphologically left ventricle.

Figure 58: Right atrial, left ventricular view demonstrating the huge atrial septal defect, fossa ovalis type, extending proximally close to the entry of the superior vena cava, the right pulmonary veins, as well as extending close to the mouth of the inferior vena cava, and small dysplastic mitral valve. ASD = atrial septal defect, atypical, huge; RAA = right atrial appendage; MV = markedly dysplastic, small mitral valve; LV = morphologically left ventricle. Arrows point to the paper-thin wall of the right atrium.

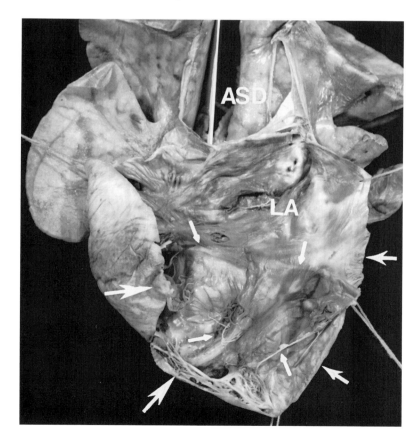

Figure 60: Left atrial, right ventricular view depicting the absent tricuspid valve with nubbins of valvular tissue with chordal extension into the inlet of the right ventricle, depicting the remnants of the valvular tissue. ASD = huge atrial septal defect; LA = left atrium. Small arrows indicate the remnant of the tricuspid valvular tissue throughout the inlet of the right ventricle, and large arrows point to the paper-thin right ventricular and left atrial walls.

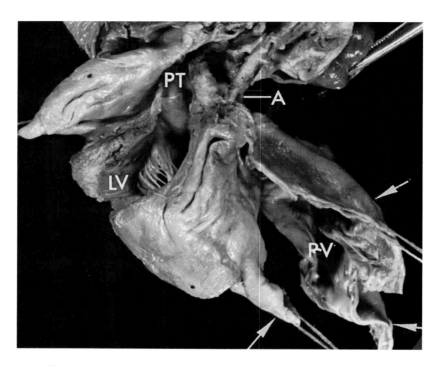

Figure 61: External view of mixed levocardia with aortic atresia and almost complete absence of the tricuspid valve with huge paper-thin right ventricle. A = small ascending aorta coming to the base without entering it; PT = pulmonary trunk; LV = left ventricle; RV = right ventricle. Arrows point to the huge right ventricle with paper-thin walls. (Used with permission from Brenner JI, et al. See Figure 64.)

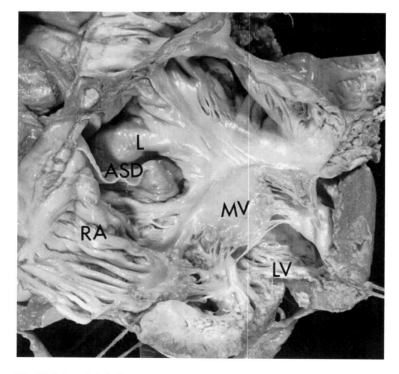

Figure 62: Right atrial, left ventricular view demonstrating a huge atrial septal defect. RA = right atrium; MV = mitral valve; LV = left ventricle; ASD = huge defect proceeding to the proximal part of the limbic margin; L = limbus. (Used with permission from Brenner JI, et al. See Figure 64.)

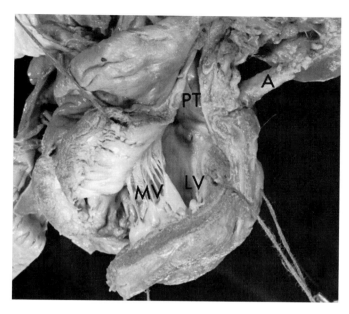

Figure 63: Outflow tract of the morphologically left ventricle. LV = left ventricle; MV = mitral valve; PT = pulmonary trunk; A = small ascending aorta. (Used with permission from Brenner JI, et al. See Figure 64.)

Figure 64: Left atrial, right ventricular view demonstrating huge opening between the atria and the ventricle with almost absent tricuspid valve, and tricuspid valve represented by chordal extensions. LA = left atrium; ASD = huge atrial septal defect; SP = septum primum; TV = remnant of the tricuspid valve in the form of strands; S = septal band; RV = paper-thin right ventricle. (Used with permission from Brenner JI, Bharati S, Winn WC, Lev M: Absent tricuspid valve with aortic atresia in mixed levocardia (atria situs solitus, L-loop): A hitherto undescribed entity. *Circulation* 1978, 57:836—840.)

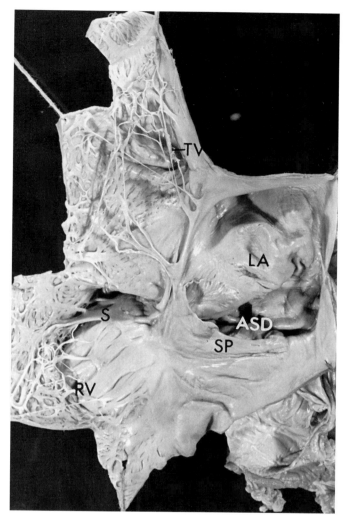

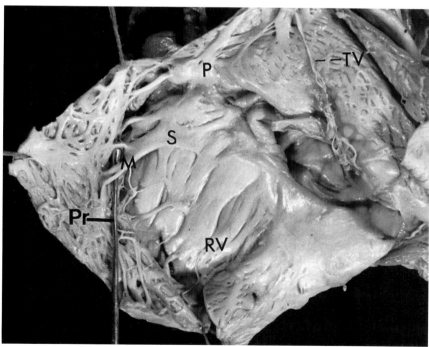

Figure 65: The outflow tract of the right ventricle. P = parietal band; S = septal band; M = moderator band; RV = right ventricle; TV = strands of tricuspid valvular tissue; Pr = Probe proceeding behind the moderator band. Note that no vessel emerges from this chamber.

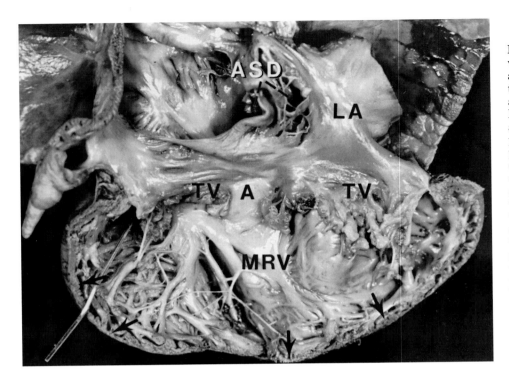

Figure 66: Mixed levocardia with ventricular inversion with partially absent tricuspid valve, significant tricuspid insufficiency, and marked aortic stenosis (functional atresia). LA = left atrium; ASD = huge atrial septal defect; MRV = morphologically right ventricle; TV = in part, markedly redundant with no clear demarcation between the tricuspid valve leaflets; A = partially absent septal leaflet of the tricuspid valve; MRV = huge right ventricle with paper-thin wall with relatively smooth architecture of the inlet or the sinus. Note the amorphous mass of irregular thickened nodular valvular tissue and almost absent papillary muscles and markedly abbreviated chordae. Note that the posterior leaflet is amorphous and displaced into the right ventricle. Arrows point to paper-thin RV. (Used with permission from Muster AJ, et al. See Figure 67.)

Marked aortic stenosis and tricuspid stenosis with marked Ebstein's anomaly of the tricuspid valve (Figs. 66, 67).

These findings suggest that there is a distinct flora of anomalies in this type of a mixed levocardia; therefore, it is possible that these anomalies are basically related to ventricular inversion with intact ventricular septum and incomplete formation of the left AV valve.

(16) *Mixed Levocardia with Ventricular Inversion and Intact Ventricular Septum.* There were only four cases and in all four the left AV valve had either a marked Ebstein-like malformation or was segmented with a large anulus, thickened leaflets with significant left AV valve insufficiency, and marked hypertrophy and enlargement of the right ventricle (Figs. 68—72). In addition, the membranous part of the ventricular septum was abnormally formed. This was quite large and extended considerably in the left ventricular aspect beneath the pulmonic valve (Fig. 73).

(17) *With AV Block and/or Preexcitation.*

Congenital AV block with preexcitation—2
Postoperative heart block—4 (1 with ventricular arrhythmia and sudden death)
Preexcitation, supraventricular arrhythmia, and sudden death—1
Postoperative ventricular arrhythmia and sudden death—1
Congenital AV block and sudden death with a familial history of VSD—1
Congenital AV block—3
Preexcitation—3

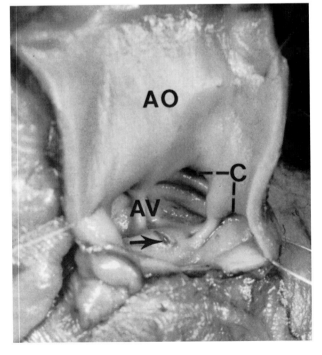

Figure 67: The fusion of the aortic cusps with a minute central opening. AV = aortic valve; AO = ascending aorta; C = coronary ostia originating in a somewhat high position. Arrow points to the central 1 mm diameter opening. (Used with permission from Muster AJ, Idriss FS, Bharati S, Riggs TW, Lev M, Culpepper WS, Paul MH: Functional aortic valvular atresia in transposition of the great arteries. *J Am Coll Cardiol* 6:630—634, 1985.)

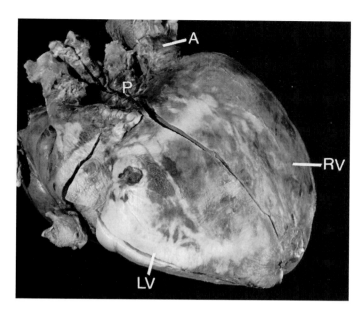

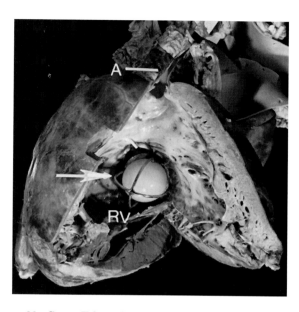

Figure 68: Mixed levocardia with ventricular inversion with marked left AV valve insufficiency and apex formed by the morphologically right ventricle. RV = right ventricle; LV = left ventricle; P = pulmonary trunk; A = aorta.

Figure 69: Starr-Edwards prosthetic valve replacing the left AV valve. A = aorta; RV = markedly hypertrophied and enlarged right ventricle. Arrow points to the Starr-Edwards valve.

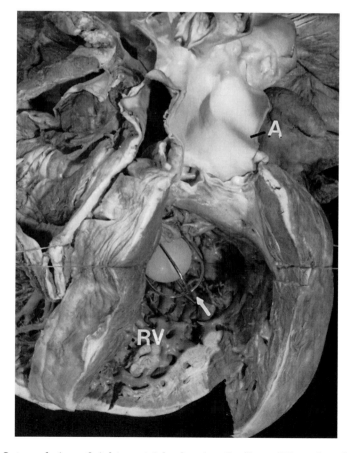

Figure 70: Internal view of right ventricle showing the Starr-Edwards valve and aorta emerging from the morphologically right ventricle. A = aorta; RV = right ventricle. Arrow points to the Starr-Edwards valve replacement for marked left AV valve insufficiency.

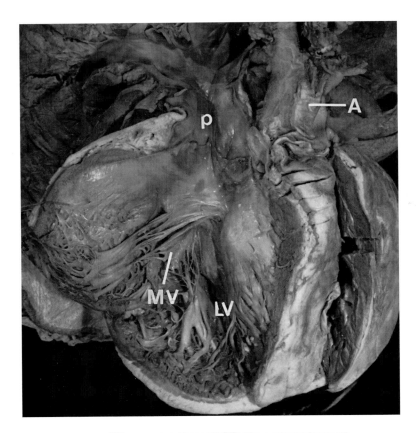

Figure 71: Mixed levocardia with ventricular inversion with intact ventricular septum. A = aorta to the left and anterior; P = pulmonary trunk; LV = left ventricle; MV = mitral valve.

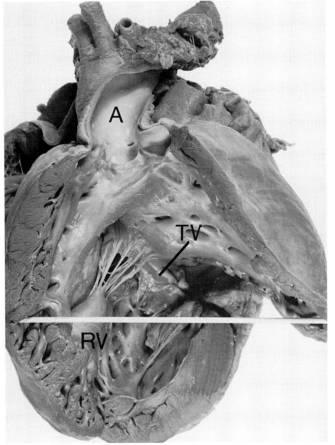

In summary, in this entity the fundamental abnormality appears to lie in the left AV valve which may be either Ebstein-like malformed or insufficient or stenosed or may present any of the above combinations from a mild to a moderate degree (Figs. 74, 75). The tricuspid valve in most cases is related to the defect (Fig. 76). Associated with this there usually is an anomaly of the inlet of the right ventricle and a large ventricular septal defect with or without pulmonary stenosis (Figs. 77—79). In addition, the aorta may override the septum simulating a picture of tetralogy of Fallot. In extreme cases, the pulmonic valve may be atretic resulting in pseudotruncus or pulmonary atresia with ventricular septal defect and this may be seen with common AV orifice. When there is DORV, the defect may be subaortic, subpulmonic, doubly committed, or noncommitted to the great arteries and, in general, the aorta is to the right of the pulmonary trunk (noninverted type of DORV). In extreme cases, the abnormal left AV valve may be associated with hypoplasia of the aorta and coarctation and rarely aortic atresia.

Figure 72: Mixed levocardia with intact ventricular septum and marked left AV valve insufficiency with huge right ventricle. Outflow tract of the right ventricle. RV = right ventricle, hypertrophied and enlarged; TV = tricuspid valve; A = aorta. Note the markedly hypertrophied and enlarged papillary muscles

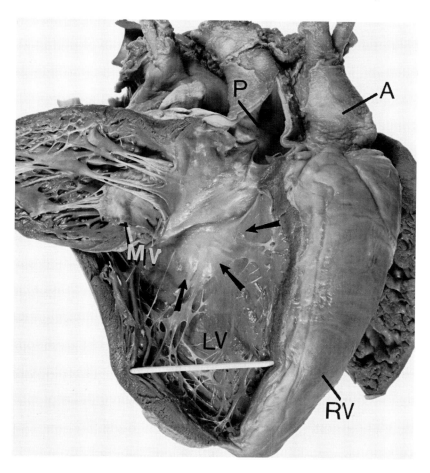

Figure 73: Outflow tract of the left ventricle demonstrating the bulge of the ventricular septum as well as aneurysm of the membranous septum with no VSD. LV = left ventricle; P = pulmonary trunk; A = aorta; RV = right ventricle; MV = mitral valve. Arrows point to the aneurysmal bulge.

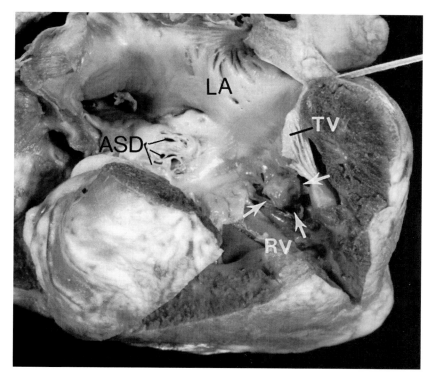

Figure 74: Left atrial, right ventricular view showing a fenestrated atrial septal defect and redundancy of the tricuspid valve with tricuspid stenosis. LA = left atrium; ASD = fenestrated atrial septal defect; TV = markedly redundant tricuspid valve with small anulus and tricuspid stenosis; RV = morphologically right ventricle. Arrows point to redundant tricuspid valve.

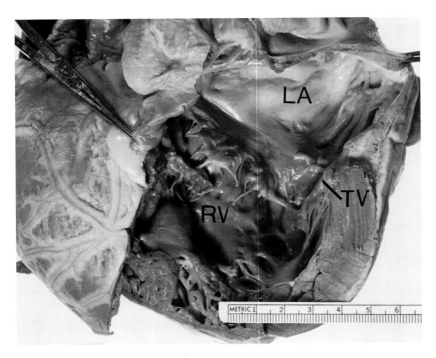

Figure 75: Markedly thickened left AV valve with mild Ebstein-like malformation and tricuspid insufficiency. LA = left atrium; RV = right ventricle; TV = mildly displaced and plastered septal leaflet of the tricuspid valve.

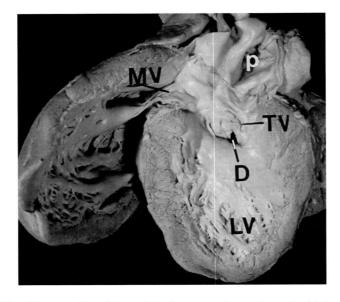

Figure 76: Mixed levocardia with ventricular inversion and marked tricuspid stenosis with basilar straddling tricuspid valve. MV = mitral valve; LV = left ventricle; P = pulmonary trunk; D = ventricular septal defect; TV = tricuspid valve. Part of the anulus, the leaflet, and the chordal extensions are beneath the pulmonic valve along the superior margin of the defect.

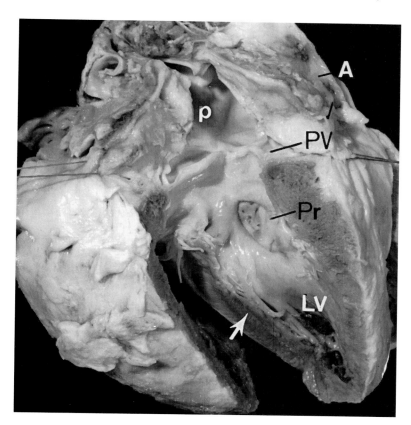

Figure 77: Corrected transposition with subpulmonary valvular stenosis and surgical closure of ventricular septal defect with postoperative AV block. Left ventricular outflow tract view. LV = left ventricle; PV = bicuspid markedly thickened, surgically altered pulmonary valve; P = pulmonary trunk; A = aorta; Pr = prosthetic closure of ventricular septal defect. Arrow points to diffuse fibroelastosis of this chamber.

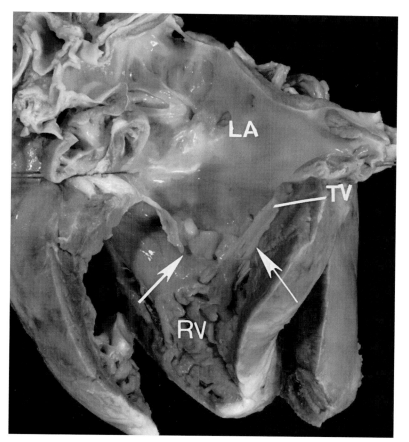

Figure 78: Left atrial view demonstrating small tricuspid valve with marked Ebstein anomaly with significant tricuspid stenosis and insufficiency. LA = left atrium; RV = right ventricle; TV = tricuspid valve with small anulus. Arrows point to the entire tricuspid valvular apparatus displaced into the inlet or the sinus of the right ventricle and is completely plastered without any chordal or papillary muscle connections.

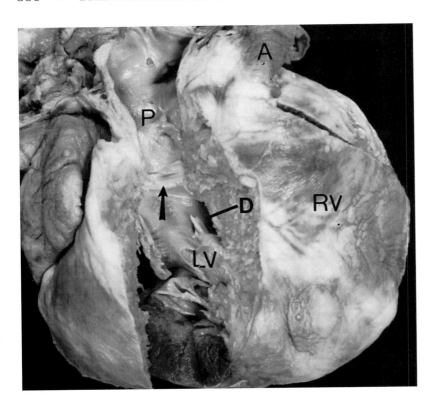

Figure 79: Outflow tract of the morphologically left ventricle demonstrating marked pulmonary valvular and subvalvular stenosis and marked left ventricular hypertrophy and ventricular septal defect. RV = right ventricle; LV = left ventricle; P = pulmonary valve; D = ventricular septal defect; A = aorta. Arrow points to subpulmonary

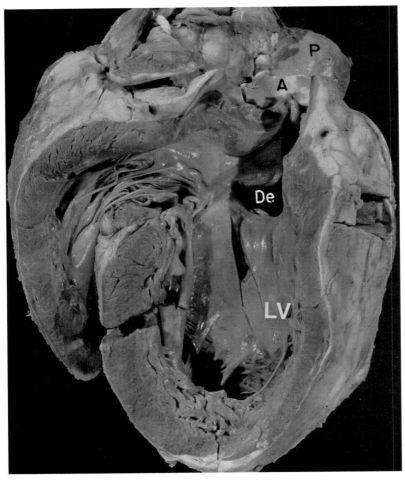

Figure 80: Aorta emerging from the morphologically left ventricle overriding a ventricular septal defect. A = aorta; De = defect; LV = left ventricle; P = pulmonary trunk. (Used with permission from Lev M, Rowlatt UF. See Figure 95.)

Type I (b). Mixed Levocardia with Ventricular Inversion and Noninverted Transposition

Here the aorta is situated to the right and somewhat anteriorly and the pulmonary trunk is situated to the left and somewhat posteriorly (as viewed from the anterior surface of the heart), as in complete transposition without ventricular inversion. Although the right-sided coronary artery forms the anterior descending branch, in contrast to type 1 (a), the right-sided coronary artery emerges from the left side of the aorta, either from the left anterior or the left sinus of Valsalva. The left-sided coronary artery emerges from the posterior or right sinus of Valsalva and passes behind the pulmonary trunk instead of in front of it as in type 1 (a). The aorta emerges either completely or almost completely from the morphologically left ventricle (Figs. 80—82) and the pulmonary trunk from the morphologically right ventricle (left-sided). In this situation, the AV valves, which in

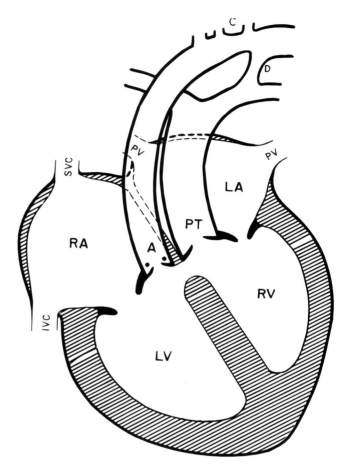

Figure 82: Diagrammatic sketch of anatomically corrected transposition with ventricular septal defect and aorta emerging from the morphologically left ventricle. SVC = superior vena cava; IVC = inferior vena cava; RA = right atrium; RV = right ventricle; LA = left atrium; LV = left ventricle; PV = pulmonary vein; A = aorta; PT = pulmonary trunk; C = coarctation; D = defect. (Used with permission from Lev M, Rowlatt UF. See Figure 95.)

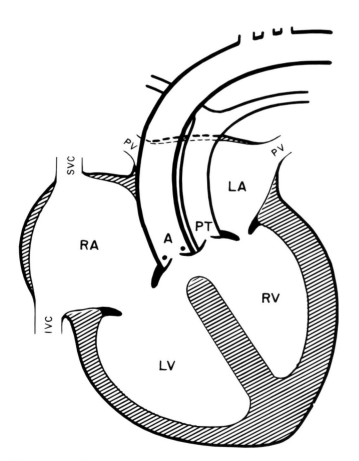

Figure 81: Diagrammatic sketch of heart seen in Figure 80. SVC = superior vena cava; IVC = inferior vena cava; RA = right atrium; RV = right ventricle; LA = left atrium; LV = left ventricle; PV = pulmonary vein; A = aorta; PT = pulmonary trunk. (Used with permission from Lev M, Rowlatt UF. See Figure 95.)

general correspond to the distal chamber, are not as altered in morphology as in the previous type.

These are rare hearts and may present as complete transposition, with ventricular septal defect and fetal coarctation, or complete transposition with ventricular septal defect and pulmonary stenosis.

Type II. Mixed Levocardia with Atrial Inversion

In general, the venous return in these cases is into the morphologically correct atrium situated in an inverted position. However, there are exceptions. In the usual cases where the venous return is to the morphologically correct atrium and the transposition is complete, then a type of corrected transposition may be

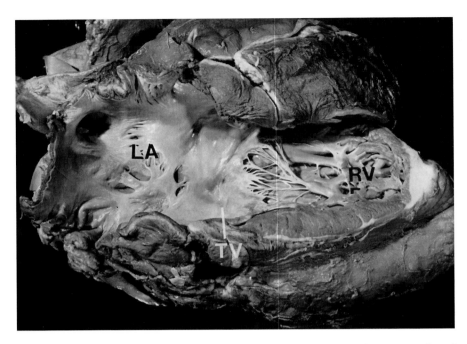

Figure 83: Mixed levocardia with atrial inversion. Left atrial, right ventricular view. LA = left atrium; TV = tricuspid valve; RV = right ventricle.

said to be present. Since atrial inversion is rare, the hearts are described in detail:

VSD, pulmonary stenosis, and subvalvular stenosis, bicuspid pulmonary valve, both coronary ostia from the left sinus of Valsalva and right aortic arch.

VSD, pulmonary stenosis, and subvalvular stenosis, right lower pulmonary vein to right atrium and right upper pulmonary vein to left atrium, inferior vena cava to right atrium and hemiazygos to left atrium and right aortic arch (Figs. 83—87).

Large ASD, double VSD, juxtaposed or displaced left-sided atrial appendage to the right, overriding aorta, and pulmonary stenosis.

Double VSD, pulmonary stenosis, tricuspid stenosis, bicuspid pulmonary valve, ASD, right aortic arch, and left PDA.

Pulmonary atresia with VSD, right aortic arch, patent foramen ovale, both coronary ostia from left sinus of Valsalva, PDA from subclavian artery.

Pulmonary atresia with VSD, right aortic arch, and right PDA and large ASD—1.

There is a distinct tendency for VSD, pulmonary stenosis or atresia and right aortic arch to occur in this entity.

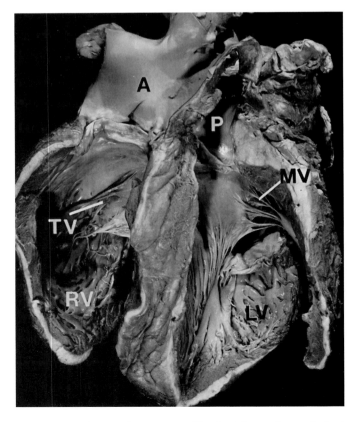

Figure 84: The outflow tracts of both right and morphologically left ventricle showing the aorta emerging from the right ventricle and the pulmonary trunk from the left ventricle. RV = right ventricle; LV = left ventricle; A = aorta; MV = mitral valve; TV = tricuspid valve; P = pulmonary trunk.

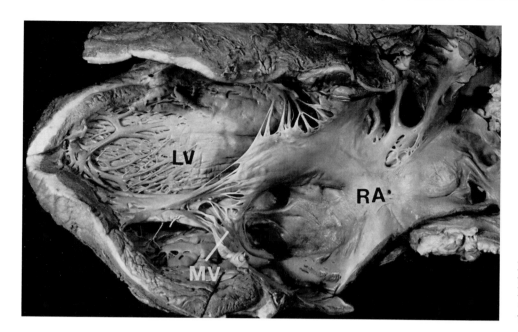

Figure 85: Right atrial, left ventricular view of same heart as in Figure 84. RA = right atrium; LV = left ventricle; MV = mitral valve.

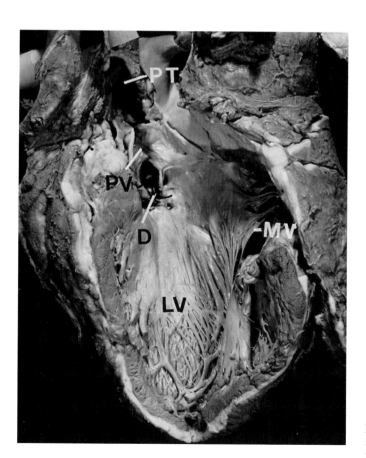

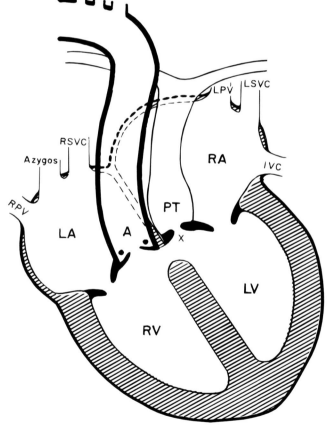

Figure 86: Outflow tract of the left ventricle depicting the subpulmonary and valvular stenosis and surgical closure of the ventricular septal defect. LV = left ventricle; MV = mitral valve; PT = pulmonary trunk; PV = bicuspid pulmonary valve; D = surgical closure of the ventricular septal defect.

Figure 87: Diagrammatic sketch of mixed levocardia with atrial inversion as seen in Figures 83—86. RSVC = right superior vena cava; IVC = inferior vena cava; RA = right atrium; RV = right ventricle; LA = left atrium; LV = left ventricle; RPV = right pulmonary vein; A = aorta; LPV = left pulmonary vein; PT = pulmonary trunk; LSVC = left superior vena cava; X = pulmonary stenosis. (Used with permission from Lev M, Rowlatt UF. See Figure 95.)

Type III. With Atria and Ventricles Relatively Normally Placed But Abnormal Connection of the AV Valves

There were two types.

Type III (a)

These are also called criss-cross or superior-inferior, or upstairs-downstairs hearts. In the majority, the atria were situated more or less in a relatively normal position but the right atrium is somewhat rotated posteroinferiorly and the left atrium anterosuperiorly, receiving their respective veins. The right atrium communicated by means of the mitral valve into the morphologically left ventricle situated to the left and posterior. The left atrium communicated by means of a tricuspid valve with the morphologically right ventricle which was situated superior and anterior and to the right. The infundibulum or the outflow tract of the right ventricle was situated where the sinus or the inlet should be, and the sinus occupied the region of the conus or the outlet.

The details of the eight hearts with mixed levocardia with relatively normal position of the chambers and criss-cross AV connection are as follows:

DORV, inverted type, subaortic VSD, pulmonary stenosis, right aortic arch, fossa ovalis defect, double superior vena cava entering the left atrium and inferior vena cava entering the left atrium and two pulmonary veins entering the right atrium (Figs. 88—91).

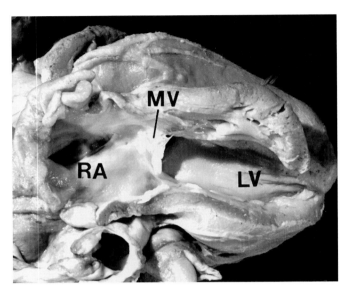

Figure 89: Right atrial, left ventricular view demonstrating the right atrium communicating by means of the mitral valve with the left ventricle situated to the left and posterior. RA = right atrium; MV = mitral valve; LV = left ventricle. (Used with permission from Lev M, Rowlatt UF. See Figure 95.)

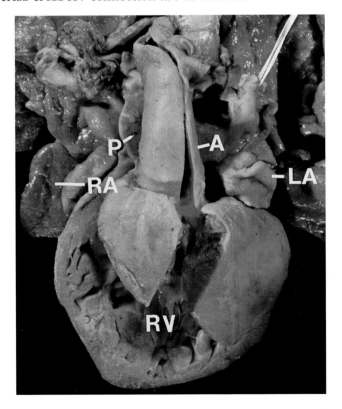

Figure 88: External view of a criss-cross heart with relatively normal position of the cardiac chambers with inverted type of DORV. RA = right atrium; LA = left atrium; RV = right ventricle; A = aorta; P = pulmonary trunk. (Used with permission from Lev M, Rowlatt UF. See Figure 95.)

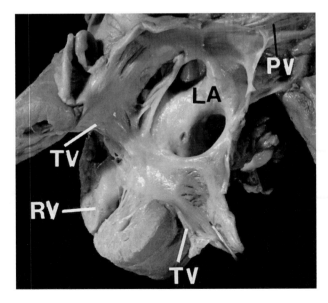

Figure 90: Left atrial, right ventricular view. Note the left atrium receiving the pulmonary veins communicating by means of a tricuspid valve with the morphologically right ventricle, which is situated anterior or superior and to the right. PV = pulmonary veins; LA = left atrium; TV = tricuspid valve; RV = morphologically right ventricle. (Used with permission from Lev M, Rowlatt UF. See Figure 95.)

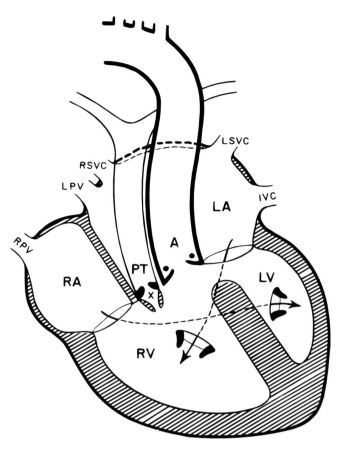

Figure 91: Diagrammatic sketch of criss-cross heart with inverted transposition is shown in Figures 88—90. RSVC = right superior vena cava; LSVC = left superior vena cava; IVC = inferior vena cava; RA = right atrium; RV = right ventricle; LA = left atrium; LV = left ventricle; RPV = right pulmonary vein; A = aorta; PT = pulmonary trunk; X = pulmonary stenosis. (Used with permission from Lev M, Rowlatt UF. See Figure 95.)

DORV, noninverted or regular type, with subpulmonary VSD, Ebstein's anomaly of the tricuspid valve and fetal coarctation of the aorta (Taussig-Bing complex) (Figs. 92—95).

Displaced tricuspid valve into the left ventricle and straddling mitral valve, with large CAVO-type VSD and pulmonary stenosis (Figs. 96—98).

DORV, noninverted type with large CAVO-type VSD, marked pulmonary stenosis with straddling right AV valve (mitral) with mild Ebstein's anomaly of the left AV valve (Figs. 99—102).

DORV, noninverted type with subpulmonary VSD (Taussig-Bing) with overriding pulmonary trunk, regular transposition type, with Ebstein's anomaly and straddling of the left AV valve, subaortic and valvular aortic stenosis, fetal coarctation PDA, and cor triatriatum sinister.

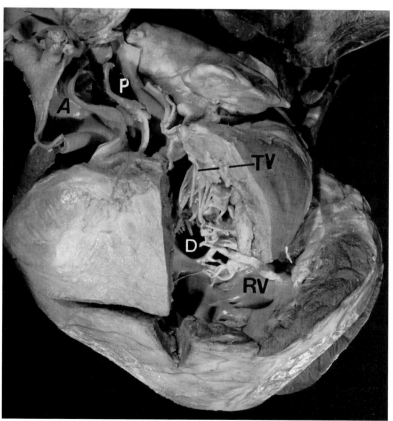

Figure 92: Corrected transposition with criss-cross AV valve connections and noninverted type of DORV, external view. A = aorta to the right; P = pulmonary to the left, both vessels side by side; TV = tricuspid valve; D = large ventricular septal defect; RV = morphologically right ventricle. (Used with permission from Lev M, Rowlatt UF. See Figure 95.)

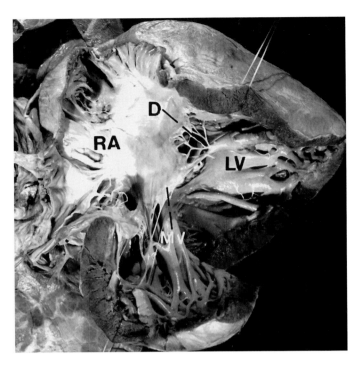

Figure 93: Right atrial, left ventricular view. RA = right atrium; MV = mitral valve; D = ventricular septal defect; LV = morphologically left ventricle. (Used with permission from Lev M, Rowlatt UF. See Figure 95.)

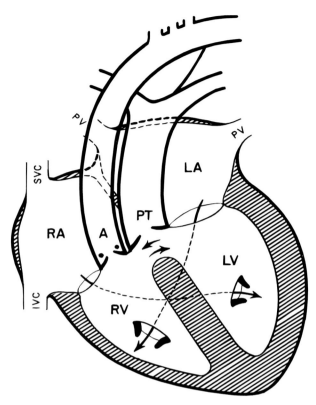

Figure 95: Diagrammatic sketch of criss-cross heart with regular transposition of heart shown in Figures 92—94. SVC = superior vena cava; IVC = inferior vena cava; RA = right atrium; RV = right ventricle; LA = left atrium; LV = left ventricle; PV = pulmonary vein; Ao = aorta; PT = pulmonary trunk. (Used with permission from Lev M, Rowlatt UF: The pathologic anatomy of mixed levocardia: A review of thirteen cases of atrial or ventricular inversion with or without corrected transposition. *Am J Cardiol* 1961, 8:216—263.)

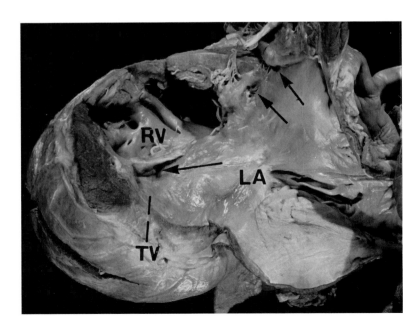

Figure 94: Left atrial, right ventricular view demonstrating Ebstein's anomaly of the tricuspid valve and anomalous attachment of the tricuspid valve. LA = left atrium; RV = right ventricle; TV = tricuspid valve. Two arrows point to the anomalous attachment of the anterior leaflet. Single arrow points to the displaced tricuspid valve into the morphologically right ventricle. (Used with permission from Lev M, Rowlatt UF. See Figure 95.)

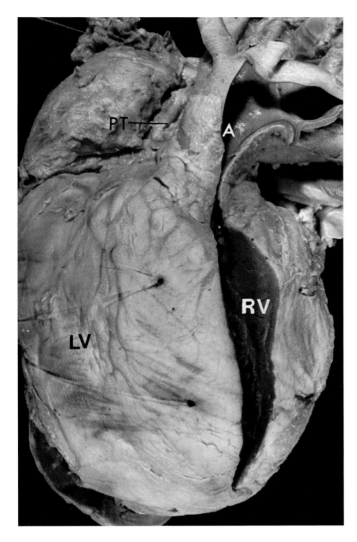

Figure 96: Mixed levocardia with ventricular inversion with anteroposterior relationship of the ventricular chambers, up-stairs/downstairs heart. External view. A = aorta; PT = pulmonary trunk; LV = morphologically left ventricle situated posterior and inferior; RV = morphologically right ventricle situated anterior and superior.

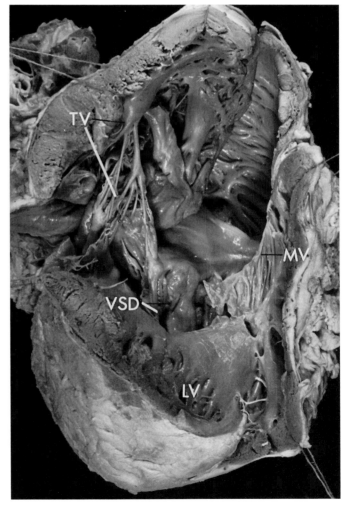

Figure 97: Displaced tricuspid valve into the posteriorly located left ventricle through a large common AV canal-type of defect. TV = displaced tricuspid valve; VSD = huge common AV canal-type of ventricular septal defect; LV = morphologically left ventricle; MV = straddling mitral valve.

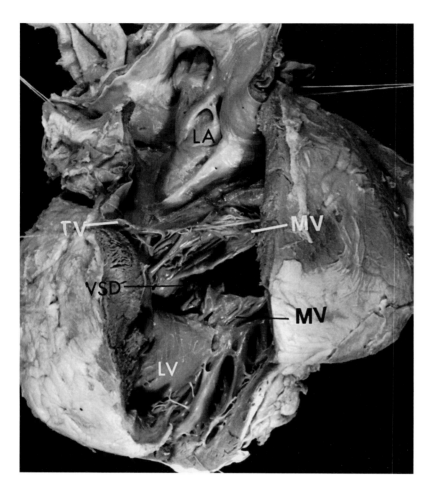

Figure 98: Left atrial, left ventricular view of the straddling mitral and displaced tricuspid valve. MV = straddling mitral valve; VSD = ventricular septal defect; LV = left ventricle; LA = left atrium; TV = displaced tricuspid valve.

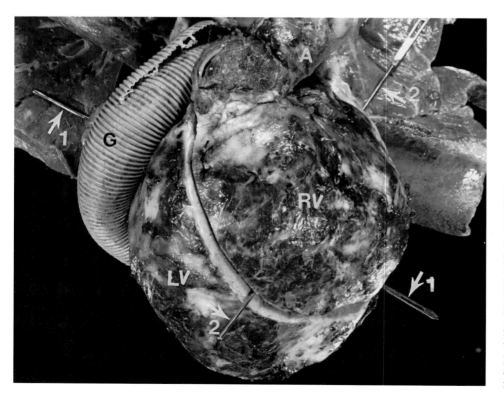

Figure 99: Mixed levocardia with criss-cross heart in relatively normally related chambers. External view of the heart with recent surgical correction. LV = morphologically left ventricle; RV = morphologically right ventricle; G = prosthetic conduit from the morphologically left ventricle to the pulmonary trunk; A = aorta. Arrow 1 indicates the probe proceeding from the right atrium into the left ventricle. Arrow 2 indicates the probe proceeding from the left atrium into the morphologically right ventricle.

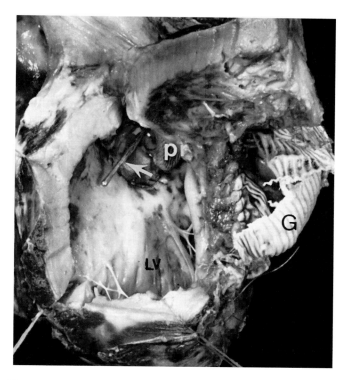

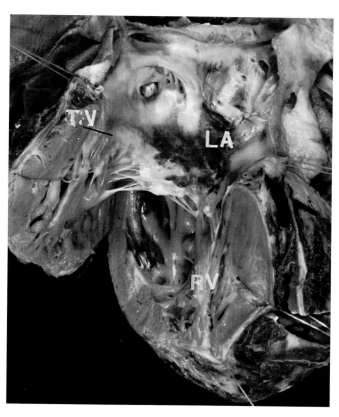

Figure 100: Left ventricular view demonstrating the patch closure of the ventricular septal defect and graft anastomosis proceeding to the pulmonary arteries. LV = left ventricle; Pr = prosthetic patch closure of the defect; G = graft extending from the morphologically left ventricle to the two pulmonary arteries. Arrow points to the probe emerging from the right atrium.

Figure 101: Left atrial, right ventricular view. LA = left atrium; TV = tricuspid valve; RV = right ventricle.

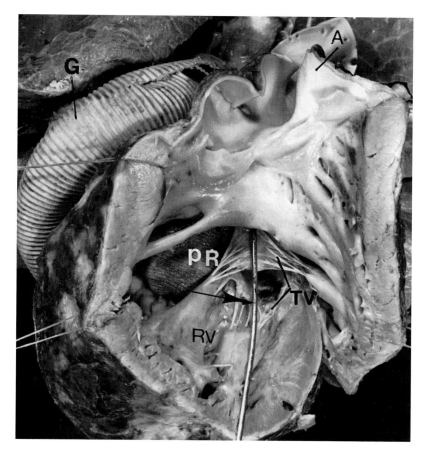

Figure 102: Outflow tract of the right ventricle depicting the aorta emerging from this chamber with patch closure of defect. The arrow points to the probe proceeding beneath the aorta to the original pulmonic trunk. This was a case of double outlet right ventricle with severe pulmonary stenosis and straddling right AV valve. A = aorta; TV = tricuspid valve; G = graft anastomosis from the morphologically left ventricle to the distal pulmonary arteries; pR = prosthetic patch closure of defect; RV = right ventricle.

DORV, noninverted type, Taussig-Bing with straddling right AV valve, Ebstein-like tricuspid valve, insufficiency of both AV valves with large atypical common AV canal type of VSD, atypical cleft-like malformation of the mitral valve.

DORV, noninverted type with subpulmonary VSD (Taussig-Bing), huge ASD, left superior vena cava entering coronary sinus, cleft-like malformation of the mitral valve with complete straddling mitral valve with tricuspid stenosis, single coronary ostium, paraductal coarctation of the aorta and PDA, and anomalous muscle bundles of the right ventricle, with arterial switch procedure (Figs. 103—107).

DORV, noninverted type, *without VSD*, with marked mitral stenosis, subaortic and subpulmonary stenosis and coarctation of the aorta, mild Ebstein-like malformation of the tricuspid valve, anomalous mus-

cle bands in the right ventricle, bicuspid aortic valve, single coronary ostium and elongated, tortuous probe PDA.

Frequently, the left AV valve (tricuspid) is an Ebstein-like malformation with or without straddling of the valve. In regard to the right AV valve, the mitral, there is a tendency for a cleft-like malformation to occur with or without straddling of the valve. Thus, both AV valves are frequently incompetent or stenotic. It is clear in criss-cross hearts that there is a greater tendency for both AV valves to be malformed. The defect, in general, was quite large and confluent with the pulmonary trunk with subaortic and/or aortic valvular stenosis and coarctation or interrupted arch. In a sense, a Taussig-Bing type of malformation was seen in 50% of the cases. Eight of the hearts were with atria

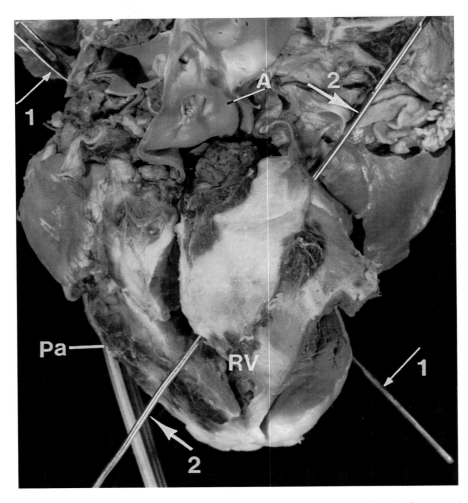

Figure 103: External view of criss-cross heart with recent arterial switch operation. Arrows marked 1 indicate the probe proceeding from the right atrium to the posteriorly located left ventricle. Arrows marked 2 indicate the probe proceeding from the morphologically left atrium into the morphologically right ventricle situated superior and anterior. A = aorta; Pa = pacemaker wire; RV = right ventricle.

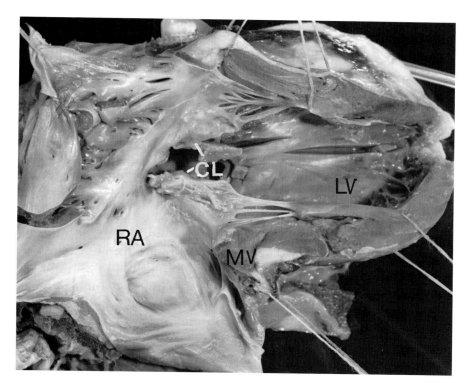

Figure 104: Right atrial, left ventricular view demonstrating the straddling mitral valve. RA = right atrium; LV = left ventricle; MV = mitral valve; CL = cleft-like formation in the mitral valve proceeding through the defect and originally attached to the opposite chamber.

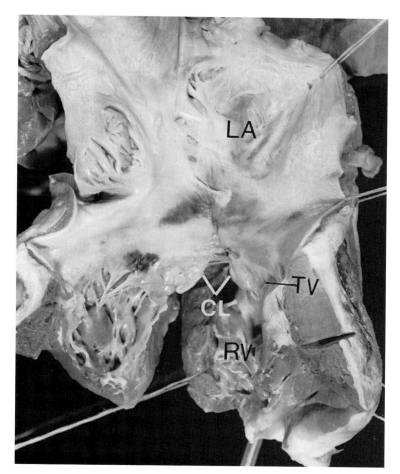

Figure 105: Left atrial, right ventricular view demonstrating the anomalous attachment of the tricuspid and incomplete cleft-like formation of the left AV valve with insufficiency. LA = left atrium; TV = redundant tricuspid valve attached to the rim of the defect; RV = right ventricle; CL = incomplete cleft-like malformation of the tricuspid valve.

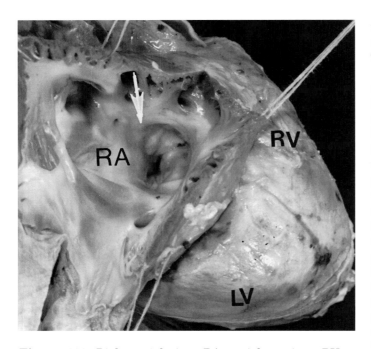

Figure 109: Right atrial view. RA = right atrium; RV = right ventricle; LV = left ventricle. Arrow points to the tricuspid valve proceeding into the morphologically right ventricle which is situated to the left and anterior.

right and posterior. Thus, there was AV concordance in a criss-cross position. Here again, the heart was of a Taussig-Bing type.

The second heart was quite bizarre in that there were three AV valves. The atria were rotated posteroinferiorly, and the right atrium communicated with the morphologically right ventricle situated to the left and anterior by means of a larger right AV valve (tricuspid). In addition, there was a smaller right AV valve (presumed mitral or a displaced accessory tricuspid) which communicated with the morphologically left ventricle situated to the right and posterior. The left atrium communicated by means of a mitral valve with the morphologically left ventricle situated to the right and posterior. Here the aorta emerged from the morphologically right ventricle, and the pulmonary trunk from the posteriorly located left ventricle. Thus, we are dealing with complete transposition and pulmonary stenosis with ventricular septal defect in AV concordant heart with criss-cross AV valve connection due to ventricular inversion. Despite ventricular inversion, the AV valve connections are concordant except for the fact that there is an additional AV valve from the right atrium connecting with the left ventricle and this is

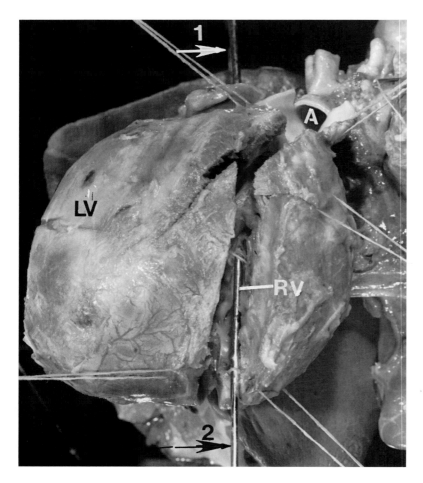

Figure 110: Probe from the right atrium emerging into the right ventricle (right to left criss-crossing), and from the right ventricle emerges the aorta. A = aorta; RV = right ventricle; LV = left ventricle. Arrows 1 and 2 point to the probe emerging from the right atrium into the right ventricle.

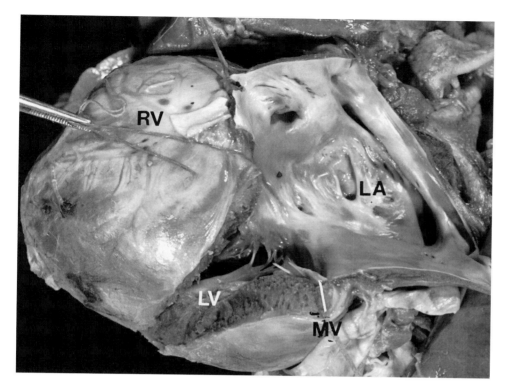

Figure 111: Heart turned backwards; left atrial view showing the mitral valve entering the morphologically left ventricle. LA = left atrium; MV = mitral valve; RV = right ventricle, left and anterior; LV = left ventricle situated right and posterior.

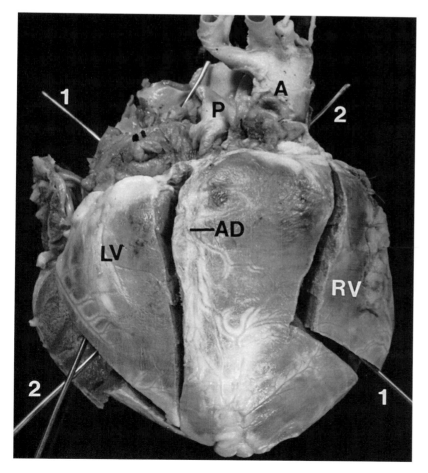

Figure 112: Criss-cross AV connection with concordant chambers, ventricles inverted. External view. A = aorta; P = pulmonary trunk; AD = anterior descending coronary artery; RV = right ventricle; LV = left ventricle. Probe labeled 1 proceeds from the right atrium into the morphologically right ventricle which is situated to the left and anterior. Probe labeled 2 indicates the left atrium situated left and posterior communicating with the morphologically left ventricle situated to the right and posterior.

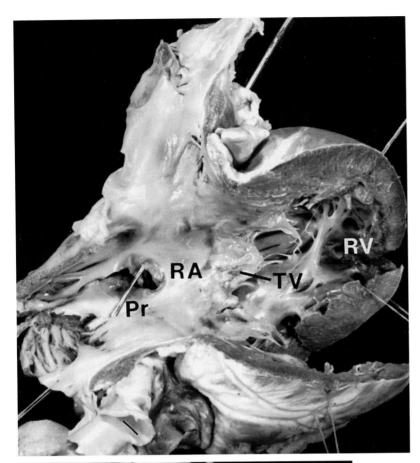

Figure 113: Right atrium communicating with the morphologically right ventricle by means of a tricuspid valve. RA = right atrium; RV = right ventricle; TV = tricuspid valve - note the tricuspid is irregularly thickened; Pr = probe passing through the atrial septal defect.

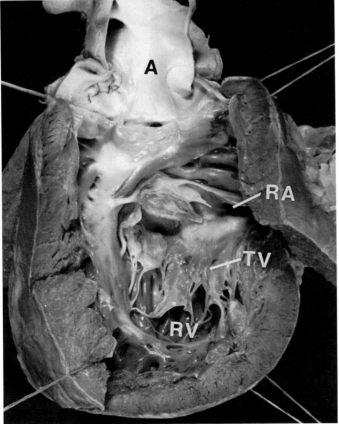

Figure 114: Outflow tract of the right ventricle from which emerges the aorta. RA = right atrium; TV = tricuspid valve; RV = right ventricle; A = aorta. Note the abnormal formation of the tricuspid valve and the right ventricle.

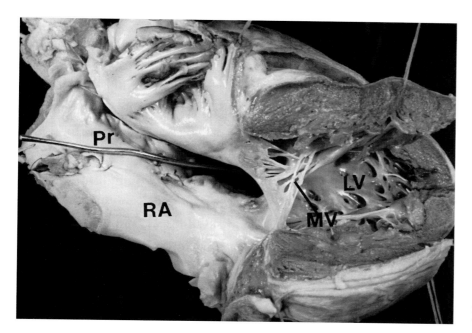

Figure 115: Right atrial, left ventricular view demonstrating the two AV valves. One valve connecting with the right ventricle and the other with the left ventricle. RA = right atrium; LV = left ventricle; MV = presumed small accessory mitral or displaced accessory tricuspid valve communicating from the right atrium with the morphologically left ventricle; Pr = probe passes through the previously demonstrated large tricuspid valve which connects with the morphologically right ventricle.

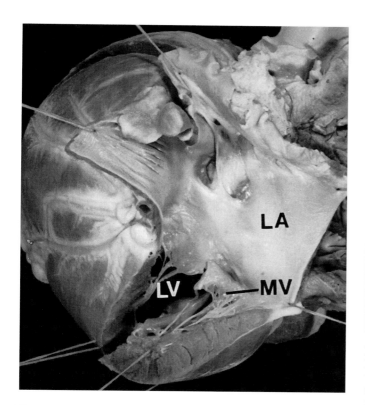

Figure 116: Left atrium communicating by means of a mitral valve with the morphologically left ventricle. LA = left atrium; MV = small mitral valve; LV = left ventricle.

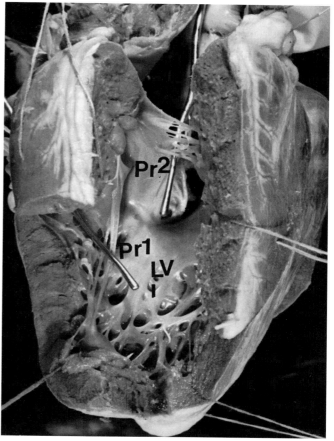

Figure 117: The two AV valves entering the morphologically left ventricle is shown by means of the probes. LV = left ventricle; Pr1 = indicates the probe passing through the presumed mitral valve or the displaced accessory tricuspid valve from the right atrium connecting with the morphologically left ventricle; Pr2 = probe 2 proceeding from the left atrium communicating with the morphologically left ventricle by means of a mitral valve.

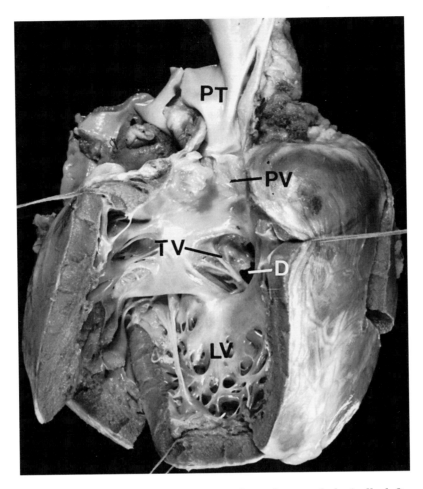

Figure 118: The pulmonary trunk emerging from the morphologically left ventricle and basilar straddling tricuspid valve. LV = left ventricle; PT = pulmonary trunk; PV = bicuspid, thickened pulmonic valve; TV = basilar straddling tricuspid valve; D = ventricular septal defect.

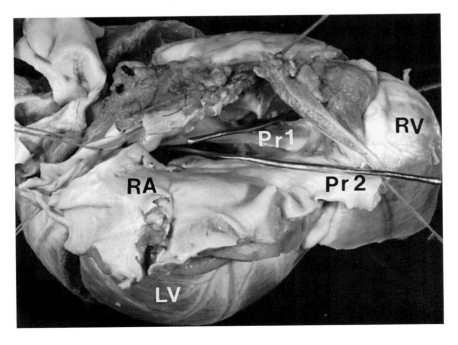

Figure 119: Superior view of the right atrium with probe 1 proceeding to the right ventricle by means of a morphologically tricuspid valve, and probe 2 proceeding from the same chamber with an accessory AV valve into the morphologically left ventricle. The valve is presumed to be a mitral valve or a displaced accessory tricuspid valve. RA = right atrium; LV = left ventricle; Pr1 = probe 1; Pr2 = probe 2; RV = right ventricle.

presumed to be a mitral valve or may be considered a displaced accessory tricuspid valve. Therefore, one may say that the AV concordance is *incomplete* because of the presence of AV discordance present in a partial form. It is not surprising that this was associated with a bizarre form of Wolff-Parkinson-White syndrome.

Comment

It is clear that mixed levocardia with ventricular inversion has proven the fact that the morphologically right ventricle cannot function as a systemic chamber. Likewise, the morphologically tricuspid valve cannot support the systemic chamber functionally for a long period of time. This is due fundamentally to the altered geometry of the right ventricle and tricuspid valve as a result of inversion of the ventricular chambers. The abnormal formation of the ventricular septum and the ventricular septal defect are a part of this complex. Rarely, the entity occurs with intact ventricular septum. The left AV valve (tricuspid) is always abnormally formed regardless of the presence or absence of a ventricular septal defect.

The morphology of the ventricular septal defect unassociated with double outlet right ventricle and other major cardiac anomalies, as well as the other associated cardiac anomalies, is given in Table 1 and 2.

Mixed levocardia with atrial inversion. This is rare and always associated with ventricular septal defect and pulmonary stenosis or atresia.

Criss-cross AV valve connections. In criss-cross AV connections with atria and ventricles in a relatively normal position or ventricles inverted, the AV valves

Table 1

The VSD in Uncomplicated Mixed Levocardia with Ventricular Inversion

	No. of Cases
Large VSD	18
Large VSD with pulmonary valvular and infundibular stenosis	5
Closing VSD with aneurysm of the membranous septum and pulmonary hypertension	2
VSD with aneurysm of the membranous septum and straddling tricuspid valve and pulmonary stenosis	1
VSD with overriding aorta	1
Double VSD	1
Double VSD with overriding aorta and pulmonary stenosis (1 defect CAVO-type) and straddling infundibulum and straddling tricuspid valve (Figs. 120—122)	1
Large VSD with overriding pulmonary trunk and pulmonary hypertension	1

Table 2

Other Associated Cardiac Anomalies

	No. of Cases
Fossa ovalis atrial septal defect	6
Patent foramen ovale	8
Common atrium	1
Aneurysm of the fossa ovalis	2
Left superior vena cava entering the coronary sinus	1
Stenosis of the coronary veins	1
PDA	4
Divided right ventricle	1
Muscular diverticulum of right ventricle	1
Anomalous muscles of the left ventricle	3
Diverticulum of left ventricle	1
Abnormal architecture of the right and left ventricles	1
Double (accessory) tricuspid orifice with insufficiency	1
Fetal coarctation with VSD and PDA	1
Single coronary artery with high origin	1
Double anterior descending coronary artery	1
Both coronary ostia from the left posterior sinus and other small coronary from right posterior sinus	1

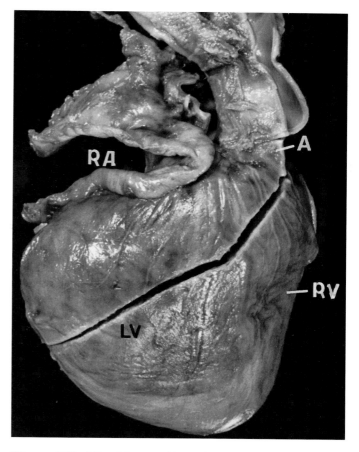

Figure 120: Mixed levocardia with overriding aorta, external view. RA = right atrium; LV = left ventricle; RV = right ventricle; A = aorta.

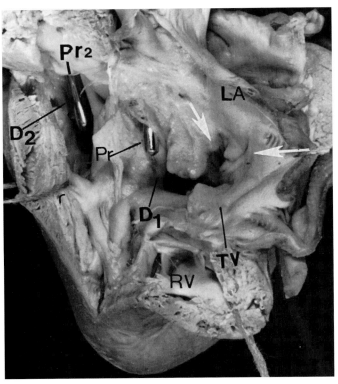

are almost always abnormally formed with a greater tendency for double outlet right ventricle to occur.

Possible Embryogenesis and Conclusion

There probably is a specific DNA marker system responsible for the normally developing cardiac tube to bend to the right and anterior during the second stage of development of the heart. This probably occurs very early during the embryogenesis (4—6 weeks of preg-

Figure 121: Left atrial, right ventricular view showing straddling tricuspid valve and double defects (one common AV canal type of atrial septal defect). LA = left atrium; TV = straddling tricuspid valve; RV = right ventricle; D_1 = common AV canal type of defect; D_2 = anteriorly located defect, the probe proceeding into the aorta; Pr = depicting the probe proceeding into the pulmonary trunk; Pr2 = points to the straddling conus. Note the markedly redundant tricuspid valve. Arrows point to the straddling of the tricuspid valve through the defect to the opposite chamber.

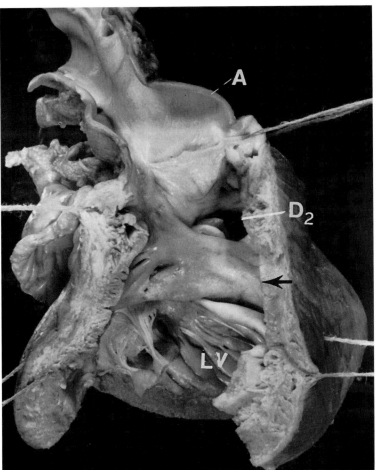

Figure 122: Outflow tract of the morphologically right ventricle showing the straddling aorta over a second U-shaped anterior defect and the straddling conus. LV = left ventricle; D_2 = anteriorly located U-shaped defect confluent with the overriding aorta; A = aorta. Arrow points to the straddling conus.

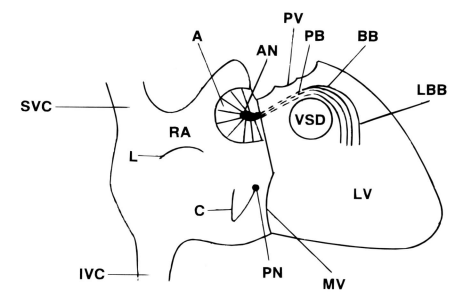

Figure 123: Schematic representation of the peripheral conduction system in a case of corrected transposition (mixed levocardia) with ventricular septal defect showing the relationship of the atrioventricular (AV) bundle to the defect. This may help the reader in understanding the anterior location of the AV bundle and its vulnerability during surgical closure of the defect, and/or while relieving the subpulmonary obstruction by surgical or other nonsurgical interventional procedures. RA = right atrium; L = limbus fossae ovalis; SVC = superior vena cava; IVC = inferior vena cava; MV = mitral valve; C = coronary sinus; PN = posterior (regular, usual AV node); A = approaches to the anterior AV node; AN = anterior AV node situated in the roof of the right atrium close to the atrial septum adjacent to the pulmonary valve; VSD = ventricular septal defect; PB = penetrating AV bundle; BB = branching bundle winds around the superolateral wall of the VSD and gives off the anterior fibers of the LBB; LBB = left bundle branch; LV = morphologically left ventricle. - - - - line represents the course of the penetrating AV bundle which emerges from the mitral pulmonic anulus and proceeds along the superior parietal (anterior wall) of the morphologic left ventricle (subendocardially-superficially) close to the base of the pulmonary valve. The superolateral rim of the defect, therefore, is vulnerable while closing the defect. In some, the posterior AV node may give rise to the posterior (usual or normal) AV bundle and both bundles may join around the superolateral and inferior margin of the VSD forming a sling. (Used with permission from Bharati S, Lev M, Kirklin JW: *Cardiac Surgery and the Conduction System.* Futura Publishing Co., Mt. Kisco, NY, 1—176, 1992.)

nancy). For whatever reason, when the cardiac tube bends to the left rather than to the right, there is a distinct associated abnormality in the movement of the atrial canal as well as in the absorption of the bulbus and the formation of the ventricular septa. It is therefore not surprising to find the ubiquitous AV valve abnormality and association of double outlet right ventricle and/or overriding of one vessel.

The Conduction System

In general, there is an anterior conduction system with AV discordance. The anterior AV node forms the anterior AV bundle at the mitral pulmonic anulus and proceeds anterosuperiorly and winds around the superolateral margin of the ventricular septal defect to become the branching bundle. Thus, the penetrating and branching bundle take a long course, making the entire superolateral margin of the defect vulnerable during surgical closure of the defect (Fig. 123).

Likewise, there is a tendency for disruption of the elongated bundle either congenitally or by acquired pathological change. Subpulmonary obstruction, either by means of endocardial ridges or tissue, or anomalous tricuspid valve in longstanding cases, may produce changes in the AV bundle producing AV block which, if not manifest at the time of birth, may manifest at the second or third decade.

The higher incidence of preexcitation in this entity is related to the higher incidence of Ebstein's malformation of the tricuspid valve. Likewise, the altered geometry of the ventricular chambers might be responsible for ventricular arrhythmias and sudden death, especially in the older age group.

58

Positional Variations of the Heart and Their Significance

Congenitally malformed hearts are usually diagnosed by referring to the situs of the atria, the type of bulboventricular loop, and the type of mutual relationships of the great arteries. In general, the direction of the base-apex axis of the heart is never mentioned. We believe that without the knowledge of the longitudinal axis or the base-axis of the heart, the description of the congenital heart malformation is deficient or incomplete. The method of describing a congenital cardiac anomaly without including the direction of the base-apex or the longitudinal axis of the heart is insufficient to indicate completely the position of the heart and its component chambers.

It is important that we indicate the position of the atria, the ventricles, and the great arteries both from the standpoint of lateral as well as anteroposterior, and, if possible, craniocaudal relationships, vis-à-vis the body of the patient. This approach will be useful in echocardiography, angiocardiography, as well as in cardiac surgery.

We believe the direction of the base-apex of the heart should first be determined. Does it point to the left or right, or does the heart point ventrally (Fig. 1)? If this direction of the base-apex axis is due to the inherent structure of the heart, levocardia, dextrocardia, or mesocardia can be diagnosed. On the other hand, if this direction results from extraneous phenomena such as diaphragmatic hernia, atelectasis, emphysema, or agenesis of the lungs, levoposition, dextroposition, or mesoposition may be diagnosed. Only then should the analysis proceed to the exact position of the atria, the venous connections, the atrioventricular connections, the position of the ventricles, the great arterial connections, and the mutual positions of the arterial trunks to themselves.

A description of the situs of the atria, in our opinion, is not sufficient; this indicates only laterality. It does not indicate anteroposterior or craniocaudal relationships. Thus, in dextroversion (Fig. 1), the atria are either side by side, with the morphologically right atrium to the right and the morphologically left atrium to the left, or the morphologically right atrium is to the right and posterior, and the morphologically left atrium is to the left and anterior. The term situs solitus for this kind of a relationship is confusing, because when the atria are in situs solitus in levocardia, the morphologically right atrium is to the right and anterior and the morphologically left atrium is to the left and posterior.

We would suggest using the term *situs solitus*, pivoted for the atrial relationship in dextroversion, although other terms may be applicable. Similarly, in one type of isolated levocardia, the morphologically right atrium is to the left and posterior and the morphologically left atrium is to the right and anterior. The term *situs inversus* for this relationship may not be sufficient or perhaps confusing. For in situs inversus atria in dextrocardia, the right atrium is to the left and anterior and the left atrium is to the right and posterior. Hence, we use the term *inversion of atria* or situs inversus, pivoted, for the relationship (Fig. 1) in the above type of isolated levocardia. Some other term that expresses both the lateral and anteroposterior relationship would also be valid.

In mesocardia, it is not sufficient to indicate only the situs of atria (Fig. 1). Here, the atria lying side by side are posterior to the ventricles whether they are in situs solitus or inversus, with the atrial septum in an anteroposterior plane. Likewise, the ventricles are anterior, more or less side by side, whether there is a dex-

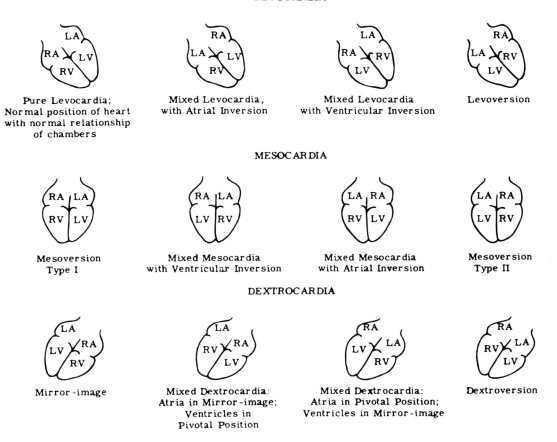

Figure 1: The position of the chambers in the various directions of the base-apex axis of the heart. RA = right atrium; RV = right ventricle; LA = left atrium; LV = left ventricle. (Used with permission from Lev M, Bharati S: Abnormal position of the heart and its chambers. In *The Heart*, edited by Edwards JE, Lev M, Abell MR, Baltimore, Williams & Wilkins, 1974, ch 16.)

tro- (D-loop) or a levo-loop (L-loop). The position of the atrial and ventricular septa are obviously important in surgical repair of defects, especially in mesocardia and dextrocardia.

The craniocaudal relationship of the atria is also important. Thus, in straddling tricuspid valve, and in criss-cross hearts, the right atrium is situated more caudally (posteriorly) to the left atrium than normal.

In describing the atrioventricular connections, concordance and discordance are good terms that indicate the correct position of the ventricles by inference. However, the terms dextro- and levo-loop *are not*, in our opinion, sufficient to indicate the position of the ventricles. In a dextro loop in levocardia (Fig. 1), the right ventricle is anterior and to the right, and the left ventricle is situated posteriorly and to the left. In D-loop dextrocardia of the dextroversion type, the right ventricle is posterior and to the right, and the left ventricle is anterior and to the left. In L-loop levocardia, the right ventricle is posterior and to the left, or situated more directly to the left, while the left ventricle is

situated anterior and to the right, or more directly to the right. In L-loop dextrocardia of the mixed (discordant) or mirror-image type, the right ventricle is situated anterior and to the left, and the left ventricle is posterior and to the right.

Regarding the ventricles, the craniocaudal relationship of the chambers may be important, especially when dealing with criss-cross hearts, and in those hearts in which the ventricular septum is in a horizontal plane or in those hearts where we have a superior-inferior relationship of the ventricles.

When dealing with ventriculoarterial connections, the terms *ventriculoarterial concordance* or *discordance* may be useful. However, in describing the mutual positions of the arterial trunks, the base-apex of the heart is also equally important. Thus, in pure (concordant) levocardia with normally related great arteries, the aortic orifice is situated posterior and to the right of the pulmonary orifice. The pulmonary trunk swings directly posteriorly to reach its bifurcations. In dextrocardia of the dextroversion type without transposition or double outlet right ventricle, the aortic orifice is likewise situated posteriorly, but lies slightly to the left or slightly to the right of the pulmonary trunk. The pulmonary trunk veers to the left, almost horizontally, and then dips posteriorly to the left of the ascending aorta to reach its bifurcation.

We believe the diagnosis of situs of atria, with dextro- or levo-loop without considering the base-apex or the longitudinal axis of the heart, does not give enough information about the position of the atria, the ventricles, and the great arteries from the standpoint of not only lateral but also anteroposterior and craniocaudal directions.

The exact location of the cardiac chambers, the great arteries, the AV valves, the entry of systemic and pulmonic veins into the heart, and their relationship to each other are of great importance in the diagnosis as well as in the clinical, interventional, and surgical management.

59

Dextroposition

The term "dextroposition" implies that the cardiac base-apex or the longitudinal axis may be pointing to the right similar to true dextrocardia, or the apex may still point toward the left but the heart may be shifted or moved to the right side due to extracardiac pathological conditions involving the lungs, pleura, diaphragm, or other neighboring structures or organs.

Analysis of Our Material

There were 11 cases: five males and six females. The youngest was a 24-weeks' gestation fetus and the oldest was a 5-month-old infant. All had severe heart disease. The complexes were

PAPVD. RPV → RA, FOD, and VSD. FC Bi AV. Wide PDA. Rt pulmonary artery smaller than Lt systemic vessel from abdomen → Rt lung	6 days M
ASD, FO type, sinus venosus type and CS type, large. DORV, subaortic VSD, TAPVD → IVC. LSVC → LA. FC. LPA from RPA. Abnormal formation of trachea, bronchi and hypoplastic Rt lung	17 days M
PAPVD—RPV → IVC. ASD, FO type. Rt small PA	5 months, 4 days M
Tricuspid atresia with PA without transposition. FOD. Minute RV and RCA. PDA. Omphalocele	7 minutes F (35-week gest.)
ASD and PDA, Bi AV. Minute RPA. LSVC → CS. Sequestrated Rt lung	10 weeks, 5 days F
FC, ASD and PDA. Minute LPA and small Rt P artery. Hypoplastic Lt pulmonary vein and small rt pulmonary vein	Stillborn M
ASD and PDA. High origin of both coronary ostia. Scoliosis, marked. Diaphragmatic hernia. Collapse of lungs—Rt	24-week gest. F
FC, ASD, FOD, LSVC → CS and Bi AV. All abdominal organs outside. Chest intact. Anencephaly	Stillborn F
TS, PS, VSD, displaced tricuspid orifice. Conus in LV, small CS. Infundibular PS. Bi PV. Divided LA. Diaphragmatic hernia	13 weeks M
Absent Rt lung with dextroposition of the heart, absence of right pulmonary artery and vein, and incomplete supravalvular mitral ridge	4 months F
Partially sequestrated Rt lung with partial resection, PAPVD, RPV → RA. ASD, FO type. Aberrant pulmonaries from subclavian artery and from subdiaphragmatic to Rt lung, and small Rt pulmonary artery. Dextroposition of the heart, and monolobate, hypoplastic Rt lung	5 months F

Comment

In eight, the major anomaly was in the lungs. The right pulmonary artery was smaller than normal in three, was minute in one, the left was minute in one and it originated from the right in one, and there was one with pulmonary atresia. In one, the right lung and

913

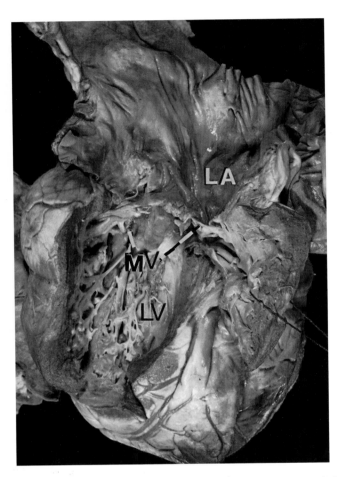

Figure 8: Rheumatic mitral stenosis in dextroversion, left anterior view. LA = left atrium; LV = left ventricle; MV = mitral valve. Note the small mitral anulus with irregularly thickened valve, chordae, and the papillary muscles.

Atypical truncus with tricuspid atresia. PDA from innominate → both pulmonaries. Juxtaposed right atrial appendage to the left. Single coronary artery — newborn M

CT with closing VSD and subpulmonary stenosis. Aneurysm of membranous septum. Juxtaposed right atrial appendage to the left. High origin of Lt coronary artery (Fig. 24) — 4 years M

Tricuspid atresia with aortic atresia without transposition and overriding pulmonary trunk. ASD combined FO and proximal, large. Aberrant Rt subclavian artery — newborn F

Common atrium. CAVO. Single ventricle, CT. TAPVD → IVC. Absent CS — 5 hours M

Tricuspid atresia with transposition. Large VSD, CAVO type. Straddling MV, MI. Subpulmonary and valvular PS. Congenital AV block. ASD, FO type. Tortuous, elongated PDA — 5 days M

Asplenia, partial visceral heterotaxy. CT with CAVO. PA. Small RSVC. Large FOD and proximal defect. Rt-sided coronary ostium small. RAA and Rt descending aorta. CS and IVC → LA. Large LSVC → LA. Unilobate, incomplete lobation both lungs. Both atrial appendages—Lt atrial morphology — 6 months M (36-wk gest.)

Ectopia cordis with DORV noncommitted. VSD and infundibular PS. Large FO and proximal ASD. TS. Bi PV. Absent PDA. Aneurysm of Lt atrial appendage — premature F

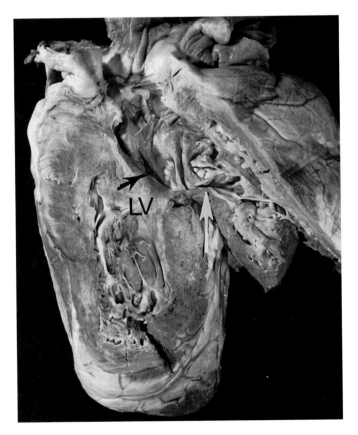

Figure 9: Dextroversion. Abnormal architecture of the left ventricle. Note the anomalous architecture of the left ventricle beneath the mitral valve and the summit of the ventricular septum. LV = left ventricle. Arrows point to the irregularly thickened mitral valve and its attachments on the septum.

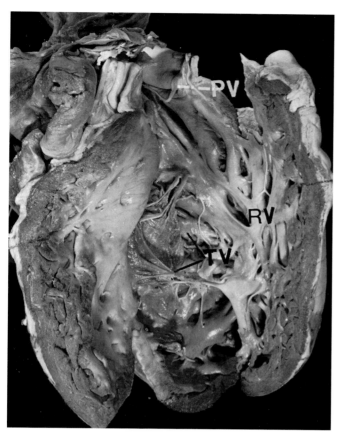

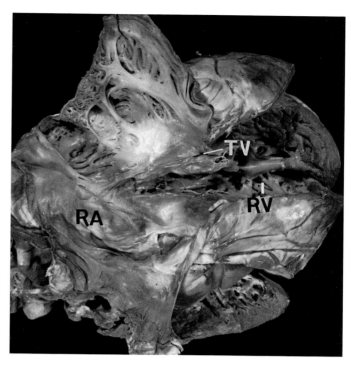

Figure 11: Right posterior view. RA = right atrium; TV = tricuspid valve; RV = right ventricle.

Figure 10: Right posterior view of morphologically right ventricle and the pulmonary trunk emerging from the right ventricle. RV = right ventricle; TV = tricuspid valve; PV = pulmonary valve.

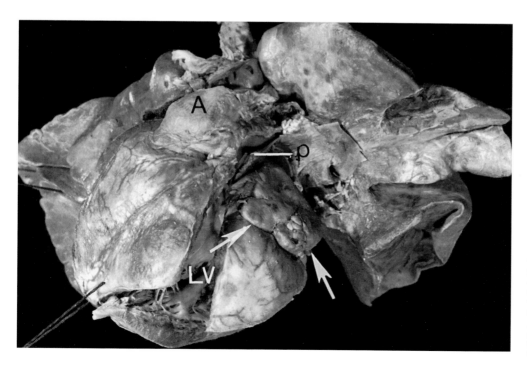

Figure 12: Dextroversion with complete transposition, ventricular septal defect, and pulmonary stenosis with juxtaposed atrial appendages. External view. LV = left ventricle; P = pulmonary trunk; A = aorta. Arrows point to juxtaposed atrial appendages to the left of the pulmonary trunk.

III. Mixed Dextrocardia, Atria–Pivotal Position, Ventricles–Mirror-Image

In this anomaly, the atria are in a pivotal position while the ventricles are in mirror-image or vice versa (Fig. 1). Two cases in our series belonged to the second group.

The one frequently seen in this series was that with the atria pivoted around and the ventricles in mirror-image. Thus, the morphologically left atrium, situated to the left and slightly anteriorly to the morphological right atrium, communicated by way of a tricuspid orifice with the morphological right ventricle present anteriorly and to the left. The morphological right atrium, situated to the right and slightly posteriorly, communicated by way of a mitral valve with the morphological left ventricle situated posteriorly and to the right.

In keeping with the position of the ventricles, there was always inverted transposition with the exception of three cases where there was situs inversus abdominalis partialis and situs inversus thoracis in two. The spleen was normal in all but four exceptional cases where there was asplenia in two (with multilobated lungs in one), polysplenia in one, and accessory spleen in one. The abdominal venous return had variations. The right superior vena cava opened normally into the right atrium in all but two cases, in which it was absent. In two, however, there was an additional left superior vena cava which opened directly into the left atrium. The pulmonary venous return was normal in all cases except in three where there was total anomalous pulmonary venous drainage. There was a tendency for the complexes to be associated with inverted transposition, with ventricular septal defect and pulmonary stenosis or atresia, or a straddling aorta and conus with pulmonary atresia.

There was a total of 31 cases. There were seven female subjects, 23 male subjects, and one unknown. The youngest were a 2-day-old, 37-weeks' gestation male infant and a 7-week-old, 35-weeks' gestation male infant, and the oldest was a 59-year-old male, with a median age of 3 years, 10 months, and 14 days. The complexes were:

Inverted transposition, VSD, and pulmonary stenosis	1 month M
Inverted transposition with VSD and PA. ASD, FOD. Absent CS. LSVC → LA (Figs. 29—32)	2½ months M
Inverted transposition. Mitral and PA. Absent IVC. ASD, FOD. LAA and Lt PDA. Azygos → RSVC → RA. Hepatic vein → RA (Figs. 33, 34)	18 hours M

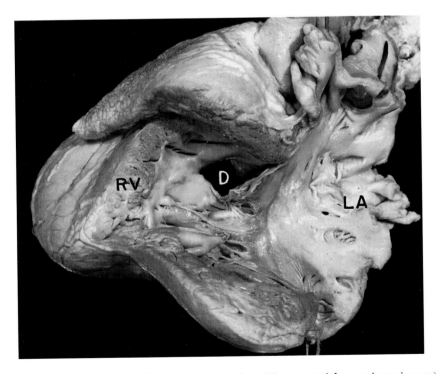

Figure 29: Mixed dextrocardia (atria—pivoted position, ventricles—mirror-image) with inverted transposition, ventricular septal defect, and pulmonary atresia. Left anterior view showing left atrium and right ventricle. LA = left atrium; RV = right ventricle; D = defect. (Used with permission from Lev M, et al. See Figure 89.)

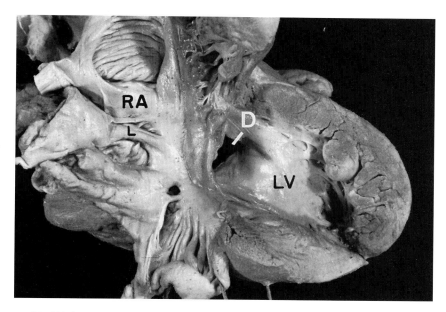

Figure 30: Right posterior view showing right atrium and left ventricle. RA = right atrium; LV = left ventricle; D = defect. (Used with permission from Lev M, et al. See Figure 89.)

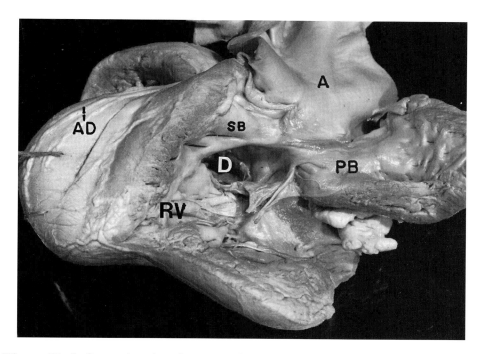

Figure 31: Left anterior view showing right ventricle. RV = right ventricle; AD = anterior descending coronary artery; SB = septal band; PB = parietal band; A = aorta; D = defect. (Used with permission from Lev M, et al. See Figure 89.)

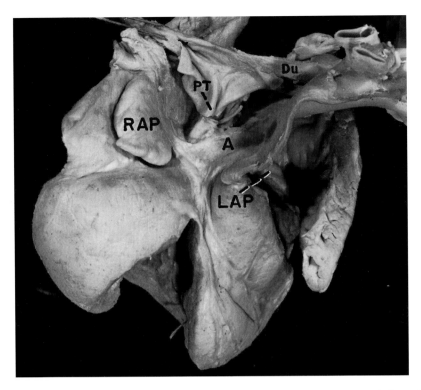

Figure 32: Right superior view. RAP = right atrial appendage; LAP = left atrial appendage; A = aorta; PT = pulmonary trunk with atresia of the pulmonic valve; Du = ductus arteriosus. (Used with permission from Lev M, et al. See Figure 95.)

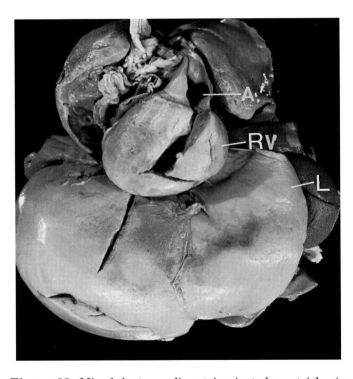

Figure 33: Mixed dextrocardia, atria pivoted, ventricles in mirror-image, with mitral and pulmonic atresia. External view. A = aorta; RV = right ventricle; L = liver.

Inverted transposition. SV and small outlet chamber, PS, LAA—Lt PDA. Unicuspid PV. ASD, FOD (Figs. 35—37)   4 years M

Inverted transposition with VSD and PA. ASD, FOD. LAA—Lt PDA (Figs. 38, 39)   7 days M

Partial visceral heterotaxy, asplenia. Thoracis inversus. Inverted transposition. CAVO. PA. ASD, FOD. Absent CS. LSVC → LA. RAA—Lt PDA (Figs. 40—42)   1 year F

Inverted overriding aorta. Straddling conus and PA (pseudotruncus). PDA. Large bronchial. Single coronary artery (Figs. 43, 44)   6 months M

Atypical inverted overriding aorta. Straddling conus with PA. ASD, FOD.   8 days M

Inverted transposition with PS and VSD.   4 days M

TAPVD → RSVC → RA. Inverted transposition and PA and MS, RAA and Lt descending aorta. LSVC and hepatic vein → LA, Liver left, trilobed both lungs   12 weeks M

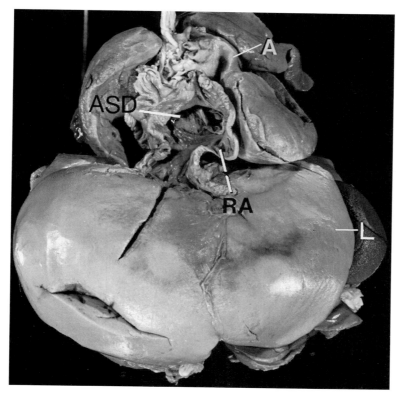

Figure 34: Mixed dextrocardia, atria pivoted, ventricles in mirror-image, inverted transposition and pulmonary atresia, right atrial view, showing huge atrial septal defect. ASD = huge atrial septal defect; RA = right atrium; L = liver; A = aorta.

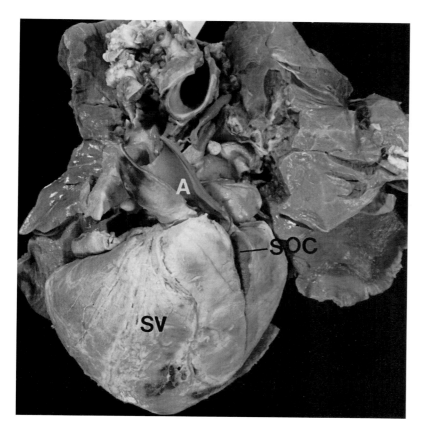

Figure 35: Mixed dextrocardia with single ventricle, small outlet chamber. External view. SV = single ventricle; SOC = small outlet chamber; A = aorta.

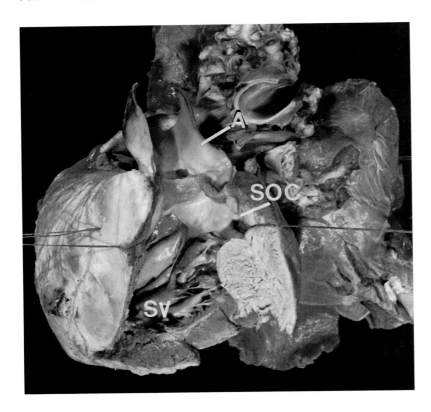

Figure 36: Single ventricle with small outlet chamber and pulmonary stenosis. Aorta emerging from the small outlet chamber. SV = single ventricle; SOC = small outlet chamber; A = aorta.

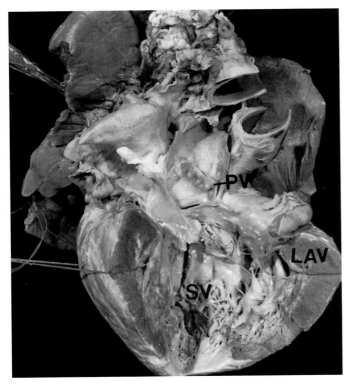

Figure 37: Pulmonary trunk emerging from the main ventricular chamber. SV = single ventricle; LAV = left AV valve; PV = pulmonary valve, bicuspid stenotic.

Criss-cross heart. Inverted DORV. TS and PS. Large VSD. Large ASD, FOD	10 years M
Inverted tetralogy with PA. RAA. ASD, FOD	5 days F
Ebstein's Lt AV with ASD and VSD and PS. Absence of proximal portion of atrial septum	13 years, sex unknown
Inverted transposition with PA and VSD (pseudotruncus). LAA	9 days M
Inverted transposition with PA and VSD	23 days M
Inverted transposition. VSD. TS and PS. Overriding PT, Taussig-Bing, LV type (Figs. 45—49)	6 months M
Inverted transposition. VSD and PA and TS. ASD, FOD. LAA	2 days M
Inverted transposition. VSD and TI	9 months, 9 days M
SV. Inverted transposition. PA and Lt AV valve atresia. RAA—double ductus. 1 RPDA → Rt lung, Lt PDA from subclavian artery → Lt lung. Premature narrowing of foramen ovale	24 hours M (37-wk gest.)
Inverted transposition. CAVO and PA. ASD, FOD. Atrophy of LV	5 days F

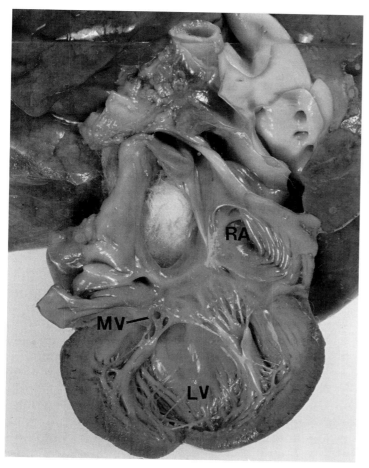

Figure 38: Mixed dextrocardia with inverted transposition, pulmonary atresia, and ventricular septal defect. Right atrial, left ventricular view. RA = right atrium; LV = left ventricle; MV = mitral valve. Note cotton plugging the large atypical ASD.

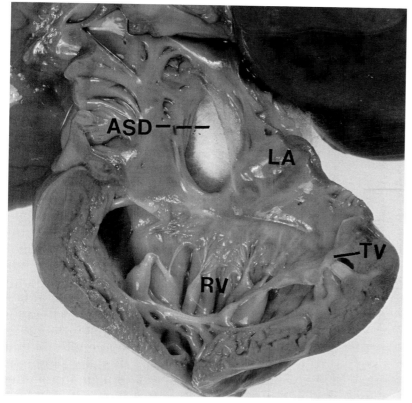

Figure 39: Left atrial, right ventricular view. LA = left atrium; RV = right ventricle; TV = tricuspid valve; ASD = atrial septal defect plugged with cotton.

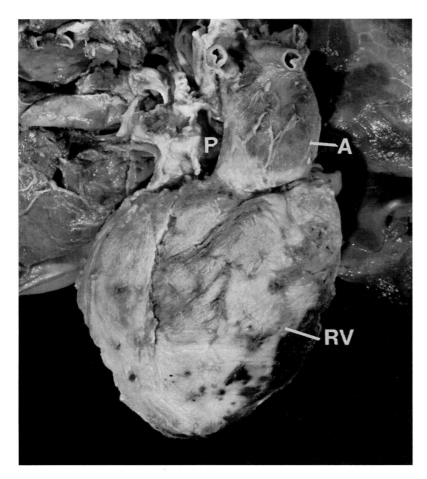

Figure 40: Mixed dextrocardia, complete inverted transposition, common AV orifice, and pulmonary atresia. RV = right ventricle; A = aorta; P = atretic pulmonary trunk.

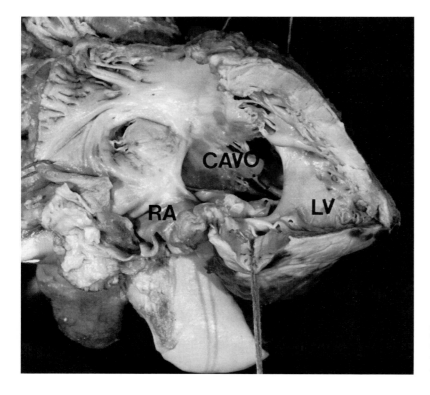

Figure 41: Right atrial, left ventricular view, and common AV orifice. RA = right atrium; LV = left ventricle; CAVO = common AV orifice, complete type.

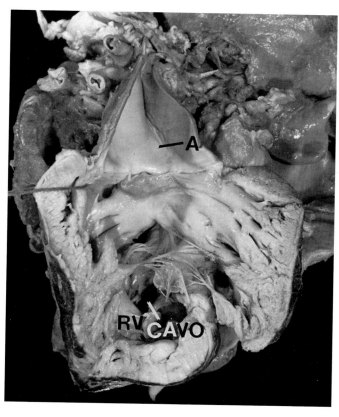

Figure 42: Aorta emerging from the morphologically right ventricle. A = aorta; RV = right ventricle; CAVO = common AV orifice, complete type.

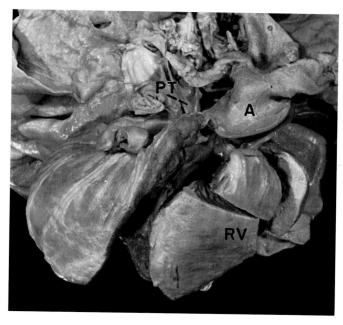

Figure 43: Mixed dextrocardia with atypical inverted overriding aorta, straddling conus, and pulmonary atresia. Anterior view. RV = right ventricle; A = aorta; PT = pulmonary trunk. (Used with permission from Lev M, et al. See Figure 89.)

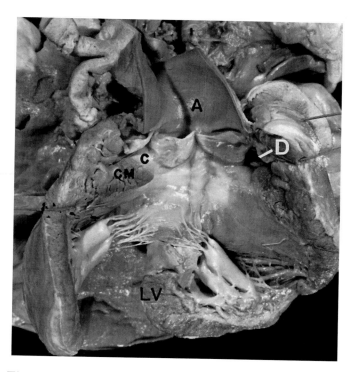

Figure 44: Right posterior view, the aorta emerging from the morphologically left ventricle but in an overriding manner through the straddling parietal band or the conus. LV = left ventricle; A = aorta; C = conus; CM = conus musculature; D = defect. (Used with permission from Lev M, et al. See Figure 89.)

VSD, overriding aorta and PS. Atypical tetralogy. ASD, CS type. ASD, FOD. LSVC and hepatic veins → LA. Bi AV. Congenital AV block	6 months M
VSD, overriding aorta and PS (atypical tetralogy) and ASD, FOD	13 years, 9 months, and 7 days M
Inverted transposition. VSD, CAVO type. Straddling TV, TI, sub PS. (Figs. 50—53)	5 years, 10 months, and 14 days M
Inverted DORV and CAVO, dominant Lt type. Marked PS. Absent IVC and azygos extension. Large ASD, FOD, PDA. Congenital AV block. LAA	9 months, 5 days F
Polysplenia, partial visceral heterotaxy. Inverted DORV, PS and CAVO. Common atrium. Absent IVC. RAA. Congenital AV block.	7 days F
Inverted transposition with mitral and PA. Large ASD, FOD. PDA. Absent LV	7 days F
Inverted transposition. Sub PS. Lt AV valve insufficiency. Spontaneously closing VSD. LSVC draining coronary veins. Absent CS. Diverticulum RV. (Figs. 54—57)	59 years, 3 months, 5 days M

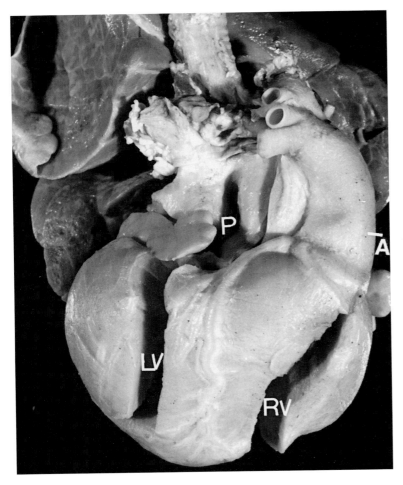

Figure 45: Mixed dextrocardia with atria pivoted and ventricles in mirror-image with inverted transposition and overriding pulmonary trunk (Taussig-Bing left ventricular type). A = aorta to the left and anterior; P = pulmonary trunk to the right and posterior; LV = left ventricle; RV = right ventricle.

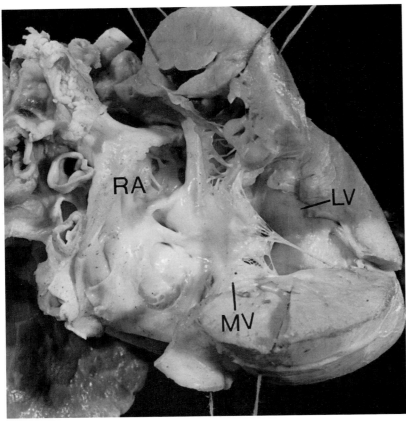

Figure 46: Right atrial, left ventricular view. RA = right atrium; LV = left ventricle; MV = mitral valve.

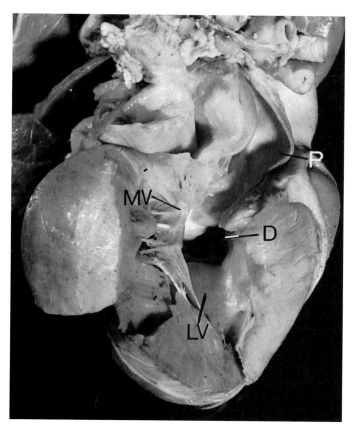

Figure 47: Overriding pulmonary trunk, left ventricular view. LV = left ventricle; MV = mitral valve; D = huge ventricular septal defect confluent with the pulmonary trunk; P = pulmonary trunk overriding the defect.

Inverted transposition. VSD and PS and total surgery, postoperative AV block — 9 years M

Asplenia, atria pivoted, total situs inversus abdominalis. 4 lobed LL and 3 lobed RL. Inverted transposition with PA and CAVO, complete type. TAPVD → RSVC with obstruction and aneurysm formation. RAA—Rt PDA. Absent CS. ASD, FOD (Figs. 58—61) — 2 days M

Inverted transposition. Mild Ebstein's type of TV. Partial absence of valve tissue. Severe TI. Paperthin enlarged RV. Marked AS and AI. Huge atypical FOD, proximal type. Aneurysm of fossa ovalis. Aneurysm of PDA. High origin of both coronary. Large blood cyst in MV (Figs. 62—67) — 12 days F

Trilobed both lungs. Accessory spleen. CAVO, complete type. TAPVD → IVC at RA junction. DORV, noncommitted type. Subpulmonary and valvular PS. ASD, FOD. Displaced CS. RAP resembling Lt. Bi PV. Rt descending aorta. LAA — 7 weeks M (35-wk gest.)

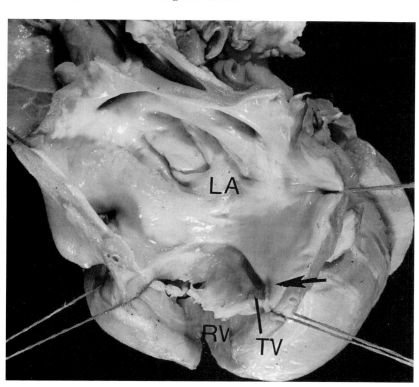

Figure 48: Ebstein's malformation of the left AV valve. LA = left atrium; TV = tricuspid valve; RV = right ventricle. Arrow points to the displaced septal and inferior leaflets.

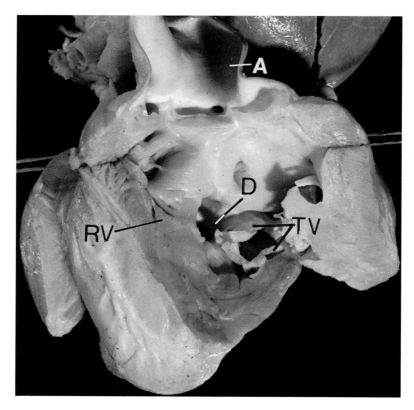

Figure 49: Aorta emerging from the morphologically right ventricle. A = aorta; RV = right ventricle; D = defect; TV = Ebstein's malformation of the tricuspid valve.

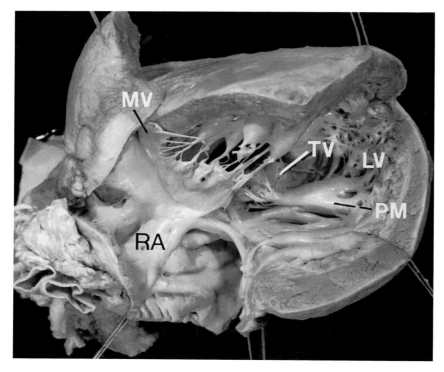

Figure 50: Mixed dextrocardia with straddling tricuspid valve. Right atrial, left ventricular view. RA = right atrium; LV = left ventricle; MV = mitral valve; TV = straddling tricuspid valve; PM = posterior or inferior papillary muscle in the morphologically left ventricle to which is connected the tricuspid valve.

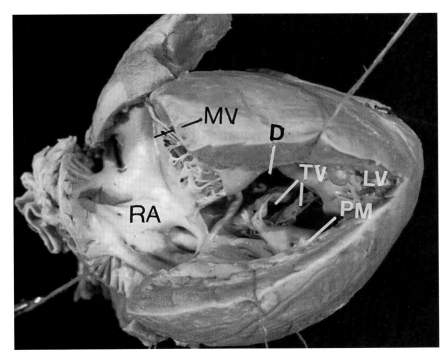

Figure 51: Straddling tricuspid valve as seen from the morphologically left ventricle. RA = right atrium; LV = left ventricle; MV = mitral valve; PM = papillary muscles; TV = straddling tricuspid valve; D = defect.

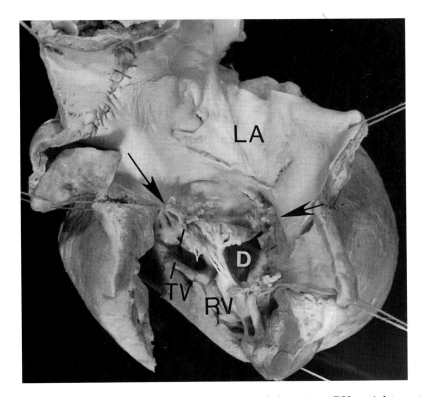

Figure 52: Left atrial, right ventricular view. LA = left atrium; RV = right ventricle; D = ventricular septal defect; TV = tricuspid valve, with recent anuloplasty. Arrows point to the anuloplasty of the tricuspid valve.

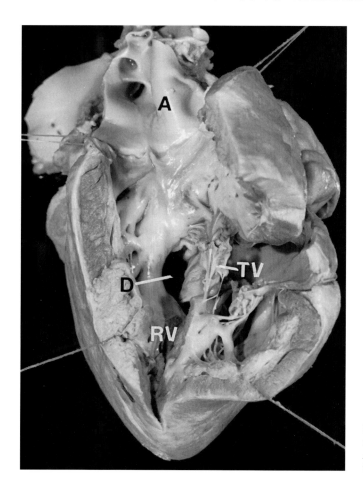

Figure 53: Aorta emerging from the right ventricle. RV = right ventricle; D = large common AV canal-type of a defect; A = aorta emerging from the right ventricle; TV = straddling tricuspid valve.

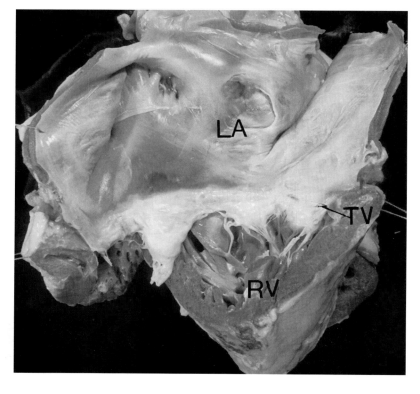

Figure 54: Mixed dextrocardia in a 59-year-old male with left AV valve insufficiency, subpulmonary stenosis and closing ventricular septal defect. Left atrial view. LA = huge left atrium; RV = right ventricle; TV = morphologically tricuspid valve. Note that the tricuspid valve is divided into several segments.

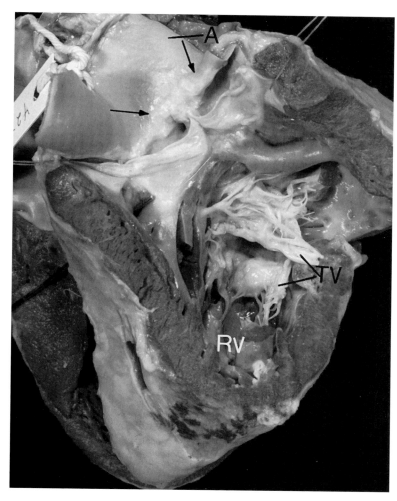

Figure 55: Aorta emerging from the outflow tract of the right ventricle. RV = right ventricle; TV = dysplastic tricuspid valve; A = aorta. Arrows point to atherosclerosis.

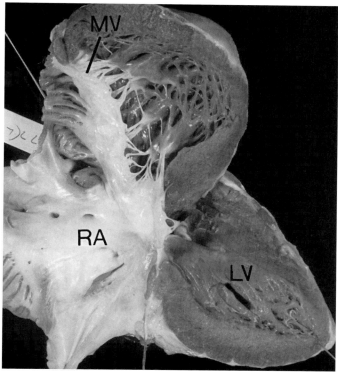

Figure 56: Right atrial, left ventricular view. RA = right atrium; LV = left ventricle; MV = mitral valve.

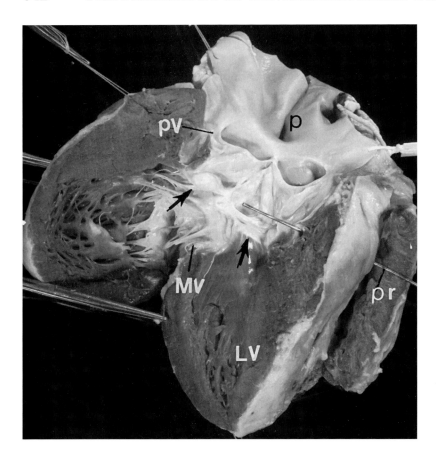

Figure 57: Subpulmonary stenosis produced by aneurysm of the membranous septum and closing ventricular septal defect. PV = pulmonary valve; P = pulmonary trunk; MV = mitral valve; Pr = probe passing through the closing ventricular septal defect; LV = left ventricle. Arrows point to the aneurysm.

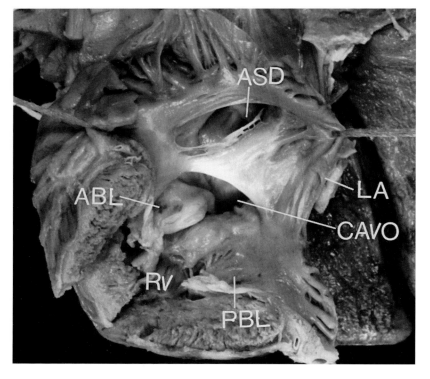

Figure 58: Mixed dextrocardia, atria pivoted, ventricles in mirror-image, with inverted transposition, common AV orifice, total anomalous pulmonary venous drainage, and pulmonary atresia. Left atrial, right ventricular view. LA = left atrium; ASD = atrial septal defect, fossa ovalis type; CAVO = common AV orifice, complete; RV = right ventricle; ABL = anterior bridging leaflet; PBL = posterior bridging leaflet. Note the dysplastic nature of the valve.

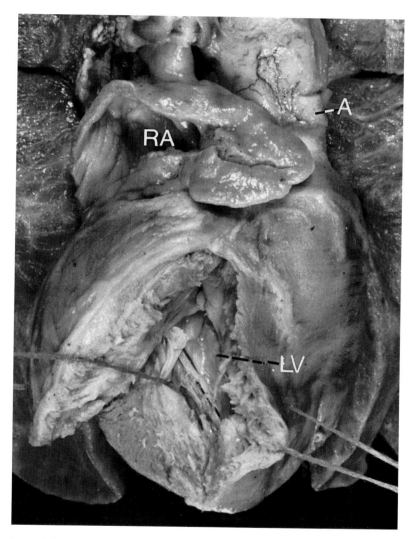

Figure 59: Right-sided view. RA = right atrium; LV = left ventricle; A = aorta.

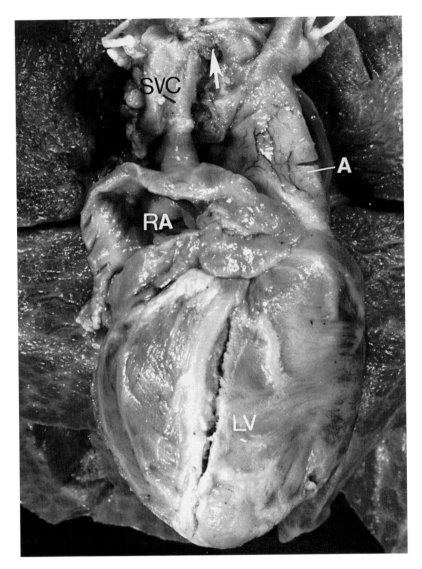

Figure 60: External view showing the obstruction of the total anomalous pulmonary venous return as the common pulmonary vein enters the superior vena cava on the right side. RA = right atrium; LV = left ventricle; A = aorta; SVC = superior vena cava. Arrow points to the obstruction of the pulmonary veins.

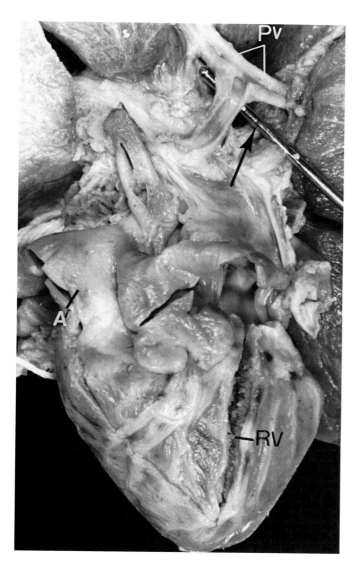

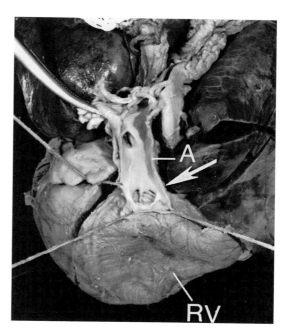

Figure 61: The pulmonary veins forming the common pulmonary vein. A = aorta; RV = right ventricle; PV = pulmonary veins. Arrow points to the probe behind the common pulmonary vein.

Figure 63: External view of the heart showing the marked aortic stenosis and the dysplastic aortic valve. RV = right ventricle; A = small aorta. Arrow points to the dysplastic, markedly stenotic aortic valve.

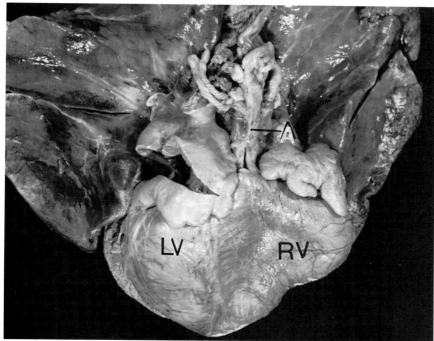

Figure 62: External view of mixed dextrocardia with marked aortic stenosis and marked tricuspid insufficiency. LV = left ventricle; RV = right ventricle; A = small aorta. Note the huge right ventricle.

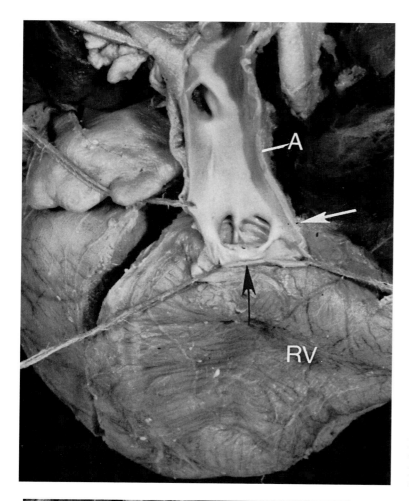

Figure 64: Close-up view of Figure 63. RV = right ventricle; A = small aorta. Arrows point to the dysplastic aortic valve with marked stenosis, almost resulting in atresia.

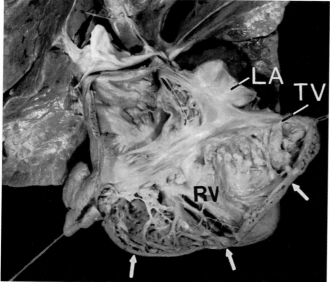

Figure 65: Left atrial, right ventricular view showing huge tricuspid orifice with partially absent leaflets and mild Ebstein-like malformation with tricuspid insufficiency and huge paper-thin right ventricle. LA = left atrium; TV = dysplastic tricuspid valve; RV = huge right ventricle with thin wall. Arrows point to the huge right ventricle with thin wall.

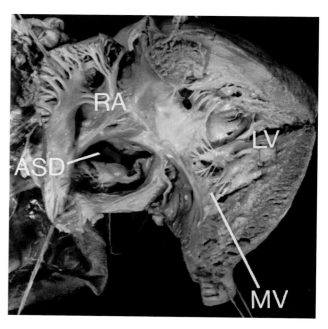

Figure 66: Right atrial, left ventricular view. RA = right atrium; LV = morphologically left ventricle; MV = mitral valve; ASD = huge atypical atrial septal defect.

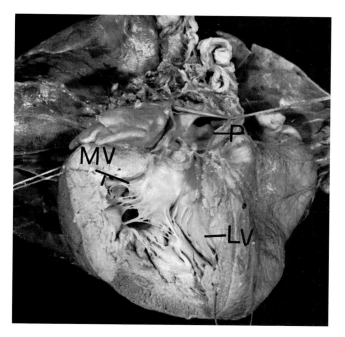

Figure 67: Pulmonary trunk emerging from the morphologically left ventricle. LV = left ventricle; MV = mitral valve; P = pulmonary trunk. Note the ventricular septal bulge.

Summarizing, the following were the complexes seen in mixed dextrocardia with ventricular inversion:

	No. of Cases
VSD and PS (1 with straddling TV)	5
CAVO, inverted DORV with PS	2
Inverted transposition with mitral and PA	2
VSD and PA	3
SV with inverted transposition and PA	1
SV with inverted transposition and PS	1
CAVO and PA	2
Atypical inverted transposition with overriding aorta	1
Overriding aorta and PA	1
TAPVD, inverted transposition, CAVO, and PA	1
TAPVD, PA, and mitral stenosis	1
TAPVD, CAVO, DORV, and PS	1
Criss-cross heart with DORV with PS and VSD	1
Tetralogy with PA or stenosis (2 with stenosis)	3
Ebstein's Lt AV valve, VSD, and PS	1
CT with PA and VSD	2
Overriding PT (Taussig-Bing) with TS and PS	1
VSD, TI	1
Ebstein's, severe, TI, thin RV (huge) with AS and AI	1

AV Block

Congenital AV block was seen in three cases and postoperative heart block in one. One had atypical tetralogy and the other two had double outlet right ventricle. One of the latter was a case of polysplenia with partial visceral heterotaxy. The postoperative heart block occurred following surgery for ventricular septal defect and pulmonary stenosis.

IV. Mixed Dextrocardia, Atria – Mirror-Image, Ventricles – Pivotal Position

There were two cases in this rare category. Here the atria were in mirror-image and the ventricles in a pivotal position. One was a male 13 years of age and the other a female 54 years of age.

The complexes were:

Asplenia. DORV regular, CAVO, PS. CS absent	13 years M
Total situs inversus. ASD, FOD, proximal and CS type. VSD and PS. Straddling CS. RAA (Figs 68-72	54 years F

V. Mirror-Image Dextrocardia

In this condition, the position of the chambers is as follows (Fig. 1): the right atrium is situated to the left and anterior, while the left atrium is situated to the right and posterior. The right ventricle is to the left and anterior and the left ventricle is to the right and posterior. If there is no transposition, the aorta is situated posteriorly and to the left, and the pulmonary orifice anterior and to the right. The pulmonary trunk dips posteriorly to the right of the aorta. If there is transposition, then it is usually of the inverted type. The anterior descending coronary artery comes off the right side of the aorta. The organs are usually in situs inversus, although there may be discordance between the situs of the chest and abdomen. The closest thing to an isolated mirror-image dextrocardia was a case with situs solitus abdominalis and bilobed lungs bilaterally. Occasionally, there is a bilobed spleen or polysplenia or asplenia. The complexes associated with this type of dextrocardia are related to varying types of transposition. In general, there is a distinct tendency for double outlet right ventricle and transposition to occur in this entity.

There was a total of 24 cases. There were 16 female subjects and eight male subjects. The youngest was a 1-hour-old, 28- to 30-weeks' gestation female fetus and the oldest a 78-year-old female, with a median age of 9 years, 10 months, and 10 days.

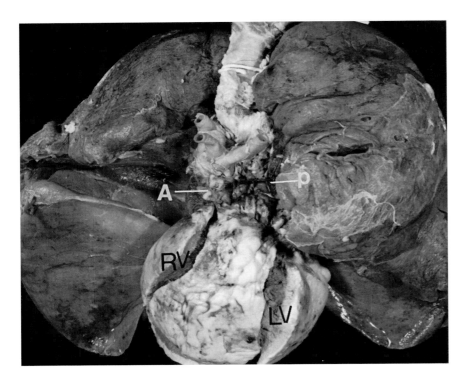

Figure 68: Mixed dextrocardia with atrial inversion and ventricles in normal position with complete transposition — corrected transposition. External view of the heart. A = aorta to the right and anterior; p = pulmonary trunk to the left and somewhat posterior; RV = right ventricle; LV = left ventricle.

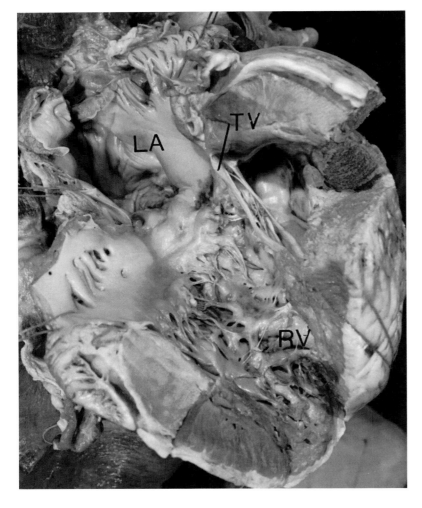

Figure 69: Left atrium situated to the right communicates with the morphologically right ventricle. Left atrial, right ventricular view. LA = left atrium receiving the pulmonary veins; RV = right ventricle; TV = tricuspid valve.

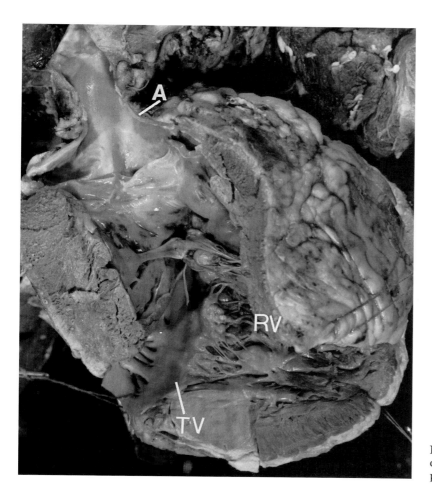

Figure 70: Aorta emerging from the right ventricle. A = aorta; RV = right ventricle; TV = tricuspid valve.

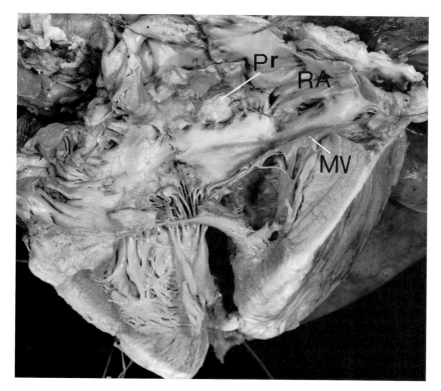

Figure 71: Morphologically right atrium situated to the left communicates with the left ventricle. RA = right atrium receiving the systemic veins; MV = mitral valve; Pr = prosthetic patch closure of the atrial septal defect.

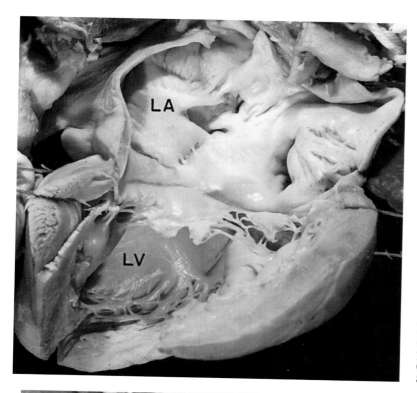

Figure 75: Right posterior view showing the left atrium and left ventricle situated to the right and posterior. LA = left atrium; LV = left ventricle. (Used with permission from Lev M. et al. See Figure 89.)

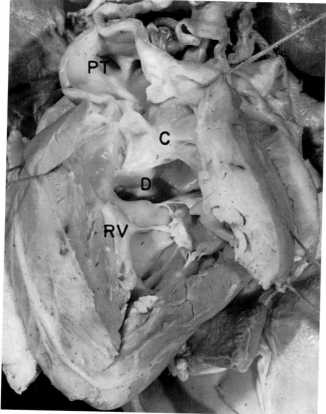

Figure 76: View of the right ventricular outflow tract into the pulmonary trunk. RV = right ventricle; D = defect; C = conus musculature; PT = pulmonary trunk. (Used with permission from Lev M. et al. See Figure 89.)

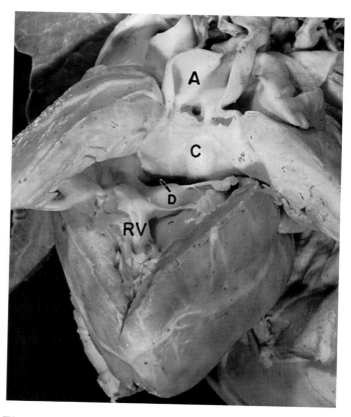

Figure 77: View of the right ventricular outflow tract into the aorta. A = aorta; C = conus musculature; RV = right ventricle; D = defect. (Used with permission from Lev M. et al. See Figure 89.)

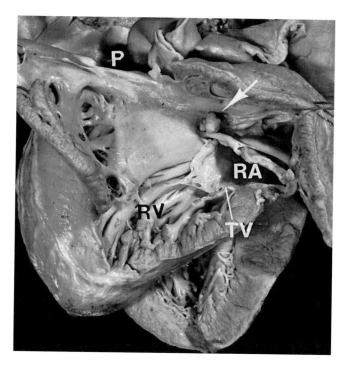

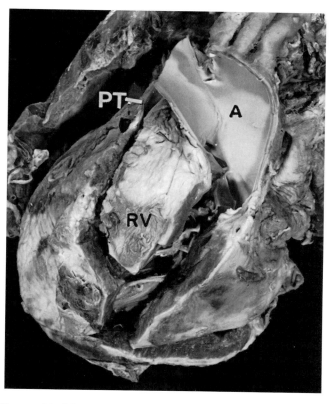

Figure 78: Mirror-image dextrocardia and aneurysm of the membranous septum and spontaneously closing ventricular septal defect. Left anterior view. RA = right atrium; RV = right ventricle; P = pulmonary trunk; TV = tricuspid valve. Arrow points to the aneurysm of the membranous septum.

Figure 80: Mirror-image dextrocardia with inverted tetralogy of Fallot. External view. RV = right ventricle; A = aorta; PT = pulmonary trunk.

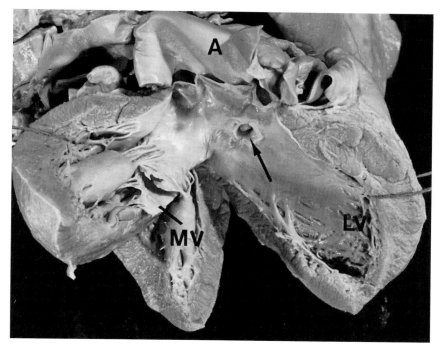

Figure 79: The aneurysm as seen from the left ventricular side showing spontaneously closing ventricular septal defect. MV = mitral valve; LV = left ventricle; A = aorta. Arrow points to the spontaneously closing ventricular septal defect.

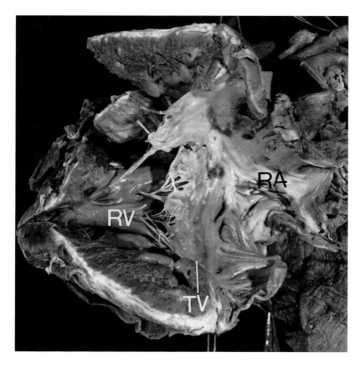

Figure 81: Left anterior view, right atrium receiving the systemic veins. RA = right atrium; TV = tricuspid valve; RV = right ventricle.

In summary, the complexes were:

DORV (1 with CAVO)	10 (41.6%)
Complete transposition	5
Tetralogy of Fallot	1
VSD	1
ASD primum	1
Coronary artery disease	1
Premature closure of foramen ovale and hypoplastia aortic tract complex, aortic and mitral atresia	1
CAVO	1
Large ASD, only IVC → LA	1
No anomaly	2

In summary, the following splenic abnormalities and visceral thoracic anomalies were noted:

	No. of Cases
Partial visceral heterotaxy—asplenia	2
Partial visceral heterotaxy—polysplenia	1
Partial visceral heterotaxy, spleen right	1
Solitus abdomen, bilobed lung	1
Inversus abdomen, thoracis solitus	1
Polysplenia, situs inversus	2
Situs inversus abdomen and thoracis, accessory spleen	1
Partial visceral heterotaxy and inversus thoracis	1

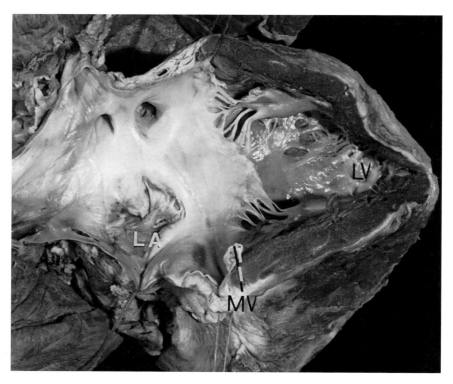

Figure 82: Right posterior view. LA = left atrium; LV = left ventricle; MV = mitral valve.

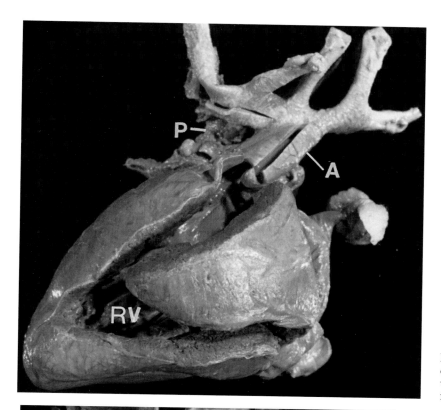

Figure 83: Mirror-image dextrocardia with complete inverted transposition. Left anterior view. RV = right ventricle; A = aorta emerging from the right ventricle; P = pulmonary trunk.

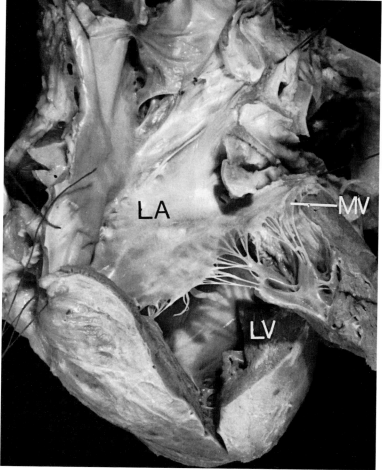

Figure 84: Mirror-image dextrocardia with inverted double outlet right ventricle and Mustard procedure and straddling of the inferior vena cava. Right posterior view. LA = left atrium; LV = left ventricle; MV = mitral valve.

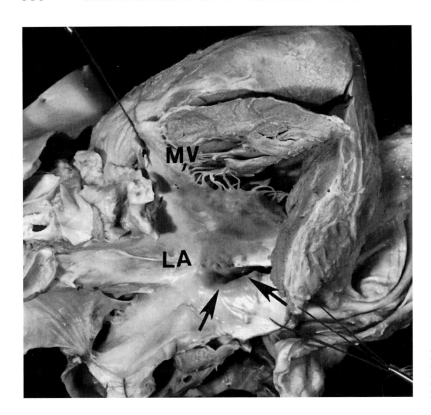

Figure 85: Same heart as in Figure 84, showing the straddling inferior vena cava. LA = left atrium; MV = mitral valve. Arrows point to the straddling inferior vena cava.

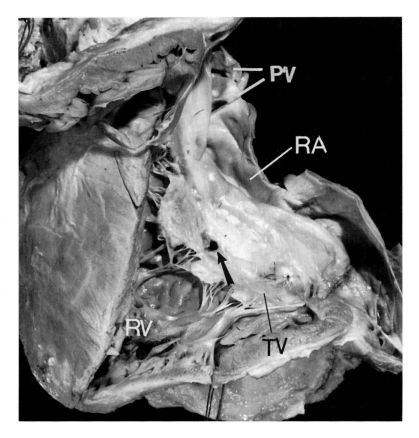

Figure 86: Left anterior view of the morphologically right atrium receiving the pulmonary veins after the Mustard procedure. RA = right atrium; TV = tricuspid valve; RV = right ventricle; PV = pulmonary veins. Arrow points to the residual atrial septal defect.

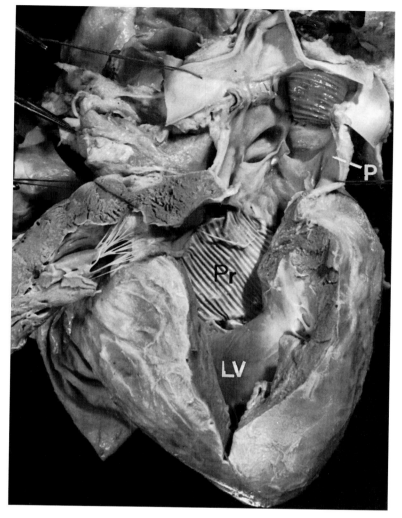

Figure 87: Right posterior view. From the morphologically left ventricle emerges the pulmonary trunk after the Hightower-Kirklin procedure—transfer of pulmonary trunk to morphologically left ventricle, and closure of the residual ventricular septal defect and Mustard procedure. LV = left ventricle; Pr = prosthetic closure of a large ventricular septal defect; P = pulmonary trunk.

VI. Presumptive Mirror-Image Dextrocardia

In this condition, the atrial septum is absent or it is not sufficiently adequate as to permit absolute identification of the morphology of the atria. Yet the position of the atria and the morphology of the atrial appendages suggest that the atria are in mirror-image position.

There was a total of 13 cases. There were six female subjects and seven male subjects. The youngest was 4 days old (one male and one female) and the oldest was an 11-year-old female. The median age was 1 year, 10 months, and 10 days.

This entity is almost invariably associated (except one in our series) with splenic abnormalities and dis-

turbed (except two) situs of organs. Thus, there was usually discordance between thoracic and abdominal viscera, or partial situs inversus abdominalis, and/or bilaterally nonlobated, bilobated, or trilobated lungs. In all cases, except two in our series, the abdominal venous return was normal if we assume the atria, whether divided or undivided, to be in mirror-image. In all cases, except three, the superior vena caval return was normal if we again assume the atria to be in mirror-image. In two of the latter three exceptional cases, bilateral venae cavae were present. In one case, only a right vena cava drained into a presumptive left atrial side of a common atrium. The pulmonary venous return was considerably disturbed. In five cases, it was normal if we assume the atria to be in mirror-image. In three cases, with the same assumption, there was total,

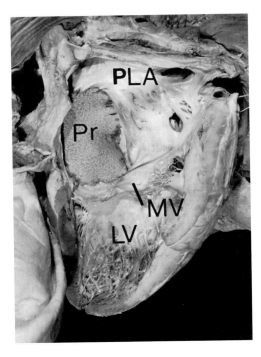

Figure 92: Right posterior view. PLA = presumptive left atrium; LV = left ventricle; MV = mitral valve; Pr = prosthetic closure of huge ASD.

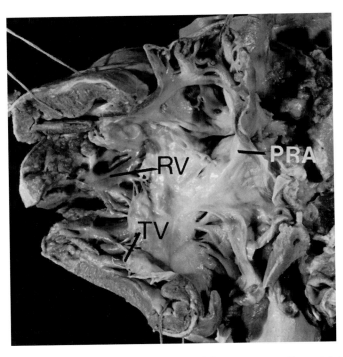

Figure 94: Left anterior view. PRA = presumptive right atrium; TV = tricuspid valve; RV = right ventricle.

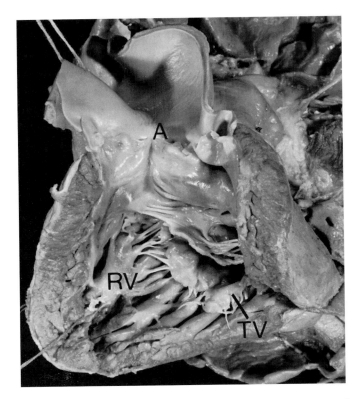

Figure 93: Presumptive mirror-image dextrocardia with complete transposition and pulmonary atresia. Left anterior view. TV = tricuspid valve; RV = right ventricle; A = aorta emerging from the right ventricle.

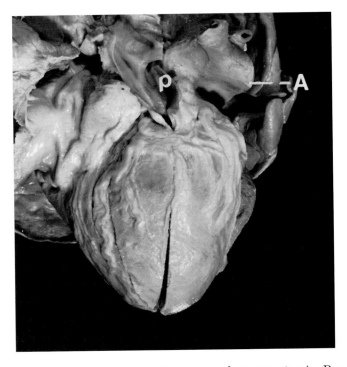

Figure 95: External view depicting pulmonary atresia. P = pulmonary trunk proceeds to the base of the heart without entering the heart; A = aorta.

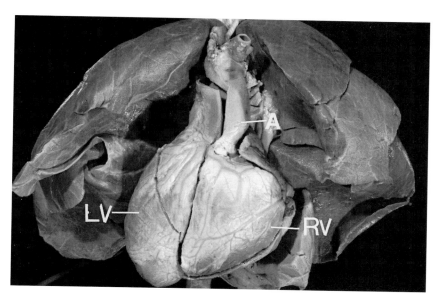

Figure 96: Presumptive mirror-image dextrocardia with double outlet right ventricle and common AV orifice. External view. A = aorta; RV = right ventricle; LV = left ventricle.

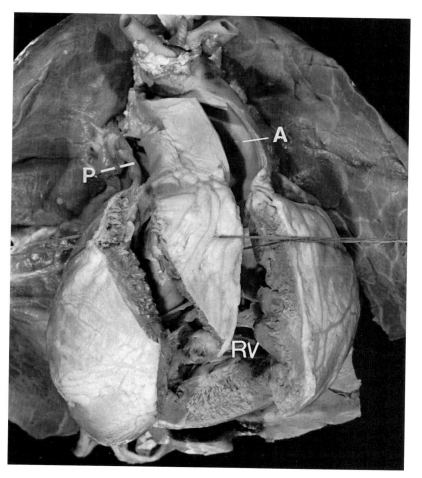

Figure 97: Close-up of Figure 96. A = aorta emerging from right ventricle; RV = right ventricle; P = pulmonary trunk emerging from right ventricle.

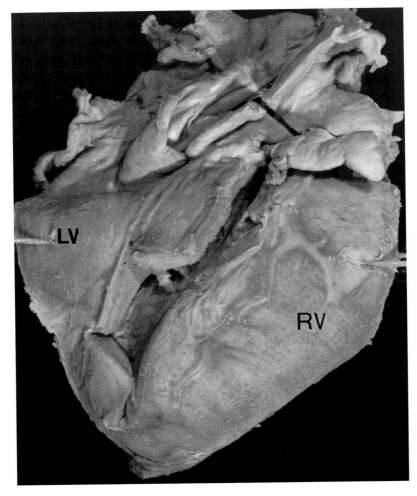

Figure 102: External view of Figure 101. RV = huge right ventricle; LV = very small left ventricle.

VII. Dextrocardia, Type Undetermined

In these cases, either the atria or both the atria and the ventricles were undiagnosable. These were associated in all cases except one with asplenia, or polysplenia, or bilateral spleens. There was either discordance of the abdominal organs with the thoracic situs, or partial situs inversus abdominalis and/or bilaterally nonlobated or bilobated lungs. The abdominal venous return was either to the right or the left side. The superior vena caval and pulmonary venous returns were either to the left or bilateral. Frequently seen in this group were a common atrium and a common AV orifice.

There was a total of 38 cases; 24 were males, 13 were females, and one was an animal. The ages ranged from newborn to 38 years with a mean age of 3 years, 4 months, and 18 days. Eleven were above 1 year of age (29%) and 17 were below the age of 1 month (45%).

Dextrocardia indeterminate type may further be subdivided into four types:

	No. of Cases
a. Atria indeterminate, ventricles mirror-image	17
b. Atria indeterminate, ventricles pivotal position	4
c. Atria pivotal, ventricles indeterminate	6
d. Atria and ventricles indeterminate	11

The complexes were:

a. Atria indeterminate, ventricles mirror-image

Situs inversus, polysplenia, atria indeterminate, ventricles in mirror-image. FC, incomplete vascular ring. LAA and Lt ligamentum

IVC, LSVC, LPV → Lt RPV → Rt side. RSVC → CS → Rt — 6 months M

Situs inversus, polysplenia, atria indeterminate, ventricles in mirror-image. Ostium primum, PAPVD, RAA. IVC, LSVC and Lt PV → Lt Rt PV → Rt. — 1 month M

Situs inversus. Bilateral bilobed lungs. Atria indeterminate, ventricles in mirror-image. Common atrium, CAVO, RAA. Lt PV → Lt. Rt PV → Rt. IVC, RSVC → Rt — 25 minutes M

Partial visceral heterotaxy. Asplenia. Atria indeterminate, ventricles in mirror-image. CAVO, CT, and PS. Absent ventricular septum, TAPVD → hemiazygos → Lt side. Hepatic vein → Lt. Absent IVC and CS. Accessory VSD, huge FOD — 5 months M

Trilobed both lungs. Asplenia, partial visceral heterotaxy. Atria indeterminate, ventricles in mirror-image. CT, PA, VSD. Large ASD. Almost common atrium. Absent IVC and CS. PV → Lt. Rt—SVC and hemiazygos extension. Straddling hepatic vein Lt and Rt side — 3 days M

Atria indeterminate. Ventricles in mirror-image. Asplenia, partial visceral heterotaxy. Truncus, common atrium, CAVO. RAA. Double SVC. Truncus completely from RV. RSVC and IVC → Rt. Absent CS. LSVC and PV → Lt — 5 days M

Atria indeterminate. Ventricles in mirror-image. Inverted DORV, PS, CAVO, dominant Rt, common atrium, Bi PV. Bilateral SVC. Atrophy of LV and Rt-sided atrium. PV, RSVC, LSVC, IVC, CS → Lt side — 5 years, 11 months, 21 days M

Atria indeterminate. Ventricles in mirror-image. Inverted DORV, CAVO, common atrium. FOD, double SVC, AS. IVC, RSVC, PV → Lt side — 12 days M

Polysplenia. Abdominal situs inversus. Atria indeterminate, ventricles presumed in mirror-image. Inverted DORV, mitral atresia. PAPVD. 2 PV → Lt LSVC → CS. Absent IVC. Azygos → RSVC → Rt hepatic vein → Rt PV and CS → Rt. Common atrium. Atrophy LV — 2 months, 18 days M

Situs inversus, polysplenia. Rt lung 3 lobes, Lt lung 2 lobes. Atria indeterminate, ventricles in mirror-image. Inverted DORV, common atrium, CAVO. Double SVC. Double CS. Azygos extension. RAA. Rt PDA. Congenital AV block. Hepatic vein and RPV → Rt side. LPV → Lt. — 1 day M

Atria indeterminate, ventricles in mirror-image. Isomerism atria. Inverted transposition. PS. Straddling conus, common atrium, mitral atresia. TI, bilateral SVC. 2 PPV → Rt. 2 PV → Lt. Absent IVC. Hepatic vein → both sides. Azygos and hemiazygos → Rt and Lt SVC separately. 2 VSDs. Bi PV. Divided LV. Atrial arrhythmias — 38 years F

Asplenia, partial visceral heterotaxy. Atria indeterminate, ventricles in mirror-image. Both lungs trilobed. CT with PA. TAPVD → abdomen → portal. CAVO. Ebstein-like malformation of CAVO leaflet into Rt side. RSVC atretic. IVC → Rt side. CS absent. ASD, FOD. LSVC → Lt side — 3 days F

Atria indeterminate, ventricles in mirror-image. Polysplenia, partial visceral heterotaxy. Bilobed both lungs. Common atrium, CAVO, complete, LV type. DORV. RSVC atresia. LSVC → Lt. Hemiazygos → Lt side. PAPVD. Rt PV → Rt side. Wide PDA. Hepatic vein and CS → Rt Doubly committed type CAVO — 1 hour F

Atria indeterminate, ventricles in mirror-image. Polysplenia, partial visceral heterotaxy. Common atrium. CAVO, complete. RAA. Rt PDA. Rt side—P vein. LSVC, IVC, CS → Lt side. — 17 days F

Atria indeterminate, ventricles in mirror-image. Lt—SVC and hepatic. TAPVD. Common atrium, CAVO, CT, PA, RAA. Rt PDA. Accessory mitral orifice and mitral insufficiency. Absent CS. Lt CC and Lt subclavian artery from innominate artery. RCC and Rt subclavian artery from transverse arch. Postoperative atrial tachycardia → AV block — 7 months F

Atria indeterminate, ventricles in mirror-image. Multilobated spleen, partial visceral heterotaxy. Tetralogy with sinus venosus, ASD. IVC, RSVC, hepatic vein and LSVC → Lt Divided RV, Bi PV. CS close to hepatic. PV → Rt side. RAA. Rt descending aorta. Single coronary.   15 years M

Asplenia. Partial visceral heterotaxy. Atria indeterminate and ventricles inverted. Inverted DORV with subpulmonary and valvular PS. TAPVD → Portal with obstruction. CAVO, Rt Absent CS, FOD. LSVC → IVC, RSVC → Rt LSVC → Lt. or SV with no small outlet chamber, both appendages resemble both   2 days M

b. Atria indeterminate, ventricals pivotal position

Partial visceral heterotaxy. Polysplenia. Atria indeterminate, ventricles pivoted. Common atrium. Absent CS and IVC. 2 Lt PV, Lt hepatic vein and hemiazygos → LSVC → Lt. Rt hepatic vein, RSVC and Rt P vein → Rt (Figs. 103—106)   6 months F

Atria indeterminate, ventricles pivoted. Absent IVC. Hemiazygos → RSVC. PAPVD. RPV → Rt Common atrium   2 years, 10 months 24 days M

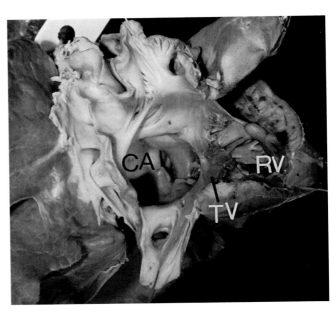

Figure 104: Common atrium, indeterminate atria. Right-sided view. CA = common atrium, huge; TV = tricuspid valve; RV = right ventricle.

Polysplenia, partial visceral heterotaxy. Bilobed lungs. Atria indeterminate, ventricles normal. Aortic and mitral atresia. Diverticulum RV   4 days F

Atria indeterminate and ventricles dextroverted (pivoted). Asplenia, partial visceral heterotaxy. CT, PA, CAVO. TAPVD → Portal with

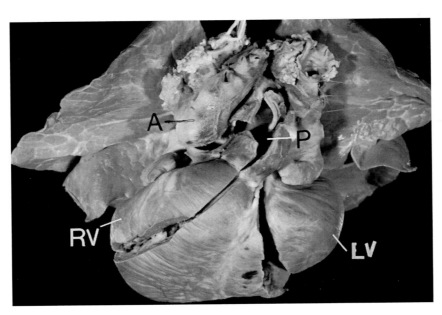

Figure 103: Dextrocardia with atria indeterminate, ventricles pivoted. External view. A = aorta; P = pulmonary trunk; LV = left ventricle; RV = right ventricle.

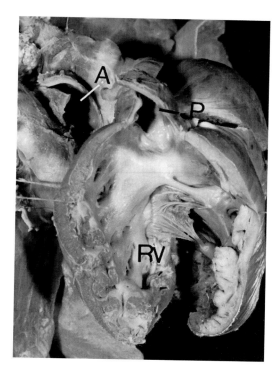

Figure 105: Pulmonary trunk emerging from the right ventricle. RV = right ventricle; P = pulmonary trunk; A = aorta.

obstruction. RSVC and IVC and LSVC → Lt. LAA Rt PDA from innominate (tortuous). Large FOD   2 days M

c. Atria pivotal and ventricles indeterminate

Atria pivoted, common ventricle, conus indeterminate. CT, CAVO and PS. LSVC and IVC Lt atrium, aneurysm of FO. RAA, Rt PDA. Absent CS   18 hours F

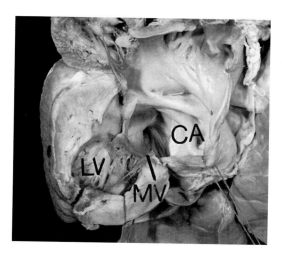

Figure 106: Left anterior view. CA = common atrium; MV = mitral valve; LV = left ventricle.

Atria pivoted, ventricular sinus indeterminate. Straddling conus. Huge ASD, VSD, CT, and PS. Juxtaposed Rt atrial appendage to the left. Bi PV. Rt AV valve atresia. RAA   2 years F

Atria pivoted, ventricles indeterminate. Straddling conus. Inverted transposition and PA. Single coronary ostium. ASD, FOD. LAA Lt PDA   3 days M

Atria pivoted, ventricles indeterminate. Truncoconal inversion. Common ventricle. CAVO and PS. FOD. RAA. Bi PV   16 years M

Asplenia. Atria indeterminate (situs solitus) and ventricles indeterminate. Common atrium, CAVO, SV inverted transposition with PA. Absent CS. SVC and IVC → Rt PV → Lt. AV block during cath and death a few weeks later.   10 months F

Situs inversus abdominalis, both lungs trilobed. Atria (situs solitus), ventricles indeterminate. Common atrium, CAVO, SV regular transposition and PA or marked PS both vessels from SV, no SOC. PV → Rt CS, SVC, IVC → Lt. VF after surgery → death   7 years M

d. Atria and ventricles indeterminate

Situs inversus. Bilobed spleen. Atria and ventricles indeterminate. Inverted transposition with PA and CAVO. IVC, LSVC, LPV → Lt. RPV → Rt side RAA (Fig. 107, 108)   5 years, 11 months M

Situs solitus. Asplenia, trilobed both lungs. Atria and ventricles indeterminate. Common atrium, CAVO, double conus. FC, RAA, Rt PDA. IVC, LSVC → Lt side. P veins → Rt side (Figs. 109—111)   3 month M

Partial visceral heterotaxy. Asplenia, inversus lungs. Atria and ventricles indeterminate. CAVO, common ventricle, inverted transposition with PS. Absent CS. PV → LSVC—Lt side. RSVC → Rt IVC both Rt and Lt sides   13 days F

Atria and ventricles indeterminate. SV inverted transposition, CAVO. Double SVC. IVC and RSVC → Rt side. P vein → LSVC and hepatic vein → Lt side. Bi PV. Common atrium. CS absent   5 months 13 days F

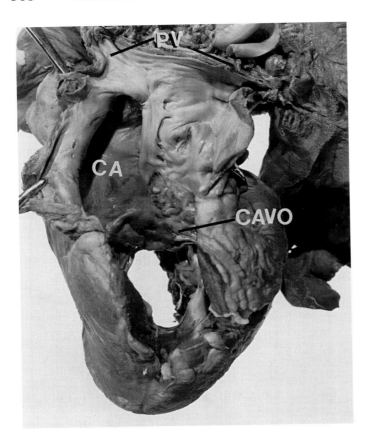

Figure 107: Dextrocardia, type indeterminate, right-sided view. Common atrium, common AV orifice, complete transposition, pulmonary atresia. CA = common atrium on the right side receiving some of the pulmonary veins; PV = pulmonary veins; CAVO = huge common AV orifice.

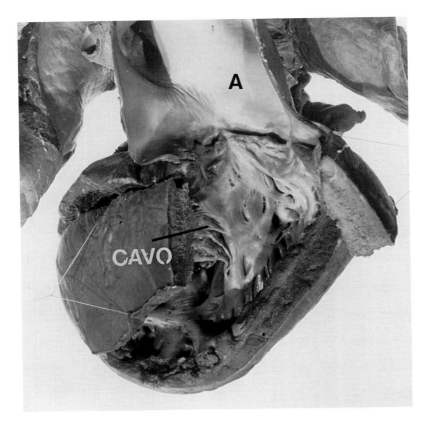

Figure 108: Dextrocardia, undetermined, aorta emerging from an indeterminate ventricular chamber left and anterior, inverted type of transposition. A = aorta; CAVO = common AV orifice.

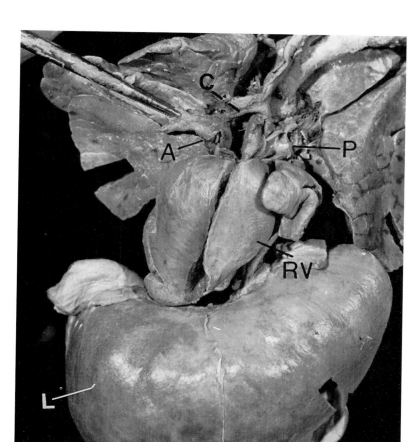

Figure 109: Dextrocardia, type indeterminate—atria and ventricles indeterminate. External view. RV = presumed right ventricle; P = pulmonary trunk; A = aorta; L = liver; C = fetal coarctation.

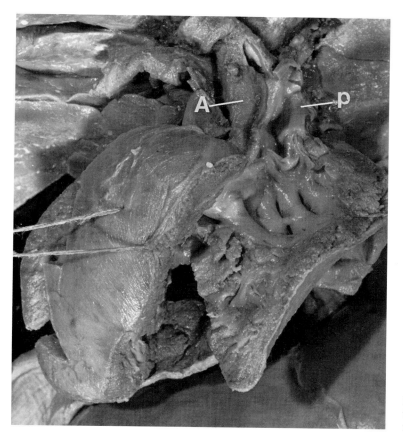

Figure 110: Double conus with aorta and pulmonary trunk emerging more or less side by side. P = pulmonary trunk; A = aorta.

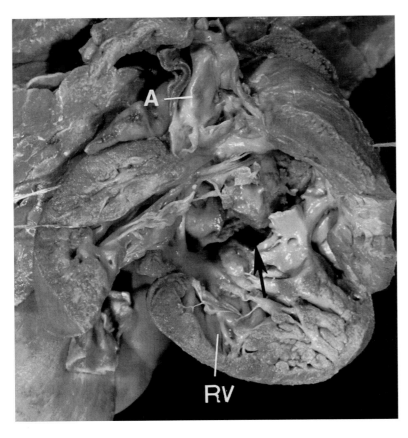

Figure 111: Double conus, atria and ventricles not determined. Aorta emerging from an indeterminate chamber and common AV orifice. A = aorta; RV = morphology resembles somewhat a right ventricle (presumed right ventricle). Arrow points to common AV orifice.

Asplenia, trilobed both lungs, partial visceral heterotaxy. Atria and ventricles indeterminate. Almost common atrium, CAVO, PS. Huge ASD. RAA. P vein → LSVC → Lt side. Inferior vena cava → Lt. Absent CS and RSVC	1 year, 5 months, 11 days M
Partial visceral heterotaxy, spleen normal. Atria and ventricles indeterminate. Common atrium, common ventricle. CT, PA, and mitral atresia. Double SVC. Hepatic vein → CA. Clinically 2 SA nodes. RAA. Rt PDA. CS, Lt 2 PV, hepatic vein, LSVC and IVC → Lt. RSVC and 2 PV → Rt side of common atrium	15 years M
Asplenia. Lt lung 5, Rt lung 4. Partial visceral heterotaxy. Atria and ventricles indeterminate. Common atrium SV, SOC. Inverted transposition. Absent CS. RAA. Rt PDA. Bi SVC each receiving 1 PV for each side (lower pulmonary veins), PAPVD → abdominal portal	1 day F
Atria and ventricles indeterminate. Common atrium, CAVO, CT and PA	Animal

Partial visceral heterotaxy. Atria and ventricles indeterminate. 3 lobed lungs both sides. SV inverted transposition, marked infundibular and valvular PS. Both vessels emerging from the main chamber, closing defect between SV and SOC. Bi PV. Absent CS. PAPVD. RAA Rt descending aorta, single coronary. PV → Rt in part and in part → a vein close to IVC (more Lt). RPV → RSVC. LPV stenotic	13 years M
Dextrocardia, type indeterminate (atria and ventricles). Common atrium, CAVO. SV without transposition. PA. Absent RPV and RPA. Almost absent right atrial appendage. Absent CS. Azygos → RSVC. LUPV → LSVC and LLPV → Lt. Absent Rt lung. CAVO related to aorta but aorta Lt and anterior. LAA Rt PDA	12 days
Asplenia. Atria and ventricles indeterminate. CAVO, common ventricle, DORV, PS, Bi PV. TAPVD → RSVC—Rt Absent PDA. LSVC, IVC and CS → Lt side atrium	2 months M

Congenital AV Block and Other Arrhythmias in Dextrocardia

II. Presumptive Dextroversion

Polysplenia, VSD, PS, TS and MI. Aneurysm of FO. Hemiazygos → LSVC → LA. CS → LA. Floppy MV. Primitive LV. Rhythm abnormalities. Absent RSVC and small RA. Spleen left. Liver midline   23 years F

III. Mixed Dextrocardia, Atria–Pivotal Position, Ventricles—Mirror-Image

VSD, overriding aorta and PS. Atypical tetralogy. ASD, CS type. ASD, FOD. LSVC and hepatic veins → LA. Bi AV. Congenital AV block   6 months M

Inverted DORV and CAVO, Dominant Lt type. Marked PS. Absent IVC and azygos extension. Large ASD, FOD, PDA. Congenital AV block. LAA (Figs. 112—115)   9 months, 5 days F

Polysplenia, partial visceral heterotaxy. Inverted DORV, PS, and CAVO. Common atrium. Absent IVC. RAA. Congenital AV block (Figs. 116—120)   7 days F

Inverted transposition. VSD and PS and total surgery. Postoperative AV block   9 years M

V. Mirror-Image Dextrocardia

Inverted tetralogy of Fallot, surgical correction, and sudden death 4 years postop   21 years F

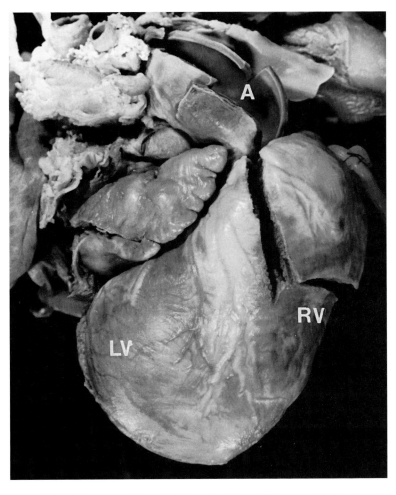

Figure 112: Mixed dextrocardia, atria in pivotal position, ventricles in mirror-image, inverted DORV, common AV orifice, and congenital AV block in a 9-month-old infant. External view of the heart. RV = right ventricle; LV = left ventricle; A = aorta.

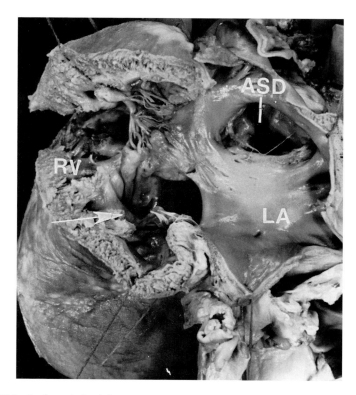

Figure 113: Left atrial, right ventricular view. LA = left atrium; ASD = large atrial septal defect; RV = right ventricle. Arrow points to the common AV orifice.

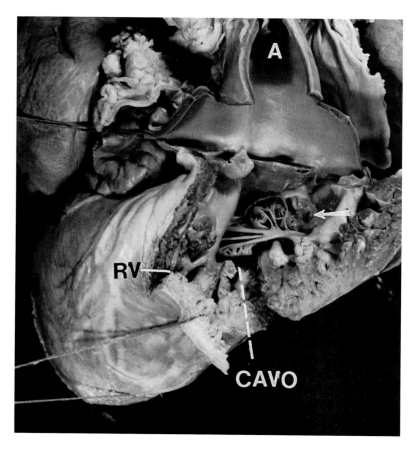

Figure 114: Left-sided view from the morphologically right ventricle emerges the aorta. A = aorta; RV = right ventricle; CAVO = common AV orifice defect confluent in part with the aorta. Arrow points to the markedly stenotic infundibulum for the pulmonary trunk.

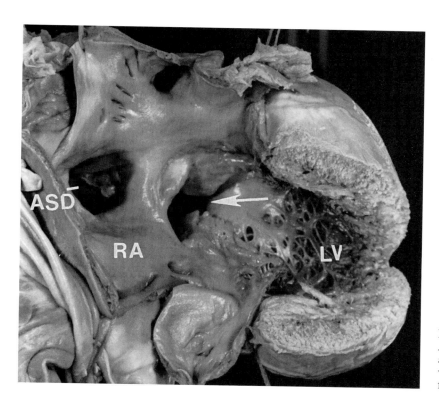

Figure 115: Right-sided view of the common AV orifice. RA = right atrium; ASD = large atrial septal defect; LV = morphologically left ventricle. Arrow points to the common AV orifice.

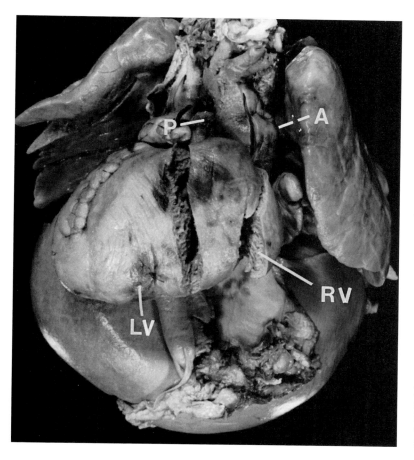

Figure 116: Dextrocardia, atria pivotal, ventricles in mirror-image, polysplenia and congenital AV block with attempted surgery, DORV, external view. RV = right ventricle; LV = left ventricle; A = aorta; P = pulmonary trunk.

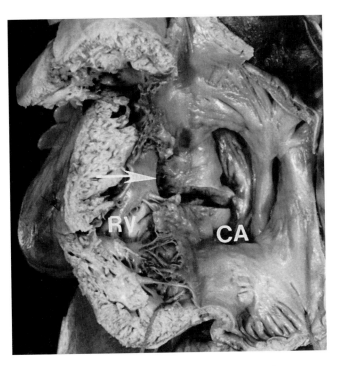

Figure 117: Common atrium, left-sided view. CA = common atrium, left side; RV = right ventricle. Arrow points to common AV orifice.

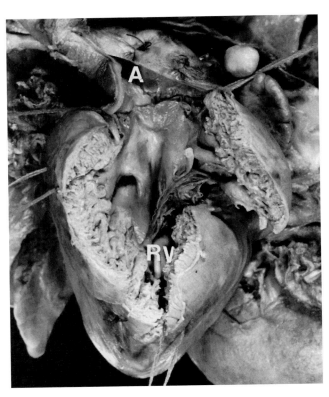

Figure 118: Left-sided view showing the inverted DORV. RV = right ventricle; A = aorta.

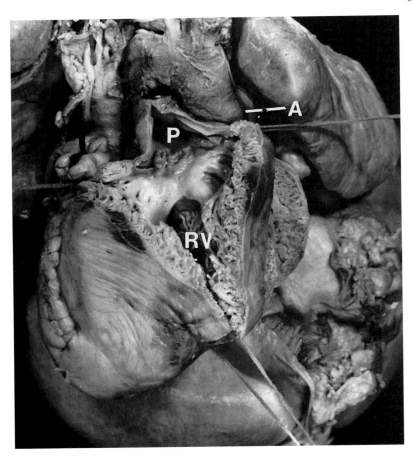

Figure 119: Infundibular and valvular pulmonary stenosis, pulmonary trunk also emerging from the right ventricle. RV = right ventricle; P = pulmonary trunk; A = aorta.

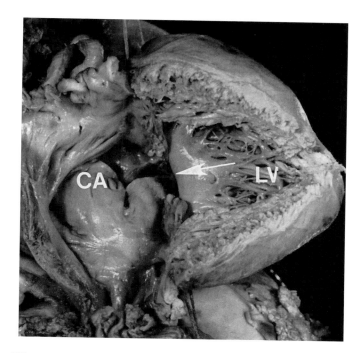

Figure 120: Right-sided view of common atrium and common AV orifice. CA = common atrium, right side; LV = left ventricle. Arrow points to common AV orifice.

VII. Dextrocardia, Type Undetermined

a. Atria indeterminate, ventricles mirror-image

Situs inversus, polysplenia. Rt lung 3 lobes, Lt lung 2 lobes. Atria indeterminate, ventricles in mirror-image. Inverted DORV, common atrium, CAVO. Double SVC. Double CS. Azygos extension. RAA. Rt PDA. Congenital AV block. Hepatic vein and RPV → Rt side. LPV → Lt. (Figs. 121—125)

1 day M

Atria indeterminate, ventricles in mirror-image. isomerism atria. Inverted transposition. PS. Straddling conus, common atrium, mitral atresia. TI, bilateral SVC. 2 PPV → Rt. 2 PV → Lt. Absent IVC. Hepatic vein → both sides. Azygos and hemiazygos → Rt and Lt SVC separately. 2 VSDs. Bi PV. Divided LV. Atrial arrhythmias

38 years F

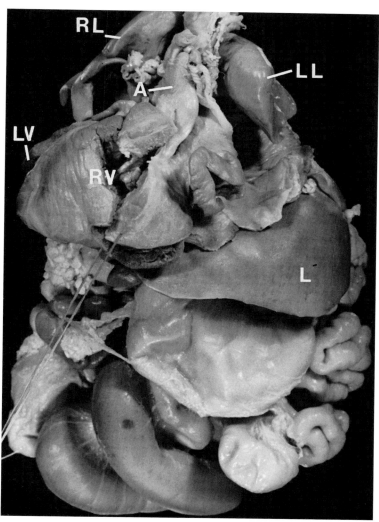

Figure 121: Dextrocardia, type undetermined, atria indeterminate, ventricles mirror-image, with situs inversus and polysplenia. External view. L = liver; RL = right lung; LL = left lung; RV = right ventricle; LV = left ventricle; A = aorta.

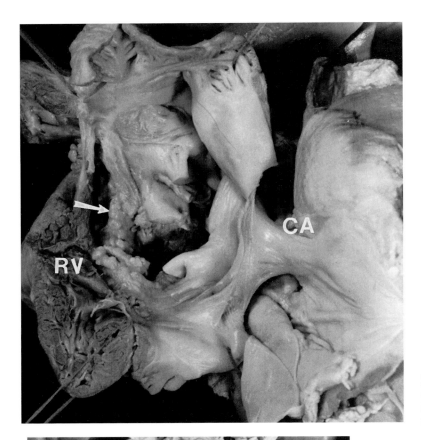

Figure 122: Left-sided view, common atrium. CA = common atrium, left side; RV = right ventricle. Arrow points to common AV orifice. Note the huge common atrium.

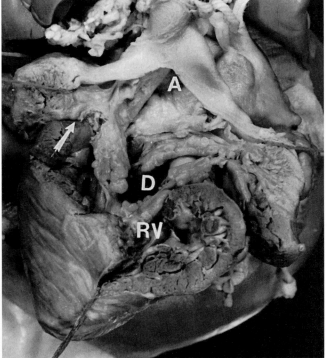

Figure 123: Left-sided view, DORV, inverted type, aorta emerging from the right ventricle. RV = right ventricle; A = aorta; D = defect of the common AV orifice. Note that the common AV defect is confluent in part with the aorta. Arrow points to the infundibulum to the pulmonary trunk.

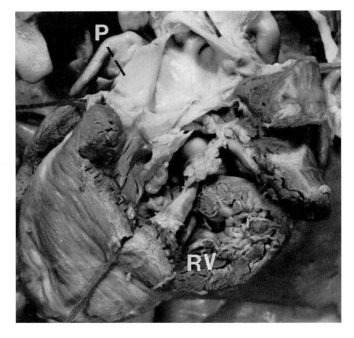

Figure 124: Outflow tract of the right ventricle, the pulmonary trunk emerging from the right ventricle. RV = right ventricle; P = pulmonary trunk;

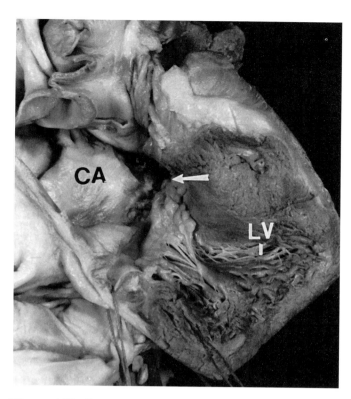

Figure 125: Common atrium as seen from the right side. CA = common atrium; LV = left ventricle. Arrow points to common AV orifice. Note the huge common atrium.

Atria indeterminate, ventricles in mirror-image. Lt—SVC and hepatic. TAPVD. Common atrium, CAVO, CT, PA, RAA. Rt PDA. Accessory mitral orifice and mitral insufficiency. Absent CS. Lt CC and Lt subclavian artery from innominate artery. RCC and Rt subclavian from transverse arch. Postoperative atrial tachycardia → AV block   7 months F

c. Atria pivoted, ventricles indeterminate

Situs inversus abdominalis, both lungs trilobed. Atria (situs solitus), ventricles indeterminate. Common atrium, CAVO, SV regular transposition and PA or marked PS both vessels from SV, no SOC. PV → Rt CS, SVC, IVC → Lt. VF after surgery → death   7 years M

d. Atria and ventricles indeterminate

Partial visceral heterotaxy, spleen normal. Atria and ventricles indeterminate. Common atrium, common ventricle. CT, PA, and mitral

atresia. Double SVC. Hepatic vein → CA. Clinically 2 SA nodes. RAA. Rt PDA. CS, Lt 2 PV, hepatic vein, LSVC and IVC → Lt. RSVC and 2 PV → Rt side of common atrium   15 years M

Comment

In dextroversion, 23 (85%) were below the age of 1 year, and although all types of complexes are seen in this type of dextrocardia, there is a tendency for transposition (partial or complete, including truncus) to occur (12 out of 27, 44%), with frequent association of tricuspid valve anomalies (6 out of 27, 22%), and juxtaposed atrial appendage (7 out of 27, 25.9%). This may explain the frequency of this anomaly in the neonatal age group.

It is of interest that there was one case of asplenia and partial visceral heterotaxy, one case of total anomalous pulmonary venous drainage, one case of ectopia cordis, and one case of congenital AV block.

In presumptive dextroversion, there were two cases (aged 23 and 27 years), one with double outlet right ventricle, the other with ventricular septal defect, with pulmonary stenosis in both. The one with polysplenia had rhythm abnormalities.

Regarding mixed dextrocardia, the one type frequently encountered in this series was that with the atria in a pivoted position and ventricles in mirror-image. Ventricular septal defect and pulmonary stenosis occurred frequently. There was one rare heart in a 12-day-old female with marked aortic stenosis, partial absence of the tricuspid valve with Ebstein-like malformation, massive tricuspid insufficiency, and huge paper-thin right ventricle.

There were two remarkable hearts with the rare type of mixed dextrocardia with atria in mirror-image and ventricles in the normal position. One was with polysplenia, regular DORV, CAVO, and pulmonary stenosis. The other was a 54-year-old female who had a large atypical ASD, VSD, and pulmonary stenosis. The anomalies are comparable to a similar setup seen in isolated levocardia with atrial inversion, obviously permitting survival to adult life.

In mirror-image dextrocardia, there is a high incidence of double outlet right ventricle followed by complete transposition. Eight were without a ventricular septal defect. The oldest, 78 years, had no anomaly, and the 70-year-old had coronary artery disease.

In general, there is a distinct tendency for transposition of the great arteries (either complete or partial, including tetralogy, double outlet, or simply overriding of the aorta or pulmonary trunk) to occur in various types of dextrocardia. Thus, it is very important to understand and identify the exact location of the cardiac chambers and their relationship to the atrioventricular valves and the semilunar valves. As seen from our material, there are many lesions that can be operated on with good success.

Presumptive mirror-image dextrocardia is usually associated with splenic abnormalities and disturbed situs of organs, but there were exceptions, rarely. Here again, there is a distinct tendency for complete transposition or DORV inverted type (10 out of 13, 77%) to be associated with disturbances in the systemic and pulmonary venous returns. The occurrence of transposition (complete or incomplete) is somewhat similar to mirror-image dextrocardia.

On the other hand, when it comes to dextrocardia undetermined type, we are dealing with a major cardiac anomaly that includes the atrial septal abnormality, ventricular septal abnormality, conotruncal abnormalities, as well as abnormalities in the systemic and pulmonic venous return. Nevertheless, some do permit survival and therefore a careful evaluation and understanding of the anatomy is very important, and in some selected cases either a total surgical correction and/or a palliative surgery may be attempted.

From the clinical as well as surgical points of view, the interrelationships between the various types of dextrocardia and the situs of viscera, splenic abnormalities, systemic and pulmonic venous returns, and the position of the great arteries are of great importance. From the anatomic data, it is clear that dextroversion and mixed dextrocardia with the atria in the pivotal position and ventricles inverted are associated with situs solitus viscera and that mirror-image dextrocardia is generally associated with situs inversus if there are no splenic abnormalities. However, it is important to remember that exceptions do occur without splenic abnormalities. Likewise, splenic abnormalities do occur with visceral heterotaxy in dextroversion and in mixed dextrocardia.

It is also clear that when there is asplenia, polysplenia, or a bilobed spleen, situs specificity of the viscera and of the atria tends to be lost. On the other hand, it should be noted and emphasized that splenic abnormalities may be encountered in cases of determined atria, both in mirror-image dextrocardia, as well as in mixed dextrocardia. There are also occasional cases of discordant thoracoabdominal situs without splenic abnormality.

In general, when the atria are determined, the systemic abdominal and thoracic venous returns are usually normal, that is, into the morphological right atrium. Discordance between the atria and abdominal venous return occurs in the presence of polysplenia. From our material, it appears that in the absence of splenic abnormalities, the entry of the inferior vena cava and of a single superior vena cava generally identifies the position of the morphological right atrium, perhaps more so than the situs of the abdominal organs. When both superior vena cava are present, the right and left superior vena cava entering an atrium directly does not necessarily help identify the atrial septal morphology.

It is also of interest that the position of the aortic and pulmonic anuli in both dextroversion and mirror-image dextrocardia without transposition may be nearly similar in that the aortic anulus in some cases of dextroversion is situated posterior and to the left, and the pulmonic anulus, anterior and to the right as in mirror-image dextrocardia. Thus, in some cases, no differentiation can be made between these two types of dextrocardia in this regard. However, the aortic orifice may be situated slightly to the right and posterior to the pulmonary orifice in dextroversion. This may constitute a point of differentiation in these cases.

The position of the pulmonary trunk also is quite different in the two types of dextrocardia without transposition. The pulmonary trunk swings to the left horizontally and dips posteriorly to the left side of the aorta in dextroversion; in mirror-image dextrocardia, it passes to the right of the aorta posteriorly. In our material, the position of the anterior descending coronary artery is also a point of differentiation. In dextroversion, where the left ventricle is anterior and to the left, it emerges from the left side of the aorta. In mirror-image dextrocardia and in mixed dextrocardia with pivotal atria, where the left ventricle is situated posterior and to the right, the anterior descending coronary artery emerges from the right side of the aorta.

Thus, the position of the ventricles, whether they are in a mirror-image position or in a pivotal position in the absence of transposition, is best indicated by the course of the pulmonary trunk and ascending aorta, as well as by that of the anterior descending coronary artery. When there is transposition and both arterial orifices are open, the right- or left-sidedness of the aortic anulus, vis-à-vis the pulmonic anulus, indicates regular or inverted transposition, respectively, thereby revealing the location of the right and left ventricles. However, where there is pulmonary atresia, the left-sidedness of the aorta may not be apparent in inverted transposition, as the small pulmonary trunk is usually hidden behind the aorta. In this respect, the convexity of the aorta may be of some help in that it tends to be directed to the left in an inverted transposition (that is, in mixed dextrocardia with pivotal atria), but the convexity of the aorta is to the right in the noninverted type (that is, in dextroversion with transposition).

It is important to remember that the abdominal visceral situs indicates the position of the atria in general, but not in all. Likewise, the position of the great arteries indicates, in general, the type of bulboventricular loop and, hence, the identity of the ventricles can be made when there is transposition and both arterial trunks emerge from the heart. However, it is important, again, to remember that when there is pulmonary atresia it will be extremely difficult to decide the type of bulboventricular loop as well as to identify the ventricular chambers. When there is no transposition, the position of the semilunar ostia may not be a reliable differentiating point between mirror-image dextrocardia and dextroversion. Here, the position of the pulmonic trunk and its relationship to the aorta and the position of the anterior descending coronary artery may be useful.

It is also important to point out that the atria in dextroversion are *not* in normal position. It is true vis-à-vis the situs, that is, the left- or right-sidedness of the atria. However, *it is not true vis-à-vis the anteroposteriority of the atria*. When the atria are in the normal position, the right atrium is situated to the right and anterior, whereas the left atrium is situated to the left and posterior. In dextroversion, the right atrium is not only situated to the right but *rotated slightly posteriorly*, and the left atrium is situated to the left and *rotated slightly anteriorly*. Thus, the position of the atria in dextroversion is as if the atria were pivoted around horizontally clockwise, looking in a direction caudad so that they are almost side by side.

Mixed dextrocardia with "pivotal" atria is usually seen with inverted transposition with VSD and pulmonary stenosis or atresia. These may be associated with a straddling conus (parietal band) and pulmonary atresia. In the presence of asplenia, there is a tendency for the occurrence of various forms of inverted transposition associated with mitral and pulmonary atresia or with common AV orifice. Our material again stresses the association of endocardial cushion defects with truncoconal anomalies in abnormalities of the spleen in positional abnormalities of the cardiac chambers.

Embryogenesis

The forces responsible for the normal shifting of the apex to the left from its more or less midline position in an earlier stage of development of the heart, and disturbance of such forces in dextroversion are as yet unknown. Likewise, the basic factors responsible for situs solitus, and the disturbance therefore of such factors in situs inversus have yet to be elucidated to explain mirror-image dextrocardia. Furthermore, still unexplained are the basic factors responsible for the genesis of the so-called levo-bulboventricular loop instead of the normal dextro-bulboventricular loop in mixed dextrocardia with "pivotal" atria. However, we hypothesize that in some it may be related to a very specific DNA marker system in the very early stages of the development of the embryo itself.

The anatomic data that will be most useful for the clinicians and surgeons in determining the identity and the position of the chambers are: (a) the site of entry of the inferior and of a single (solitary) superior vena cava for the determination of atria; (b) the course of the anterior descending coronary artery, with or without transposition, for the determination of ventricular morphology; (c) the position and course of the pulmonary trunk when there is no transposition, for the identification of the ventricles; (d) the position of the pulmonic and aortic anuli when there is transposition, and both of these orifices are patent (open) for the identification of ventricles.

The occurrence of congenital AV block in mixed dextrocardia with ventricular inversion is similar to mixed levocardia with ventricular inversion (corrected transposition heart). When there is indeterminate atria in dextrocardia, undetermined type, there is a tendency for arrhythmias to occur, similar to isolated levocardia with partial visceral heterotaxy, common atrium, and polysplenia. There is a distinct tendency for congenital AV block to occur with polysplenia in dextrocardia similar to mesocardia and isolated levocardia.

Postoperative heart block and supraventricular arrhythmias following surgery are also noted. Likewise, sudden death several years following surgery in "asymptomatic and healthy young adults" also occurs in this entity.

Differentiation Between Dextroversion and Criss-Cross Hearts

Is there a relationship between hypoplastic or small right ventricle and dextroversion? The frequent association of tricuspid valve anomalies in this type of dextrocardia suggests that there probably is a relationship between the two entities, at least in some. The heart in dextroversion is rotated horizontally on its axis to the right, resulting in a horizontal septum mimicking or simulating a criss-cross or upstairs-downstairs heart (Figs. 126—128). It is important to understand that dextroverted hearts *are not* true criss-cross hearts.

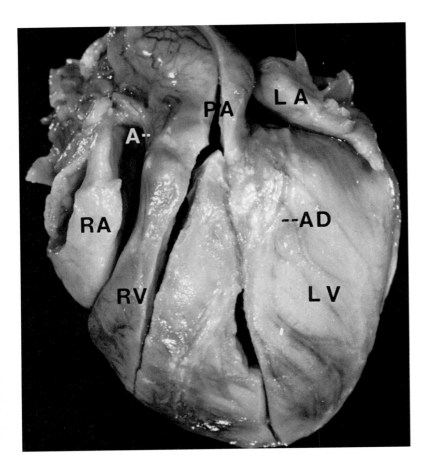

Figure 126: External view of the heart in dextroversion with tricuspid atresia and aortic atresia. RA = right atrial appendage; LA = left atrial appendage; RV = right ventricle; LV = left ventricle; PA = pulmonary artery; A = aorta; AD = anterior descending coronary artery. (Used with permission from Thilenius et al. See Figure 128.)

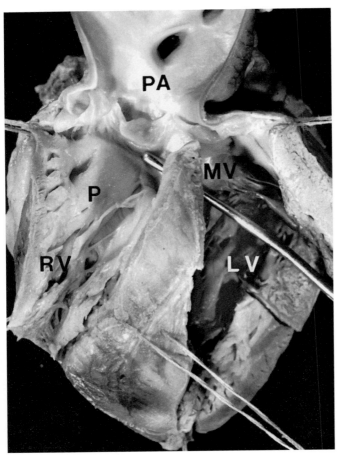

Figure 127: Right ventricular view of heart shown in Figure 126. LV = left ventricle; RV = right ventricle; MV = mitral valve; PA = pulmonary artery overriding the defect; P = parietal band straddling or passing through the VSD. Probe passing through the U-shaped VSD. (Used with permission from Thilenius, et al. See Figure 128.)

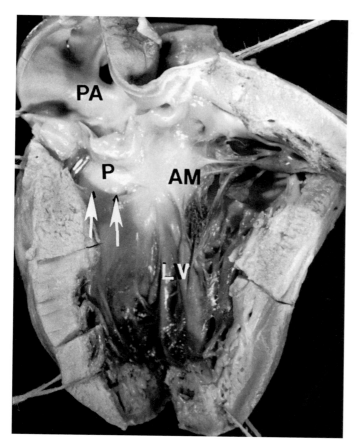

Figure 128: Left ventricular view of heart shown in Figures 126 and 127. LV = left ventricle; PA = pulmonary artery overriding the defect; P = straddling parietal band; AM = anterior mitral leaflet. Arrows point to the straddling parietal band and the probe passing through the U-shaped VSD. (Used with permission from Horizontal ventricular septum with dextroversion hearts with and without aortic atresia. Thilenius, et al., *Pediatr Cardiol* 8:187—193, 1987.)

There probably are several genes responsible for the positional abnormalities of the heart and its chambers. In some, this may occur during the early stages of the development of the embryo itself. This may explain the complicated congenital cardiac anomalies that are usually encountered in dextrocardia associated with splenic anomalies, anomalies in the visceral situs, anomalies in the lungs, and venous anomalies. This area needs a great deal of attention in the future.

Abbreviations:

FO = fossa ovalis; FOD = fossa ovalis defect; PS = pulmonary stenosis; TI = tricuspid insufficiency; TS = tricuspid stenosis; CS = coronary sinus; CT = complete transposition; CAVO = common atrioventricular orifice; BiPV = bicuspid pulmonary valve; TI = tricuspid insufficiency; Rt = right side; MS = mitral stenosis; Lt = left side; LAA = left aortic arch; RAA = right aortic arch; RPDA = right patent ductus arteriosus; RSVC = right superior vena cava; RAP = right atrial appendage; PA = pulmonary atresia; AS = aortic stenosis; AI = aortic insufficiency; LP = left pulmonary vein; VS = ventricular septum; RtSVC = right superior vena cava; LtSVC = left superior vena cava; AV = atrioventricular; LLPV = left lower pulmonary vein; CC = common cartoid artery; RCC = right common cartoid artery; LtAA = left aortic arch; LtPV = left pulmonary vein.

61

Isolated Levocardia

In isolated levocardia, the base apex or the longitudinal axis of the heart points to the left, while there is partial or complete situs inversus abdominalis. The organs in the thorax may show symmetrical likeness, with trilobated lungs on both sides and two superior vena cavae, or there may be situs inversus thoracis. There is often an associated asplenia or polysplenia.

General Statement

In this entity, the atria are usually presumptively in the normal position. That is, usually an absolute diagnosis of the position of the atria cannot be made because of the absence of or defective atrial septum. However, the morphology of the atrial appendages would indicate that they are in the normal position. When that is the case, there may be two superior vena cavae, one entering each atrium or the left may enter a coronary sinus, or there may be only a right superior vena cava entering the presumptive right atrium. The inferior vena cava, when present, may enter the left atrium. Often there is absence of the inferior vena cava and then the azygos may constitute the venous return from the abdomen and enter the right superior vena cava or the hemiazygos may enter the left superior vena cava. The right and left hepatic veins may enter the right and left atrium, respectively. When there is a left superior vena cava, the coronary sinus may be absent. The pulmonary veins very often open into the systemic venous circuit, either completely or partially.

When the atria are in the presumptively normal position, the ventricles are usually also in the normal position. Under these circumstances, it is not unusual to have a common AV orifice with complete noninverted transposition with pulmonary stenosis or atresia. In fewer cases, there is no transposition. Rarely, complete transposition with aortic atresia and fetal coarctation with ventricular septal defect may occur.

In some cases, the atria are presumptively in the normal position but the ventricles are inverted. In two cases, the atria and ventricles were relatively in the normal position, but they abnormally connected the right atrium to the left ventricle and the left atrium to the right ventricle. In two such cases, there was an associated common AV orifice in one case with inverted transposition and pulmonary atresia, and in another there was noninverted transposition.

In a small number of cases, the atria may be inverted. The veins then enter normally. Generally, where the ventricles were noninverted, there was complete noninverted transposition with ventricular septal defect and pulmonary stenosis. In one case, there was common AV orifice with pulmonary stenosis.

Definition of Terminology

"Isolated levocardia" falls under the broader classification of levocardia with visceral heterotaxy and is defined as that condition in which the heart is normally located. That is, the heart is in the left hemithorax with its base-apex pointing to the left but the remainder of the body viscera are situated in varying degrees of situs inversus or heterotaxia. A true "isolated levocardia" is the extreme form in which the viscera are in complete situs inversus, the mirror-image of the normal, and there is a normal spleen located in the right upper abdomen. In the less extreme form, levocardia is associated with only partial situs inversus of the abdominal viscera, where some of the abdominal organs may be completely inverted, or some only mildly rotated, and some in normal situs solitus position.

Thus, in order to clarify the partial visceral heterotaxy from complete situs inversus, both the thoracic and the abdominal viscera must be carefully evaluated. The situs of the thorax is determined by lobation of the lungs and by the bronchial branching pattern. In thoracis situs inversus, there is a bilobed lung on the right and a trilobed lung on the left. Thoracic symmetry implies bilateral bi-, tri-, or quadrilobated lungs. The location of the superior vena cava (SVC) and its entry into a chamber varies considerably in isolated levocardia and therefore may not be useful as a determinate of thoracic situs. The situs of the abdomen is defined by the position or location of the major organs.

The term "complete inversion" implies the mirror-image of normal. Partial abdominal situs inversus or heterotaxy is that condition in which only some of the abdominal organs are inverted or in an abnormal position, especially those derived from the superior tract of the developing digestive system, that is, the stomach, duodenum, liver, biliary passages, pancreas, and spleen. Those developed from the lower gastrointestinal tract, that is, the cecum and the distal abdominal structures, may be either in a normal position or malrotated.

The Spleen

Of major significance in evaluating the situs is determination of the status of the spleen. Polysplenia is defined as that condition when there are two or more nearly equal-sized splenic masses. The term "asplenia" implies that there is complete absence of splenic tissue. In accessory spleen, a nearly normal-sized splenic mass is associated with one or more additional small spleens.

Identification of Chambers

The cardiac chambers are identified by their morphological characteristics. If atrial and ventricular septa are present, a positive identification of the chamber can be made. If the septa were absent or not well defined, the chambers are classified as indeterminate. In some cases, however, with indeterminate atria, a presumptive diagnosis could be made on the basis of atrial appendages where the septa was not diagnostic. The venous connections are too inconsistent and not reliable for chamber diagnosis.

The right atrium is diagnosed by the presence of the limbus fossae ovalis, and the left atrium by the presence of the upturned arch of the derivative of the septum primum. The right ventricle is identified by the presence of the inlet or the sinus, the apical recess and the conus or the outflow tract or the infundibulum characterized by the septal and parietal bands forming an arch beneath the efferent vessel. The left ventricle is identified by its smooth outflow tract and finely trabeculated apical portion.

The term "inversion of the ventricles" implies that the morphologically right ventricle is situated on the left side and the morphologically left ventricle is situated on the right side. The term "situs" is used to refer to the position of the abdominal viscera, and to the position of the cardiac atria. It is not used to refer to cardiac ventricles or to the position of the heart in the chest.

The term "mixed levocardia" refers to the relationship of the atria and ventricles to one another and does not imply the relationship regarding body situs, which may be situs solitus or inversus. In "mixed levocardia," the atria and ventricles are discordant. That is, the morphologically right atrium enters the morphologically left ventricle, and the morphologically left atrium enters the morphologically right ventricle. Thus, levocardia with visceral heterotaxy includes some cases with "mixed levocardia."

The term "transposition" in levocardia refers to: (1) the abnormal anteroposterior relationship of the great arteries to one another, and/or (2) the abnormal origin of the great vessels from the chambers from which they emerge, and/or (3) the abnormal relationship of the great vessels to the atrioventricular valves. Regular (noninverted) transposition indicates that the aorta is to the right of the pulmonary trunk (d-transposition). In inverted transposition, there is an abnormal relationship of the great arteries from the standpoint of laterality in that the aorta lies to the left of the pulmonary trunk. It is, however, emphasized that there are exceptions to this differentiation.

The venous drainage is considered to be normal when the systemic veins enter the morphologically right atrium and the pulmonary veins enter the morphologically left atrium.

Analysis of Our Material

There was a total of 79 cases; 47 were male subjects and 32 were female subjects. The youngest was a 25-weeks' gestation stillborn fetus and the oldest was a 58-year-old male. The median age was 3 years, 6 months.

Isolated levocardia with partial visceral heterotaxy may be classified as follows:

I. Isolated levocardia with visceral heterotaxy and situs solitus atria   18

II. Isolated levocardia with visceral heterotaxy, situs solitus atria, and ventricular inversion   2

III. Isolated levocardia with visceral heterotaxy, situs inversus atria, and ventricles normal   11

IV. Isolated levocardia with visceral heterotaxy, indeterminate atria, and ventricles in normal position   41

V. Isolated levocardia with visceral heterotaxy, indeterminate atria, and ventricular inversion   7

I. Isolated Levocardia with Visceral Heterotaxy and Situs Solitus Atria

In this group, the morphological right atrium was on the right side and the morphological left atrium on the left. There were 18 cases in this category. All had varying degrees of partial visceral heterotaxy and splenic abnormalities.

Eleven were male subjects and seven were female subjects. The ages ranged from a 1½-hour-old newborn infant to 37 years, with a mean age of 4 years, 9 months. It is of interest that 11 (61%) were below the age of 1 month.

The splenic abnormalities were:

Asplenia	9
Polysplenia	5
Accessory spleen	3
Heterotopic splenic mass in pancreas and heterotopic pancreatic mass in spleen	1

Pulmonary Venous Abnormalities

Total anomalous pulmonary venous drainage	4

In others, varying types of partial anomalous and systemic venous anomalies were present. The complexes in this entity were:

Complete transposition with PA, CAVO, PAPVD—RPV → RA, LSVC → CS, RAA, left ductus, single coronary and accessory mitral orifice, and congenital AV block—polysplenia	3 days M
Huge ASD, FOD proximal type, and PDA Accessory spleen	8 days M
Complete transposition with PA, CAVO dominant Lt, FOD, LSVC → LA, small CS—asplenia	7 months M
Complete transposition with PA and multiple VSDs, restrictive subaortic VSD, and FOD, RA—hepatic vein and LSVC → CS—polysplenia	11 days M
Complete transposition, PA, mitral atresia, PDA, ostium primum and FOD, absent CS—asplenia (Figs. 1, 2)	6 mo, 26 days M

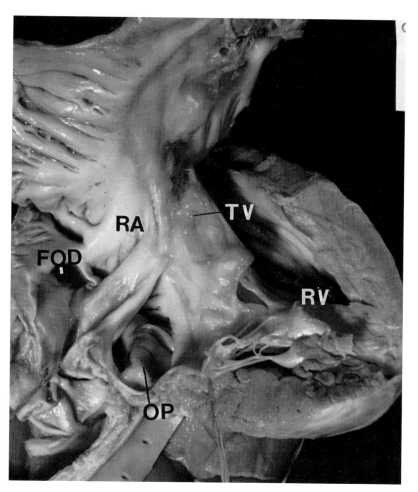

Figure 1: Isolated levocardia, visceral heterotaxy, atria situs solitus with asplenia, complete transposition, and mitral atresia, with ostium primum and fossa ovalis defect. Right atrial, right ventricular view. FOD = fossa ovalis defect; RA = right atrium; RV = right ventricle; TV = tricuspid valve; OP = ostium primum defect.

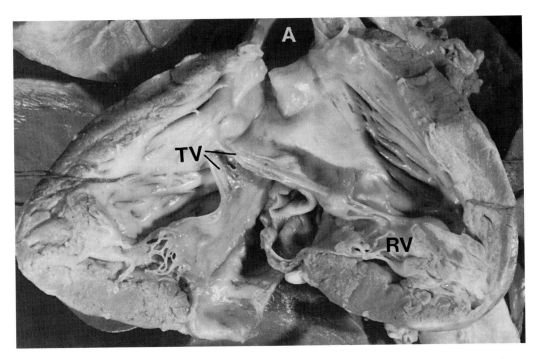

Figure 2: Outflow tract of the right ventricle from which emerges the aorta. RV = right ventricle; TV = tricuspid valve; A = aorta.

Complete transposition with mitral and PA, tortuous, elongated PDA, FOD, large single left coronary ostium, absent SVC, hepatic veins → the RA, LSVC → CS. CS displaced to central fibrous body, wandering pacemaker—asplenia   3 days F

CT with PA and mitral atresia, TAPVD → RA, PDA from innominate artery and absent CS—asplenia   2 days F

Common ventricle, CAVO, CT atypical, overriding aorta, straddling conus, TAPVD → RA. Large FOD, absent CS, hepatic veins → RA, IVC → LA—asplenia   2 months F (twin 39-wk)

Single ventricle with regular transposition, CAVO, TAPVD and pulmonary atresia—asplenia   15 years M

DORV, CAVO dominant right, FC, aortic valvular and sub AS, hepatic vein → RA and absent IVC. Hemiazygos → RSVC, polysplenia and congenital AV block   1 day F

DORV, CAVO noncommitted type, infundibular valvular PS, atypical FO and proximal type ASD, bicuspid PV, hepatic vein → the RA, IVC → LA, LSVC and coronary veins → LA, CS absent—asplenia   30 years M

Paraductal coarctation with VSD, aortic and mitral stenosis, bicuspid aortic valve and absent IVC, hemiazygos → LSVC → CS → RA Rt hepatic vein → RA. Lt hepatic vein → LSVC → CS → RA—accessory spleen Rt   17 days F

Aortic stenosis, mitral atresia, and cor triatriatum, fossa ovalis defect, IVC straddling RA → LA, hepatic vein → RA, polysplenia   1½ hours M

Aneurysm of pars membranacea with VSD, fenestrated aortic valve, overriding aorta, absent IVC, hemiazygos → LSVC → CS → RA. Hepatic vein → RA—accessory spleen Rt (Figs. 3—5)   37 years M

Tricuspid atresia with pulmonary stenosis without transposition, TAPVD → Lt gastric vein, ASD fossa ovalis and primum types, bicuspid aortic valve and cleft in anterior leaflet of the mitral valve, IVC → RA Lt hepatic vein → LA—asplenia   15 days F

Absent IVC, hepatic veins into the right atrium, azygos extension → RSVC—polysplenia   2 years F

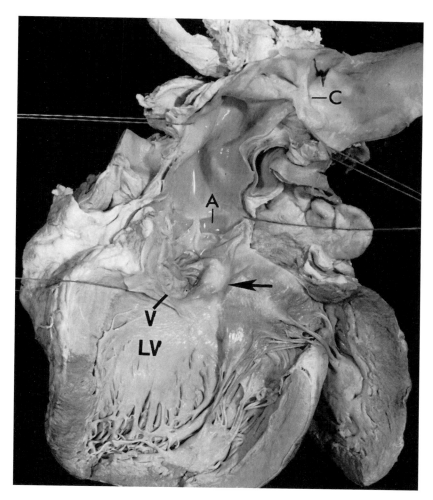

Figure 3: Levocardia with visceral heterotaxy and situs solitus atria, aneurysm of the membranous septum with surgical closure of ventricular septal defect, and anatomic coarctation of the aorta in a 37-year-old male, left ventricular view. LV = left ventricle; V = surgical closure of the defect; A = aorta; C = coarctation. Arrow points to the aneurysm of the membranous septum. (Used with permission from Liberthson RR, et al. See Figure 34.)

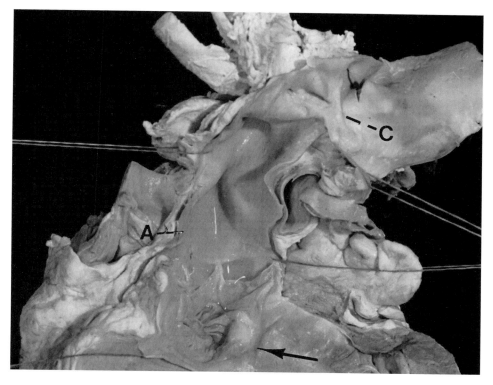

Figure 4: Close-up view of the aneurysm. A = aorta; C = coarctation. Arrow points to the aneurysm of the membranous septum.

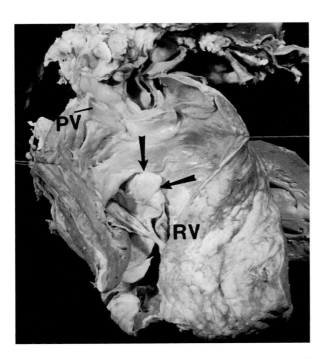

Figure 5: Aneurysm of the pars membranacea as seen from the right ventricle. RV = right ventricle; PV = pulmonary valve. Arrows point to the aneurysm of the membranous septum at the junction of the anterior and septal leaflets of the tricuspid valve.

ASD, fossa ovalis type, PDA, quadricuspid pulmonic and aortic valves and anomalous vein entering the coronary sinus, and trisomy D syndrome—heterotopic splenic tissue in pancreas and vice versa	27 days F
CAVO indeterminate, DORV, pulmonary stenosis, CS → LA, atypical ASD, anomalous vein → LA, bicuspid PV—asplenia (Figs. 6, 7)	25 days M

One polysplenia with complete transposition, pulmonary atresia, CAVO, and partial pulmonary venous drainage and another polysplenia, CAVO and DORV had congenital AV block. There was one remarkable heart; a 2-year-old female with polysplenia who had atresia of the portal vein and absent IVC with hepatic veins entering the right atrium and azygos extension into the right SVC with no other anomalies in the heart. This child had several liver transplantations.

Seven had CAVO. In seven with transposition and pulmonary atresia, there were three with mitral atresia. One had straddling conus with overriding aorta. There were three with double outlet right ventricle. Six had no transposition but one in this group had overriding aorta.

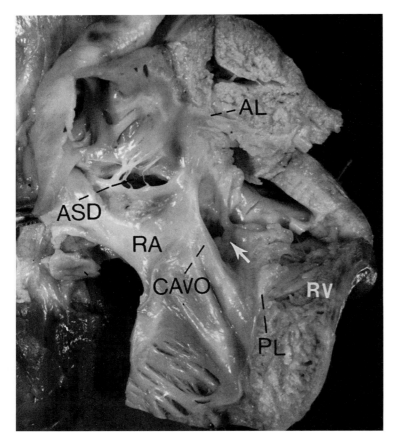

Figure 6: Isolated levocardia visceral heterotaxy, situs solitus, atria, with common AV orifice, intermediate type. RA = right atrium; ASD = atrial septal defect, fossa ovalis type; AL = anterior bridging leaflet; PL = posterior bridging leaflet; CAVO = common AV orifice; RV = right ventricle. Arrow points to the intermediate type of common AV valve.

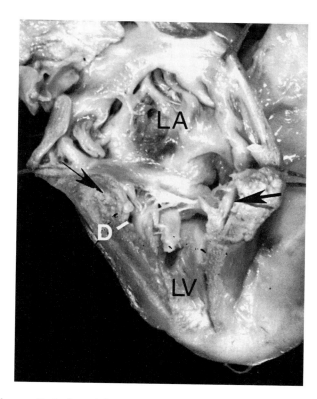

Figure 7: Left atrial aspect of the common AV orifice. LA = left atrial aspect of the common AV orifice; LV = left ventricle; D = accessory VSD. Arrows point to the connections of the common AV valve on the left side.

II. Isolated Levocardia with Visceral Heterotaxy, Situs Solitus Atria, and Ventricular Inversion

In this rare group, although the atria were in the normal position, the ventricles were inverted or in mirror-image of the normal. The left ventricle was on the right and anterior and the right ventricle was on the left and posterior. Both had asplenia and both lungs were symmetrical; however, one had partial visceral heterotaxy and the other complete situs inversus abdomen.

There were two cases: one male aged 15 days, and one female aged 2 months, 20 days.

The complexes were:

Asplenia with partial visceral heterotaxy, CAVO, pulmonary atresia, TAPVD → portal vein, FOD, LAA, and Rt PDA from innominate. RA—hepatic vein and absent RSVC. Azygos extension of IVC → LSVC → CS → LA, accessory VSD   2 mo, 20 days F

Asplenia with complete situs inversus abdomen, CAVO, SV inverted ventricular mass and regular transposition and coarctation of the aorta, TAPVD → RSVC → RA. Hepatic vein → RA. Absent CS. LSVC and IVC → LA (Figs. 8, 9)   15 days M

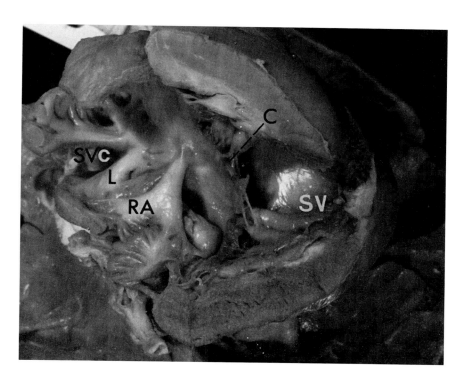

Figure 8: Isolated levocardia with situs solitus atria, single ventricle and inversion of the ventricular mass (L loop), regular (noninverted) double outlet right ventricle and common AV orifice. Right atrial view and view of the main ventricular mass. RA = right atrium; C = common AV valve; SVC = superior vena cava; L = limbus fossa ovalis; SV = single ventricle. (Used with permission from Liberthson RR, et al. See Figure 34.)

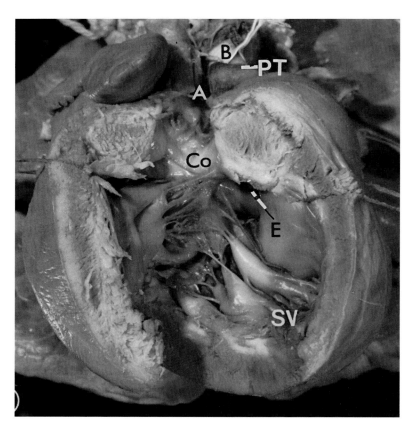

Figure 9: View of the main ventricular mass. SV = single ventricle; E = entry into the small outlet chamber; Co = conus of aorta; PT = pulmonary trunk emerging from the small outlet chamber; A = aorta; B = banding of the main pulmonary trunk. (Used with permission from Liberthson RR, et al. See Figure 34.) Note the double coni and the aorta situated to the right and the pulmonary trunk to the left—regular transposition.

III. Isolated Levocardia with Visceral Heterotaxy, Situs Inversus Atria and Ventricles Normal

In all cases the morphologically right atrium and right ventricle were lateral to the left atrium and left ventricle, and the ventricles were in the normal position. That is, the atria were inverted and ventricles noninverted, resulting in "mixed levocardia" in all.

There was a total of 11 cases; six females and five males. The ages ranged from 3 weeks to 58 years, with an average age of 11 years, 4 months, 22 days. The 3-week-old had CAVO and pulmonary stenosis, and the oldest had mild subpulmonary stenosis, tricuspid insufficiency, and acquired AV block. Seven out of 11 were above 1 year of age, and only one was below the age of 1 month.

Eight had complete situs inversus, seven had right aortic arch, nine had normal spleens (located on the right side), and two had accessory spleens. The three that did not have complete situs inversus differed in that two had symmetrical and one solitus lungs. One

had a persistent right superior vena cava and hemi-azygos veins, both of which entered the left atrium, as well as partial pulmonary venous drainage. In one, the morphologically left atrium also received a persistent small right superior vena cava and the coronary sinus, and in the third, the coronary veins entered both the atria.

The complexes present were:

Regular noninverted complete transposition with VSD, pulmonary stenosis and tricuspid stenosis and RAA (Figs. 10, 11)	4 months M
Regular noninverted complete transposition with VSD and pulmonary atresia, both coronary from left sinus and RAA	20 months F
Regular noninverted complete transposition with CAVO and pulmonary atresia, left aortic arch	8 months F
Regular noninverted complete transposition with VSD and PS, 2 PV →	

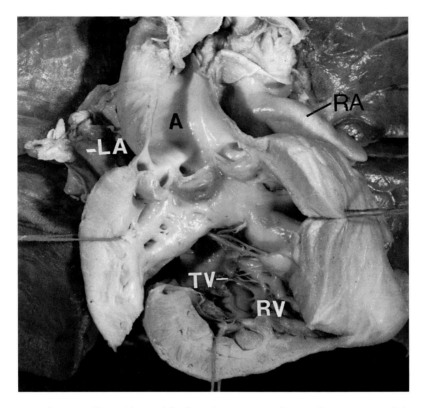

Figure 10: Levocardia with atrial situs inversus and complete transposition, right ventricular view. RV = right ventricle; TV = tricuspid valve; A = aorta emerging from the right ventricle; LA = left atrium situated to the right and anterior communicates with the morphologically right ventricle from which emerges the aorta; RA = right atrium situated to the left and posterior communicates with the morphologically left ventricle situated to the left and posterior.

RA and 2 PV → LA, and hemiazygos → LA and RAA (Fig. 12)	19 years M
Regular noninverted complete transposition with VSD and PS, bicuspid PV, both coronary arteries emerged from the left sinus, and RAA (Figs. 13—17)	30 years F
DORV, VSD, with pulmonary stenosis and sinus venosus ASD, RA—LSVC and IVC, LA—RSVC, CS and P veins and left aortic arch	2 years F
Complete transposition (noninverted) with overriding pulmonary trunk and pulmonary valvular, and infundibular stenosis, large VSD, straddling MV, right aortic arch, fossa ovalis defect, bicuspid pulmonary valve, (Figs. 18—21)	19 months F
Subpulmonary stenosis, tricuspid insufficiency, RAA acquired complete AV block	58 years M
ASD, VSD, mild Ebstein's anomaly with tricuspid insufficiency, bicuspid PV with valvular and infundibular stenosis and straddling conus, small LSVC → CS and coronary vein → RA and LA, marked fat in LV and RV, RAA, and sudden death	11 years M
Single ventricle small outlet chamber, noninverted regular complete transposition with common AV orifice RAA, and pulmonary stenosis and accessory spleen	3 weeks M
Single ventricle, regular transposition, pulmonary atresia, right aortic arch, ASD fossa ovalis type, left patent ductus, juxtaposition of the right atrial appendage above the left and diverticulum of single ventricle, Lt AV valve stenosis, LSVC, IVC and CS → RA, and accessory spleen	11 mo, 13 day F

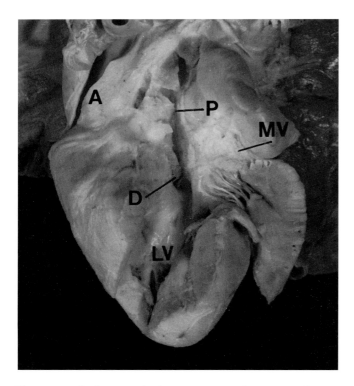

Figure 11: Left ventricle demonstrating the ventricular septal defect, pulmonary valvular and subpulmonic stenosis. LV = left ventricle; D = ventricular septal defect; P = pulmonic valve; MV = mitral valve; A = aorta. Note the bicuspid pulmonic valve with infundibular and valvular stenosis.

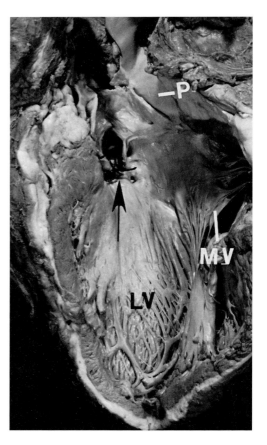

Figure 12: Pulmonary trunk emerging from the left ventricle and surgical closure of the ventricular septal defect in a 19-year-old male. MV = mitral valve; LV = left ventricle; P = pulmonary valve, bicuspid with stenosis. Arrow points to surgical closure of the defect.

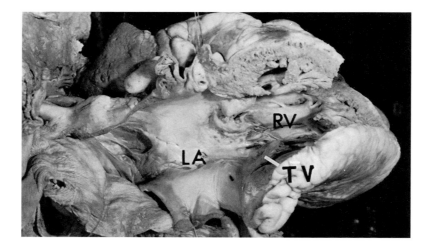

Figure 13: Isolated levocardia with situs inversus atria — mixed levocardia or AV discordance and regular noninverted complete transposition with VSD and pulmonary stenosis (corrected transposition in a 30-year-old female). Left atrial, right ventricular view. LA = left atrium; RV = right ventricle; TV = tricuspid valve. (Used with permission from Liberthson RR, et al. See Figure 34.)

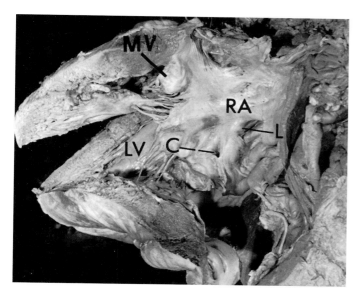

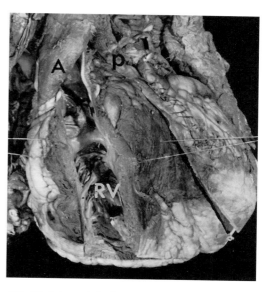

Figure 14: Right atrial, left ventricular view. RA = right atrium situated to the left; LV = left ventricle; C = coronary sinus; L = limbus fossae ovalis; MV = mitral valve. (Used with permission from Liberthson RR, et al. See Figure 34.)

Figure 15: Right ventricular view showing the aorta emerging from the morphologically right ventricle but the circulation is physiologically corrected. RV = right ventricle; A = aorta; P = pulmonary trunk. (Used with permission from Liberthson RR, et al. See Figure 34.)

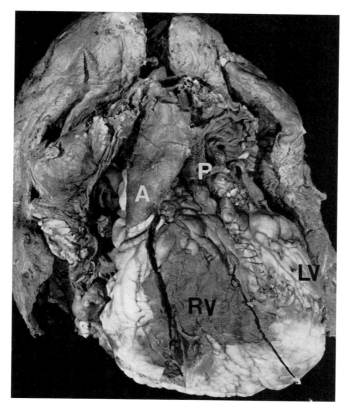

Figure 16: External view of levocardia with atrial inversion. RV = right ventricle; LV = left ventricle; A = aorta; P = pulmonary trunk. Note the aorta emerging from the morphologically right ventricle but the circulation is physiologically corrected.

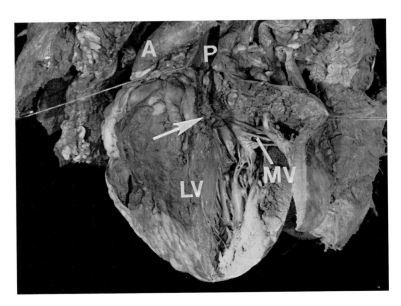

Figure 17: Pulmonary trunk emerging from the left ventricle. P = pulmonary trunk; LV = left ventricle; MV = mitral valve; A = aorta. Arrow points to the surgical closure of the ventricular septal defect.

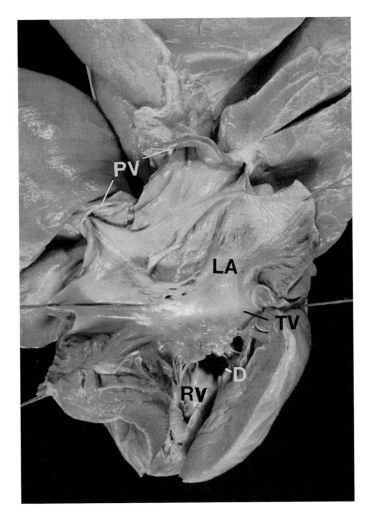

Figure 18: Atrial situs inversus in levocardia — corrected transposition in a 19-month-old female child with left AV valve insufficiency. Left atrial, right ventricular view, left atrium receiving the pulmonary veins. LA = left atrium; PV = pulmonary veins; RV = morphologically right ventricle; D = defect; TV = tricuspid valve.

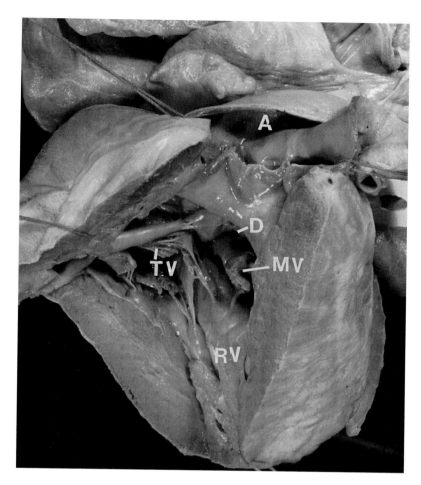

Figure 19: Outflow tract of the right ventricle showing the aorta emerging from this chamber; A = aorta; D = ventricular septal defect; TV = tricuspid valve; RV = right ventricle; MV = mitral valve straddling through the defect.

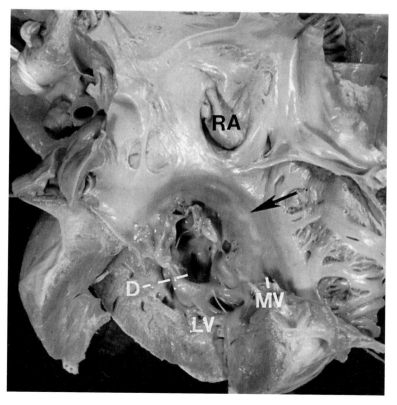

Figure 20: Right atrial, left ventricular view. Right atrium receiving the systemic veins. Note the large ventricular septal defect with straddling mitral valve. RA = right atrium situated to left; LV = left ventricle; D = defect; MV = straddling mitral valve. Arrow points to the straddling mitral valve.

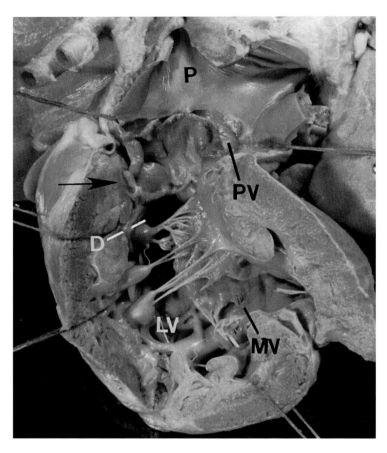

Figure 21: From the left ventricle emerges the pulmonary trunk with valvular and subpulmonary stenosis. PV = bicuspid pulmonic valve; MV = mitral valve, straddling; LV = left ventricle; D = defect, huge; P = pulmonary trunk. Arrow points to the subpulmonary stenosis. Note the huge ventricular septal defect, almost a common ventricle.

Eight had pulmonary and subpulmonary stenosis, and three had pulmonary atresia. Six had VSD, two with single ventricle, and two with common AV orifice. The oldest had subpulmonary stenosis and tricuspid insufficiency with intact ventricular septum. This was the only case with intact ventricular septum. There were nine with right aortic arch and two with a left aortic arch.

IV. Isolated Levocardia with Visceral Heterotaxy, Indeterminate Atria, and Ventricles in Normal Position

In this group, there was a common atrium, mostly associated with a common AV orifice in almost all, making it difficult to establish the situs solitus; however, the ventricles were in the normal position.

There was a total of 41 cases in this group; 24 were males and 17 were females. The youngest was a 25-

weeks' gestation stillborn fetus, and the oldest was 12 years with a mean age of 1 year, 3 months, 10 days. Twenty-two (53.6%) were below the age of 1 month.

All had varying degrees of visceral heterotaxy and although some had abdominal situs inversus, the lungs were either multilobated or bilobed. Thus, none had complete situs inversus and all had splenic abnormalities, although in three the status of the spleen was unknown. The most distinguishing feature in this group is the presence of a common atrium or almost a common atrium in all.

The complexes were:

Asplenia, almost common atrium, CT, CAVO, PA, TAPVD → portal vein, absent PDA, absent CS. LSVC → LA   13 days M

Polysplenia, common atrium, CT with aortic atresia with VSD, overriding PT, aberrant Lt subclavian artery, SVC, IVC, and P veins → LA   1 hour F

Situs inversus abdominalis, spleen Rt, common atrium, CT, CAVO, PS, RAA, Lt PDA, bicuspid PV, absent CS, Rt side—small RSVC and P vein, LSVC → Lt side — 16 days M

Asplenia, common atrium, SV, CT with PA, PDA → Lt lung, LSVC and IVC → Lt. RSVC and hepatic vein → Rt side, probable TAPVD — 5 mo, 14 days M

Asplenia, common atrium, CAVO, SV, CT and PA, bronchials → lungs, and absent CS — 12 days M

Polysplenia, common atrium, SV, transposition, straddling Lt AV valve, FC, PDA, single coronary and juxtaposed atrial appendages to the left, P veins → Rt. Systemic veins → Lt — Stillborn (32-wk gest.) M

Polysplenia, common atrium, CAVO indeterminate, subaortic stenosis, Rt—RSVC, hepatic vein and 2 P veins. Lt—CS and LSVC and congenital AV block — 15 days M

Polysplenia, common atrium, CAVO, CT and PA, Rt—RSVC, hepatic vein, LSVC, small CS and 2 P veins. Lt—2 PV and congenital AV block — newborn M

Asplenia, common atrium, DORV, CAVO, dominant Rt, bicuspid PV with infundibular and valvular stenosis, absent CS, common P vein in part → LA, with stenosis, and in part → LSVC—innominate → RSVC — 19 days M

Spleen unknown, common atrium, common ventricle, CAVO, CT with PA, PAPVD, 2 PV → RA, absent CS. RAA and Lt PDA — 2 days M

Asplenia, common atrium, CAVO, common ventricle, CT with PA, LAA and Rt PDA, single coronary artery, TAPVD → Rt, Small CS → Rt. LSVC → Lt — 10 months F

Polysplenia, common atrium, CAVO, TAPVD → Rt Absent IVC, hepatic vein, CS, RSVC → Rt. Hepatic veins, azygos and LSVC → Lt — 1 month F

Asplenia, common atrium, CAVO, CT, PA, accessory VSD, TAPVD → RSVC. CS → Lt — 9 months M

Small spleen on Rt, common atrium, CAVO, SV, CT with PA, large bronchial → Rt lung, TAPVD →

portal. Rt—RSVC, LSVC, IVC, and small CS — 1 month M

Polysplenia, common atrium, cleft in anterior leaflet of the MV, absent IVC Rt—hepatic vein and azygos → RSVC. Lt—LSVC, CS, and P veins — 4½ months F

Spleen unknown, almost a common atrium, partial visceral heterotaxy, DORV with mitral atresia with no VSD, FC, bicuspid AV and PAPVD, Lt PV → LSVC → innominate vein — 2 weeks F

Abdominal situs inversus except spleen on Lt, common atrium, CAVO, SV, both vessels from SOC, and no transposition. RAA—Rt PDA, bicuspid PV, PAPVD, Rt PV → Rt, absent IVC and CS and azygos → RSVC. Lt-Lt PV and LSVC, and supraventricular arrhythmia — 10 years F

Polysplenia, common atrium, CAVO, PAPVD, Rt—Rt PV and coronary vein. Lt—Lt PV, LSVC and RSVC, hemiazygos → SVC, hepatic vein and coronary veins and arrhythmias — 4½ months M

Polysplenia, common atrium, CAVO indeterminate, bicuspid AV, probable TAPVD and absent CS (Fig. 22) — 4 months M

Spleen on Rt, partial visceral heterotaxy, common atrium, CAVO indeterminate, vertebral from transverse arch, muscular diverticulum RV. Lt-PV, Rt—absent IVC, hemiazygos → RSVC and hepatic vein and CS — 1 year F

Abdominal sinus inversus, common atrium, CT, CAVO, marked PS (almost atresia), Lt—hepatic vein, IVC, CS, LSVC, and all P veins. Rt—RSVC. 2 coronary ostia from Rt posterior cusp, Rt and Lt circumflex, stenosis of Rt PV — 7 years M

Polysplenia, almost a common atrium, spontaneously closed VSD, FC, PAPVD → RSVC and LSVC → CS → Rt. Lt—Lt PV. Bicuspid AV and wide PDA — 13 days F

Asplenia, common atrium, CAVO dominant left, mitral insufficiency, PAPVD—RPV → Rt, absent IVC, azygos → RSVC, hepatic vein → Rt, Lt—Lt PV, sub AS — 3 months F

Hypoplastic spleen Rt, common atrium, tetralogy with CAVO, bicuspid PV, spongy ventricular mass, atresia of Rt PV, LSVC → CS → Lt. RSVC and IVC → Rt — stillborn (25-weeks' gest.)

Asplenia, CT with CAVO, common atrium, PA, common ventricle, PAPVD → 1 small PV → LSVC → Lt. Common PV → RSVC → Rt (Figs. 23—25) — 4 weeks M

Asplenia, almost a common atrium, CT with CAVO, PS, common ventricle, large ASD, proximal and distal defect, absent CS, PAPVD, 1 RPV → Rt. 3 PV → Lt LSVC → Lt — 2 years F

Asplenia, atypical truncus, CAVO, common atrium, SV with SOC, TAPVD → below diaphragm, pulmonary artery from innominate, LSVC → Rt — 1 month F

Accessory spleen, DORV, PS, CAVO, TAPVD, Rt RAA, CS and LSVC → Lt — 3 years M

Polysplenia, CAVO dominant Lt, coarctation of aorta, almost common atrium, absent CS and IVC. LSVC → Lt — 3 months F

Asplenia, CAVO dominant Lt, PS, common atrium, TAPVD → Rt. RAA — 1 day M

Spleen unknown, spontaneously closed VSD, PS, and TS — several days F

Polysplenia, ostium primum, cleft in the anterior leaflet of the MV, TAPVD—Rt PV → Rt, LPV → LSVC → CS → Rt — 12 years M

Spleen Bilobed right side, CAVO, FC, common atrium, high origin of coronary, absent CS, LSVC → Lt, 2 PV → Rt (Figs. 26—28) — 1 day F

Asplenia, CAVO intermediate type, dominant Lt, isolated ventricular inversion, and no transposition, common atrium, bicuspid PV, PV → LSVC → innominate → Lt, LSVC → Lt (Figs. 29—32) — 20 months M

Accessory spleen on Rt, common atrium, CT with CAVO, PA, RAA, absent IVC. LSVC → Lt — 2½ years M

Polysplenia, common atrium, CAVO, DORV, PS, TAPVD → below diaphragm → systemic vein, RAA, LSVC → CS → Rt — 18 days F

Asplenia, common atrium, CT, CAVO, TAPVD → portal vein, absent CS. RSVC and hepatic veins → Rt. IVC, LSVC → Lt (Figs. 33—35) — 5 months M

Accessory spleen Rt, common atrium, CAVO, CT, PA, anoma-

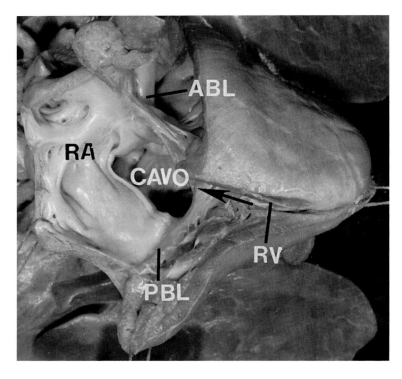

Figure 22: Polysplenia, common AV orifice, intermediate type, and common atrium. CAVO = common AV orifice, intermediate type; ABL = anterior bridging leaflet; PBL = posterior bridging leaflet; RV = right ventricle; RA = right side of the common atrium. Arrow points to the intermediate type of common AV orifice.

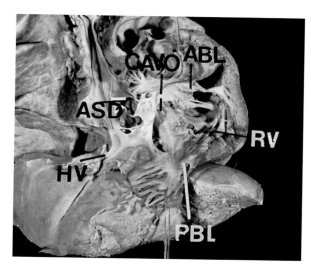

Figure 23: Four-week-old male infant, levocardia with atria indeterminate, almost a common atrium, complete transposition, common AV orifice, right side of the heart. ASD = fenestrated fossa ovalis defect, almost a common atrium; HV = hepatic veins entering the right side of the common atrium; CAVO = common AV orifice; ABL = anterior bridging leaflet; PBL = posterior bridging leaflet; RV = right ventricle.

lous band from PV → common atrium, RAA	10 days	M
Accessory spleen Rt, common atrium, CAVO, CT, PA, absent IVC, PAPVD, 2 PV → Rt, LSVC → Lt and RAA	3 days	M
Accessory spleen Rt, common atrium, CT, PA, CAVO indeterminate, TAPVD → Rt, LSVC → Lt	5 weeks	F
Asplenia, common atrium, CT with CAVO, PA, TAPVD, Rt AA, Rt PDA, straddling IVC (Figs. 36—38)	1 year, 7 mo	F

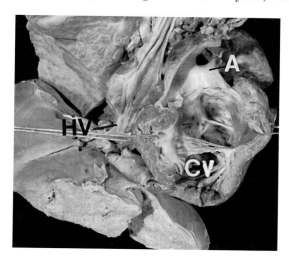

Figure 24: From the common ventricle emerges the aorta. CV = common ventricle; HV = hepatic veins entering the right side of the common atrium; A = aorta.

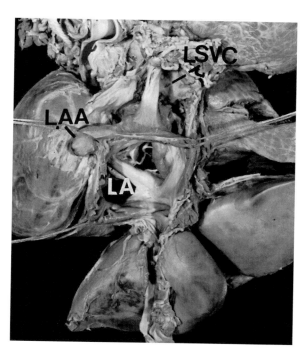

Figure 25: Left side of the common atrium demonstrating the entry of left superior vena cava. LA = left side of the common atrium; LSVC = left superior vena cava; LAA = left-sided appendage resembling left atrial morphology. Note that the left-sided atrial chamber cannot be stated definitively whether it's a left or a morphologically right atrium. It is an indeterminate atrium.

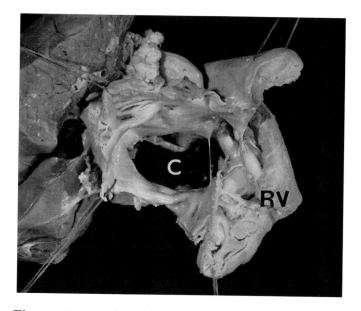

Figure 26: One-day-old female with isolated levocardia, common atrium, common AV orifice, preductal coarctation, and subaortic stenosis. C = common atrium combined with common AV orifice; RV = right ventricle. Note the huge common atrium.

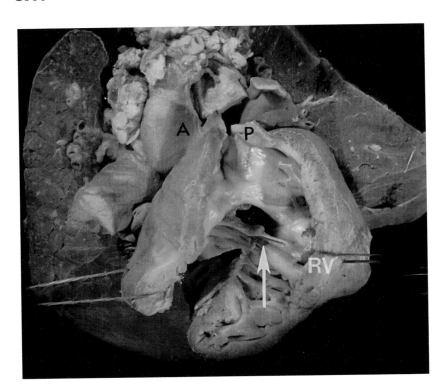

Figure 27: Right ventricular outflow tract showing the normally related vessels. Aorta to the right and posterior, pulmonary trunk emerging from the morphologically right ventricle. RV = right ventricle; P = pulmonary trunk; A = aorta. Arrow points to the common AV orifice.

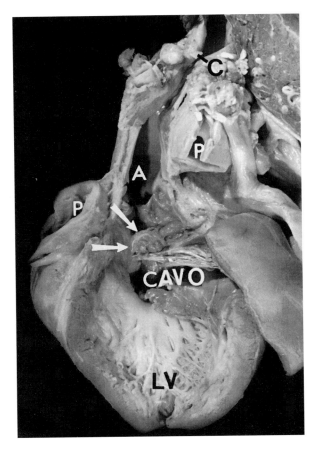

Figure 28: Outflow tract of the left ventricle showing subaortic stenosis produced by endocardial tissue and coarctation of the aorta. CAVO = common AV orifice; LV = left ventricle; P = pulmonary trunk; A = aorta; C = coarctation. Arrows point to the subaortic stenosis.

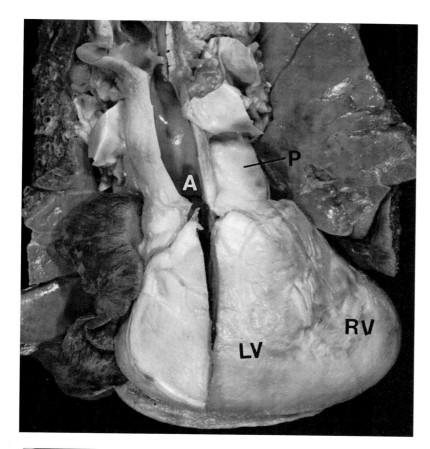

Figure 29: Common AV orifice with isolated ventricular inversion (sinus) and no transposition. External view. A = aorta; P = pulmonary trunk; LV = left ventricle; RV = right ventricle.

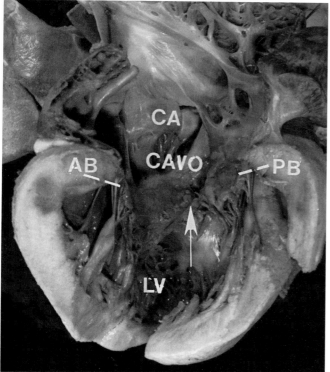

Figure 30: Right side of the common atrium, common AV orifice and morphologically left ventricle. CA = common atrium; CAVO = common AV orifice; AB = anterior bridging leaflet; PB = posterior bridging leaflet; LV = morphologically left ventricle. Arrow points to common AV orifice, intermediate type.

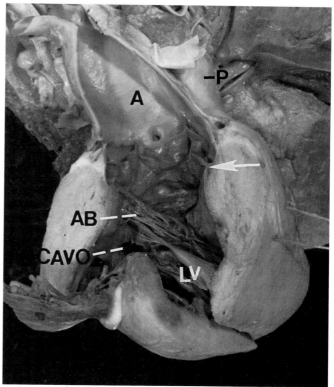

Figure 31: Outflow tract of the morphologically left ventricle, the aorta emerging from this chamber. A = aorta; P = pulmonary trunk; LV = left ventricle; CAVO = common AV orifice; AB = anterior bridging leaflet. Arrow points to the straddling conus.

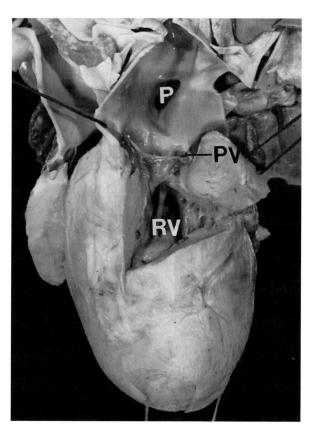

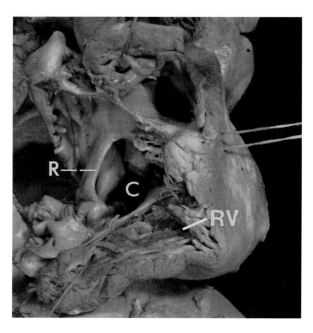

Figure 33: Levocardia with visceral heterotaxy and indeterminate atria, regular complete transposition with common AV orifice and pulmonary atresia. C = combined atrial and ventricular septal defect – CAVO; R = remnant of the atrial septum; RV = right ventricle. (Used with permission from Liberthson RR, et al. See Figure 34.)

Figure 32: Conus-like chamber on the left side for the morphologically right ventricle, and pulmonary trunk emerging from this chamber. RV = small right ventricle; PV = bicuspid pulmonic valve; P = pulmonary trunk.

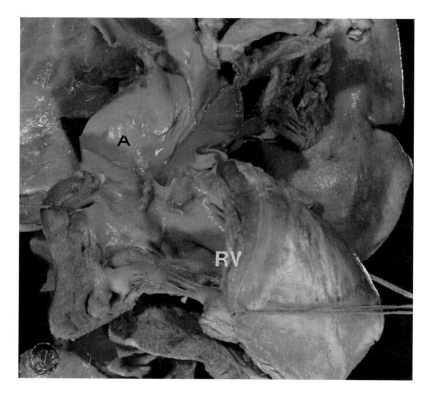

Figure 34: Aorta emerging from the morphologically right ventricle. RV = right ventricle; A = aorta. (Used with permission from Liberthson RR, Hastreiter AR, Sinha SN, Bharati S, Novak GM, Lev M: Levocardia with visceral heterotaxy—isolated levocardia: pathologic anatomy and its clinical implications. *Am Heart J* 1973, 85:40–54.)

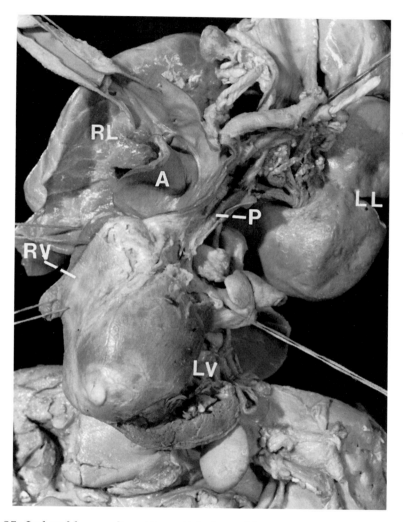

Figure 35: Isolated levocardia with partial visceral heterotaxy. External view of the heart from a case of asplenia in a 5-month-old infant. Regular complete transposition and pulmonary atresia and common AV orifice. RL = right lung; LL = left lung, quadrilobed, both lungs; RV = right ventricle; LV = left ventricle; A = aorta; P = pulmonary trunk.

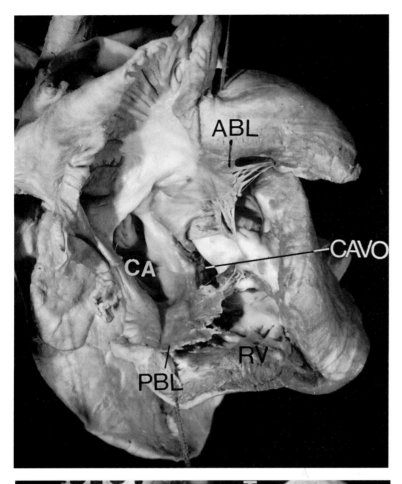

Figure 36: Isolated levocardia, common atrium, atria indeterminate and ventricles in normal position CAVO. Right-sided view. CA = common atrium; CAVO = common AV orifice; RV = right ventricle; PBL = posterior bridging leaflet; ABL = anterior bridging leaflet.

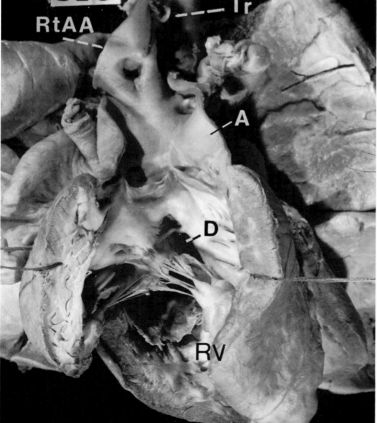

Figure 37: Complete transposition, aorta emerging from right ventricle, right aortic arch. Tr = trachea; RV = right ventricle; A = aorta; D = defect of common AV orifice; RtAA = right aortic arch.

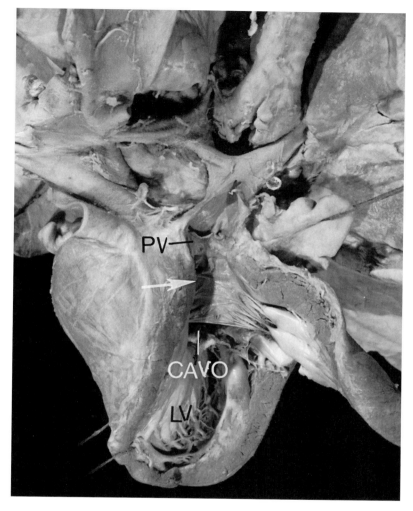

Figure 38: Left ventricular view demonstrating the subpulmonary stenosis. PV = bicuspid pulmonary valve; CAVO = common AV orifice; LV = left ventricle. Arrow points to subpulmonary stenosis.

In summary, the abnormalities in the spleen were:

	No. of Cases
Asplenia	14
Polysplenia	12
Situs inversus abdominalis with spleen on right	3
Hypoplastic or very small spleen	2
Unknown	3
Spleen on right (bilobed)	2
Accessory spleen	5

The complexes were:

Common atrium or almost a common atrium	39
CAVO	32
Complete transposition, usually with pulmonary stenosis (4) or atresia (11)	15
DORV	4
Tetralogy	1
Single ventricle with atypical truncus	1
Single ventricle with transposition	4
Single ventricle with no transposition	1
Complete transposition with aortic atresia	1
TAPVD	15
PAPVD	14
Atresia of right pulmonary veins	1
LSVC → LA	22
LSVC → RA	7

V. Isolated Levocardia, Visceral Heterotaxy, Indeterminate Atria and Ventricular Inversion

In this group there was a common atrium or almost a common atrium with splenic abnormalities in all, except in one where the spleen was on the right with situs inversus abdominalis. Thus, the atria were indeterminate and the ventricles were inverted.

There were seven cases: five males and two females and their ages ranged from 5 days to 15½ years, with a mean age of 2 years, 4 months, 4 days.

The splenic and venous anomalies were:

Asplenia	4
Polysplenia (situs inversus abdominalis)	1
Spleen right (situs inversus)	1
Spleen bilobed	1
TAPVD	3
PAPVD	2
1 PV → Rt. IVC → Lt.	1

The complexes were:

Asplenia, inverted transposition, pulmonary atresia, CAVO dominant Lt, ASD FO type, RAA, TAPVD → RSVC → Rt, absent CS	2 months M
Asplenia, overriding aorta, inverted conus and ventricular mass, CAVO dominant Lt, pulmonary atresia, PAPVD, ASD, Rt—IVC and 2 PV. Lt—2 PV and LSVC	24 months M
Spleen bilobed Rt, inverted DORV and PS, valvular and infundibular PS VSD, Bi-PV, RAA, Rt—1 PV, Lt—IVC and 2 PV	1 month M
Asplenia with common atrium, CAVO dominant Lt, TAPVD → gastric vein, RAA, inverted transposition with pulmonary atresia, Rt—absent CS, Lt—LSVC	5 days M
Polysplenia, congenital AV block, common atrium, double VSD, overriding aorta and PS, Lt AV valve atresia, single coronary, PAPVD, cleft in MV, Lt—Lt PV and LSVC, Rt—2 PV, hepatic vein, RSVC, and CS	29 days F
Asplenia, common atrium, CAVO, infundibular PS, TAPVD → RSVC. CS → left side	4 months F
Ventricular inversion with overriding aorta, PA, RAA and Rt PDA, regular transposition, CAVO type VSD, straddling TV and accessory MV, LSVC → CS → Rt situs inversus abdominalis, and bilobed both lungs, spleen Rt	15½ years M

(*Note:* Rt implies right side of the common atrium; Lt implies left side of the common atrium.)

The major anomalies in addition to the common atrium were:

Common AV orifice	4
CAVO type VSD	1
Pseudotruncus or overriding aorta, inverted transposition and PA	1
Pseudotruncus, overriding aorta inverted transposition and PS	1
Inverted transposition and PA	2
Inverted transposition and PS	1
Ventricular inversion and regular transposition	1
Inverted DORV and PS	1
Left AV valve atresia	1

The oldest, 15½ years, had isolated ventricular inversion and regular transposition.

Other Associated Cardiac Anomalies

These included single coronary, bicuspid pulmonary valve or aortic valve, double ventricular septal defect, juxtaposed atrial appendages, cleft in the anterior leaflet of the mitral valve, and spontaneously closed ventricular septal defect. Rarely, a left aortic arch with a right ductus arteriosus was seen.

Congenital AV Block

It is not surprising to find congenital AV block and/or supraventricular arrhythmias in this entity. This was seen in five. All were associated with polysplenia and partial visceral heterotaxy except one was with total situs inversus. The ages were 15 days, newborn, one day, 3 days, and 29 days; two were males and three were female subjects.

The complexes were:

Isolated Levocardia, Atria Situs Solitus and Ventricles Normal

Complete transposition with PA, CAVO, PAPVD, RPV → RA, LSVC → CS. RAA Lt PDA. Single coronary, accessory mitral orifice, with AV block, polysplenia in a 3-day-old male (Figs. 39–41)

DORV, CAVO, dominant Rt. Preductal coarctation, aortic and subaortic stenosis. Absent IVC, hepatic veins → RA and hemiazygos → RSVC. Atypical ASD, FOD. Polysplenia, partial visceral heterotaxy in a 1-day-old female (Figs. 42–46)

Isolated Levocardia, Atria Indeterminate with Ventricles Normal

Common atrium, common AV orifice—intermediate type, subaortic stenosis, and hepatic veins entering the right side with absent IVC and 2 pulmonary veins entering the right side with LSVC and CS entering the left side of the common atrium, and polysplenia in a 15-day-old male (Figs. 47–51)

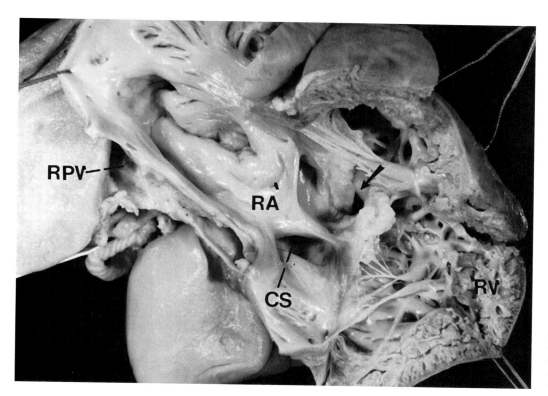

Figure 39: Isolated levocardia, atria situs solitus, ventricles normal. Complete transposition and pulmonary atresia and congenital AV block in a 3-day-old infant. Right side of the heart. RA = right atrium; RV = right ventricle; CS = large coronary sinus receiving a left superior vena cava; RPV = right pulmonary vein entering right atrium. Arrow points to common AV orifice.

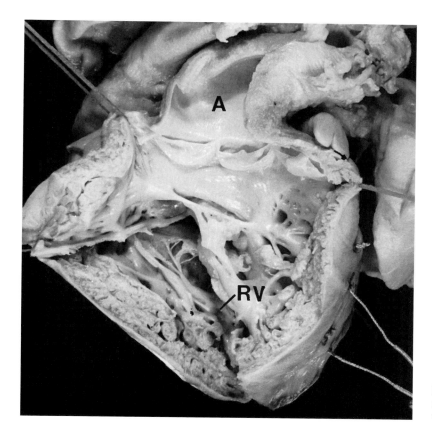

Figure 40: Complete transposition and pulmonary atresia. Aorta emerging from the right ventricle. A = aorta; RV = right ventricle.

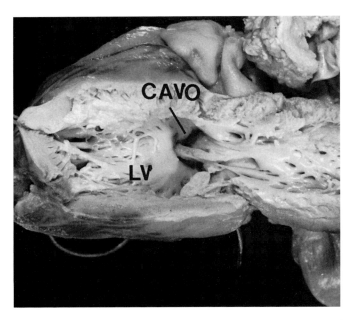

Figure 41: Outflow tract of left ventricle showing no vessel emerges from this chamber. LV = left ventricle; CAVO = common AV orifice.

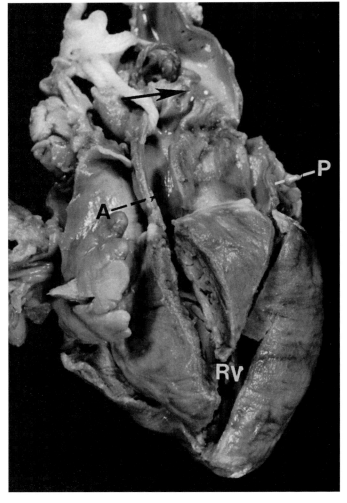

Figure 42: Isolated levocardia. CAVO, dominant right, double outlet right ventricle and congenital AV block. RV = right ventricle; A = aorta; P = pulmonary trunk. Arrow points to coarctation.

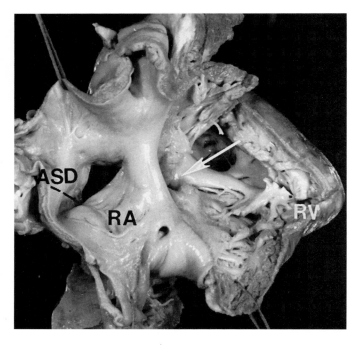

Figure 43: Huge atypical fossa ovalis defect extending proximally, CAVO. RA = right atrium; ASD = huge atypical defect; RV = right ventricle. Arrow points to CAVO.

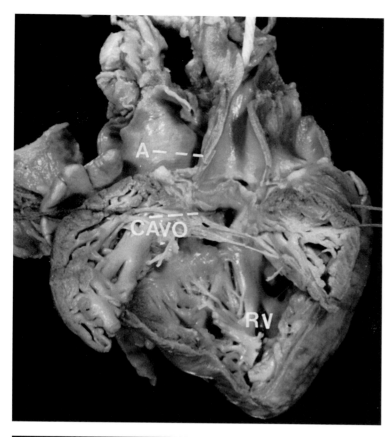

Figure 44: CAVO defect confluent with the aorta. RV = right ventricle; A = aorta emerging from the right ventricle; CAVO = common AV orifice defect extending beneath the aorta.

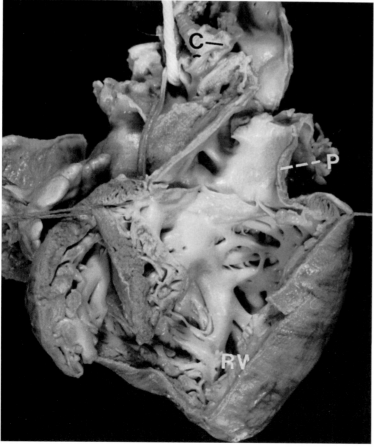

Figure 45: Pulmonary trunk emerging from right ventricle. RV = right ventricle; P = pulmonary trunk; C = coarctation of the aorta.

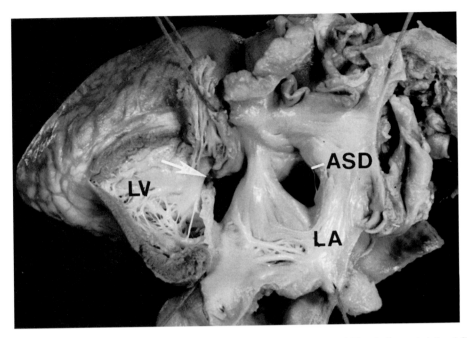

Figure 46: Left atrial, left ventricular view. LA = left atrium; LV = left ventricle; ASD = large atrial septal defect. Arrow points to common AV orifice.

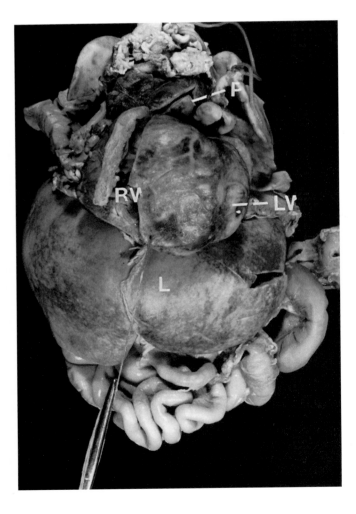

Figure 47: Isolated levocardia, atria indeterminate, ventricles normal. Polysplenia with congenital AV block. RV = right ventricle; LV = left ventricle; P = pulmonary trunk; L = liver.

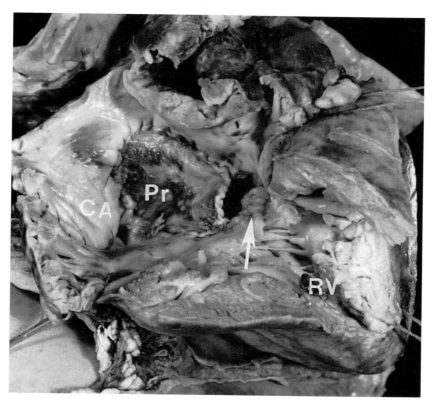

Figure 48: Congenital AV block, CAVO intermediate type, operated. CA = right side of common atrium; RV = right ventricle; Pr = prosthesis closing the defect. Arrow points to the intermediate type of CAVO.

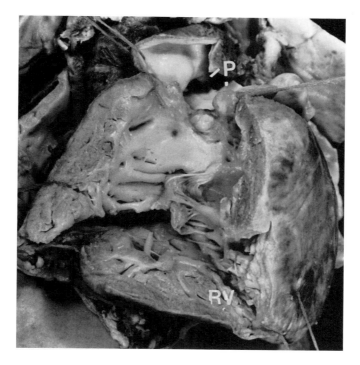

Figure 49: Pulmonary trunk also emerging from right ventricle. RV = right ventricle; P = pulmonary trunk.

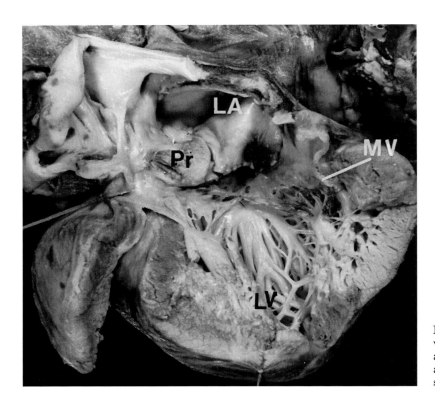

Figure 50: Left side of common atrium. Left ventricular view. LA = left side of common atrium; LV = left ventricle; MV = newly created mitral valve; Pr = prosthetic patch closure of the defect.

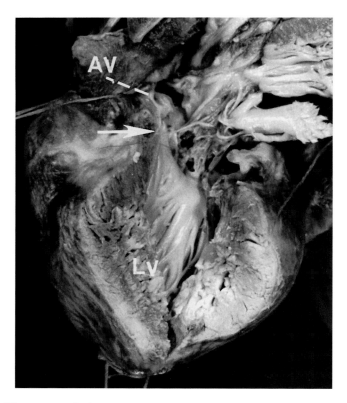

Figure 51: Left ventricular outflow tract showing subaortic stenosis. LV = left ventricle; AV = aortic valve. Arrow points to subaortic stenosis.

Common atrium, common AV orifice, complete transposition, pulmonary atresia, absent IVC, hepatic veins and 2 pulmonary veins into the right side of the common atrium with LSVC entering the right side of the common atrium with small CS and only 2 pulmonary veins entering left side of the common atrium, and polysplenia in a newborn male (Figs. 52–55)

Isolated Levocardia, Atria Indeterminate with Ventricles Inverted

Total situs inversus, ventricular inversion, left AV valve atresia, common atrium, partial anomalous pulmonary venous drainage, double VSD, overriding aorta, single coronary, left side of common atrium receiving the left pulmonary veins and LSVC, the right side receiving the right SVC, right 2 pulmonary veins, hepatic veins and CS, and polysplenia in a 29-day-old female

Supraventricular Arrhythmias

Total situs inversus, common atrium, CAVO, SV both vessels from SOC, PAPVD, RAA, Rt PDA, absent IVC and CS, azygos → RSVC, RPV → Rt. Lt P vein and LSVC → Lt in a 10-year-old female child

Polysplenia, common atrium, CAVO, PAPVD, Rt P vein and coronary vein → Rt and Lt P vein, LSVC, hemiazygos → RSVC, hepatic vein and coronary vein → Lt in a 4 1/2 month-old male child

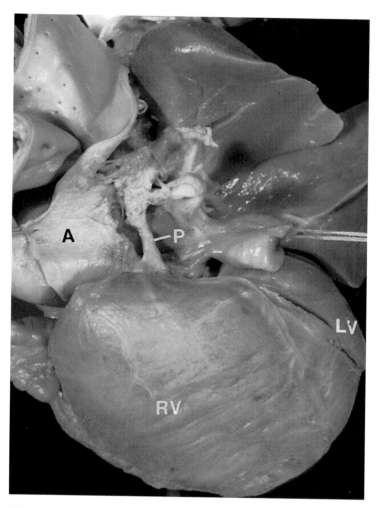

Figure 52: Isolated levocardia with indeterminate atria, complete transposition with pulmonary atresia and congenital AV block. External view. A = aorta; P = atretic pulmonary trunk; RV = right ventricle; LV = left ventricle.

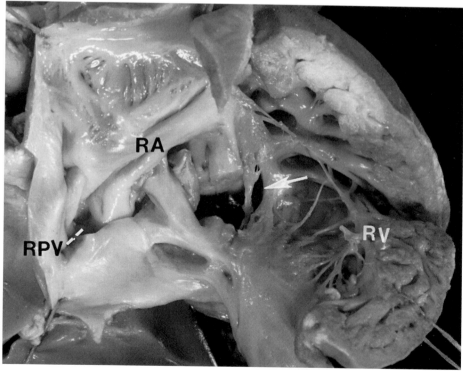

Figure 53: Common atrium, right side. RA = common atrium, right side; RV = right ventricle; RPV = entry of right pulmonary veins. Arrow points to common AV orifice.

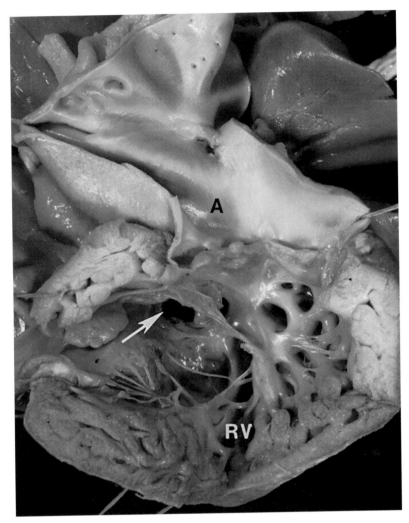

Figure 54: Aorta emerging from right ventricle. RV = right ventricle; A = aorta. Note the defect of CAVO in part beneath the aorta. Arrow points to the defect.

Comment

Although isolated levocardia is a rare anomaly, it is important to recognize this entity since some of them permit survival to adult life.

We were able to extend our previous classification into five main types: (1) with situs solitus atria, (2) with solitus atria and ventricles inverted, (3) with atrial inversion and total situs inversus, (4) atria indeterminate with ventricles in the normal position, and finally, (5) atria indeterminate and ventricles inverted.

In the first group, with atrial situs solitus, there is a tendency for left-sided lesions to occur both with and without transposition and a left superior vena cava to enter the right atrium. There is also a tendency for transposition, either complete or partial or simply an overriding aorta with pulmonary stenosis or atresia, and total or partial anomolous pulmonary venous drainage and CAVO.

The second group, with atria situs solitus and ventricles inverted, is a new group added to the old classification. These are rare hearts. It is of interest that though both had asplenia, one was partial and the other total abdominal situs inversus. Both had total anomalous pulmonary venous return; one with single ventricle with inverted mass had regular transposition.

In the third group there was total situs inversus of the abdominal viscera, the atria inverted, in general receiving their respective veins with minor variations. The ventricles were in the normal position and the aorta emerged from the right ventricle and the pulmonary trunk from the morphologically left ventricle, thus, the circulation was physiologically corrected provided there were no major associated cardiac anomalies. In general, in this entity, there was a ventricular septal defect and pulmonary stenosis or atresia and tricuspid valve abnormalities in the form of Ebstein's anomaly or insufficiency and stenosis of the valve.

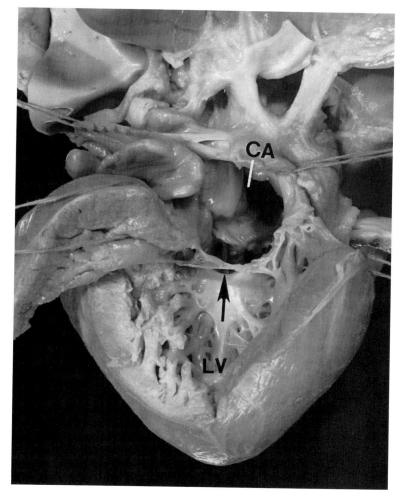

Figure 55: Common atrium from left side. CA = left side of common atrium; LV = left ventricle. Arrow points to the deficient mitral valve tissue to the common AV orifice leaflet, intermediate type.

Thus, the associated anomalies are somewhat similar to corrected transposition or AV discordant heart (mixed levocardia with ventricular inversion).

In the fourth group, with atria indeterminate, although somewhat similar to the situs solitus atria category, there was almost always a common atrium accompanied by common AV orifice, usually of a complete type, making it difficult to establish the identity of the atria (Fig. 36). In this group, 21 of them had transposition of the great vessels, usually of the complete regular type. Included in this group are four cases of single ventricle and one case of single ventricle with truncus. Four had double outlet right ventricle and one had tetralogy of Fallot. Fifteen (36%) had no transposition but two had overriding aorta. In general, in this group there was common AV orifice and pulmonary stenosis (Figs. 37, 38) and/or atresia.

It is of interest that in the first group the oldest was 37 years of age, in the second 2 months, in the third group 58 years (with situs inversus atria), in the fourth 12 years, and in the fifth 15½ years

It is also of interest to note that in the fourth group there two remarkable cases; one was a single ventricle in which both vessels emerged in a more or less normally related position from the small outlet chamber with no transposition, and one had complete transposition with aortic atresia.

The fifth group is another new addition to the previous classification where the ventricles are inverted but the atria are indeterminate. Although anomalies in pulmonary venous return, common atrium, common AV orifice, and inverted transposition are almost always present with splenic anomalies, there was one with regular transposition.

Although practically all had some kind of an anomalous systemic or pulmonic venous return, and 45% were below the age of 1 month, some do permit survival to adult life. In some selected cases, a total surgical correction of the anomaly or a palliative procedure may be attempted. It is of interest that in the first group with atria situs solitus there was a 2-month-old twin. One remarkable heart with atrial inversion (morphological right atrium situated on the left), had its appendage displaced above the morphological left atrial appendage situated on the right side.

There are probably multiple genes responsible for the situs of the abdominal organs as well as the atria. Their relationship to conotruncal anomalies and anomalies in the systemic and pulmonary venous returns deserves future research at the molecular and genetic levels.

Abbreviations:

PA= pulmonary atresia; CAVO = common AV orifice; PAPVD = partial anomolous pumonary venous drainage; RPV = right pulmonary vein; RA = right atrium; LSVC = left superior vena cava; CS = coronary sinus; RAA = right aortic arch; AV = atrioventricular; ASD = atrial septal defect; FOD = fossa ovalis defect; PDA = patent ductus arteriosus; LA = left atrium; VS = ventricular septal defect; SVC = superior vena cava; CT = complete transposition; TAPVD = total anomalous pumonary venous drainage; LA = left atrium; IVC = inferior vena cava; DORV = double outlet right ventricle; FO = fossa ovalis; PV = pulmonary valve; RSVC = right superior vena cava; FC = fetal coarctation; AS = aortic stenosis; LAA = left aortic arch; SV = single ventricle; RAA = right aortic arch; 2PV = 2 pulmonary veins; RPV = right pulmonary vein; LPV = left pulmonary vein; SOC = small outlet chamber.

62

Mesocardia

Mesocardia is that condition in which the longitudinal axis of the heart lies in the midsagittal plane, with the heart having no distinct apex, and this is due to an inherent abnormality in the development of the heart (Fig. 1).

Definition of Terms

Situs solitus means normal position of the viscera from the standpoint of right- and left-sidedness, and *situs inversus* implies the mirror image of that position. These terminologies will pertain to visceral organs and atria but do not apply to the heart in general nor to the ventricles. In the case of the ventricles, the term "inverted" is used, implying that the chambers are in the mirror-image relationship of the normal. This distinction is necessary because of the difference in the development of the atria and viscera on the one hand, and the ventricles on the other, from the standpoint of their laterality. *Transposition of the great arteries*, as used here, implies abnormal position of the great arteries in relation to each other, the chambers from which they emerge, or the atrioventricular (AV) orifice, or all three. Regular transposition implies that the aorta is situated distinctly to the right, as well as anterior to the pulmonary trunk in the great majority of cases. In most cases, in this type of transposition, the bulboventricular loop is normally formed (dextro-loop).

The term "inverted transposition" implies that the aorta is situated distinctly to the left as well as anterior to the pulmonary trunk in the great majority of cases. Here, in most cases, the loop is formed in the opposite direction to the normal (levo-loop). The systemic venous return is considered to be normal if the veins enter the morphologically right atrium, present on the right in situs solitus viscerum and on the left in situs inversus viscerum. The pulmonary venous return is considered to be normal if the pulmonary veins enter the morphologically left atrium, situated on the left in situs solitus viscerum and on the right in situs inversus viscerum. The term "polysplenia" as used here implies that the splenic tissue is divided into two or more discrete, nearly equal-sized masses. The term "accessory spleen" implies that in addition to one approximately normal-sized spleen, there are one or more smaller splenic masses.

Analysis of Our Material

There was a total of 55 cases, and the ages ranged from a 24-weeks' gestation fetus to 49 years, with a mean age of 1 year, 2 months, and 20 days. There were 26 male subjects and 29 female subjects.

Classification

Mesocardia may be classified as follows:

		No. of Cases
I.	Mesoversion with atrial situs solitus and normal ventricles	29
II.	Presumptive mesoversion with atrial situs solitus and normal ventricles	10
III.	Mixed mesocardia with atrial situs solitus and ventricular inversion	6
IV.	Presumptive mixed mesoversion with atrial situs inversus and normal ventricles	1
V.	Mesocardia, atria indeterminate, and ventricles in normal position	7
VI.	Mesocardia, atria indeterminate, and ventricular inversion	2
		55

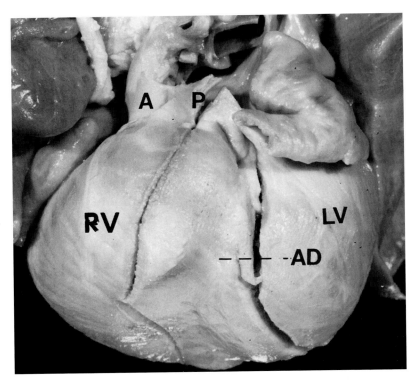

Figure 1: Mesoversion, common AV orifice, anterior view. A = aorta; P = pulmonary trunk; RV = right ventricle; LV = left ventricle; AD = anterior descending coronary artery. (Used with permission from Lev M, et al. See Figure 34.)

General Examination – External Configuration of the Heart

The heart had no apex (Fig. 1). The anterior descending coronary artery proceeded ventrally from the base, veering slightly to the right or the left, with asymmetrical bulges of the heart on each side of it, the greater bulge usually being toward the right (Fig. 1). The ventricular septum was likewise close to the sagittal plane, shifting or veering slightly to the left. In one case, both the anterior descending coronary artery and the ventricular septum veered or shifted considerably to the left. If there was no transposition of the great arteries, then the arterial trunks were in the normal position, or the pulmonary trunk lay directly anterior to the aorta and the former swung to the left to give off the two pulmonary arteries. The atria in general were side by side but more posteriorly situated.

I. Mesoversion with Atrial Situs Solitus and Normal Ventricles

There was a total of 29 cases; 15 were females and 14 males. The ages ranged from a 34-weeks' gestation fetus to 15 months with a mean age of 1 month, 23 days. Nineteen were below the age of 1 month.

In this type of mesoversion, the atria and the ven-

tricles were side by side with the right to the right, and the left to the left. There was a left aortic arch. The atria were situs solitus in all, and the spleen was normal in all but one. This unique case was a 34-weeks' gestation fetus who had polysplenia. Likewise, the lungs were normal in all except two where the lungs were polylobated, both sides in one and, in the other, both lungs were bilobed (polysplenia).

The complexes associated with this lesion were as follows:

	No. of Cases
Tetralogy of Fallot	5
Atrial septal defect, fossa ovalis type	3
Double outlet right ventricle (Figs. 2, 3) (2 with MS and 1 with mitral atresia)	3
Preductal coarctation of the aorta (2 with AS and MS and 1 with VSD)	3
Hypoplasia of aortic tract complex with aortic and mitral atresia	1
Absent transverse arch, straddling conus, subaortic stenosis	1
Congenital polyvalvular disease (1 with CAVO-type VSD and straddling TV)	2
Ebstein's anomaly with marked pulmonary, valvular, and infundibular stenosis	1

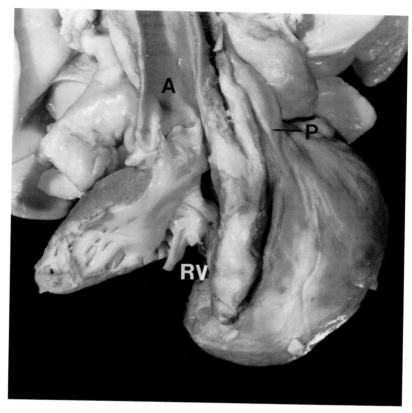

Figure 2: Mesocardia, double outlet right ventricle with mitral stenosis, right ventricular view. RV = right ventricle; A = aorta; P = pulmonary trunk.

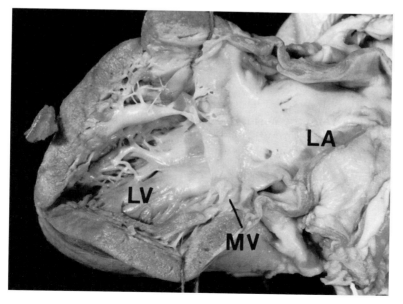

Figure 3: Mesocardia, double outlet right ventricle with mitral stenosis. LA = left atrium; MV = mitral valve; LV = left ventricle.

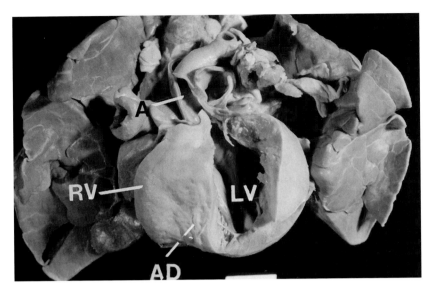

Figure 4: External view of mesocardia with tricuspid stenosis, large left side. LV = left ventricle; RV = small right ventricle; A = aorta; AD = anterior descending coronary artery.

ASD, VSD, aortic and pulmonic stenosis, and congenital AV block	1
VSD with overriding aorta	1
Atypical tricuspid stenosis (Figs. 4, 5)	1
ASD, VSD, and PDA (Fig. 6)	1
Common AV orifice (Figs. 1, 7–9)	1
Complete transposition with pulmonary atresia	1
Complete transposition with characteristics of Taussig-Bing and fetal coarctation and tricuspid stenosis (Figs. 10–12)	1
Single ventricle with regular transposition, both vessels emerging from the small outlet chamber, pulmonary stenosis, and juxtaposed, right atrial appendage to the left (Figs. 13–15)	1
Complete transposition with infundibular, and valvular, pulmonary, and tricuspid stenosis	1
Complete transposition with tricuspid atresia, preductal (fetal) coarctation, juxtaposed right atrial appendage to the left, and double VSD	1

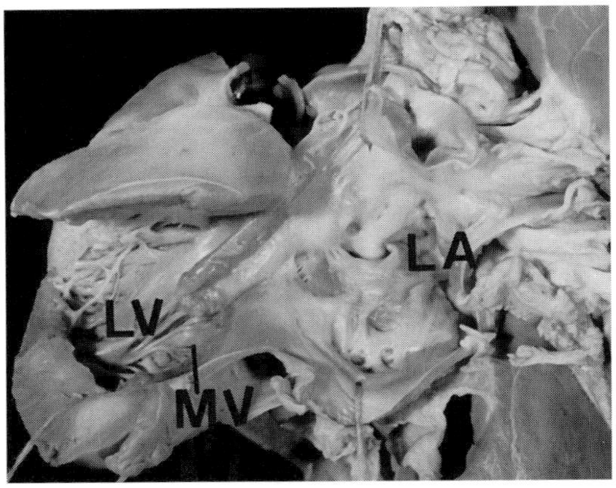

Figure 5: Left side of the heart in tricuspid stenosis showing the large atrium. LA = left atrium; LV = left ventricle; MV = mitral valve.

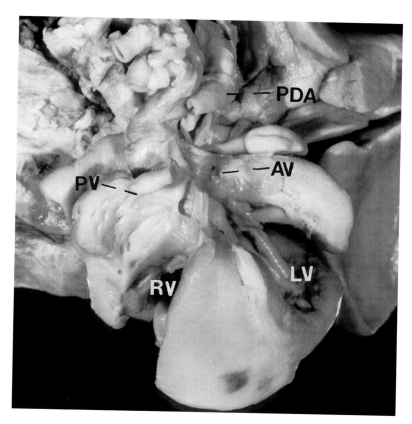

Figure 6: Mesocardia with large patent ductus arteriosus with ASD and VSD, external view. RV = right ventricle; LV = left ventricle; AV = aortic valve; PV = pulmonary valve; PDA = patent ductus arteriosus, large.

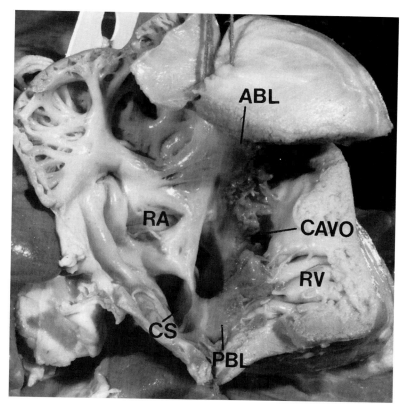

Figure 7: Mesoversion, common AV orifice, right atrial, right ventricular view. RA = right atrium; RV = right ventricle; CS = coronary sinus; CAVO = common AV orifice; ABL = anterior bridging leaflet; PBL = posterior bridging leaflet. (Used with permission from Lev M, et al. See Figure 34.)

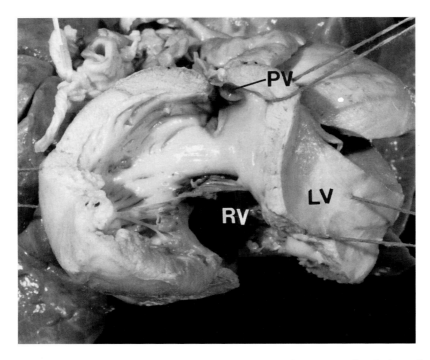

Figure 8: Mesocardia with common AV orifice, ventricles situated side by side, and right ventricular hypertrophy. RV = right ventricle; PV = pulmonary valve; LV = left ventricle.

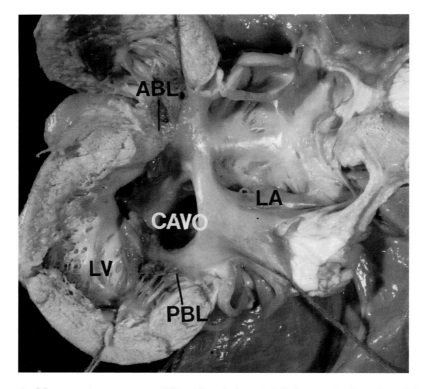

Figure 9: Mesoversion, common AV orifice, left atrial, left ventricular view. LA = left atrium; LV = left ventricle; CAVO = common AV orifice; ABL = anterior bridging leaflet; PBL = posterior bridging leaflet. (Used with permission from Lev M, et al. See Figure 34.)

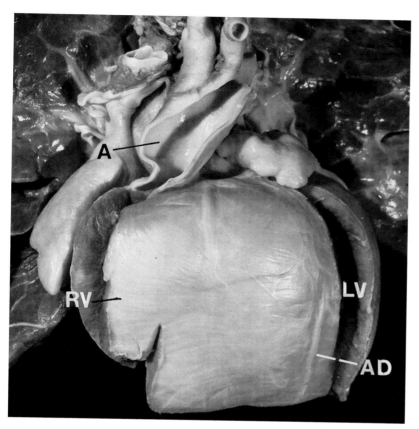

Figure 10: External view of mesocardia with complete transposition with characteristics of Taussig-Bing and preductal coarctation of the aorta. RV = right ventricle; LV = left ventricle; A = aorta; AD = anterior descending coronary artery.

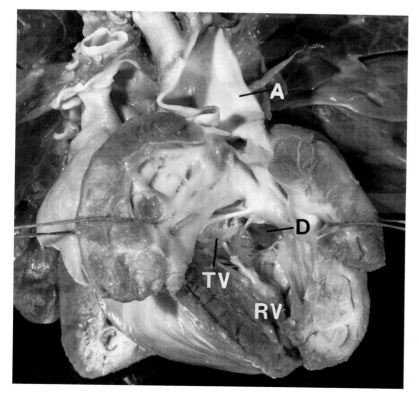

Figure 11: Right ventricular outflow tract demonstrating the aorta emerging from the right ventricle and the ventricular septal defect unrelated to the aorta. TV = tricuspid valve; RV = right ventricle; D = ventricular septal defect covered by excess of endocardial tissue of the tricuspid valve and the membranous septum; A = aorta.

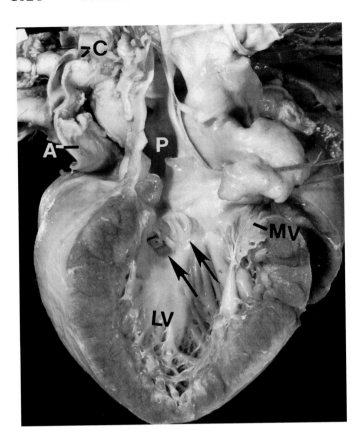

Figure 12: Left ventricular outflow tract demonstrating the ventricular septal defect confluent with the pulmonary trunk and the pulmonary trunk in part overriding the defect. LV = left ventricle; MV = mitral valve; A = aorta; P = pulmonary trunk; C = coarctation of the aorta. Arrows point to the aneurysmal bulge of the membranous septum and the tricuspid valvular tissue bulging through the defect and in part closing the VSD and producing subpulmonary obstruction.

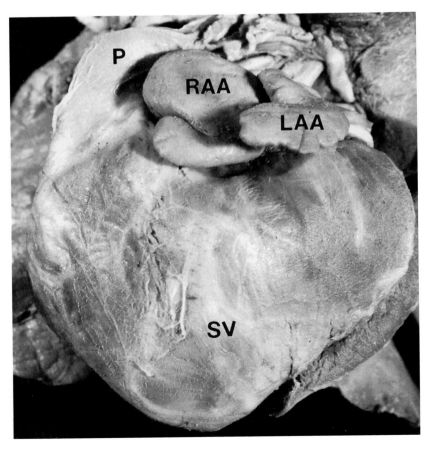

Figure 13: Mesocardia with single ventricle with regular transposition and pulmonary stenosis and juxtaposed right atrial appendage to the left; external view. SV = single ventricle; RAA = right atrial appendage; LAA = left atrial appendage; P = pulmonary trunk.

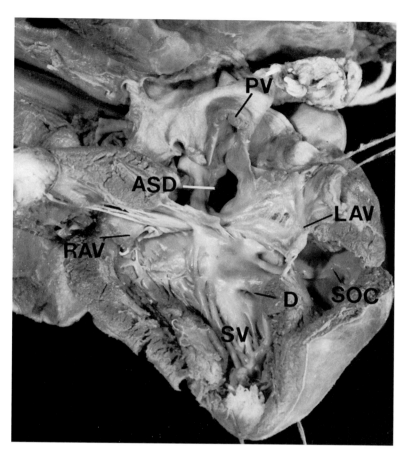

Figure 14: Single ventricle and small outlet chamber with small defect between the two chambers. RAV = right AV valve; LAV = left AV valve; SV = single ventricle; SOC = small outlet chamber; D = small defect between the main chamber and the small outlet chamber; PV = pulmonary vein; ASD = atrial septal defect, fossa ovalis type.

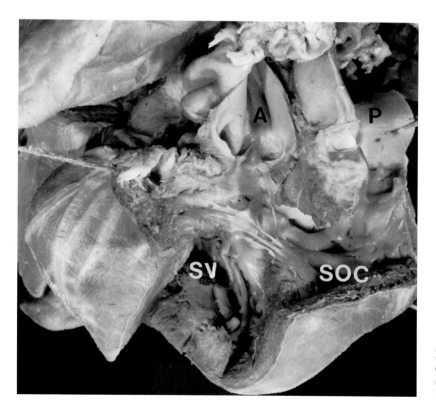

Figure 15: Single ventricle with both vessels emerging from the small outlet chamber. SV = single ventricle; SOC = small outlet chamber; P = pulmonary trunk; A = aorta.

Significant associated cardiac abnormalities were:

	No. of Cases
Left superior vena cava entering coronary sinus	8 (27.5%)
Bicuspid pulmonary valve	7
Bicuspid aortic and pulmonic valves	3
Absent pulmonary valve	2
Bicuspid aortic valve	1
Unicuspid aortic valve	1
Diverticulum of the right ventricle	4
Single left coronary, high origin	2
High origin of left coronary	1
High origin of right coronary	1

II. Presumptive Mesoversion with Atrial Situs Solitus and Normal Ventricles

There was a total of 10 cases; five were males and five were females. The ages ranged from a 24-weeks' gestation fetus to 6½ years old, with a median age of 10 months, 13 days. Six were below the age of 1 month (three were stillborn).

In this type, the atrial septum was either deficient or septum primum and septum secundum components could not be ascertained (Fig. 16). However, the atrial appendages were typical of right and left atria, and were thus presumptively in a position of mesoversion (Fig. 17). The ventricles were clearly in mesoversion (Figs. 16–18).

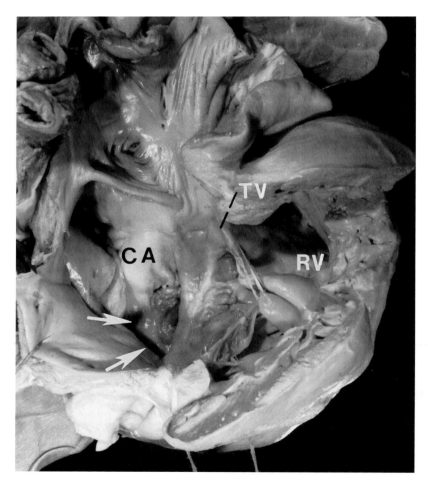

Figure 16: Right-sided view demonstrating common atrium, tricuspid and mitral valve. CA = common atrium; TV = tricuspid valve; RV = right ventricle. Arrows point to the mitral valve.

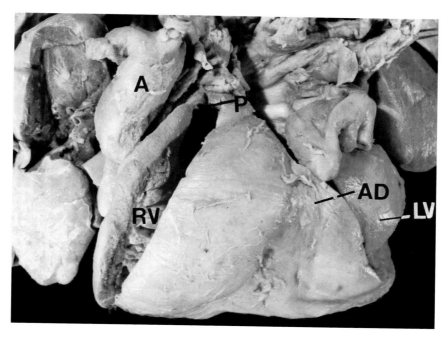

Figure 17: Presumptive mesoversion with atrial situs solitus and ventricles in normal position with abdominal situs inversus. External view of the heart. RV = right ventricle; LV = left ventricle; A = aorta; P = pulmonary trunk; AD = anterior descending coronary artery.

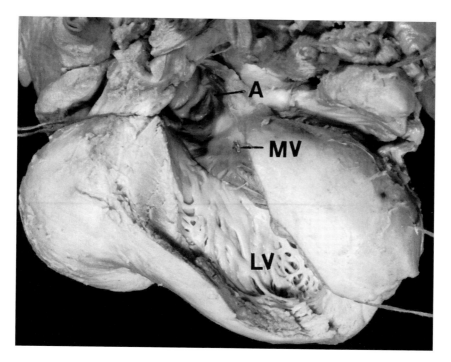

Figure 18: Left ventricular outflow tract view. LV = left ventricle; MV = anterior leaflet of the mitral valve; A = aorta.

The Status of Spleen and Abdominal Organs

There were two cases of asplenia with partial visceral heterotaxy, two with polysplenia, and one was associated with accessory spleen. One had partial visceral heterotaxy with a spleen on the right, and one with polysplenia also had partial visceral heterotaxy. In the other three, the status of the spleen was not known. The one associated with polysplenia and the other with accessory spleen were cases of situs inversus abdominalis and abnormal lobation of the lungs. The lungs were bilobed in one case of polysplenia and in one with accessory spleen. One with polysplenia had a trilobed left lung.

The venous anomalies were:

	No. of Cases
Absent right superior vena cava	2
Absent coronary sinus	4
Coronary sinus entered the presumptive left atrium	1
Left superior vena cava entered the presumptive left atrium	5
Left superior vena cava entered the presumptive right atrium	1
Hepatic vein entered the presumptive left atrium	2
Hepatic vein entered the presumptive right atrium	2
Absent inferior vena cava	3
Entry of inferior vena cava into the presumptive left atrium	1
Partial anomalous pulmonary venous drainage	3

In a case of asplenia, both appendages resembled left atrial appendage.

Congenital AV Block and Other Arrhythmias

There were three with congenital AV block. One was a stillborn 34-weeks' gestation female fetus with polysplenia, common atrium, and CAVO. The other with polysplenia and partial visceral heterotaxy was a 4-day-old female infant who also had common atrium, double outlet right ventricle, CAVO, and severe pulmonary stenosis. The third was a 3-day-old male infant who had accessory spleen, CAVO, double outlet right ventricle, and absent transverse arch. The 6½-year-old male had common atrium, common AV orifice, and atrial flutter.

The complexes associated with this type of mesocardia were as follows:

	No. of Cases
Common atrium with common AV orifice	1
Common atrium, common AV orifice, patent ductus arteriosus	2
Common atrium with cleft in the anterior leaflet of the mitral and divided right ventricle	1
Common atrium, common AV orifice, divided right ventricle and accessory mitral orifice and atrial flutter	1
Common atrium, common AV orifice, total anomalous pulmonary venous drainage to right superior vena cava with obstruction by pulmonary artery, infundibular pulmonary stenosis	1
Common atrium with mitral atresia, straddling tricuspid valve, common AV canal type of VSD, and double outlet right ventricle	1
Common AV orifice, double outlet right ventricle, and absent transverse arch	1
Common atrium with cleft in the anterior leaflet of the mitral valve	1
Common atrium, common AV orifice, double outlet right ventricle, and pulmonary stenosis	1

III. Mixed Mesocardia with Situs Solitus Atria (Atria Pivotal and Ventricles Inverted)

There was a total of six cases; four were females and two were males. The ages ranged from newborn to 49 years, with a median age of 8 years, 8 months.

In these six cases, the right and left atria and ventricles were side by side, with the right atrium entering into the left ventricle on the right, and the left atrium entering into the morphologically right ventricle on the left. The pulmonary trunk emerged from the morphologically left ventricle and the aorta from the right ventricle (Figs. 19, 20).

The Status of Spleen and Abdominal Organs

These cases were associated with situs solitus organs. Two had normal spleens, two had accessory spleens, and one had asplenia. In the sixth, multilo-

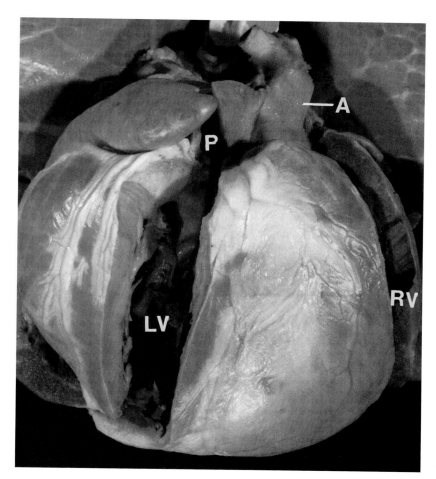

Figure 19: Mixed mesocardia, external view. LV = left ventricle; RV = right ventricle; A = aorta to the left and anterior; P = pulmonary trunk to the right and posterior.

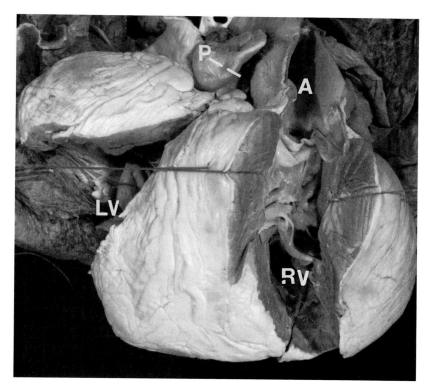

Figure 20: External view of mixed mesocardia. LV = left ventricle to the right and anterior; RV = right ventricle to the left and posterior; A = aorta emerging from the right ventricle; P = pulmonary trunk emerging from the left ventricle.

bated spleen and pancreas with atypical lobulation of the lungs were present.

The Venous Return

The venous return was normal in four, and in one case with accessory spleen there was partial anomalous pulmonary venous drainage. In the other with asplenia, there was absent inferior vena cava and the coronary sinus, and the hepatic veins, right pulmonary veins, and right superior vena cava entered the right atrium, and the left pulmonary veins were stenotic and entered the morphologically left atrium.

AV Dissociation

This was present in a 2-year-old female with ventricular septal defect and Ebstein's anomaly of the left AV valve.

The complexes were as follows:

	No. of Cases
Ebstein's anomaly of the tricuspid valve with tricuspid insufficiency	1
VSD and left AV valve stenosis and insufficiency	1
VSD, Ebstein's anomaly of the left AV valve with insufficiency (Figs. 21–24)	1
VSD, straddling conus, overriding aorta, pulmonary atresia, tricuspid stenosis, atypical ostium primum, and atypical fossa ovalis defect	1
CAVO, inverted double outlet right ventricle, infundibular pulmonary stenosis (Figs. 25–28)	1
VSD, subpulmonary stenosis, accessory tricuspid orifice, right aortic arch forming partial vascular ring with left ligamentum arteriosum and left subclavian from descending aorta	1

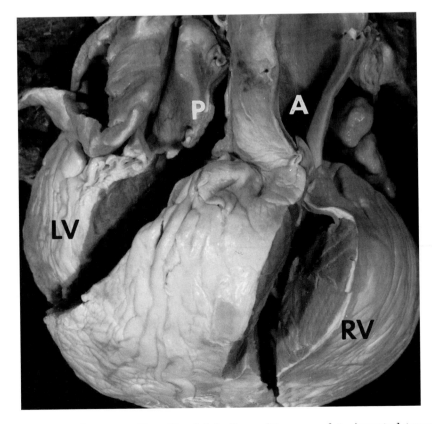

Figure 21: Mixed mesocardia with atrial situs solitus, complete inverted transposition, and Ebstein's anomaly. External view. LV = left ventricle; RV = right ventricle; A = aorta; P = pulmonary trunk. (Used with permission from Lev M, et al. See Figure 34.)

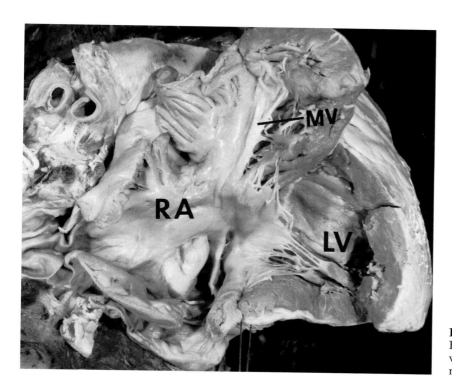

Figure 22: Right atrial, left ventricular view. RA = right atrium; LV = morphologically left ventricle; MV = mitral valve. (Used with permission from Lev M, et al. See Figure 34.)

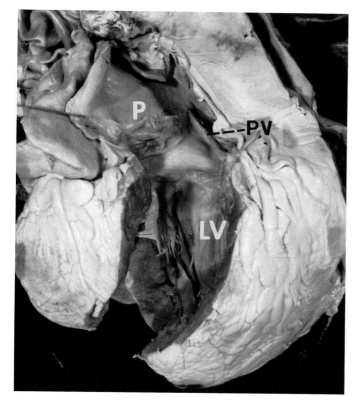

Figure 23: Left ventricular outflow tract demonstrating the pulmonary trunk emerging from this chamber. LV = morphologically left ventricle; PV = pulmonary valve; P = pulmonary trunk. (Used with permission from Lev M, et al. See Figure 34.)

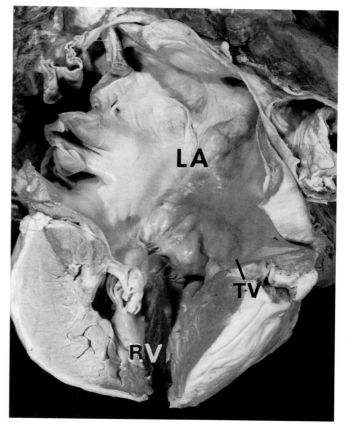

Figure 24: Left atrial, right ventricular view. LA = left atrium; RV = morphologically right ventricle; TV = Ebstein's anomaly of the tricuspid valve. (Used with permission from Lev M, et al. See Figure 34.)

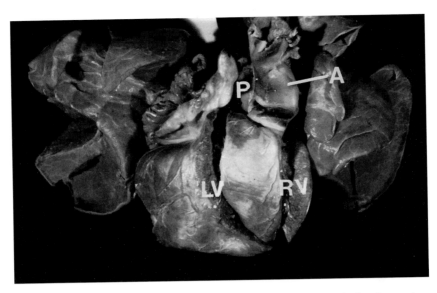

Figure 25: Mixed mesocardia with atrial situs solitus and ventricular inversion, common AV orifice, and double outlet right ventricle. External view of the heart. RV = right ventricle; LV = left ventricle; A = aorta to the left and anterior; P = pulmonary trunk to the right and posterior.

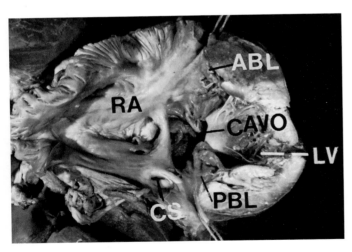

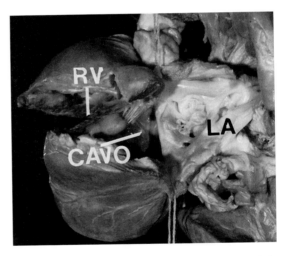

Figure 26: Right atrial, left ventricular view demonstrating complete type of common AV canal. RA = right atrium; LV = morphologically left ventricle; ABL = anterior bridging leaflet; PBL = posterior bridging leaflet; CAVO = common AV orifice, complete; CS = coronary sinus.

Figure 27: Left atrial, right ventricular view. LA = left atrium; CAVO = common AV orifice; RV = morphologically right ventricle.

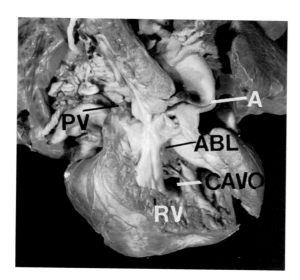

Figure 28: Outflow tract of the right ventricle demonstrating both the aorta and the pulmonary trunk emerging side by side. RV = right ventricle; CAVO = common AV orifice, complete type; ABL = anterior bridging leaflet; A = aorta; PV = pulmonary valve. Note that the aorta and pulmonary trunk are side by side, emerging from the morphologically right ventricle and the aorta is to the left of the pulmonary trunk.

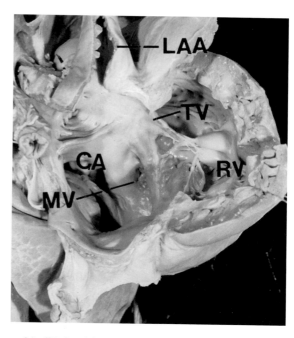

Figure 30: Right side of the common atrium. CA = common atrium, pulmonary veins entering the right side; MV = mitral orifice in the left side of the common atrium; RV = right ventricle; TV = tricuspid valve; LAA = atrial appendage resembling the left atrial appendage.

IV. Mixed Mesocardia with Presumed Situs Inversus Atria

There was one case in this group where the atrial septum was defective and therefore a definitive identification of the atria could not be made but a presumptive diagnosis of the atria was made on the basis of the atrial appendages. The presumptive left atrium that was present on the right entered the morphologically right ventricle present on the right, whereas the presumptive right atrium present on the left side emptied into the morphologically left ventricle present on the left. The venous return was normal. This case was associated with situs inversus of the organs with a normal spleen and was with regular complete transposition and pulmonary stenosis and right aortic arch (physiologically corrected transposition). This was a 3-month-old female child (Figs. 29–31).

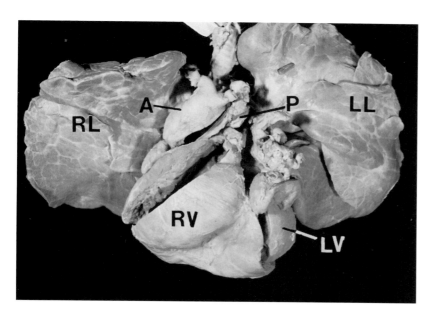

Figure 29: Presumptive mixed mesocardia with atrial situs inversus and normal ventricles. External view. RV = right ventricle; LV = left ventricle; RL = right lung; LL = left lung; A = aorta; P = pulmonary trunk.

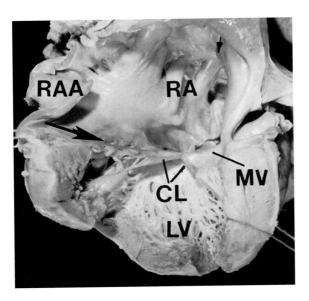

Figure 31: Left side of the common atrium receiving the systemic veins, presumptive right atrium. RA = presumptive right atrium on left side; MV = mitral valve; LV = left ventricle; CL = cleft in anterior leaflet of the mitral valve; RAA = atrial appendage resembling the right atrial appendage. Arrow points to the accessory opening in the anterior leaflet of the mitral valve.

V. Mixed Mesocardia, Atria Indeterminate with Ventricles in Normal Position

There was a total of seven cases: five females and two males. Ages ranged from stillborn to 1 year, 9 months with a median age of 4 months, 7 days. Four were below the age of 1 month.

In this group, the atrial septum was markedly defective, and neither the atrial septum nor the atrial appendages were diagnostic as to right or left. The ventricles, however, were in normal position, but the myocardium was made up mostly of spongiosa (Figs. 32–34).

The Status of Spleen and Abdominal Organs

Five were associated with polysplenia, one with accessory spleen, and one was unknown. The one with accessory spleen and the one with polysplenia were associated with situs inversus abdominalis and abnormal lobation of both lungs.

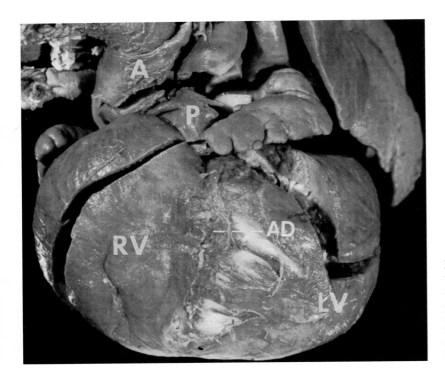

Figure 32: Mesocardia, atria indeterminate, ventricles in normal position with common atrium and common AV orifice, and pulmonary stenosis. External view. RV = right ventricle; LV = left ventricle; A = aorta; P = pulmonary trunk; AD = anterior descending coronary artery. (Used with permission from Lev M, et al. See Figure 34.)

The complexes associated with this type of mesocardia were:

	No. of Cases
Almost absent atrial septum, CAVO, tetralogy of Fallot	1
CAVO, intermediate type, common atrium and subaortic stenosis, and congenital AV block	1
Common atrium with CAVO, intermediate type with infundibular pulmonary stenosis, and congenital AV block	1
Almost common atrium, total anomalous pulmonary venous drainage, mitral stenosis, infundibular pulmonary stenosis	1
Common atrium, CAVO, total anomalous pulmonary venous drainage, complete transposition, pulmonary stenosis, accessory VSD, and right aortic arch with double conus (Figs. 35–37)	1
Common atrium, CAVO with pulmonary stenosis, and congenital AV block (Figs. 32–34)	1
Common atrium, CAVO, double outlet right ventricle, right aortic arch, right descending aorta and coarctation posteriorly in the descending aorta, right PDA, aortic stenosis, and congenital AV block (Figs. 38, 39)	1

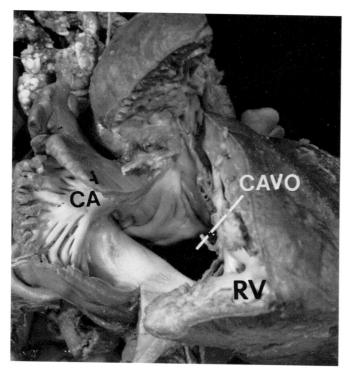

Figure 33: Right-sided view of common atrium and right ventricle. CA = common atrium; RV = right ventricle; CAVO = common AV orifice. (Used with permission from Lev M, et al. See Figure 34.)

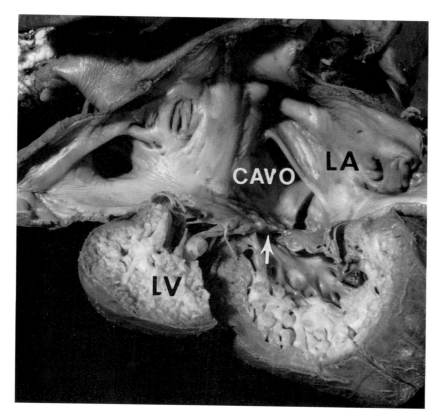

Figure 34: Left side of common atrium, left ventricular view. LA = left atrial side of common atrium; LV = left ventricle; CAVO = common AV orifice, intermediate type. Arrow points to the anterior and posterior bridging leaflets joining together, intermediate form. (Used with permission from Lev M, Liberthson RR, Golden JG, Eckner FAO, Arcilla RA: The pathologic anatomy of mesocardia. *Am J Cardiol* 1971, 28:428–435.)

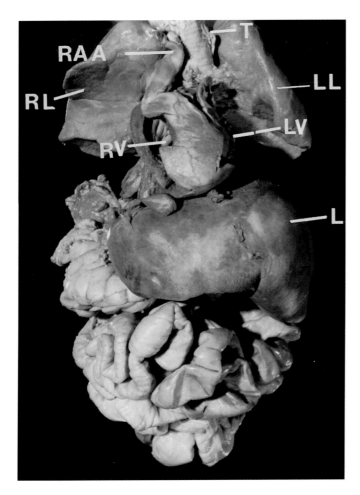

Figure 35: Mesocardia, atria indeterminate and ventricles normal with visceral situs inversus, complete transposition with pulmonary stenosis. L = liver on the left side; RV = right ventricle; LV = left ventricle; RL = right lung; LL = left lung; T = trachea; RAA = right aortic arch.

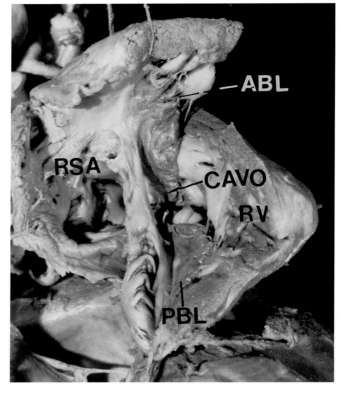

Figure 36: Common atrium, common AV orifice. RSA = right side of common atrium; CAVO = common AV orifice, complete type; PBL = posterior bridging leaflet; ABL = anterior bridging leaflet; RV = right ventricle.

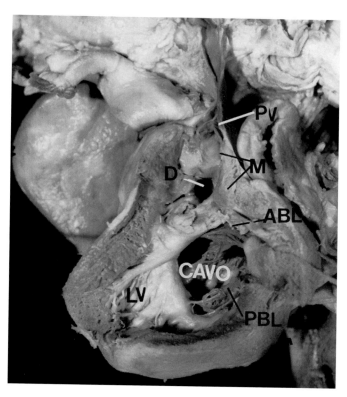

Figure 37: Outflow tract of the left ventricle demonstrating straddling conus and accessory ventricular septal defect. LV = left ventricle; CAVO = common AV orifice, complete type; ABL = anterior bridging leaflet; PBL = posterior bridging leaflet; M = conal muscle extension; PV = bicuspid pulmonic valve with stenosis; D = accessory anterior defect.

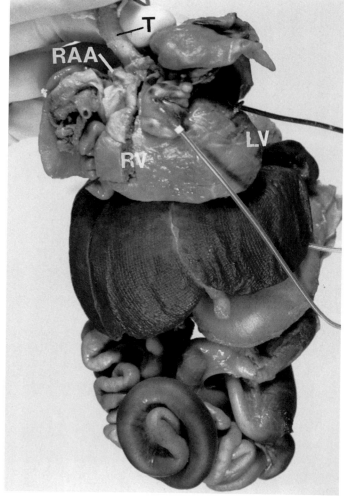

Figure 38: Mesocardia, atria indeterminate, ventricles normal, with right aortic arch, right descending aorta, and posteriorly situated coarctation. External view of the heart. RV = right ventricle; LV = left ventricle; RAA = right aortic arch; T = trachea.

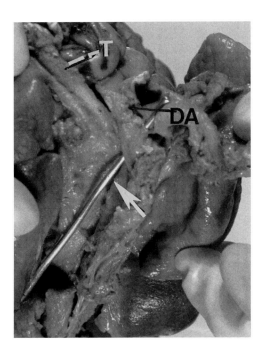

Figure 39: Posterior aspect of trachea and lungs showing the right descending aorta and coarctation. T = trachea; DA = descending aorta to right of trachea and probe passing through the coarcted area. Arrow points to the probe passing through the coarcted area.

The Venous Return

In two, the venous return was normal, in one, the left side of the common atrium also received the left superior vena cava. In one, the left side of the common atrium received the inferior vena cava and the left superior vena cava, and there was total anomalous pulmonary venous drainage into the portal system. In one, the right side of the common atrium received the pulmonary veins, the hepatic veins with absent inferior vena cava and superior vena cava, and the left side received the left superior vena cava, the coronary sinus, and partly the hepatic veins. The azygos vein entered the left superior vena cava. In the sixth, the right-side of the common atium received the two hepatic veins, coronary sinus, and the right pulmonary veins with absent inferior vena cava, and the left side received the left pulmonary veins. In the last case, there was an absent inferior vena cava and coronary sinus with hemizygous extension into the right superior vena cava; and the hepatic vein entered the right side of the common atrium and the left side received the pulmonary veins and a large left superior vena cava.

In two, both lungs were bilobed and the atrial appendages resembled the left atrial appendage. In one, there was absence of one kidney, and in one with polysplenia and partial visceral heterotaxy, the mother was hypothyroid and treated for goiter.

Congenital AV Block

One with accessory spleen and three with polysplenia (two with partial visceral heterotaxy) also had congenital AV block. Their ages were: stillborn, newborn, and a 7-day-old female whose mother was treated for hypothyroid, and a 1-year, 9-month-old child.

VI. Mesocardia, Atria Indeterminate with Ventricles Inverted

There were two cases, both were males. One was a stillborn, 32-weeks' gestation fetus, and the other a newborn, 1 hour, 37 minutes old.

One was a case of polysplenia with diaphragmatic hernia on the right side and part of the liver was on the left chest. The right lung was hypoplastic, the left di-

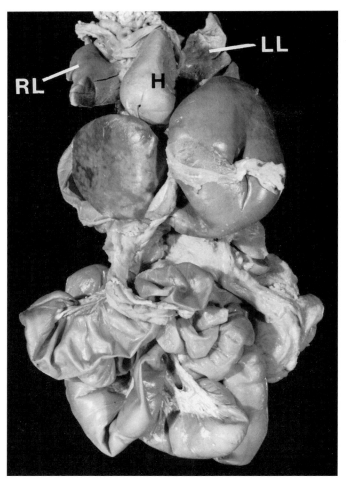

Figure 40: Mixed mesocardia, atria indeterminate, and ventricles inverted. External view of the probable visceral heterotaxy with complete transposition, pulmonary atresia, and total anomalous pulmonary venous drainage. H = heart in the mid-line; RL = right lung; LL = left lung.

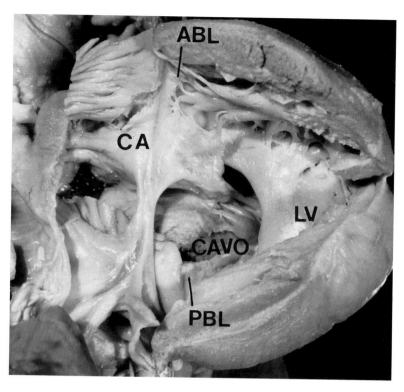

Figure 41: Right-sided view showing the common atrium and the morphologically left ventricle and common AV orifice, complete type. CA = common atrium, atria indeterminate; LV = left ventricle; PBL = posterior bridging leaflet; ABL = anterior bridging leaflet; CAVO = common AV orifice.

vided into three, and there was partial visceral heterotaxy.

The complexes associated with this type of mesocardia were: common AV orifice, complete transposition, pulmonary atresia, common atrium, and total anomalous pulmonary venous drainage into the left superior vena cava and right aortic arch and double patent ductus arteriosus (Figs. 40–42). The other had common atrium, common AV orifice, intermediate type, aortic stenosis, juxtaposition of atrial appendages to the left without transposition, primitive spongy ventricular mass, and bicuspid pulmonary valve.

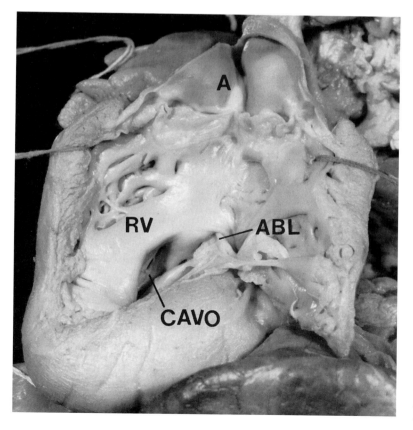

Figure 42: The aorta situated to the left and anterior and emerging from the morphologically right ventricle. RV = morphologically right ventricle; ABL = anterior bridging leaflet; CAVO = common AV orifice; A = aorta.

Comment

In mesocardia, the shape of the heart is remarkable, regardless of the type of mesocardia we are dealing with, in that there is no apex. Instead, the heart is oriented ventrally.

The classification of mesocardia given here corresponds to that in the literature except for certain aspects of nomenclature. This classification is primarily based on the atrial situs and the position of the ventricles. The term "mixed mesocardia" is used by us to indicate that the atria and ventricles do not correspond. This may be due either to atrial situs inversus or ventricular inversion. In either case, it is noted that corrected transposition usually ensues.

As seen from our material from the standpoint of the relationship of the atria to the ventricles, the hearts in mesocardia, in general, correspond to the hearts in levocardia and dextrocardia. Thus, mesoversion corresponds to dextroversion and levoversion, and mixed mesocardia corresponds to mixed dextrocardia and mixed levocardia or corrected transposition. It is of interest that there were six types of mesocardia present in this series.

Splenic Abnormalities

Our material indicates that mesoversion was associated with situs solitus organs and normal spleen and rarely with polysplenia. Presumptive mesoversion was associated with polysplenia, asplenia, or accessory spleens and with or without situs inversus abdominalis and either bilaterally bilobed lungs or multilobulation of lungs. On the other hand, mixed mesocardia with situs solitus atria and inverted ventricles was also associated with situs solitus organs if the spleen was normal. When the spleen was abnormal (accessory spleen), in one case there was situs inversus abdominalis and situs solitus thoracis, and in the other, situs solitus abdominalis with atypical lobulation of lungs. The situs was solitus in one with asplenia. Mixed mesocardia with presumed situs inversus atria and ventricles in normal position was associated with situs inversus organs and normal spleen. Although in general there was no discordance between the situs of atria and that of the organs and the venous return when the spleen was normal, there were a few exceptions.

The splenic abnormalities present in this series included accessory spleens, polysplenia, and asplenia.

Associated Congenital Anomalies

The complexes associated with mesoversion do not, in general, appear to be specific for this entity. However, there appears to be a greater tendency for the left superior vena cava to persist than in congenital heart disease with pure levocardia (normal position of the heart and normal relation of chambers). Likewise, there appears to be a tendency for dominance of the left coronary artery. Further, multiple extracardiac congenital malformations frequently occurred in this group. This is probably the reason for the high incidence of this anomaly below the age of 1 month (32 out of 55–58%). The complexes associated with mixed mesocardia with atria situs solitus and inverted ventricles were inverted transposition, left AV valve anomalies, and ventricular septal defect. These are similar to those found in mixed levocardia with ventricular inversion or corrected transposition hearts.

Embryogenesis

The fundamental embryological problem associated with mesocardia is the absence of the apex. Normally, after the heart is formed at the end of approximately 20 to 25 mm in fetal length, there is no real apex, and the heart looks like the heart in mesocardia. After this stage, the heart either points to the left or to the right, giving it an apex. The reason why the heart points to the left normally has not been explained embryologically as of this date. It is very likely that there is a specific DNA marker system that may be responsible for the heart pointing to the left during a particular stage of development of the heart.

There were three cases of mesocardia in this series that had the typical shape of mesocardia (mesoversion) but were associated with diaphragmatic hernia and one with partial absence of the diaphragm. In addition, two other cases, one with hypoplastic right, middle, and upper lobes of the lung, and the other with ectopia cordis and a defective pericardium were not added in this series. However, it is possible that mesocardia, or lack of apicality, may occur by itself or may be related to certain associated abnormalities that may prevent the formation of an apex. Hence, the associated extracardiac abnormalities that may prevent the formation of the apex are to be taken into account. This again may be related to abnormalities in several genes.

Congenital AV Block

It is significant that mesocardia was frequently seen in the neonatal period and there appears to be a greater tendency for congenital AV block to occur in this entity (16%). This occurred predominantly when associated with polysplenia (six out of nine cases of congenital AV block). It is of interest that in contrast to corrected transposition in levocardia with ventricular inversion where there is a greater tendency for AV block to occur, there was only one case of AV dissociation in mesocardia with situs solitus atria and ventricular inversion. Thus, when there is levocardia with ventricular inversion, there is a tendency for AV block to occur. On the other hand, when the atria are indeterminate with ventricles in the normal position, there is a greater tendency for AV block to occur in mesocardia.

In mesocardia, in addition, there is a high inci-

dence of common atrium (29%) and common AV orifice (23.6%). The above findings suggest that the abnormal development of atria as such may indeed be the force in the formation of mesocardia in contrast to corrected transposition in levocardia or mixed levocardia with ventricular inversion, where the fundamental problem is the shifting or movement of the cardiac tube to the left side. This again suggests the possibility of multiple genetic abnormalities, especially those related to the development of the atria and the AV valves (endocardial cushions) may be the primary factors responsible for mesocardia in some. Because of the high incidence of AV block or atrial arrhythmias in mesocardia, they are listed below:

Congenital AV Block or AV Dissociation or Atrial Flutter in Mesocardia

Age	Sex	Status of Spleen	Arrhythmias	Cardiac Anomalies
I. Mesoversion with atrial situs solitus and normal ventricles				
34-wk gest.	F	Polysplenia	CAV block	ASD, VSD, PS, AS. Overriding aorta. Spongy ventricle.
II. Presumptive mesoversion with atrial situs solitus and normal ventricles				
Stillborn 34-wk gest.	F	Polysplenia	CAV block	Common atrium, CAVO
3 days	M	Accessory spleen	CAV block	CAVO, DORV, absent transverse arch (Figs. 43–45)
4 days	F	Polysplenia Partial visceral heterotaxy	CAV block	Common atrium CAVO, DORV and PS
6½ years	M	Spleen unknown	Atrial flutter	Common atrium, CAVO, divided RV, accessory MO
III. Mixed mesocardia with atrial situs solitus and ventricular inversion				
2 years	F	Normal	AV dissociation	Ebstein's anomaly, VSD
V. Mesocardia, atria indeterminate, and ventricles in normal position				
Stillborn	F	Polysplenia Partial visceral heterotaxy	CAV block	Common atrium, CAVO (Figs. 46–49)
8 hours	F	Accessory spleen	CAV block	Common atrium, CAVO and PS (Figs. 32–34)
7 days	F	Polysplenia Partial visceral heterotaxy	CAV block	Common atrium, CAVO
1 year, 9 months, 19 days	F	Polysplenia	CAV block	Common atrium, CAVO intermediate, subaortic stenosis (Figs. 50–54)

(CAV = congenital atrioventricular; MO = mitral orifice)

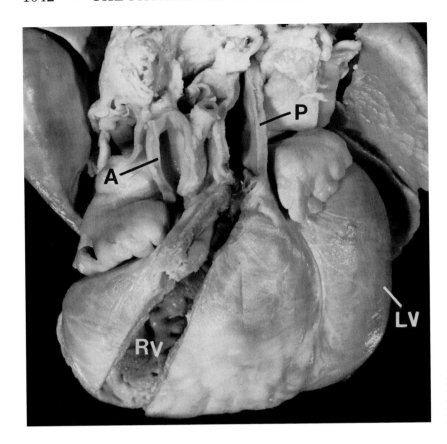

Figure 43: Congenital AV block in presumptive mesoversion in a 3-day-old infant with double outlet right ventricle and absent transverse arch. External view. A = aorta; P = pulmonary trunk; RV = right ventricle; LV = left ventricle.

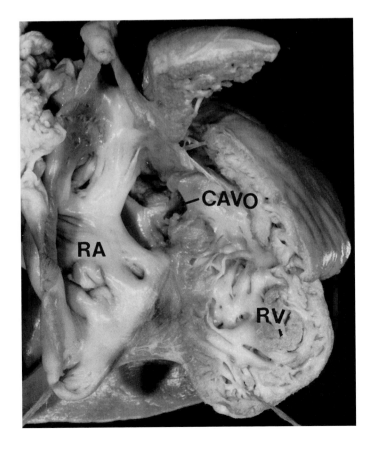

Figure 44: Right-sided view. RA = right atrium; RV = right ventricle; CAVO = common AV orifice.

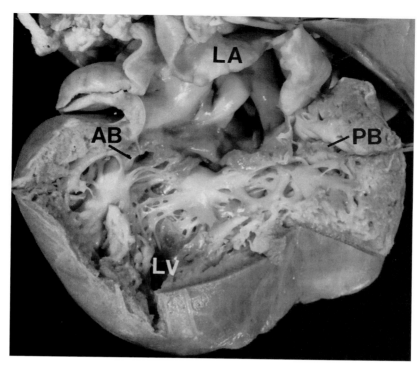

Figure 45: Left-sided view. LA = left atrium; LV = left ventricle; AB = anterior bridging leaflet; PB = posterior bridging leaflet.

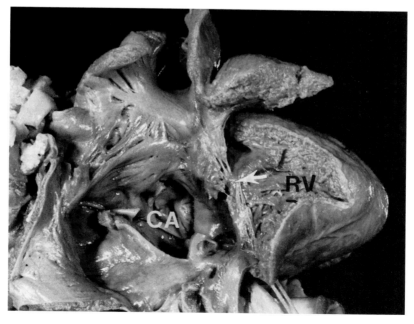

Figure 46: Congenital AV block in a stillborn, common atrium, common AV orifice. CA = common atrium; RV = right ventricle. Arrow points to the small ventricular component and the intermediate type of CAVO.

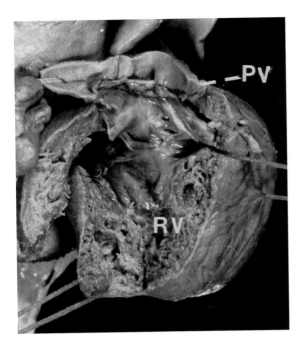

Figure 47: Pulmonary trunk emerging from the right ventricle. RV = right ventricle; PV = pulmonary valve.

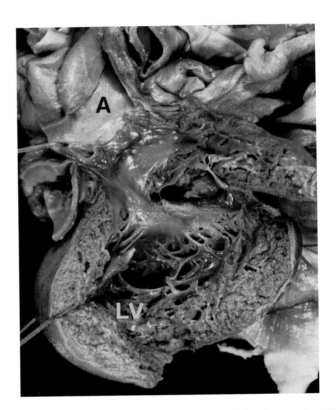

Figure 49: Outflow tract of the left ventricle. A = aorta; LV = left ventricle. Note the spongy ventricular mass.

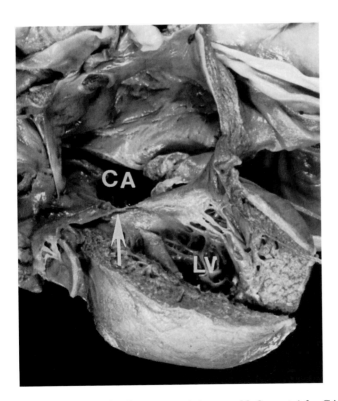

Figure 48: Left side of common atrium and left ventricle. CA = common atrium, left side; LV = left ventricle. Arrow points to the small ventricular component to intermediate type of CAVO.

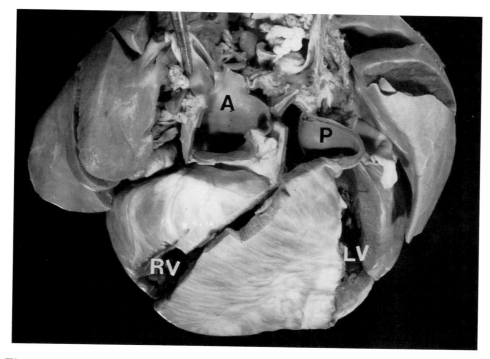

Figure 50: Mesocardia, atria indeterminate, ventricles inverted, and congenital AV block in a 1-year-old child. External view. P = pulmonary trunk; A = aorta; RV = right ventricle; LV = left ventricle.

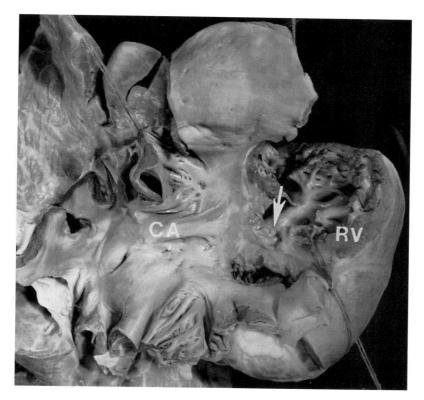

Figure 51: Right-sided view. CA = common atrium, right side; RV = right ventricle. Arrow points to intermediate type of common AV orifice.

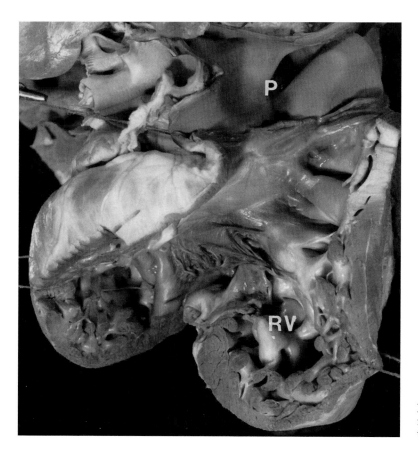

Figure 52: Pulmonary trunk emerging from the right ventricle. RV = right ventricle; P = pulmonary trunk.

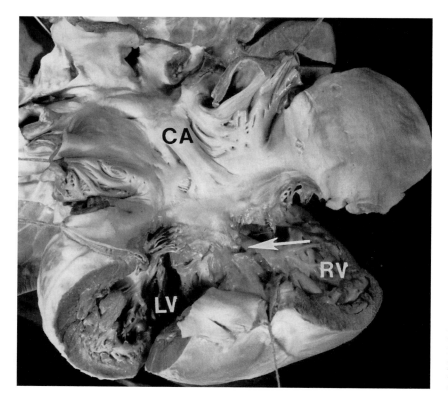

Figure 53: Common atrium as seen from superior aspect showing both ventricles. CA = common atrium; RV = right ventricle; LV = left ventricle. Arrow points to the common AV orifice with no ventricular component.

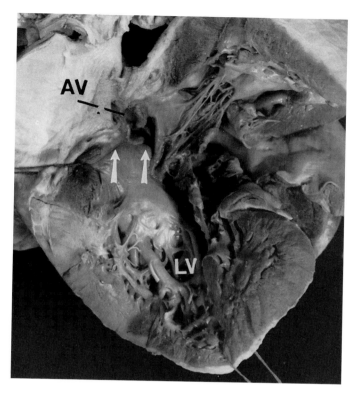

Figure 54: Left ventricular outflow tract showing subaortic stenosis. LV = left ventricle; AV = aortic valve. Arrows point to subaortic stenosis.

Anatomical Location of the Chambers and Great Vessels and Their Clinical and Surgical Significance

The exact location of the atria and the ventricles is of great importance to the clinicians and surgeons. More posterior location of the atria may create problems in identifying veins as well as defects in the atrial septum. More importantly, surgical creation of adequate new tricuspid and mitral valves in the repair of common AV orifice may be difficult. In one particular heart with a right aortic arch, a coarctation was present in the right descending aorta posteriorly. Thus, a right aortic arch with a right descending aorta and coarctation and a right ductus located posteriorly may cause a problem for the clinical diagnosis and surgical correction.

63

Single Ventricle with Small Outlet Chamber

Single ventricle is that entity in which both the atrioventricular (AV) orifices or a common atrioventricular orifice (CAVO) enter a single (primitive) ventricular chamber or a sinus or an inlet from which both arterial trunks emerge with their coni. One or both of these coni are sufficiently well developed so as to constitute a small outlet chamber, or a conus may form simply an outflow tract to the main ventricular chamber (or the single ventricle). The ventricular mass may have originated from a dextro (D-) or a levo (L-) loop. Neither conus may be said to be related directly to an individual AV orifice. The efferent vessels may be transposed or normally related. If transposed, the type of transposition usually follows the type of bulboventricular loop, and so is either a regular (D-) or inverted (L-) transposition. On gross examination, the outflow chamber is considered to consist of only the abnormally developed conus of the right ventricle, without possessing a sinus or an inlet of the right ventricle (Figs. 1–5). Single ventricle has also been called double inlet left ventricle by others.

Definition of Terms

Common ventricle is that condition in which both AV orifices enter or a common AV orifice enters two sinuses slightly subdivided by a remnant of the posterior ventricular septum. Each of these two sinuses is related to an individual conus. A portion of anterior ventricular septum is usually present (Fig. 6). Thus, in common ventricle we are basically dealing with a large ventricular septal defect. The arterial trunks arise again either in a normal or in a transposed position.

The diagnosis of atria and ventricles is made on the septal morphology. If the presence of a septum is

questionable, as in the ventricular mass in single ventricle, the diagnosis of the identity of a chamber is not justifiable. The sinus of a ventricle is that portion which normally contains the tensor apparatus of the AV valves, including the papillary muscles and chordae. If the tensor apparatus resembles the normal tricuspid apparatus, it is then the right sinus and if it resembles the mitral valvular apparatus, it is then the left sinus. If such a tensor apparatus is not present, the presence of a sinus may be inferred if the area is demarcated by a well-recognized posterior portion of the ventricular septum. We believe that there is not sufficient evidence or proof that the trabecular structure of a parietal (anterior or superior) wall provides an adequate basis for identifying the right or left ventricular sinus.

The term *common sinus* implies that the tensor apparatus of both AV valves is included in that sinus.

The term *conus* is used to indicate that an outflow tract, which, as is known embryologically, is derived from the bulbus. It is understood that every arterial trunk, both normally as well as abnormally, has a conus or an outlet, however abbreviated or one-sided it may be. The conal or infundibular septum is the muscular septum that forms a separation between the two coni. The position of the coni vis-à-vis the septum may aid in the diagnosis of regular and inverted transposition.

The term *small outlet chamber* implies that the conus or infundibulum giving rise to a certain vessel is clearly demarcated, and its size approaches that of the normal right ventricular outflow tract or conus. It is emphasized, however, that the small outlet chamber is an abnormally developed infundibulum.

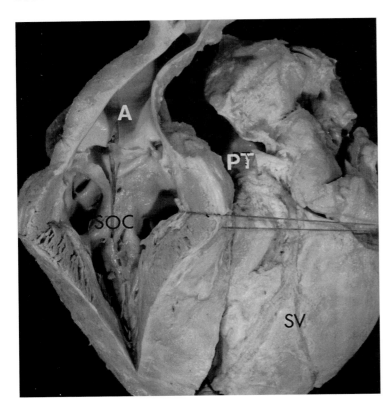

Figure 1: Single (primitive) ventricle with regular transposition in levocardia. Anterior view of the heart with the small outlet chamber opened. A = aorta situated anterior and to the right emerging from the small outlet chamber; SOC = small outlet chamber; PT = pulmonary trunk situated to the left and posterior emerging from the single ventricle; SV = single ventricle. (Used with permission from Lev M, et al. See Figure 109.)

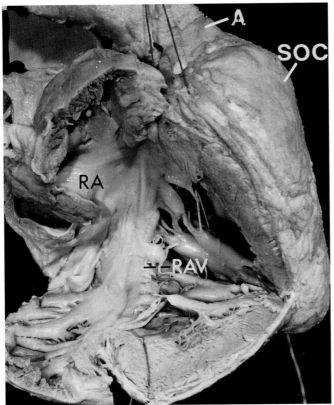

Figure 2: Internal view of Figure 1 as seen from the right side. RA = right atrium; RAV = right atrioventricular valve; SOC = small outlet chamber; A = aorta. (Used with permission from Lev M, et al. See Figure 109.)

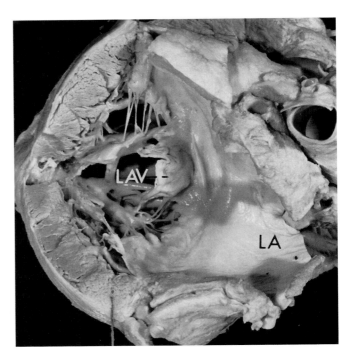

Figure 3: Left atrial view into the single ventricle. LA = left atrium; LAV = left atrioventricular valve. (Used with permission from Lev M, et al. See Figure 109.)

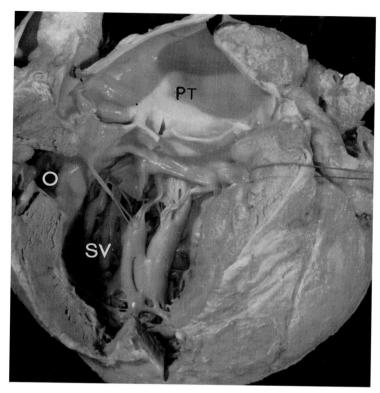

Figure 4: Pulmonary trunk emerging from the single ventricular chamber between the two AV valves. PT = pulmonary trunk; SV = single ventricle; O = opening of the defect into the small outlet chamber. (Used with permission from Lev M, et al. See Figure 109.)

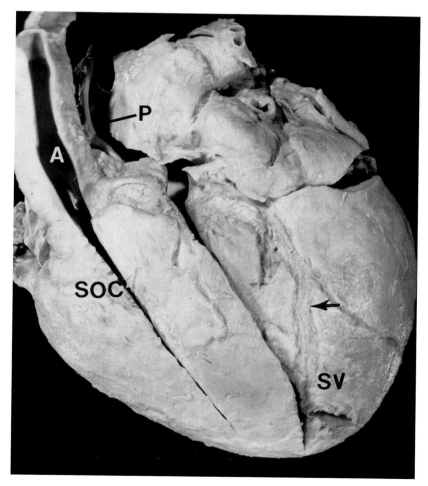

Figure 5: External view of single ventricle with small outlet chamber with regular (noninverted) transposition in an adult. A = aorta emerging from the small outlet chamber; SOC = small outlet chamber situated to the right shoulder or the right base of the heart, superior and anterior; P = pulmonary trunk situated to the left and posterior emerging from the main chamber; SV = single ventricle. Arrow points to the left-sided delimiting artery which is quite large.

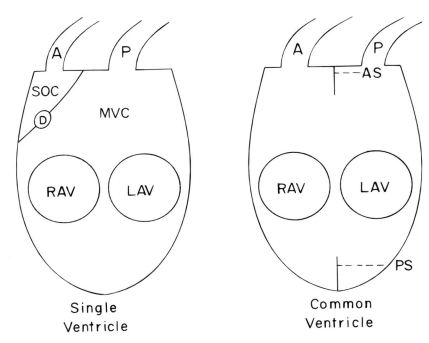

Figure 6: Diagrammatic sketches of the difference between single and common ventricle. No distinction is made in the diagram between inverted and noninverted loop or inverted and noninverted transposition. MVC = main ventricular chamber; SOC = small outlet chamber; A = aorta; PS = posterior ventricular septum; P = pulmonary trunk; AS = anterior ventricular septum; RAV = right atrioventricular valve; LAV = left atrioventricular valve; D = defect between the main or the single ventricular chamber and the small outlet chamber. (Used with permission from Bharati S, Lev M. See Figure 126.)

The term *transposition* implies an abnormal relationship either between the arterial trunks from the standpoint of anteroposterior relationships, or between the arterial trunks and the AV orifices. Reference to the origin of the great vessels from specific chambers, used by us ordinarily in describing transposition, cannot be made in single ventricle since the identity of the chambers is in question. The term *inverted transposition* implies that in addition to the disturbance in the anteroposterior relationship of the bulbotruncal area, there is a disturbance in lateralness (laterality). The point of reference for judgment of the position of the arterial trunks is the normal position in the great arteries seen in levocardia.

The terms *right* and *left delimiting coronary arteries* refer to those coronary arteries that demarcate the small outlet chamber. This terminology is necessary, especially in single ventricle, because the term *anterior descending coronary artery* cannot be applied to these vessels. An anterior descending coronary artery by definition is that artery that lies or enters the anterior interventricular sulcus or supplies the anterior two-thirds of the ventricular septum. Since there is doubt as to what constitutes a ventricular septum and whether a ventricular septum is actually present in single ventricle, the term *anterior descending coronary artery* is not used in this discussion.

Classification

The classification of the types of single ventricle is made on the basis of the direction of the base-apex axis of the heart, the presence or absence of transposition, and the type of transposition. The judgment as to the type of transposition, whether regular or inverted, is made on the basis of the following group of factors:

1. the position of the outlet chamber and its relationship to the right and left AV valve
2. the prominence of the left or right delimiting coronary artery
3. the relative position of the aorta and the pulmonary trunk to each other
4. the relationship of the atrioventricular valves to the aorta and the pulmonary trunk and
5. the position of the conal septum vis-à-vis the pulmonary trunk.

All types of single ventricles show the following characteristics (Figs. 1–5): (1) the mitral and tricuspid valves are usually not readily diagnosable, with one posteromedial and one anterolateral or anterior group of papillary muscles being usually attached to each valve. There is a tendency for one of the anterolateral papillary muscle groups to be small, or at times absent, (2) the posterior wall of the sinus of the single ventricle may be divided by a longitudinal ridge passing from the base of the pulmonary trunk to the apical region in some, (3) where there is transposition, regular or inverted, and the pulmonary orifice is not atretic, there is usually continuity between one aspect of the anulus of the pulmonary valve with both AV orifices, or with a common AV orifice, but there are exceptions; (4) there is a tendency for the left AV orifice to be smaller than normal with anomalous connections of this valve leaflet resulting in stenosis or insufficiency or both; (5) there is a small outlet chamber in the majority of the cases which communicates with the single ventricle by means of a defect or an opening.

Although the above characteristics are seen in most cases of single ventricle, there are exceptions. The exceptions include absence of a small outlet chamber with double coni or overriding of one or both vessels. The exception in general occurs with marked left AV valve stenosis or atresia of one of the semilunar valves. It is emphasized that by our definition we have excluded atresia of the right or the left AV valve which may occur with or without transposition. We will deal with single ventricle with atresia of one of the AV orifices separately.

Single ventricle may broadly be classified into the following:

1. with regular (noninverted, D-) transposition in levocardia
2. with inverted loop and inverted transposition in levocardia (L-)
3. with normal position of the vessels in levocardia (with no transposition)
4. with transposition, type undetermined, in levocardia
5. in dextrocardia
6. in mesocardia
7. in isolated levocardia with partial visceral heterotaxy and asplenia or polysplenia syndromes.

1. With Regular (Noninverted) Transposition in Levocardia (Figs. 1–5)

In this type (1) the outlet chamber is situated to the right base of the heart (superior) or the shoulder of the heart and is closer to the right AV valve than to the left, (2) the left delimiting coronary artery is more prominent than the right, (3) the left atrial appendage is visible from the anterior view of the heart, (4) the aorta is situated anteriorly and to the right and the pulmonary trunk posteriorly and to the left, (5) the atrial septum has a tendency to be in a more sagittal position than in the cases with inverted transposition, (6) the conal septum lies to the right of the pulmonary trunk, and (7) the anterior papillary muscle of the right

AV valve has a tendency to be attenuated. It is emphasized, however, that rarely exceptions do occur to the above descriptions especially when there is atresia or marked stenosis of one semilunar valve, the other dominant vessel almost always is situated anteriorly and the atretic or stenotic vessel in most cases is situated posteriorly (Fig. 7) or sometimes the vessels may be side by side. Likewise, the left delimiting artery may not be more prominent than the right.

The coronary artery distribution is as follows (Fig. 8): The right-sided coronary artery comes off from the posterior sinus of Valsalva. It gives off the right delimiting branch and continues as the right circumflex to supply the right lateral and posterior walls of the sin-

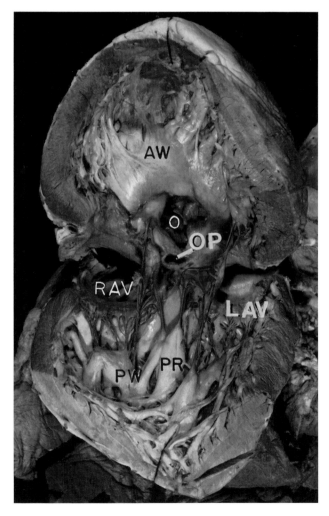

Figure 7: Single (primitive) ventricle with regular (noninverted) transposition in levocardia with pulmonary stenosis. View of single ventricle looking into the base. PW = posterior wall of single ventricle; AW = anterior wall of single ventricle; PR = posterior group of papillary muscles; OP = opening into stenotic pulmonary conus; O = opening into the small outlet chamber; RAV = right AV valve; LAV = left AV valve. (Used with permission from Lev M, et al. See Figure 109.)

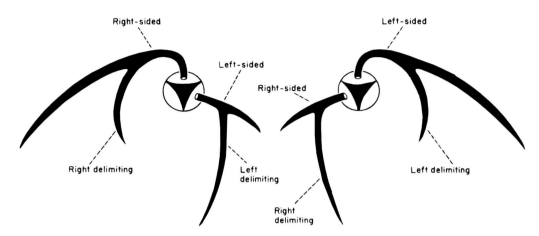

Figure 8: Coronary artery circulation in single (primitive ventricle with regular and inverted transposition in levocardia. (Used with permission from Lev M, et al. See Figure 109.)

gle ventricle. The left-sided coronary artery comes off the left anterior sinus of Valsalva. It gives off the left delimiting coronary artery, and then continues as the left circumflex to supply the left lateral and posterior walls of single ventricle.

2. With Inverted Loop and Inverted Transposition in Levocardia (Figs. 9–13)

In this type (1) the outlet chamber is situated to the left base of the heart or shoulder of the heart (anterior and superior) and is closer to the left AV orifice than the right, (2) the right delimiting coronary artery is more prominent than the left, (3) the left atrial appendage is buried behind the aorta when viewed from the anterior surface of the heart, (4) in most cases the aorta is situated anteriorly and to the left and the pulmonary trunk posteriorly and to the right, (5) the atrial septum has a tendency to be in a more frontal position than in the previous type, (6) the conal septum lies to the left of the pulmonary trunk, and (7) the anterior papillary muscles of the left AV valve is attenuated or absent and there is a distinct tendency for the left AV valve to be small with anomalous connections resulting in stenosis or insufficiency or both.

The origin and distribution of the coronary arteries is a mirror-image of that found in a noninverted type where there were two coronary arteries (Fig. 8). A single coronary artery is not an uncommon finding in this group.

It is again emphasized that exceptions to the above characteristics do occur in this entity. Although in most cases the aorta is situated to the left and anterior and

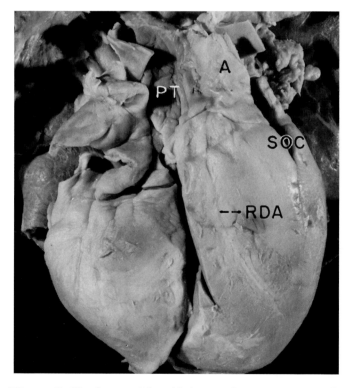

Figure 9: Single ventricle with inverted transposition in levocardia, external view. PT = pulmonary trunk; A = aorta; SOC = small outlet chamber situated to the left base or the shoulder of the heart; RDA = right delimiting artery situated to the right side of the aorta. Note that the aorta is distinctly situated to the left and anterior and the pulmonary trunk to the right and posterior. (Used with permission from Lev M, et al. See Figure 109.)

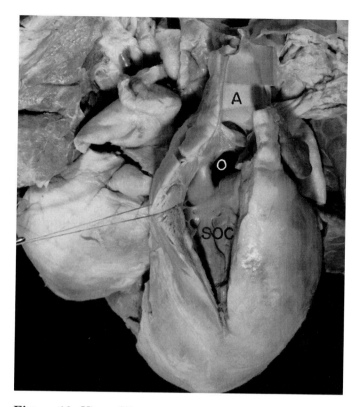

Figure 10: View of the aorta emerging from the small outlet chamber over a defect confluent with the base of the aortic valve. A = aorta; O = opening or defect with aorta overriding the defect; SOC = small outlet chamber. (Used with permission from Lev M, et al. See Figure 109.)

the pulmonary trunk to the right and posterior, where there is atresia of one of the semilunar valves or marked stenosis especially of the pulmonary valve, the dominant vessel is distinctly anterior and the atretic or markedly stenotic vessel either posterior or the vessels may be side by side. The right delimiting artery, which is prominent in most cases, may show variation. The right delimiting coronary artery may give off several prominent branches in the anterior surface of the heart or the right delimiting coronary artery may not be prominent. The small outlet chamber may not be situated exactly to the left base of the heart anteriorly and superiorly, it may be situated in the center of the heart or the middle part of the heart in a horizontal position situated transversely or in extreme cases may be situated superoposteriorly to the left side.

In both of the above types (with regular and inverted transposition), the aorta emerges from the small outlet chamber. Rarely, there are two outlet chambers with a vessel arising from each in regular transposition.

In both types, the situs of the viscera is in general solitus, although an occasional case with malrotation of the intestine is found. The spleen is usually normal, although occasionally asplenia, bilobed spleen, or multiple spleens are noted.

A small defect between the single ventricle and small outlet chamber, hypoplasia of the transverse arch with coarctation (fetal or preductal type), or segmental coarctation (adult type of coarctation) are com-

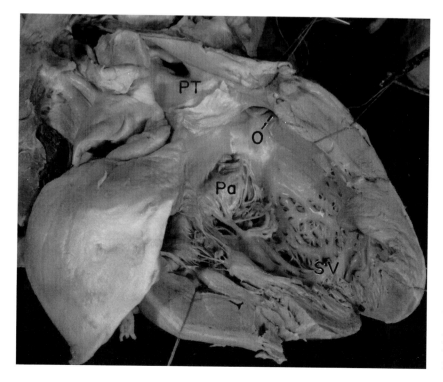

Figure 11: Internal view of single ventricle showing stenotic left AV orifice – parachute type of a valve. O = defect or opening into the small outlet chamber with subaortic stenosis; Pa = parachute left AV valve; SV = single ventricle; PT = pulmonary trunk. (Used with permission from Lev M, et al. See Figure 109.)

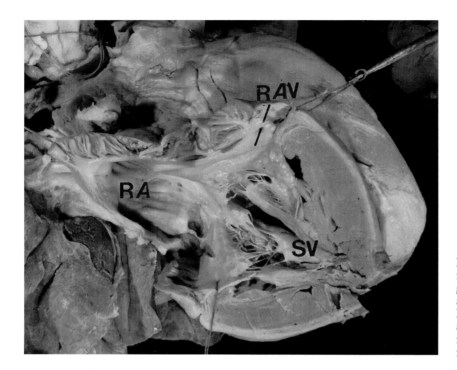

Figure 12: Right atrial view showing the right AV valve and its connection into the single ventricle. RA = right atrium; RAV = right atrioventricular valve; SV = single ventricle. Note that the right AV valve does not resemble a tricuspid or a mitral valve and the papillary muscles are situated in the anterior and posterior walls of the single ventricle.

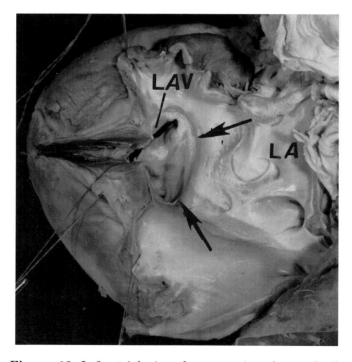

Figure 13: Left atrial view demonstrating the markedly stenotic left AV valve with tremendous hypertrophy and enlargement of the left atrium. LA = hypertrophied and enlarged left atrium; LAV = stenotic small left AV valve. Arrows point to the small anulus of the left AV valve.

mon in both groups but have a tendency to occur more frequently with regular transposition than the inverted type.

A left common pulmonary vein or occasionally a right common pulmonary vein may be seen.

In most cases, there is bi-atrial hypertrophy and enlargement and hypertrophy and enlargement of the single ventricular mass. This is seen in infant hearts as well.

3. With Normal Position of the Arterial Trunks in Levocardia–Holmes Heart (Figs. 14–16)

In this type (1) the pulmonary trunk emerges from the small outlet chamber, and (2) the aortic anulus is continuous with the left AV or common AV anulus or the aorta may be in continuity with both AV valves. There is a tendency for pulmonary valvular and infundibular stenosis to occur in this entity more so than with transposition.

4. Type Undetermined, with or without Transposition, in Levocardia

In this group, although the diagnosis of single ventricle was clear, according to our definition, it is not

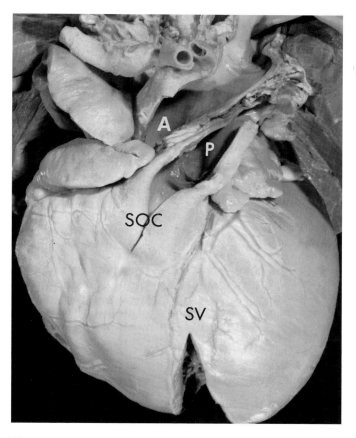

Figure 14: Single ventricle with normal position of arterial trunks in levocardia, with pulmonary stenosis; external view of the heart. A = aorta; P = pulmonary trunk; SOC = small outlet chamber situated to the left and anterior; SV = single ventricle. Note the normal position of the great arteries. (Used with permission from Lev M, et al. See Figure 109.)

possible to classify the type of transposition present because of insufficient anatomic data. That is, the relationship of the arterial trunks to each other, the position or the absence of the outlet chamber, and the size of the delimiting arteries are not sufficiently distinctive as to yield a distinct diagnosis. All had a common denominator, ie, one AV valve was markedly abnormally formed or with a common AV orifice, or there were anomalies in the pulmonary venous return, or either the aorta or the pulmonary trunk was small.

Single Ventricle in Dextrocardia, Mesocardia, and Isolated Levocardia

We have intentionally not included those single ventricles when seen with abnormal position of the heart and its chambers in this particular section because these will be dealt with in detail later. We take exception to the rule in one case where a single ventricle was seen in a case of dextrocardia with truncus.

Analysis of Our Material

There was a total of 101 cases: 66 males, 31 females, and four unknown. The youngest was a 31-weeks' gestation fetus, the oldest was 43 years, with a mean age of 3 years, 9 months, 28 days. This includes an 11-day-old male antelope.

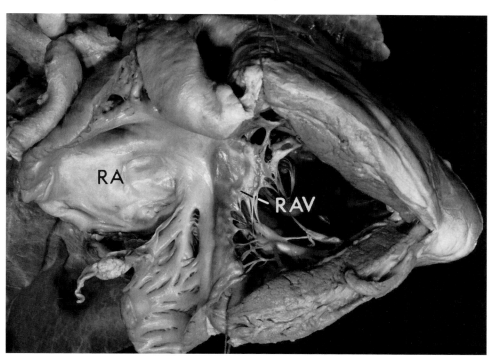

Figure 15: Internal view of the single ventricle from the right side. RA = right atrium; RAV = right AV valve. Note the poorly developed anterior group of papillary muscles. (Used with permission from Lev M, et al. See Figure 109.)

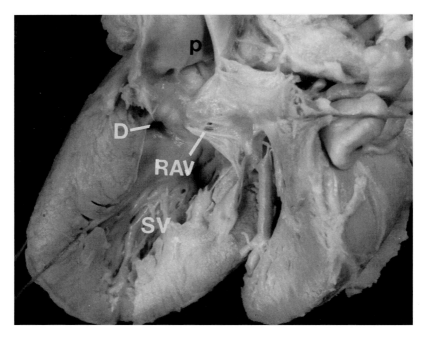

Figure 20: Single ventricle showing the main pulmonary trunk emerging from the single ventricle and a small defect between the single ventricle and the small outlet chamber. SV = single ventricle; RAV = right AV valve; D = small defect; P = pulmonary trunk.

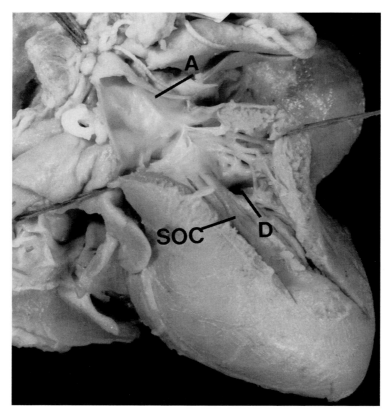

Figure 21: Aorta emerging from the small outlet chamber from the right base of the heart with a small defect and coarctation of the aorta. SOC = small outlet chamber; D = small closing defect; A = aorta.

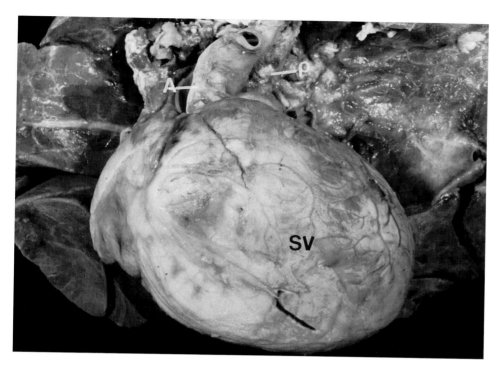

Figure 22: Single ventricle with regular transposition, coarctation of the aorta, and banding of the main pulmonary trunk; external view. SV = single ventricle; A = aorta; P = pulmonary trunk with the band. (Used with permission from Lev M, et al. See Figure 55.)

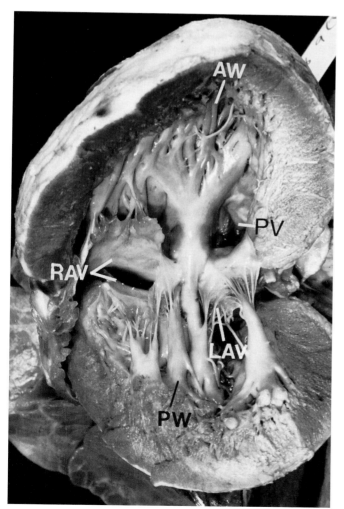

Figure 23: Single ventricle with regular transposition demonstrating the entry of both AV valves into the main chamber with the pulmonary trunk not in continuity with the AV valves. PW = posterior wall of the single ventricle; AW= anterior wall of the single ventricle; RAV= right AV valve; LAV = left AV valve; PV = pulmonary valve emerging somewhat closer to the left AV valve but not in continuity with the left and right AV valves. (Used with permission from Lev M, et al. See Figure 55.)

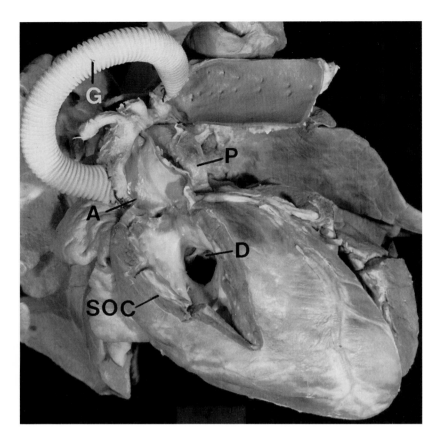

Figure 24: Single ventricle with small outlet chamber with regular transposition and fetal coarctation and surgical repair; external view. SOC = small outlet chamber; D = defect between the main chamber and the small outlet chamber; A = aorta situated to the right and anterior, pulmonary trunk to the left and posterior; P = pulmonary trunk; G = graft proceeding from the ascending aorta to the descending aorta.

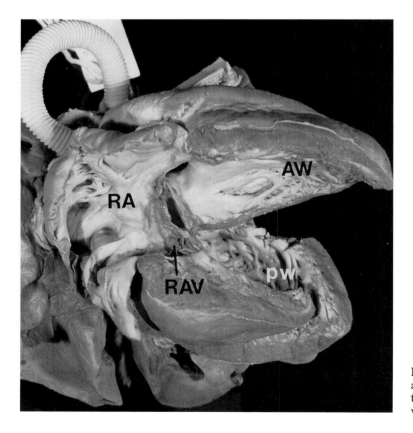

Figure 25: Right-sided view of Figure 24. RA = right atrium; RAV = right AV valve; PW = posterior wall of the single ventricle; AW = anterior wall of the single ventricle. Note the intact atrial septum.

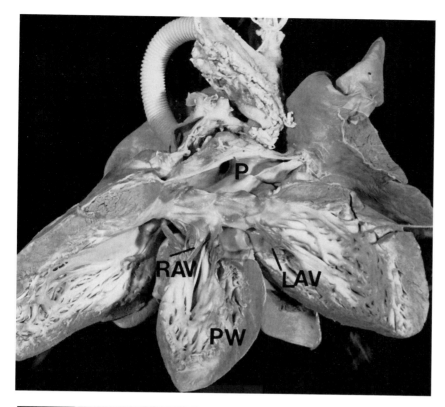

Figure 26: The large pulmonary trunk emerging from the main ventricular chamber confluent with both the AV valves. RAV = right AV valve; LAV = left AV valve; PW = posterior wall of the single ventricle; P = main pulmonary trunk.

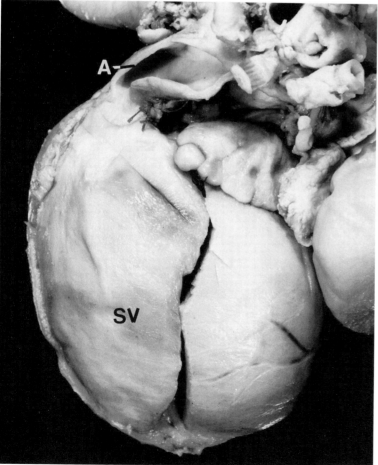

Figure 27: Single ventricle with regular transposition and double conus; external view. SV = single ventricle; A = aorta emerging from the right base of the heart.

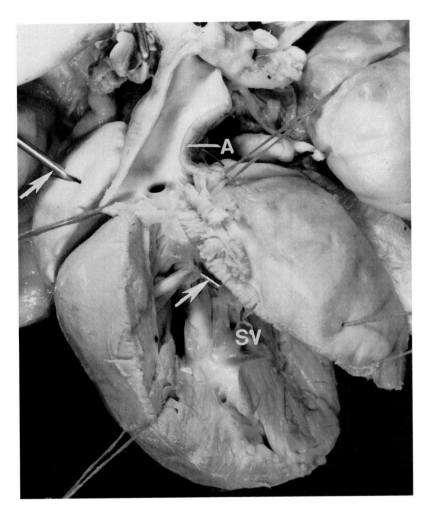

Figure 28: Aorta emerging from the single ventricle unrelated to the AV valves with no outlet chamber. SV = single ventricle; A = aorta. Arrows point to the probe showing the connection of both AV valves to the same papillary muscle. Note coarctation of the aorta, conus beneath the aorta and subaortic stenosis.

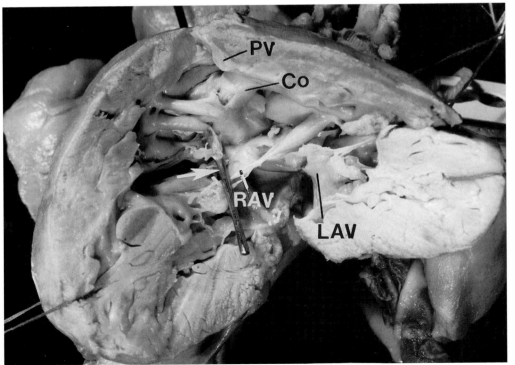

Figure 29: Pulmonary trunk emerging from single ventricle but unrelated to the AV valves and muscle bundles separating the pulmonary valve from the AV valves. RAV = right AV valve – note the bizarre connections; LAV = left AV valve; PV = pulmonary valve; Co = conus muscle beneath the pulmonary valve separating the pulmonary from the AV valves. Arrow points to the probe passing from the aorta to the main ventricular chamber.

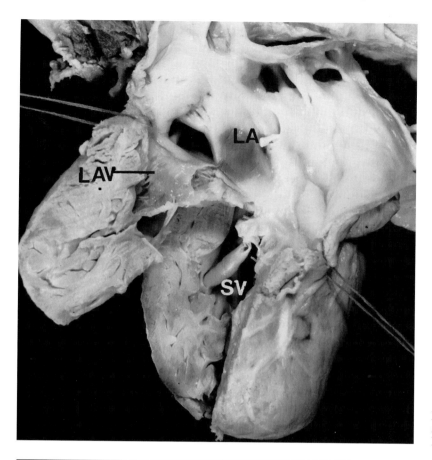

Figure 30: Single ventricle as seen from the left side with small left AV valve. LA = left atrium; LAV = left AV valve; SV = single ventricle.

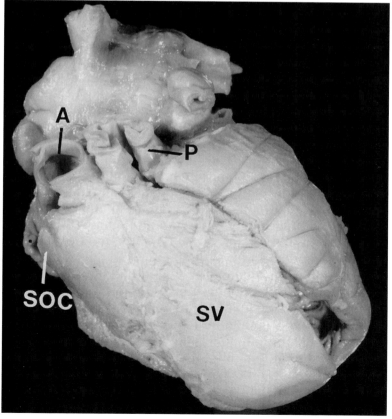

Figure 31: Single ventricle with regular transposition and small outlet chamber situated to the right base of the heart; external view of the heart. SV = single ventricle; SOC = small outlet chamber giving rise to a small aorta; A = aorta, small; P = pulmonary trunk.

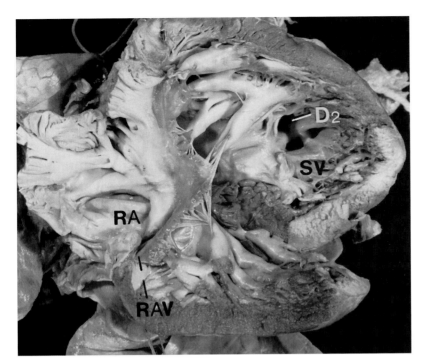

Figure 36: Internal view of the single ventricle from the right side. RA = right atrium; RAV = large right AV valve; SV = hypertrophied and enlarged single ventricle; D$_2$ = the second defect communicating with the main ventricular chamber.

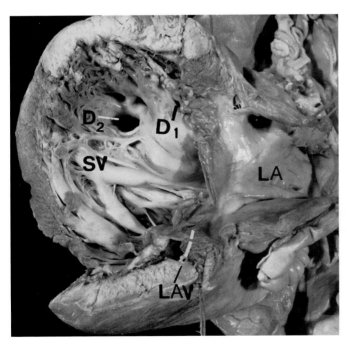

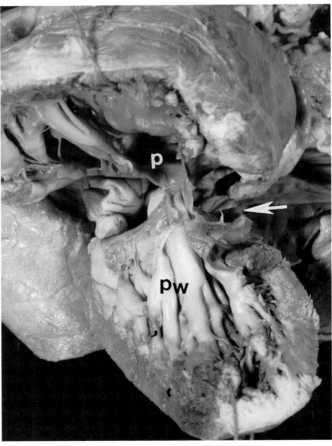

Figure 37: Internal view of the single ventricle from the left side. LA = left atrium; LAV = left AV valve with stenosis; D$_2$ = the second defect entering the single ventricle at its lower third; D$_1$ = the first defect – note the anterior leaflet of the LAV obstructing the defect; SV = single ventricle. Note the poorly developed papillary muscle for the left AV valve in the anterior wall.

Figure 38: Single ventricle demonstrating the entry of both AV valves into the single chamber. Note that the papillary muscles in the posterior wall connect with both the AV valves, and the papillary muscles in the anterior wall connect only with the right AV valve. PW = posterior wall of the single ventricle; P = pulmonary trunk emerging between the two AV valves with stenosis of the left AV valve. Arrow points to the stenotic left AV valve.

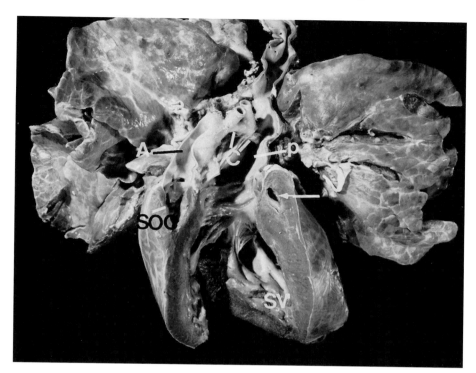

Figure 39: Single ventricle with small outlet chamber with regular transposition and hypoplasia of transverse arch and coarctation of the aorta resulting in atresia – absent transverse arch. A = small aorta emerging from the small outlet chamber; SV = single ventricle; SOC = small outlet chamber; P = main pulmonary trunk emerging from the single ventricle; C = hypoplasia of the transverse arch with coarctation resulting in atresia. Arrow points to the small defect.

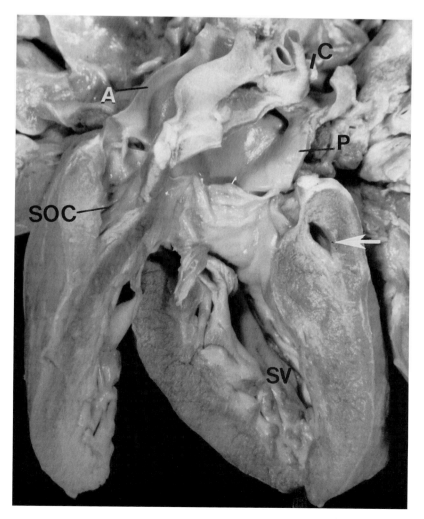

Figure 40: A close-up view of Figure 39 demonstrating the small defect with the small outlet chamber and coarctation of the aorta. SV = single ventricle; SOC = small outlet chamber; A = aorta; C = coarctation; P = pulmonary trunk. Arrow points to the small defect between the main chamber and the small outlet chamber.

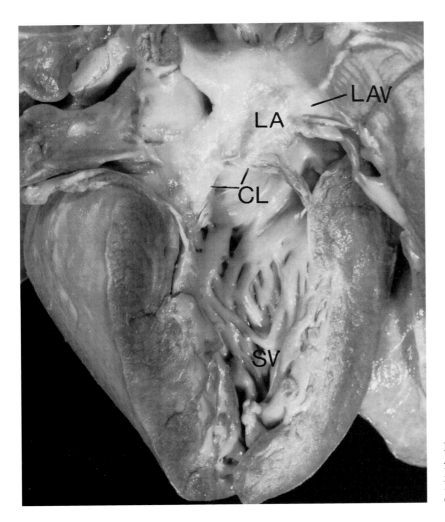

Figure 41: Cleft in the left AV valve with left AV valve stenosis. LAV = left AV valve, small; LA = left atrium; CL = cleft in the anterior leaflet of the left AV valve; SV = single ventricle.

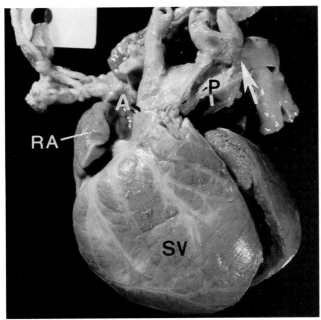

Figure 42: Single ventricle with no outlet chamber with aortic atresia; external view. P = pulmonary trunk; A = aorta; SV = single ventricle; RA = right atrium. Arrow points to the anomalous origin of the subclavian arteries at the junction of the ductus arteriosus as it forms the descending aorta.

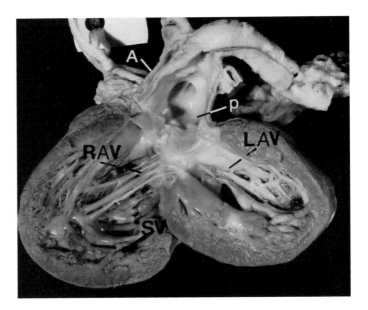

Figure 43: Single ventricle without an outlet chamber, internal view demonstrating both AV valves entering the same chamber and the pulmonary trunk between the two AV valves. RAV = right AV valve; LAV = left AV valve; A = small aorta; p = larger pulmonary trunk; SV = single ventricle.

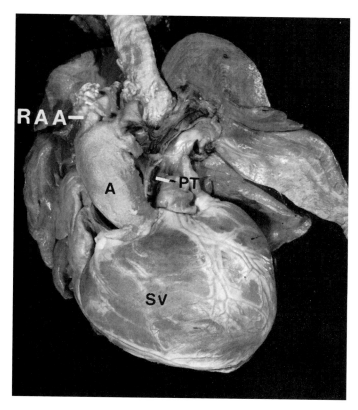

Figure 44: External view of single ventricle and small outlet chamber with regular transposition and pulmonary atresia in a newborn infant with premature closure of the foramen ovale. A = huge aorta situated to the right and anterior; SV = single ventricle; PT = minute pulmonary trunk situated to the left and posterior; RAA = right aortic arch.

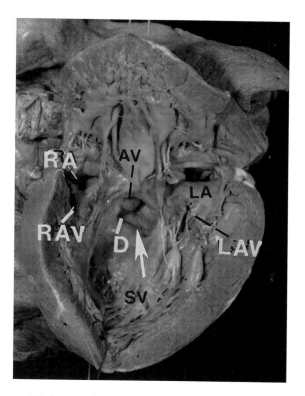

Figure 45: Internal view of single ventricle showing the entry of both AV valves and the aorta emerging from the small outlet chamber and is not in direct continuity with the AV valves but overrides the defect. RAV = right AV valve; LAV = left AV valve; SV = single ventricle; RA = right atrium; LA = left atrium; AV = aortic valve; D = large defect between the SV and the SOC with overriding aorta. Note that the aortic valve is not in direct continuity with the AV valves but overrides the large defect. Arrow points to the SOC.

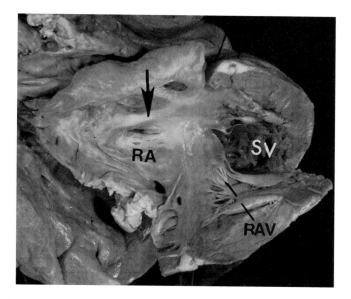

Figure 46: Single ventricle, same heart as shown in Figures 44 and 45, as seen from the right atrial view in a newborn infant with premature closure of the foramen ovale. RA = hypertrophied and enlarged right atrium; SV = single ventricle; RAV = markedly enlarged right AV valve. Arrow points to the premature closure of the foramen ovale.

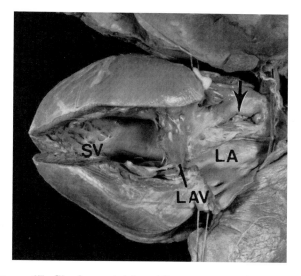

Figure 47: Single ventricle with premature closure of the foremen ovale as seen from the left side. LA = left atrium; LAV = small left AV valve; SV = single ventricle. Arrow points to the closure of the foreman ovale.

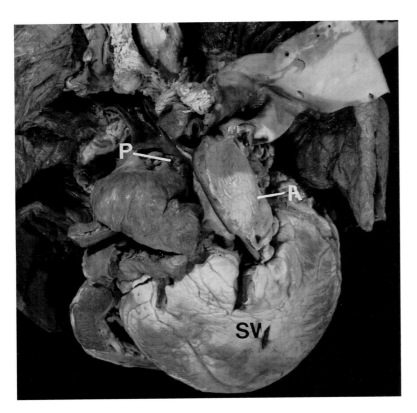

Figure 48: Single ventricle with small outlet chamber with regular transposition. External view of the heart showing the aorta slanting slightly to the left and anterior and a very small pulmonary trunk posterior and somewhat to the right. SV = single ventricle; P = very small pulmonary trunk; A = huge aorta anterior and slanting somewhat to the left.

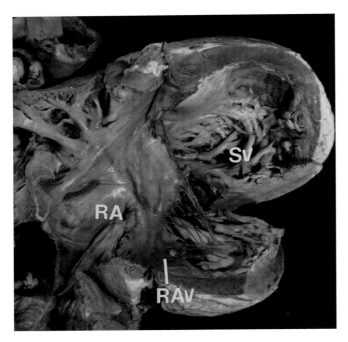

Figure 49: Internal view of single ventricle from the right side demonstrating the connections of the right atrioventricular valve almost exclusively to the inferior wall. RA = right atrium; SV = single ventricle; RAV = right AV valve. Note that practically all of the papillary muscles are in the inferior wall of the single ventricle.

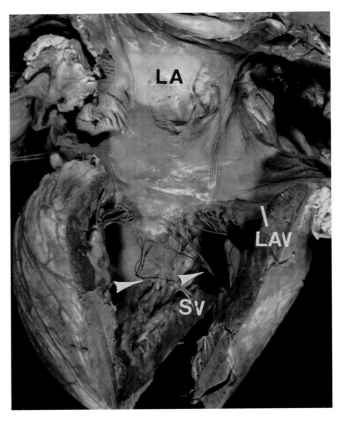

Figure 50: Single ventricle as seen from the left side demonstrating the elongated chordal connections of the left AV valve to the inferior group of papillary muscles. LA = hypertrophied and enlarged left atrium; LAV = left AV valve; SV = single ventricle. Arrowheads point to the elongated chordae.

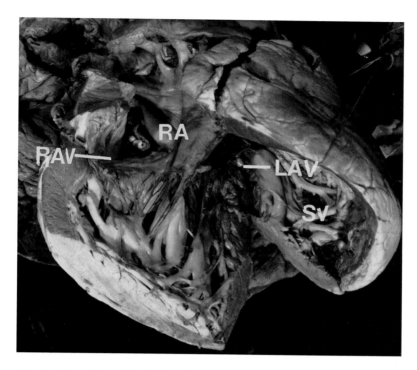

Figure 51: Another view of the internal anatomy of the single ventricle demonstrating that the architecture of this chamber does not resemble either a morphologically right or a left ventricle. RA = right atrium; LAV = left AV valve; RAV = right AV valve; SV = single ventricle. Note that the posterior wall is filled with well-developed papillary muscles and markedly trabeculated anterior wall.

The above clearly demonstrates that there is a distinct tendency for hypoplasia of the transverse arch with coarctation (fetal coarctation) or paraductal coarctation (segmental) or interrupted aortic arch and rarely aortic atresia to occur in this entity. This was seen in 17 (56%). The second important factor is the equal incidence (56%) of AV valve abnormalities. Anomalies of both AV valves in seven (23%), left AV valve in five (16.5%) and right AV valve in five (16.5%) were present. The anomalies included right or left AV valve stenosis with small anulus, absence of one or both papillary muscles in the anterior or posterior walls, and anomalous insertion of the anterior leaflet of the left or the right AV valve at the junction of the defect with the small outlet chamber and restricting the defect to a varying extent. Six (20%) were with CAVO. Thus, only seven (23%) had "normal AV valves." Where there was coarctation of the aorta, it was most frequently associated with a small defect and a very small outlet chamber (11 out of 17–65%), and subaortic stenosis.

It is also of interest that hypoplasia of the aorta is frequently associated with an oblique patent foramen ovale, and varying types of anomalies of the remnants of the sinus venarum valves in the right atrium. One was with premature closure of the foramen ovale with a large defect between the single ventricle and the small outlet chamber with overriding aorta.

Pulmonary atresia was seen in six and common atrioventricular orifice in six.

2. Inverted Transposition with Presumed Inverted Loop

There was a total of 46 cases in this group. Fifteen were female, 29 were male, and two were unknown. The youngest was a 31-weeks' gestation fetus, and the oldest was 43 years with an average age of 5 years, 11 months, 16 days. Pertinent details of the cases are as follows:

FC, PFO, PDA, and *small defect* with small SOC	6 weeks M
FC, PDA, PFO, subaortic stenosis, bicuspid AV, and PM to base of right AV, *large defect*	2½ months F
PFO, FC, PDA, *small defect*, subaortic stenosis, double ductus (right ductus–right subclavian) and large left ductus forming descending aorta and partial absence of the aortic valve (Figs. 52–55)	14 days M
FC, PDA–closing, RAA, PFO, and *small defect* and parachute left AV valve with stenosis (Figs. 56–60)	1 month, 17 days M
FC, subaortic stenosis, PDA—closing, no distinct PM to RAV with marked RAV stenosis and *small defect*	21 days F
FC, subaortic stenosis, wide PDA and *small defect*—aneurysm of the aortic sinus of Valsalva and stenotic left AV valve (Figs. 61, 62)	4 days M
FC, PDA, left AV stenosis, PFO, and small defect (Figs. 63–65)	21 days F
FC, AS, subaortic stenosis, PDA–several *small defects* between the main chamber (MC) and SOC, unicuspid aortic valve and two coronary sinus ASDs	4 weeks M
FC, PDA, ASD, basilar straddling left AV valve with stenosis and obstructing the defect between SOC and MC, banding of PT and residual coarctation and *small defect*, bicuspid aortic valve with aneurysm of the ascending aorta and poorly developed PPM for RAV	2 months F
FC repair and ligation of PDA, PA banding, spontaneous *closure of the defect* following banding, sub-AS, residual coarctation, PFO, left AV valve stenosis (parachute, no APM), bicuspid aortic valve with aneurysm of posterior sinus	2½ months M
Coarctation, banding–old, with spontaneous *closure of the defect*, closed defect confluent with aortic valve and AA outpouched and both lungs bilobed, supravalvular PS following banding and elongated chordae for RAV, PFO, aneurysm of fossa ovalis	6 months M
Coarctation, repair, banding with spontaneous *closing of the defect* with restriction, small aneurysm of fossa ovalis, large right coronary with double delimiting arteries, PFO, left AV valve insufficiency (accessory openings) and anterior leaflet attached to the defect and no APM, right AV sheet of tissue, abbreviated and thickened chordae	3 months M
Marked coarctation (almost atresia), PDA, recent banding, combined eustachian and thebesian valve, oblique PFO, redundant septum primum, three large delimiting arteries–right, aortic valvular and subaortic stenosis, *slit-like closing defect*, high origin of both coronary ostia, unicuspid aortic valve with shallow aneurysms, left AV, valve parachute (completely anchored to PPM with short chordae) and right AV valve stenosis, atypical parachute (anchored completely to anterior PM with short chordae)	2 months M, (premature twin)
Coarctation, repair, banding producing subaortic obstruction with *closing defect*, left AV valve insufficiency (anterior leaflet directly anterior wall at the junction of the defect with the main chamber), both AV valves connected to the same PPM, PFO, septostomy	21 months M
Coarctation, PDA, left AV valve stenosis (anomalous connections), and accessory PM in posterior wall for RAV (Figs. 66–69)	10 weeks M
Coarctation, PDA, left AV valve stenosis and insufficiency (double orifice), adequate sized defect (both vessels slightly to left) SOC anterior and superior. Both coronary ostia from the right posterior sinus	1 month M
Paraductal coarctation, old surgery, debanding, *restrictive defect* between MC and SOC, left AV insufficiency (both AV valves inserted into PPM, PPM base of the valve with incomplete supravalvular ridge), defect confluent with the aortic valve and overriding AO, origin of the left subclavian artery away and pericarditis, bicuspid aortic valve with fenestrations and insufficiency	7 years M
FC, subaortic stenosis, ASD, FOD, *small defect*	unknown
Absent transverse arch, wide PDA, SOC with *small defect*, blood cysts in RAV, and aneurysm of sinus of Valsalva of the aortic valve	21 days M
Absent transverse arch with AS and subaortic stenosis, wide PDA, left AV valve stenosis, and *small defect* with large ASD	19 days M

Absent transverse arch repair, banding, *closing defect* following banding, PDA, probe patent, posterior defect, left AV valve stenosis (parachute, no APM), RAV hypoplastic with abbreviated chordae, unequal size of pulmonic valve cusps–one larger than the other two	4 months M
Subaortic stenosis, common conus, common Lt and Rt P vein	5 years M
Subaortic stenosis, prominent eustachian valve, common Lt P vein	unknown
Lt AV valve stenosis and PS, PDA, absent eustachian and thebesian valves, common Lt P vein, bilobed spleen	4 months M
PS, PFO, endocardial band in RA, large defect, cleft in RAV and single PPM to LAV (parachute) (Figs. 70–74)	15 years F
Large ASD, subpulmonary stenosis, bicuspid PV with SBE, parachute right AV (no APM) with SBE stenosis, Rete chiari and *large defect* and fenestrations of aortic valve	26 years M
PS, ASD, PDA, *small defect*, and bicuspid PV	12 days M
PS with heart block, pacemaker, PFO, *large defect*, RAV stenosis (no PPM, anomalous muscle to base of valve), no APM to LAV, with accessory opening and LAV insufficiency	16 years F
Rt AV valve stenosis with thrombosis of RAV almost occluding, bicuspid pulmonic valve, and PS (Figs. 75, 76)	4 years, 8 months F
Single coronary artery, both vessels mildly overriding a large U-shaped defect, bicuspid PV, PS, and aneurysm of aortic sinus of Valsalva (Figs. 77–79)	5 years, 3 months M
Two defects between MC and SOC (one between A and P and the other close to the superior wall) single coronary artery, SBE of RAV, bicuspid PV, and atherosclerosis (Figs. 80–84)	35 years F
Intermittent spontaneous AV block, single coronary, pulmonary hypertension, large defect, overriding AO and left AV valve stenosis and insufficiency–mostly PPM (atypical parachute) and accessory opening	19 years M
Large ASD, LSVC into CS, pulmonary hypertension, and large defect	43 years, 7 months F
Parachute LAV with stenosis, pulmonary hypertension, and wide commissures of the aortic valve	26 years M
Pulmonary hypertension with aneurysmal dilatation of MP and PA with thrombus formation, dissection and rupture, left AV valve stenosis (parachute, no APM) and large defect, and subaortic stenosis	22 years F
Oblique PFO, pulmonary atresia, small PDA, two coronary ostia from aortic sinus of Valsalva, 4 brachiocephalic vessels, *small defect*, and AO from MC	10 months M
Pulmonary atresia, PDA, PFO, SOC–large (superior and posterior) (Figs. 85–87)	5½ months F
PFO, pulmonary atresia, marked stenosis of LAV, aneurysm of fossa ovalis, PDA, *small defect* (very small left AV valve) (Figs. 88–91)	1 month, 15 days F
Pulmonary atresia, overriding aorta, adequate sized defect, and subacute bacterial endocarditis of the left AV valve with insufficiency	15 years F
Large ASD, small PDA, almost absent APM for left AV valve, absent coronary sinus, and 2 defects between SV and SOC and very small SOC (Figs. 92–94)	22 days F
Double large orifice in LAV valve with insufficiency, AL joining the SOC and the large defect with congenital AV block (Figs. 95–97)	8 years, 11 months M
Aneurysm of fossa ovalis, ASD, PDA, *small defect* and accessory muscle bundle to RAV and LAV	6 days F
Both AV valves join PPM and RAV insufficiency and left AV obstructing the defect (AL at junction of MC and SOC) with no APM and insufficiency, LAV producing subaortic obstruction	7 years M
CAVO with PA, conal truncal inversion, SOC–small, posterior and large defect with atrial inversion, SVC and hepatic veins to LA, and some PV and IVC into RA and one vein indeterminate–TAPVD–mixed	1½ months M
CAVO, dominant–right AV valve, PA, absent PDA, enlarged bronchials, LSVC to LA, large ASD; right 2 PV into RSVC, SOC superior and posterior with chord-like PT	2 months M
Common atrium, CAVO, pulmonary stenosis, stenosis of pulmonary veins, absent coronary sinus, absent ductus, overriding aorta, huge atrial appendages, spongy SV, small SOC and overriding pulmonary trunk with heart block and both atrial appendages resembling left, normal spleen, and normal viscera	12 hour, (31-wks gest.) M

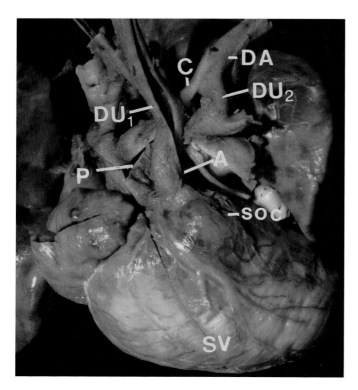

Figure 52: Single ventricle with inverted transposition with hypoplasia of the transverse arch and coarctation and double ductus arteriosus in a 14-day-old infant; external view. SV = single ventricle; soc = small outlet chamber situated to the left anterior; A = aorta emerging from the small outlet chamber; P = pulmonary trunk situated to the right and posterior, large; DU_1 = right sided ductus arteriosus, large, giving rise to one of the subclavian arteries; DU_2 = left sided ductus arteriosus forming the descending aorta; DA = descending aorta; C = markedly narrowed transverse arch with coarctation of the aorta. (Used with permission from Lev M, et al. See Figure 55.)

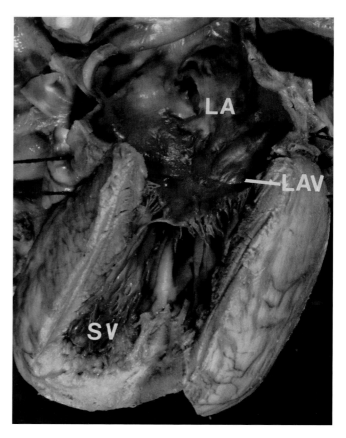

Figure 54: Single ventricle as seen from the left side; internal view. LA = left atrium; LAV = left AV valve; SV = single ventricle. Note the small left AV valve and the papillary muscles proceeding to the undersurface of the valve in the posterior wall. (Used with permission from Lev M, et al. See Figure 55.)

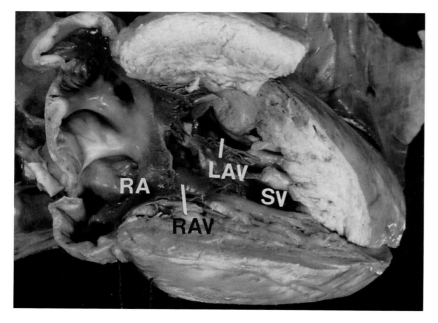

Figure 53: Internal view of single ventricle, right atrial view. Note the aneurysm of the fossa ovalis with no atrial septal defect. RA = right atrium; SV = markedly hypertrophied single ventricle; RAV = right AV valve; LAV = left AV valve. (Used with permission from Lev M, et al. See Figure 55.)

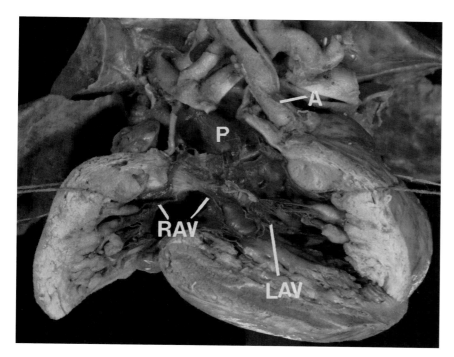

Figure 55: Single ventricle giving rise to the pulmonary trunk. Note that the pulmonary trunk is confluent with both the right and the left AV valves and the small aorta situated to the left and anterior. A = aorta; RAV = right AV valve entering the single ventricle; LAV = left AV valve; P = larger pulmonary trunk. (Used with permission from Lev M, Bharati S: Transposition of arterial trunks in levocardia. In *Cardiovascular Pathology Decennial 1966–1975*, Ed. SC Sommers, Appleton-Century Crofts, NY, 1975, pp. 1–46.)

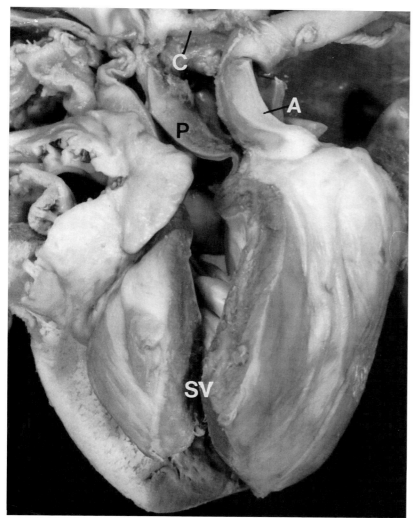

Figure 56: External view of single ventricle with inverted transposition and hypoplasia of the transverse arch with coarctation of the aorta. SV = single ventricle; P = pulmonary trunk; A = aorta; C = hypoplasia of transverse arch with coarctation.

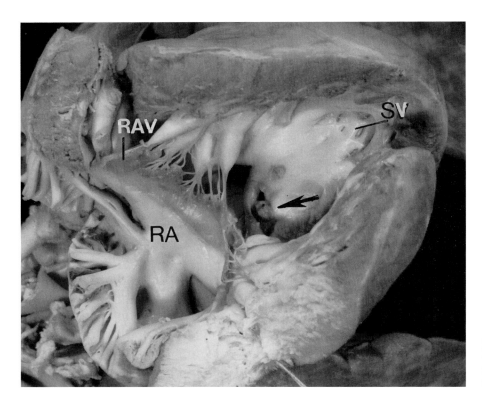

Figure 57: Right atrial view of single ventricle. RA = right atrium; RAV = right AV valve; SV = single ventricle. Arrow points to the left AV valve.

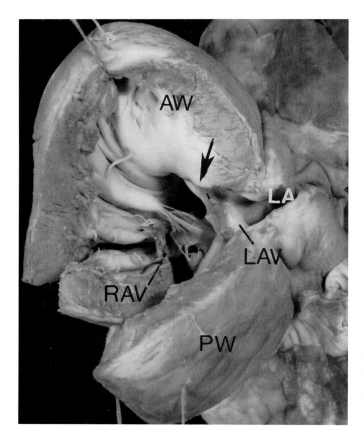

Figure 58: Both AV valves entering the small chamber with left AV valve stenosis and almost absent anterior papillary muscle for the left AV valve. AW = anterior wall of the single ventricle; PW = posterior wall of the single ventricle; RAV = right AV valve; LAV = left AV valve; LA = left atrium. Arrow points to the hypoplastic left anterior papillary muscle in contrast to the well-developed muscles of the right AV valve.

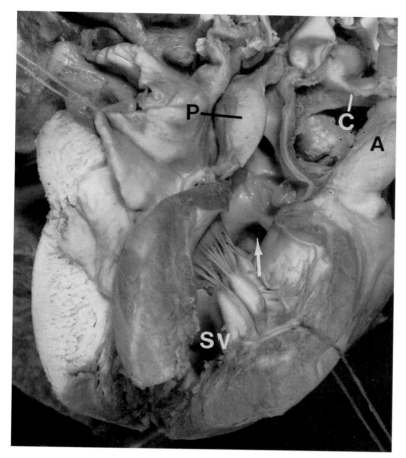

Figure 59: Pulmonary trunk emerging from the main ventricular chamber unrelated to the AV valves, and a small opening (defect) between the main chamber and the small outlet chamber. SV = single ventricle; P = larger pulmonary trunk; A = aorta; C = hypoplasia of the transverse arch with coarctation of the aorta. Arrow points to the small defect as seen from the single ventricle.

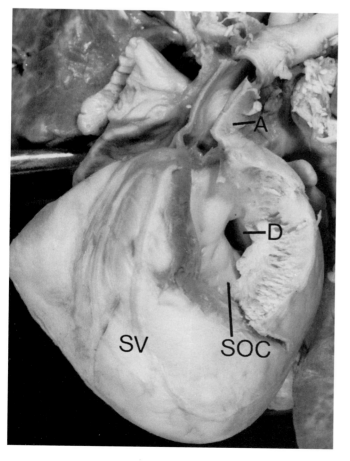

Figure 60: Defect as seen from the small outlet chamber with aortic stenosis. SV = single ventricle; SOC = small outlet chamber; D = defect located at the midpart of the small outlet chamber in an oblique manner; A = aorta. Note that the defect appears to be larger in the small outlet chamber. Also note the small bicuspid aortic valve.

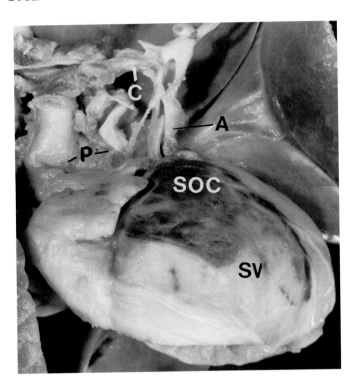

Figure 61: Single ventricle with inverted transposition with a markedly hypoplastic transverse arch and coarctation. SOC = small outlet chamber; SV = single ventricle; A = small aorta; C = markedly hypoplastic transverse arch with coarctation; P = pulmonary trunk, large.

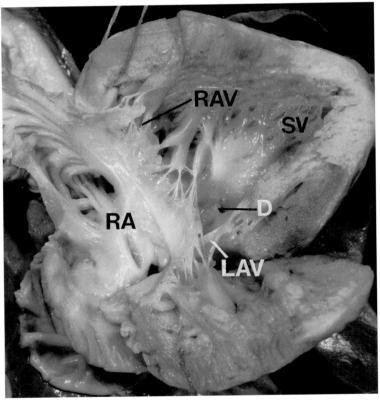

Figure 62: Internal view of single ventricle demonstrating the intact atrial septum, minute defect between the single ventricle and the small outlet chamber, and stenotic left AV valve in an infant. RA = hypertrophied and enlarged right atrium – note that the atrial septum is intact; RAV = large right AV valve; SV = single ventricle; LAV = small left AV valve; D = minute defect. Note both AV valves inserted into the same papillary muscle in the anterior wall.

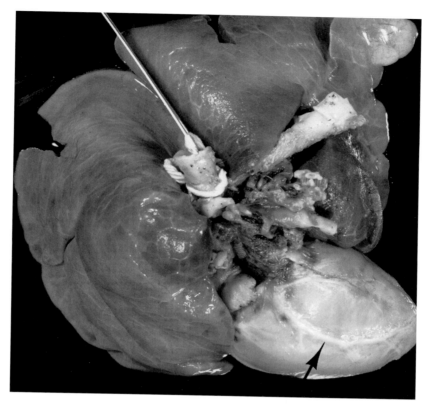

Figure 63: External view of single ventricle with small outlet chamber and inverted transposition with recent surgical intervention. Arrow points to the large right delimiting artery.

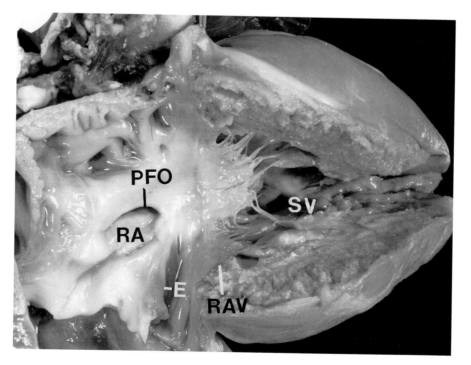

Figure 64: Right side of the heart demonstrating the hypertrophied and enlarged eustachian valve and patent foramen ovale in a newborn infant. RA = right atrium; PFO = patent foramen ovale; E = eustachian valve; RAV = right AV valve; SV = single ventricle. Note the markedly hypertrophied single ventricular mass.

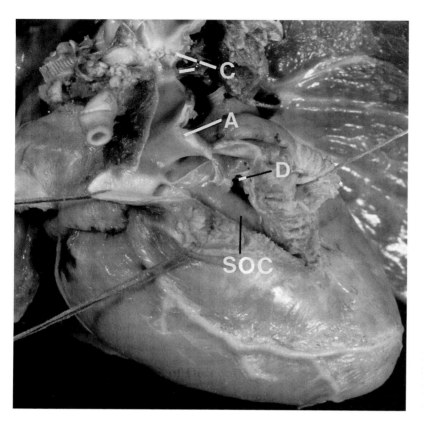

Figure 65: Small outlet chamber with a small defect and coarctation of the aorta. SOC = small outlet chamber; D = small defect somewhat confluent with the aortic valve; A = aorta; C = coarctation with recent surgery.

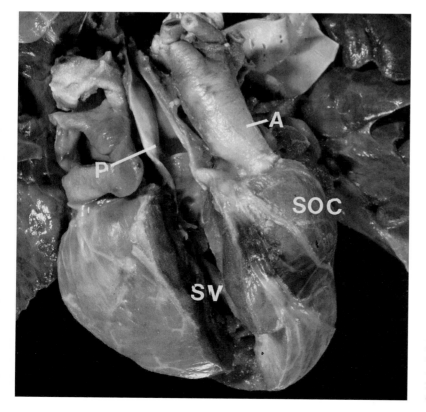

Figure 66: Single ventricle with small outlet chamber with inverted transposition, coarctation, and left AV valve stenosis, external view. p = pulmonary trunk; A = aorta; SOC = small outlet chamber; SV = single ventricle.

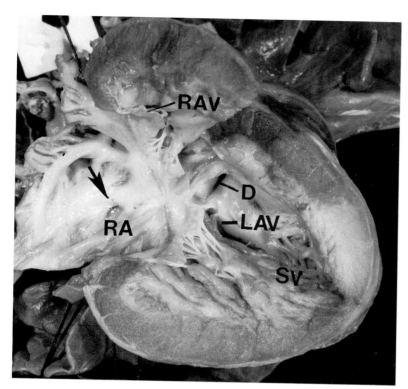

Figure 67: Right-sided view of the single ventricle demonstrating probe patent foramen ovale and a small defect between the single ventricle and the small outlet chamber in a 10-week-old infant. RA = right atrium; SV = single ventricle; RAV = right AV valve; D = small defect between the single ventricle and the small outlet chamber; LAV = stenotic left AV valve. Arrow points to the probe patent foramen ovale.

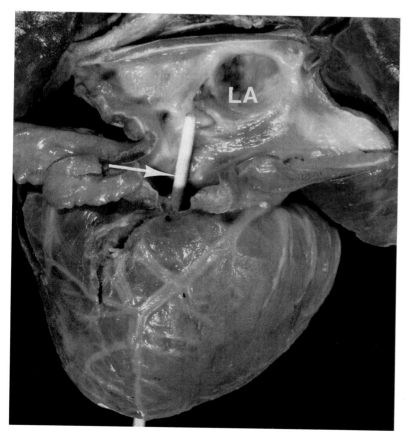

Figure 68: Left atrial view of Figure 67 demonstrating the marked left AV valve stenosis. LA = left atrium. Arrow points to the probe passing through the stenotic left AV valve into the single ventricle.

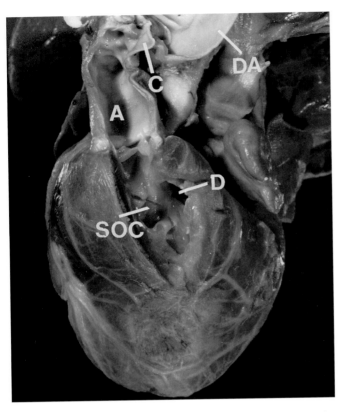

Figure 69: Small defect entering the small outlet chamber in an oblique manner with coarctation of the aorta. SOC = small outlet chamber; D = small defect situated in an oblique angle; A = aorta emerging from the small outlet chamber; C = marked coarctation of the aorta; DA = descending aorta.

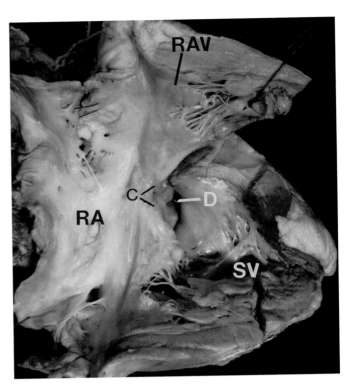

Figure 71: Internal view of the single ventricle from the right side demonstrating the large cleft in the anterior leaflet of the right AV valve with right AV valve insufficiency. RA = hypertrophied and enlarged right atrium; RAV = right AV valve; C = cleft in the anterior leaflet of the right AV valve; SV = single ventricle; D = defect between the main chamber and the small outlet chamber.

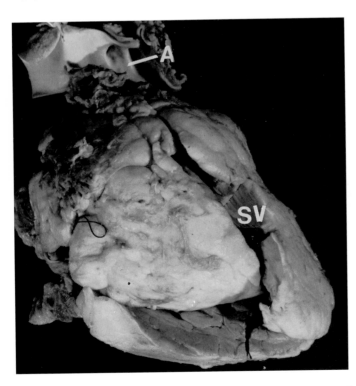

Figure 70: External view of single ventricle with inverted transposition with pulmonary stenosis in a 15-year-old. SV = single ventricle; A = aorta emerging left and anterior.

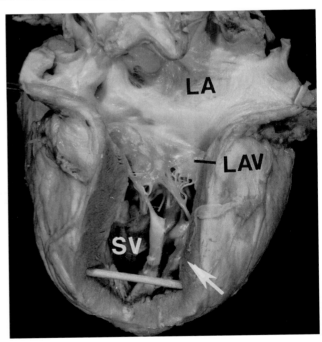

Figure 72: Single ventricle from the left side demonstrating a single papillary muscle connection to the left AV valve in the inferior wall of the single ventricle. LA = hypertrophied and enlarged left atrium; LAV = left AV valve; SV = single ventricle. Arrow points to the single papillary muscle in the inferior wall (parachute left AV valve) with stenosis.

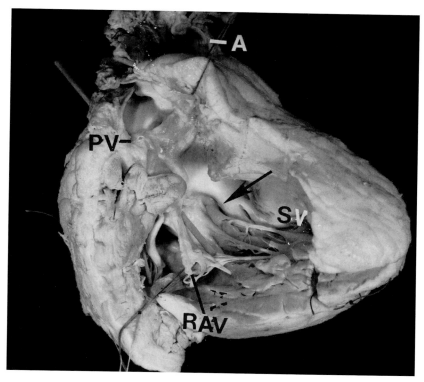

Figure 73: The pulmonary trunk emerging from the main ventricular chamber but unrelated to the AV valves with stenosis. PV = pulmonary valve; SV = single ventricle; RAV = right AV valve. Arrow points to the parachute left AV valve.

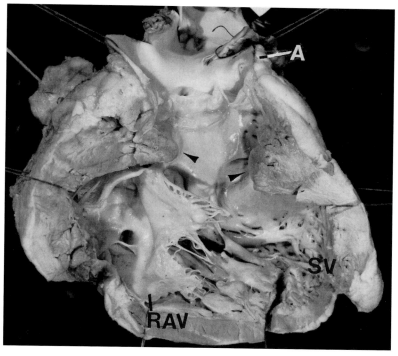

Figure 74: The aorta emerging from the small outlet chamber. The two small arrowheads indicate the cut end of the small outlet chamber and the large defect that was situated underneath this muscle. A = aorta; RAV = right AV valve; SV = single ventricle.

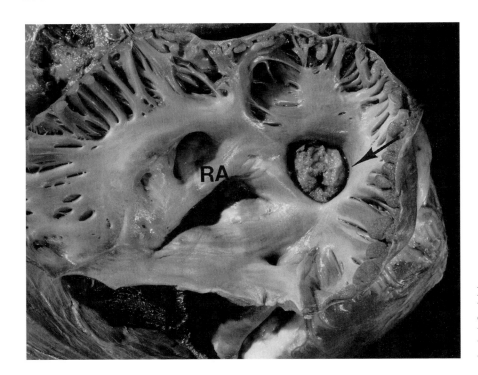

Figure 75: Single ventricle with inverted transposition with right AV valve almost occluded by thrombic material; right atrial view. RA = right atrium. Arrow points to the irregular thrombic material almost occluding the right AV orifice.

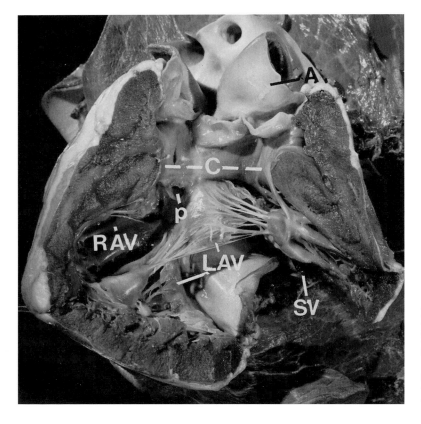

Figure 76: Internal view of single ventricle depicting the markedly stenotic pulmonic orifice between the two AV valves and the aorta emerging from the small outlet chamber. RAV = right AV valve; LAV = left AV valve; SV = single ventricle; A = aorta; p = pulmonary trunk; C = cut ends of small outlet chamber with a large opening beneath this muscle.

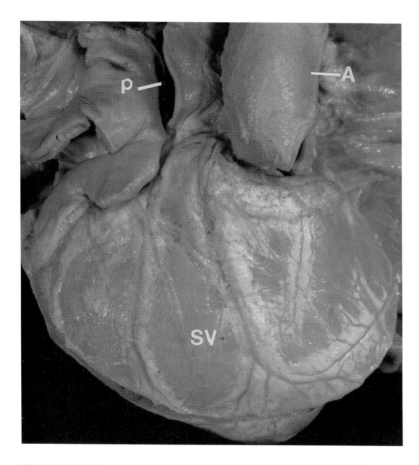

Figure 77: Single ventricle with inverted transposition; external view of the heart. SV = single ventricle; A = aorta; P = pulmonary trunk.

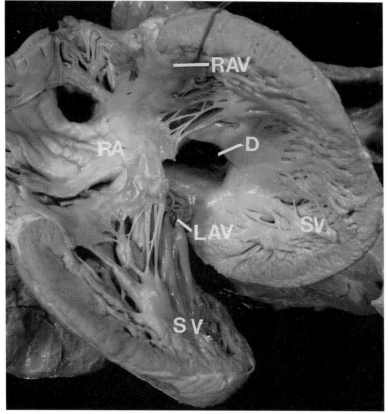

Figure 78: Single ventricle as seen from the right side. RA = right atrium; SV = single ventricle; RAV = right AV valve; LAV = left AV valve; D = U-shaped deficiency in the anterior wall of the single ventricle confluent in part with the aortic valve.

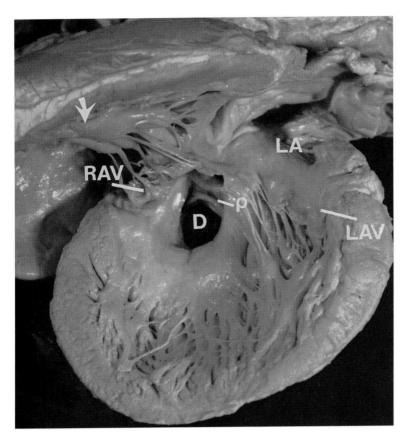

Figure 79: Left-sided view of the single ventricle demonstrating the same U-shaped deficiency (defect) and the pulmonary trunk emerging somewhat confluent with the deficiency (defect) and the AV valves. LA = left atrium; LAV = left AV valve; RAV = right AV valve; P = pulmonary trunk emerging confluent with the U-shaped deficiency or defect (D). Note both the AV valves are inserted to the same papillary muscle. Arrow points to the insertion of both of the AV valves into the same papillary muscle.

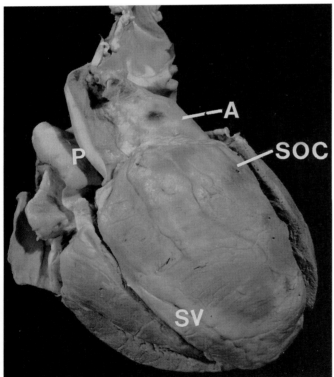

Figure 80: Single ventricle with inverted transposition in a 35 year old; external view of the heart. A = aorta situated to the left and anterior emerging from the small outlet chamber; P = pulmonary trunk situated to the right and posterior; SV = single ventricle; SOC = small outlet chamber. (Used with permission from Bharati S, Lev M. See Figure 84.)

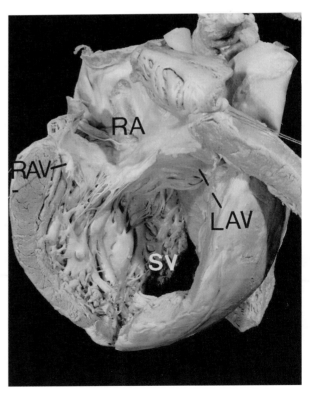

Figure 81: Right atrial view of the single ventricle. RA = right atrium; RAV = right AV valve showing thickening, old infective endocarditis; LAV = left AV valve entering the single ventricle; SV = single ventricle. (Used with permission from Bharati S, Lev M. See Figure 84.)

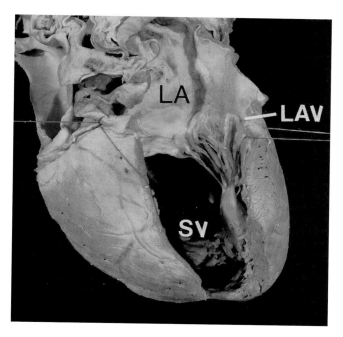

Figure 82: View of the single ventricle from the left side. LA = left atrium; LAV = left AV valve; SV = single ventricle. (Used with permission from Bharati S, Lev M. See Figure 84.)

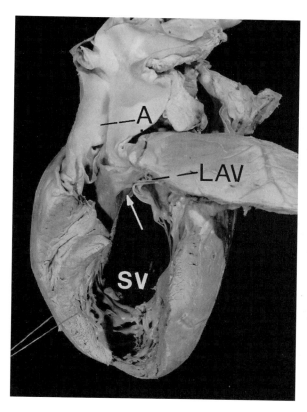

Figure 84: Aorta emerging from the small outlet chamber and emerging in a somewhat overriding manner. Arrow points to the first defect confluent with the left AV valve and the pulmonary trunk. A = aorta; SV = single ventricle; LAV = left AV valve, (Used with permission from Bharati S, Lev M: The relationship between single ventricle and small outlet chamber and straddling and displaced tricuspid orifice and valve. *J Herz* 1979, 4:176–183.)

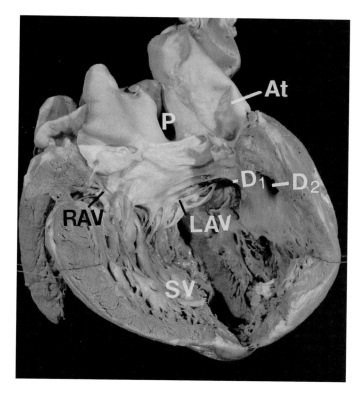

Figure 83: Huge pulmonary trunk emerging from the single ventricle with marked pulmonary hypertension, atherosclerosis of the main pulmonary trunk. and double defects. RAV = right AV valve; SV = single ventricle; LAV = left AV valve; P = huge pulmonary trunk; At = atherosclerosis of the main pulmonary trunk; D_1 = defect confluent with the base of the pulmonary and the aorta; D_2 = second defect between the main chamber and the small outlet chamber. (Used with permission from Bharati S, Lev M. See Figure 84.)

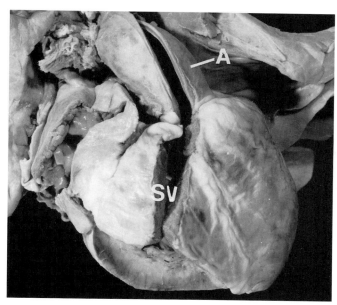

Figure 85: Single ventricle with inverted transposition with pulmonary atresia and overriding aorta; external view. A = aorta; SV = single ventricle.

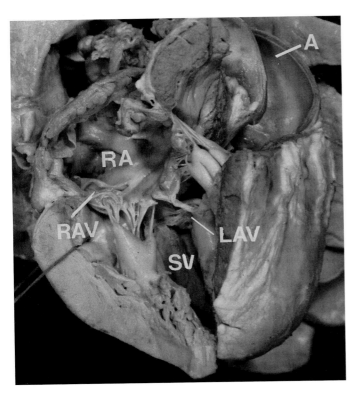

Figure 86: Single ventricle as seen from the right side. RA = right atrium; SV = single ventricle; RAV = right AV valve; LAV = left AV valve; A = aorta emerging in part from the single ventricle.

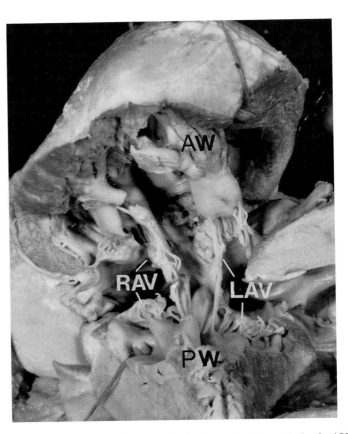

Figure 87: Internal view of single ventricle with both AV valves entering the same chamber. Note that no vessel emerges between the two AV valves. RAV = right AV valve; LAV = left AV valve; AW = anterior wall; PW = posterior wall of the single ventricle merging between the two AV valves.

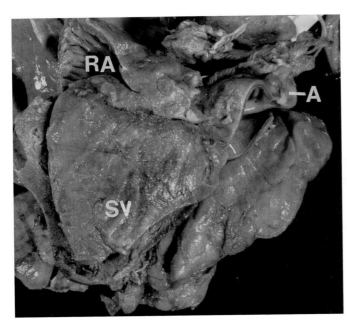

Figure 88: Single ventricle with inverted transposition with pulmonary atresia and marked left AV valve stenosis; external view of the heart. RA = right atrium; SV = single ventricle; A = aorta.

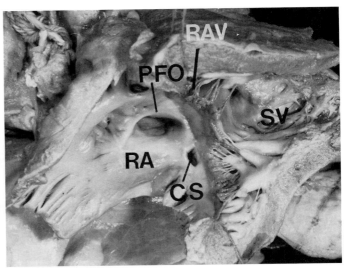

Figure 89: Single ventricle as seen from the right side. Note the marked abnormalities in the right atrium; the deep fossa ovalis with oblique foramen ovale and the coronary sinus displaced close to the anulus of the right AV valve. RAV = right AV valve; SV = single ventricle; CS = coronary sinus; PFO = patent foramen ovale; RA = right atrium.

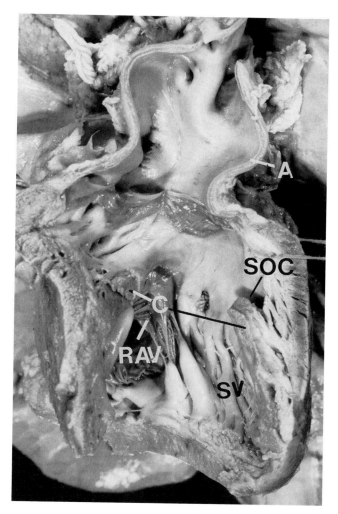

Figure 90: Aorta emerging from the main chamber and the small outlet chamber in an overriding manner. RAV = right AV valve; A = aorta; SOC = small outlet chamber; SV = single ventricle; C = cut ends of the small outlet chamber.

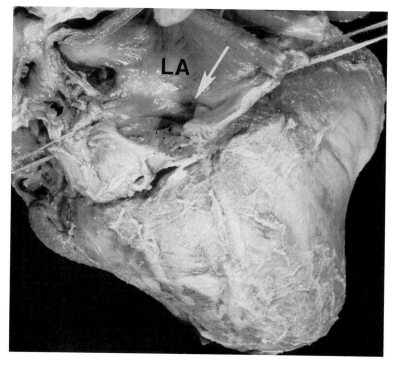

Figure 91: Left atrial view demonstrating marked left AV valve stenosis. LA = left atrium. Arrow points to the marked stenosis.

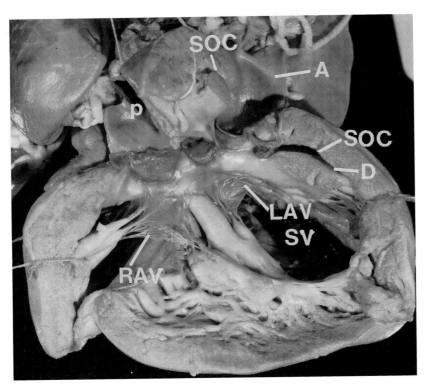

Figure 92: Single ventricle with inverted transposition and small outlet chamber, slit-like defect with two openings: one close to the base of the aorta and pulmonary trunk and the other towards the apex of the small outlet chamber. RAV = right AV valve; LAV = left AV valve; p = pulmonary trunk; A = aorta; SOC = small outlet chamber; D = the distal defect close to the apex of the small outlet chamber.

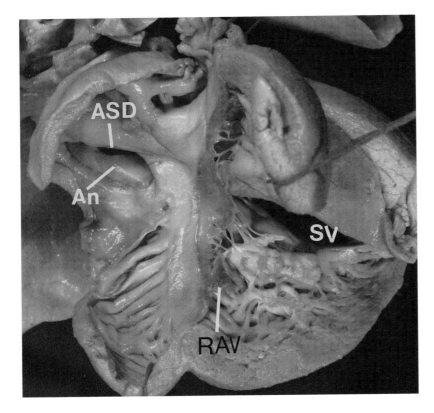

Figure 93: Single ventricle as seen from the right side. An = aneurysm of the fossa ovalis; ASD = atrial septal defect, fossa ovalis type, large; RAV = enlarged right AV valve; SV = single ventricle. Note the hypertrophied and enlarged right atrium, absent coronary sinus, and direct entry of one coronary vein near the eustachian valve.

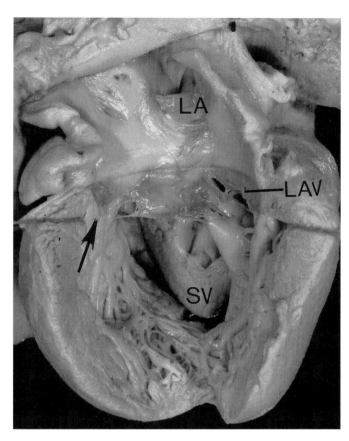

Figure 94: Single ventricle as seen from the left side demonstrating almost absent anterior papillary muscle for the left AV valve. LA = left atrium; LAV = left AV valve; SV = single ventricle. Arrow points to the almost absent left anterior papillary muscle for the AV valve.

Figure 96: As in Figure 95, single ventricle seen from the right side. RA = right atrium; RAV = right AV valve; SV = single ventricle.

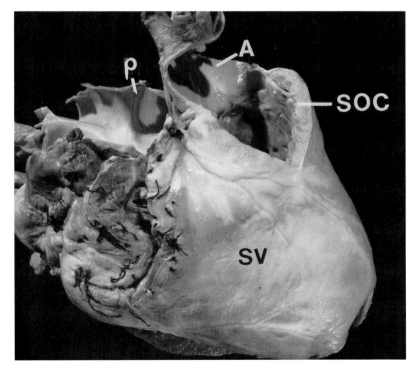

Figure 95: Single ventricle with inverted transposition and congenital AV block; external view of the heart. P = pulmonary trunk; A = aorta; SOC = small outlet chamber; SV = single ventricle.

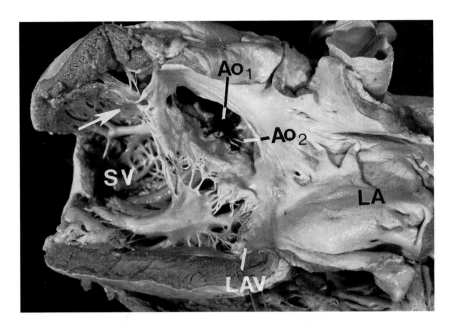

Figure 97: Left atrial view demonstrating accessory large openings for the left AV valve with left AV valve insufficiency. LA = hypertrophied and enlarged left atrium; LAV = left AV valve; SV = single ventricle; AO₁, AO₂ = accessory openings in the left AV valve with marked insufficiency. Note the poorly developed anterolateral papillary muscles for the left AV valve. Arrow points to the abbreviated chordae.

Here again, there appears to be some common denominators in this entity similar to the previous group with regular transposition. Frequently, fetal coarctation or paraductal type of coarctation was present with associated left AV valve stenosis. Hypoplasia of the aorta with coarctation (18) or absent transverse arch (3) was present in 21 (45.6%). In most cases (15 of 18–83%) associated with coarctation, there was a small defect between the main chamber and the small outlet chamber with subaortic stenosis, and restriction at the level of the defect with the main chamber. In cases where banding procedure was performed, there was a distinct tendency for closing of the small defect (spontaneously) or the defect actually closed. Subaortic stenosis without coarctation was seen infrequently.

Malformation of AV valves (31 out of 46–67%) either in the form of parachute (frequent absence of anterior papillary muscle or hypoplastic anterior papillary muscle), accessory openings, anomalous connections of the valvular tissue straddling through the small outlet chamber and/or connected to the margins of the defect, thus restricting the defect occurred in this entity. Abnormalities of the right AV valve were seen in seven (15%), and 14 (30%) were associated with left AV valve anomalies, 10 (22%) with anomalies of both the AV valves, and three had CAVO. The AV valves were "normal" (without obvious anomalies) only in 12 (26%).

Remnants of the sinus venarum valves and frequent association of oblique patent foramen ovale was also noted with coarctation. The incidence of AV valve abnormalities is similar to single ventricle with regular transposition. However, there is a lesser incidence of coarctation with inverted transposition. In five, there was catheter-proven, documented closing or closed defect between the main chamber and the small outlet

chamber following banding procedure in coarctation. Interrupted aortic arch was present in three. There were eight (17%) with pulmonary stenosis which was often infundibular and valvular in nature with occasional infective endocarditis, and six with pulmonary atresia (13%).

Spontaneous heart block was observed in two. Three had postoperative heart block.

There were five cases aged 35 years, 19 years, 43 years, 26 years, and 22 years. Four of them had pulmonary hypertension. The defect was large in all and in one there were two defects and the aorta overrode the defect in one. Pulmonary atresia was present in four and in one it permitted survival to 15 years where the defect was large and the aorta overrode the septum. Common atrioventricular orifice was seen in three. Eleven were below 1 month of age and 28 were below the age of 1 year (63%).

Similar to the previous group, the common denominators are coarctation of the aorta, a small defect between the main chamber and the small outlet chamber with subaortic obstruction in infancy, and in the older age group, usually the defect is large with pulmonary hypertension or pulmonary stenosis. Regardless of the fact whether there is coarctation or not, there is a distinct increase in atrioventricular valve abnormalities, especially left AV valve stenosis and/or insufficiency. The left AV valve may have double orifice and one orifice may point towards the small outlet chamber or both AV valves may have anomalous connections and straddling of the one AV valve to the small outlet chamber. Both AV valves may be inserted into the same papillary muscle in the inferior wall (Figs. 98, 99). The defect in the small outlet chamber in some may be present at two locations: one close to the base of the aortic valve and the other towards the apex. And, if a

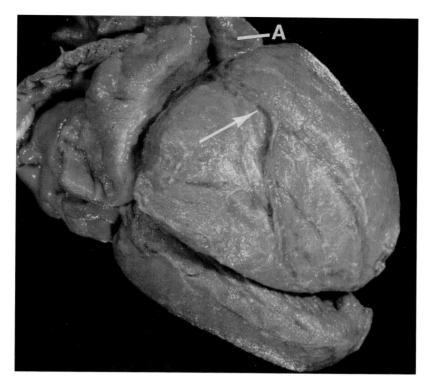

Figure 98: External view of the heart demonstrating a large delimiting artery bifurcating into two large branches. A = aorta. Arrow points to the delimiting artery.

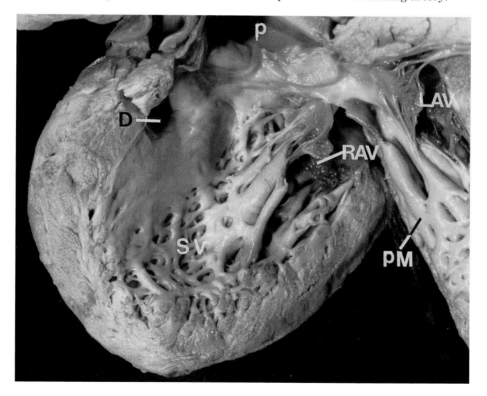

Figure 99: Single ventricle with inverted transposition with both AV valves inserted into the inferior group of papillary muscles which fuse together. LAV = left AV valve; RAV = right AV valve; SV = single ventricle; PM = fusion of the two papillary muscles; P = larger pulmonary trunk; D = defect. (Used with permission from Bharati S, Lev M. See Figure 126.)

defect is situated confluent with the aortic valve in a U-shaped fashion, the aorta may override, emerging from both chambers.

3. Single Ventricle with No Transposition–Holmes Heart

There was a total of 13 cases: nine male subjects and four female subjects. The youngest in this group was a stillborn and the oldest was 7 years old, with an average age of 1 year, 3 months, 23 days. In this entity the small outlet chamber is situated where the infundibulum is normally present in an otherwise normal heart. Thus, the position of the vessels is normal. The aorta is situated to the right and posterior, emerging between the two AV valves and the pulmonary trunk left and anterior with frequent association of infundibular pulmonary stenosis.

Pulmonary valvular and infundibular stenosis with several small defects between the small outlet chamber and the main chamber, some to the left and some to the right side of the single ventricle and absent anterolateral papillary muscle for the right AV valve, stenosis of CS	7 years F
RAV stenosis	9 months M
Pulmonary stenosis, left AV valve stenosis, small PDA, LSVC → CS, *small defect* between the main chamber and the SOC, marked thickening and irregularity of the right AV valve, and postoperative AV block	2 years, 24 days F
Left supravalvular ridge with stenosis of the left AV valve and pulmonary atresia (Figs. 100–102)	3 years, 8½ months M
Left AV valve stenosis (no anterior papillary muscle, parachute), ASD–large, both AV valves join together anteriorly with three defects between the main chamber and the small outlet chamber (two basal and one apical) with overriding pulmonary trunk (Figs. 103–106)	animal (antelope), 11 days M
Double conus, left AV valve (parachute and supravalvular) stenosis, and infundibular pulmonary stenosis	3 years M
CAVO, large ASD, right aortic arch, infundibular pulmonary stenosis with small SOC, bicuspid pulmonary valve, valvular and infundibular stenosis, dominant right type CAVO with very small left AV valve (Figs. 107–109)	2 months M
CAVO, probe PDA, double conus	4 months, 15 days F
CAVO, Ebstein-like right AV valve, hypoplasia of the transverse arch with coarctation, PDA, ASD, double conus, LSVC → CS	6 hours M
CAVO, common atrium, aortic atresia, PDA–wide, double conus	2 days M
CAVO, bicuspid pulmonary valve with stenosis, ASD, PDA	stillborn M
CAVO, subaortic stenosis, ASD, FOD, PDA, bicuspid aortic valve, common eustachian and thebesian valves	1 day M
Common conus, no transposition, tri-atrial heart, LSVC → CS, PV → indeterminate chamber, preductal coarctation (FC), juxtaposed Rt atrial appendage to Lt, Rt AV valve stenosis, both vessels from SOC, double defect	5 weeks F

In this entity, in contrast to the other two, there is either pulmonary stenosis (5), valvular, infundibular, or atresia (1), with AV valve abnormalities in all. Both AV valves were abnormal in two, the left valve was abnormal in two, and the right valve was abnormal in three. There were six cases of atrioventricular orifice. Thus, all had abnormalities in the AV valves. There were unique cases, one with aortic atresia, two with subaortic stenosis, and one with preductal coarctation. Multiple defects were observed in this entity in three cases, and overriding of the pulmonary trunk in one. A double conus was seen in three, and a common conus in one.

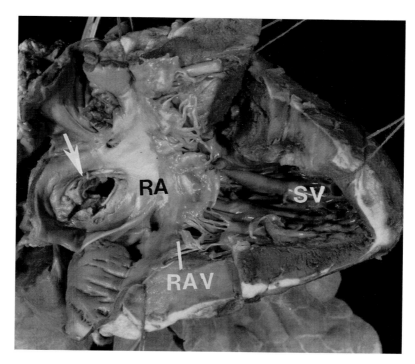

Figure 100: Single ventricle with no transposition (Holmes heart) with left AV valve stenosis and pulmonary atresia, right atrial view. RA = right atrium; RAV = enlarged right AV valve; SV = single ventricle. Note the tremendously hypertrophied and enlarged right atrium. Arrow points to the atrial septectomy that had resulted in a good-sized atrial septal defect.

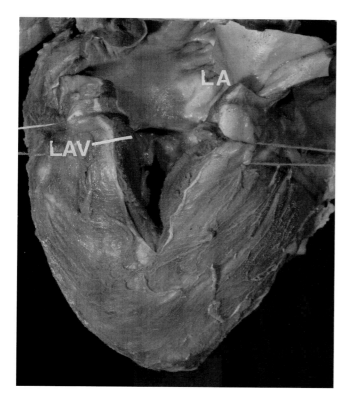

Figure 101: Left-sided view demonstrating the marked left AV valve stenosis. LA = left atrium; LAV = left AV valve, markedly redundant but small anulus with stenosis.

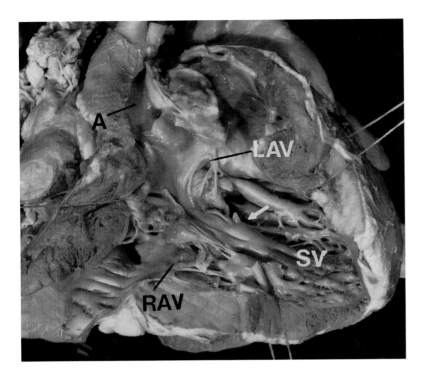

Figure 102: Aorta emerging from the single ventricle between the two AV valves. Note that both AV valves are inserted into the same papillary muscle in the posterior wall of the single ventricle. A = aorta emerging between the AV valves; RAV = right AV valve; LAV = left AV valve; SV = single ventricle. Arrow points to the papillary muscle to which both AV valves are attached.

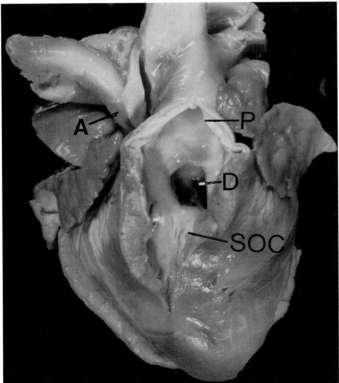

Figure 103: Single ventricle with no transposition in an antelope with a large U-shaped defect confluent with the pulmonary trunk and overriding pulmonary trunk; external view. A = small aorta situated to the right and posterior; P = larger pulmonary trunk situated to the left and anterior overriding a U-shaped defect; D = large U-shaped defect confluent with the pulmonary trunk; SOC = small outlet chamber situated anterior and superior.

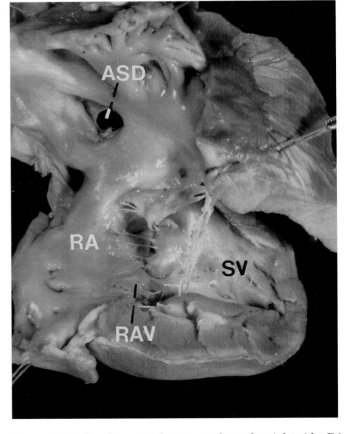

Figure 104: Single ventricle as seen from the right side. RA = right atrium; SV = single ventricle; RAV = right AV valve; ASD = atrial septal defect fossa ovalis type.

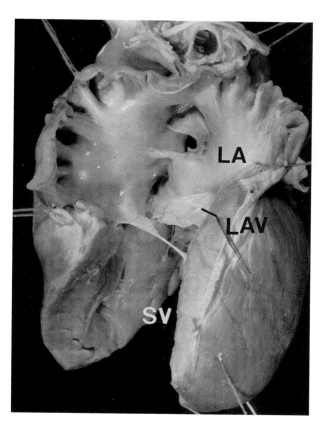

Figure 105: Same as in Figure 104 from the left side. LA = left atrium; LAV = left AV valve; SV = single ventricle. Note that there is no anterolateral papillary muscle for the left AV valve.

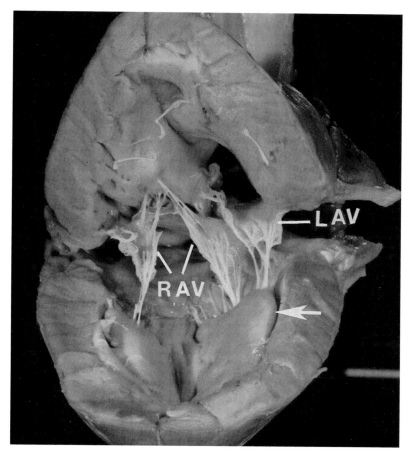

Figure 106: Internal view of a single ventricle demonstrating the small left AV valve and insertion of both AV valves into the same papillary muscle in the posterior wall. LAV = left AV valve; RAV = right AV valve. Arrow points to the insertion of the left AV valve into the same papillary muscle.

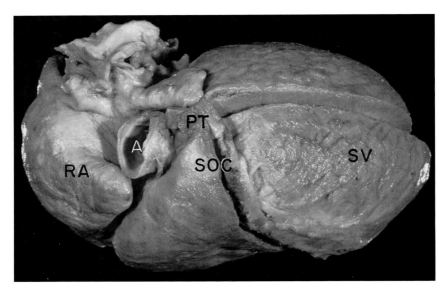

Figure 107: Single ventricle with normal position of the arterial trunk and levocardia with common AV orifice and pulmonary stenosis. Antero-superior view of the heart. RA = right atrium; SOC = small outlet chamber; A = aorta; PT = pulmonary trunk; SV = single ventricle. (Used with permission from Lev M, et al. See Figure 109.)

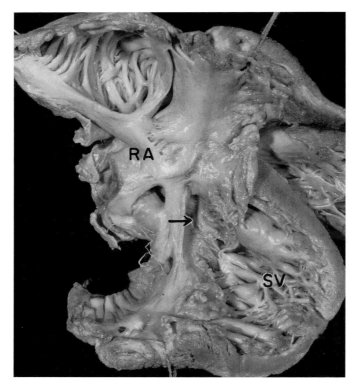

Figure 108: Internal view of the heart from the right side. RA = right atrium; SV = single ventricle. Arrow points to opening of left atrium into single ventricle. (Used with permission from Lev M, et al. See Figure 109.)

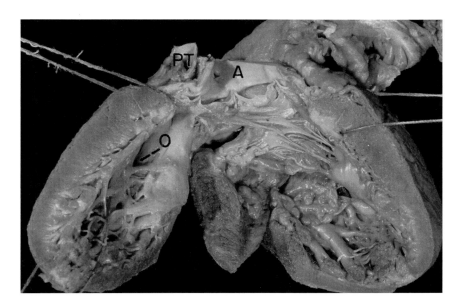

Figure 109: View of the single ventricle with the aorta emerging confluent with the common AV valve. O = opening into the small outlet chamber; A = aorta; PT = pulmonary trunk. (Used with permission from Lev M, Liberthson RR, Kirkpatrick JR, Eckner FAO, Arcilla RA: Single (primitive) ventricle. *Circulation* 1969, 39:577–591.)

4. Single Ventricle Indeterminate Types

In this group there were 12 cases, and all showed varying degrees of abnormalities in the AV valves.

Truncus

Truncus, common atrium, CAVO, straddling conus, double conus, dextrocardia, and absent right lung	2 hours M

Position of the Vessels – Anteroposterior – Aorta Anterior and Pulmonary Trunk Posterior

FC, PDA, peripheral PS, attenuated RAV with stenosis, and small defect	25 days M
Probable inverted transposition, old banding, recent surgical intervention, juxtaductal coarctation, restrictive small defect, parachute left AV valve with supravalvular ridge and stenosis (no APM), thrombosis in right atrium, RAV, small APM, and supravalvular ridge for aortic valve	8 years 9 months M
FC, wide PDA–short, window type, straddling right AV valve into SOC with small APM and large curtain of tissue obstructing SOC	10 years, 12 weeks M
CAVO, total anomalous pulmonary venous drainage, LSVC, pulmonary atresia, right aortic arch, large defect, ASD	14 days M

CAVO, PA, TAPVD → Lt gastric vein, minute LA	Newborn F
Transposition, CAVO, PS, TAPVD → SVC, ASD, FOD, ASD, coronary sinus type	1 year, 2 months F

There were six cases in this group with anteroposterior position of the great vessels; three out of six were with coarctation and small defects between the single ventricle and small outlet chamber with associated AV valve abnormalities restricting the defect. Three were with common AV orifice and total anomalous pulmonary venous drainage.

Position of the Vessels–Side by Side

DORV type, noninverted type with left AV valve stenosis, PDA, and double conus (no SOC) (Figs. 110–114)	3 months F
DORV type, noninverted type, interrupted aortic arch, interruption beyond left common carotid, left AV valve stenosis, aneurysm of fossa ovalis, PFO, double conus and no SOC, LAV shrunken tissue, and RAV only with PM in posterior wall (Figs. 115–119)	13 days M
Atypical regular transposition, RAV stenosis, and LAV cleft, insufficiency with accessory opening in LAV with attachment at the junc-	

tion of SOC with MC, PDA ligated, old banding (with marked fenestrations), remnants of the venous valves in the right atrium, ASD, U-shaped basal large defect with straddling parietal band and overriding of both aorta and pulmonary trunk with left AV restricting the defect   7 years M

Asplenia, symmetrical lungs, midline liver, situs inversus, regular transposition with CAVO, coarctation, PDA, LSVC–LA, IVC–LA, right hepatic veins–RA, ASD, SOC, small and to the left and superior with small defect   15 days M

No SOC, both vessels from main chamber, CAVO, TAPVD → RA, Lt atrial atrophy, ASD, FOD, absent CS, solitus, asplenia (Figs. 120–122)   11 months M

Here there were five cases, three of double outlet right ventricular type with double conus. The oldest in this group was of 7 years of age with right AV valve stenosis and left AV valve insufficiency with a large U-shaped defect and straddling parietal band with overriding of both the aorta and the pulmonary trunk. One was associated with situs inversus and asplenia with anomalies in the systemic venous return.

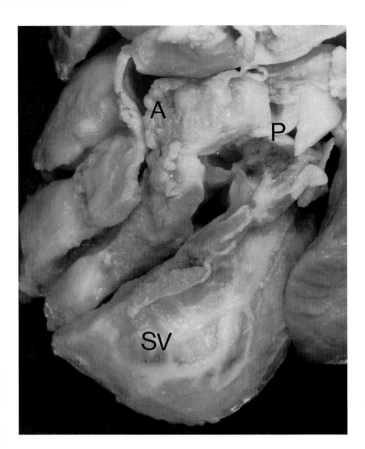

Figure 110: Single ventricle with no outlet chamber with both vessels emerging from the single ventricle side by side; external view. SV = single ventricle; A = aorta; P = pulmonary trunk. Note both vessels are side by side.

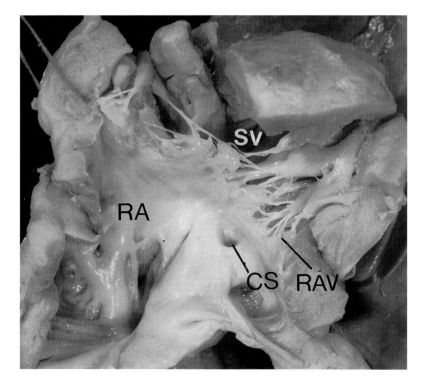

Figure 111: Single ventricle showing the hypertrophied and enlarged right atrium. RA = right atrium; CS = coronary sinus; RAV = right AV valve; SV = single ventricle. Note the profuse connections of the right AV valve to both the posterior and the anterior group of papillary muscles.

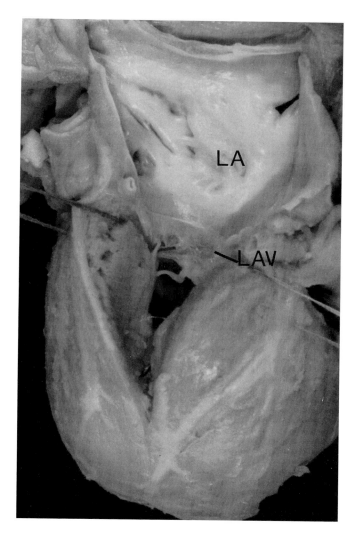

Figure 112: Marked left AV valve stenosis; left-sided view. LA = left atrium; LAV = shrunken left AV valve with small anulus.

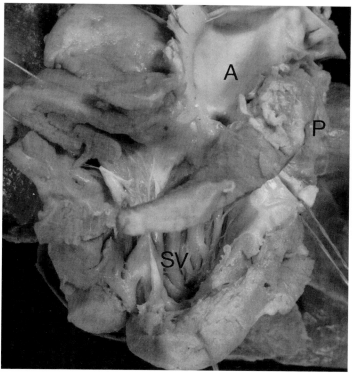

Figure 113: Aorta and pulmonary trunk emerging from single ventricle side by side. A = aorta; P = pulmonary trunk; SV = single ventricle.

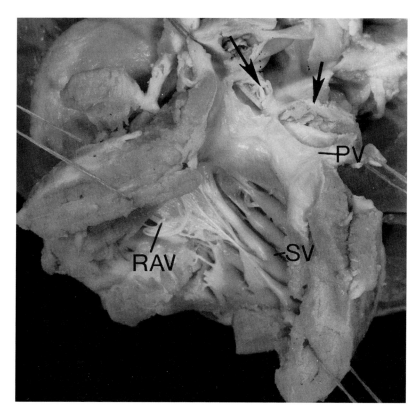

Figure 114: Pulmonary trunk emerging from single ventricle unrelated to the right AV valve with old banding procedure with erosion of the band into the lumen of the pulmonary trunk with rupture. RAV = right AV valve; SV = single ventricle; PV = large pulmonary valve. Arrows point to the erosion of the banding procedure with rupture of the pulmonary artery.

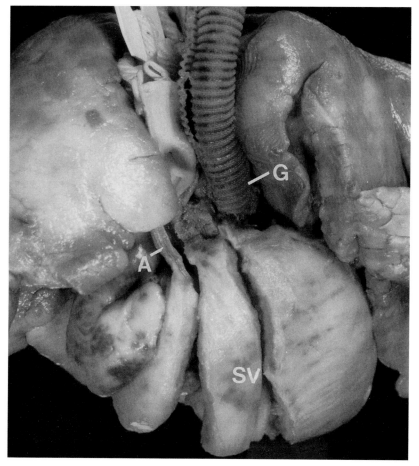

Figure 115: Single ventricle with side-by-side vessels and no outlet chamber, both vessels emerging from the single ventricle, with surgery; external view. SV = single ventricle; A = aorta. Repair of interrupted aortic arch by means of a graft from the main pulmonary trunk to the descending aorta.

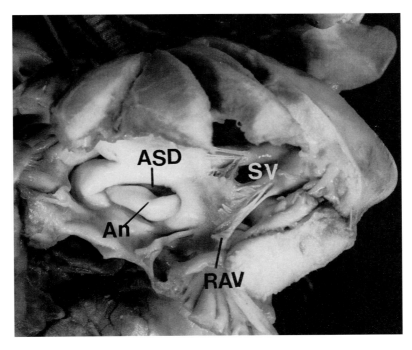

Figure 116: Single ventricle with no outlet chamber as seen from the right side. ASD = atrial septal defect; An = aneurysm of the fossa ovalis; RAV = right AV valve; SV = single ventricle. Note the papillary muscle connection present only in the posterior wall.

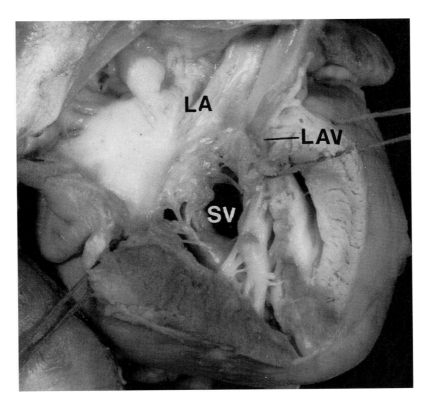

Figure 117: Single ventricle as seen from the left side of the heart. LA = left atrium; LAV = small anulus and thickened leaflets with shrunken valvular tissue; SV = single ventricle. Note the papillary muscles proceeding to the base of the posterior leaflet.

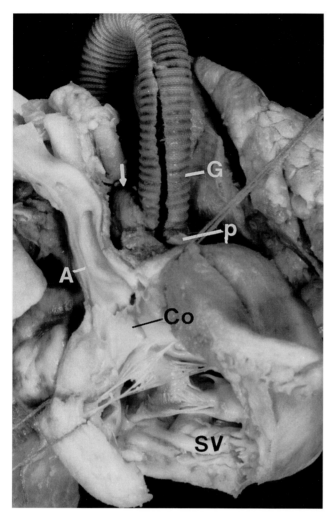

Figure 118: Aorta emerging from the single ventricle with a distinct conus separating the AV valves without a small outlet chamber. SV = single ventricle; A = aorta; P = pulmonary trunk; G = graft anastomosis from the main pulmonary trunk to the descending aorta; Co = conus muscle separating the aorta from the AV valve; SV = single ventricle. Arrow points to the interrupted aortic arch.

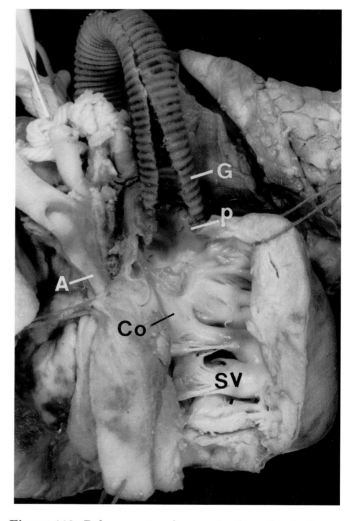

Figure 119: Pulmonary trunk emerging from the single ventricle with a distinct conus separating the pulmonary valve from the AV valves. SV = single ventricle; Co = conus muscle separating the pulmonary from the AV valves; P = pulmonary trunk; G = graft anastomosis from the main pulmonary trunk to the descending aorta; A = aorta.

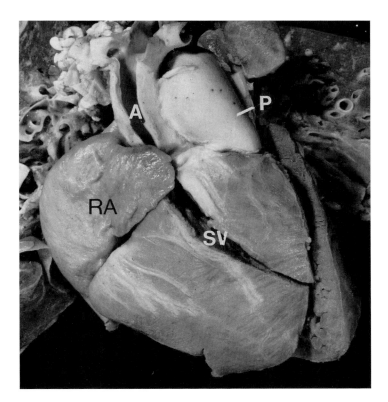

Figure 120: Single ventricle with no small outlet chamber; external view of the heart. P = pulmonary trunk; RA = right atrium; A = aorta; SV = single ventricle.

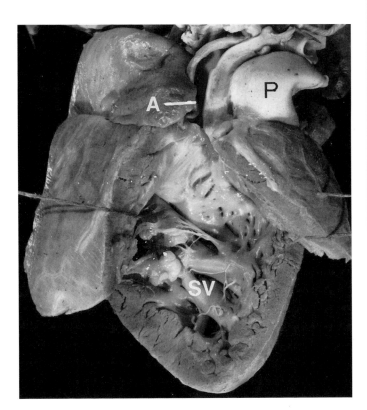

Figure 121: Aorta emerging from the single ventricle unrelated to common AV valve. A = aorta; P = pulmonary trunk; SV = single ventricle.

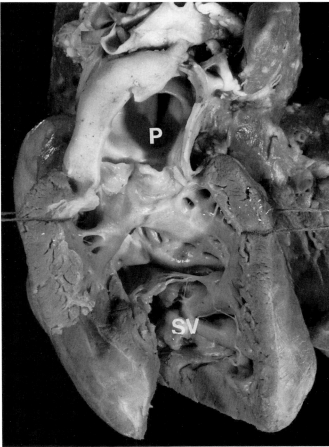

Figure 122: Pulmonary trunk emerging from the single ventricle unrelated to CAVO. P = pulmonary trunk; SV = single ventricle.

Comment

Single ventricle is usually associated with a small outlet chamber and the small outlet chamber may be situated either to the right or to the left of the base of the heart. Uncommonly, single ventricle may occur with no transposition. Likewise, there are hearts where the type of transposition cannot be made accurately due to the major intracardiac anomalies.

Our material clearly brings out some common denominators in this entity, especially in the very young. These denominators are (1) abnormal formation of the atrial septum with oblique patent foramen ovale and remnants of the sinus venarum, (2) frequent occurrence of both AV valve anomalies with stenosis or insufficiency or both, (3) a small defect between the small outlet chamber and the main chamber with hypoplasia of the transverse arch and coarctation or in extreme cases absent transverse arch and subaortic stenosis. Aortic arch anomalies were seen in 44 (43.5%). This type of single ventricle, regardless of whether it has regular or inverted transposition, is seen frequently in infancy. And if a banding procedure was done, the small defect closes spontaneously with time. Twenty-five (24.7%) were below the age of 1 month, and 59 (58%) were below the age of 1 year.

On the other hand, single ventricle with small outlet chamber may permit survival to adult life provided the defect between the two chambers is large and/or confluent with the aortic valve and/or if the aorta overrides the U-shaped defect. This has permitted survival to adult life with the development of pulmonary hypertension and in some there was associated pulmonary stenosis.

In a broad sense, one may therefore classify single ventricle into two distinct groups:

1. in infancy—below the age of 1 year (58%)
2. above the age of 1 year (42%).

Regardless of whether it is seen in the younger or in the older age group, there is a distinct increase in the incidence of AV anomalies (82–81%) with a slight increase or a tendency for left AV valve anomalies, such as a parachute type of valve, accessory openings in the valve, anomalous connections from the anterior leaflet to the defect, and/or straddling of the AV valve to occur in this entity.

Embryology

Normally during the second phase of development of the heart, as the bulbus moves or shifts to the left side and is absorbed into the ventricles, the auricular (atrial) canal shifts or moves to the right, and this movement makes it possible for the expansion of the tricuspid orifice and elaboration of the sinus or the in-

let of the right ventricle. Thus, it is conceivable that varying degrees of abnormal movements associated with the auricular canal to the right may result in either complete placement of both AV valves into the primitive ventricle or may result in a straddling tricuspid orifice entering into both ventricular chambers. Therefore, one may consider that persistence of the primitive state of the buboventricular loop, whether inverted or noninverted, is due fundamentally to improper expansion and movement or shift of the atrial canal to the right (or left, when inverted) during the process of absorption of the bulbus into the heart as a cause for single ventricle with or without transposition.

It is very likely that the genes responsible for the movement of the atrial canal to the right may be fundamentally defective or altered to a varying degree due to infective or other factors that might altered the hemodynamics of the heart.

The fact that single ventricle is seen frequently in infancy with abnormal formation of the septum secundum and septum primum suggests that there may be an additional hemodynamic factor in the embryogenesis of this entity. The left AV valve anomalies also favor this theory. One may therefore hypothesize that there are several types of etiology in the embryogenesis of single ventricle. The altered hemodynamics theory at the atrial level may not have played a significant role in the embryogenesis of single ventricle when seen in older age groups.

Morphology of the Main Ventricular Chamber

In our material, we are unable to identify the main ventricular chamber from the morphology. In general, there are groups of papillary muscles for both AV valves in the posterior wall of the main ventricular chamber. The superior wall of the main ventricular chamber in general may be smooth, to some extent. Because of the smooth nature of the superior wall of this chamber, many authors would like to call this chamber the left ventricle. We do not agree with this concept because we believe that embryologically the descending limb (proampulla) gives rise to the sinuses of both ventricles and the ascending limb (metaampulla and bulbus) to the coni of both ventricles and in part to the sinus of the right ventricle. We therefore believe that single ventricle is *not* a definitive left ventricle but includes in its composition a portion of the sinus of the right ventricle. Because of this, we believe that the geometry of the single ventricular mass would react differently to altered hemodynamics starting from intrauterine life. Thus, we believe hypertrophy of the main ventricular mass occurs in the majority of the cases in fetal and/or in neonatal life which is carried over later on.

The AV Valves

Although we have discussed the anomalies of the AV valves individually, the various anomalies of the right and the left AV valves may be grouped as follows:

Anomalies of the AV Valve in Various Types of Single Ventricle

	Left AV Valve	Right AV Valve	Both AV Valves	CAVO
Regular transposition	5	5	7	6
Inverted transposition	14	7	10	3
Holmes heart (no transposition)	2	3	2	6
Indeterminate type	1	2	3	6
	22	17	22	21

Hypoplasia of the Aorta with Coarctation or Interrupted Aortic Arch

The summary of coarctation or hypoplasia of the transverse arch in various types of single ventricle is given below:

Regular type	17
Inverted type	21
Holmes heart	2
Indeterminate type	4
	44

The right and the left AV valves, as seen from the material, are frequently abnormally formed (82–81%). We believe that the abnormal development of the AV valves is fundamentally related to the abnormally developed single ventricular chamber. Varying degrees of straddling of the left or right AV valve into the small outlet chamber may restrict the defect between the two chambers. A frequent occurrence of parachute AV valve, especially the left, suggests an abnormal hemodynamic pattern at the atrial level in intrauterine life, especially when seen in neonates.

Only in less than 20% of the cases are the AV valves "relatively normally" formed. However, it is emphasized that the right and the left AV valves cannot be morphologically identified as to whether they are tricuspid or mitral valves.

The abnormally developed AV valves adapt to the altered geometry of the single ventricular mass and perhaps may function "relatively normally" for a specific period of time. However, when the single ventricular mass reaches a critical stage of hypertrophy, the function of the AV valve correspondingly changes. This may not be significant from the standpoint of hemodynamics in the early stages, but following surgery, either septation or modified Fontan or any type of palliative surgery, the insufficiency of the valve becomes evident sooner or later. It is important to note that common AV orifice was present in 21 cases (20.7%).

The Defect and the Small Outlet Chamber

The defect between the single ventricle and the small outlet chamber deserves attention.

Because of the variations in the size, shape, number, and location of the opening between the single ventricle and the small outlet chamber, we do not use the term "bulboventricular foramen" to describe the anatomy of this opening. Since there is no anatomically identifiable ventricular septum, we prefer to call the opening between the single ventricle and small outlet chamber a "defect."

The defect was small in 12 (40%) with regular transposition, and in 22 (48%) with inverted transposition, and one in the former and six in the latter group closed following banding procedure (Figs. 123–125). There are infants who are born with a small defect between the main chamber and the small outlet chamber with associated coarctation of the aorta and large pulmonary trunk. The small outlet chamber, when it is small and the defect to start with is less than 3 to 5 mm in size, there is a tendency for the defect to close spontaneously with or without a banding procedure. This is frequently associated with an oblique patent foramen ovale and anomalies of the remnants of the sinus venarum valves in the right atrium.

The association of remnant of the sinus venarum valves, oblique patent foramen ovale, abnormal forma-

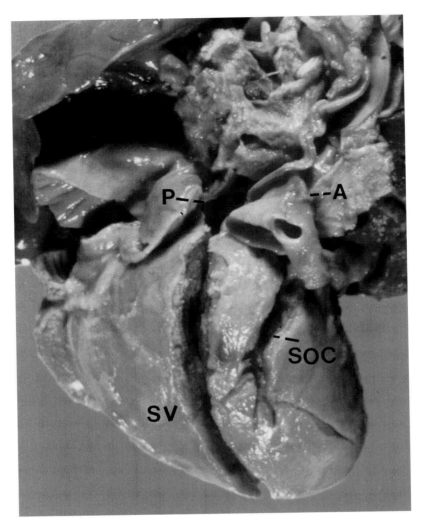

Figure 123: External view of single ventricle with inverted transposition, preductal coarctation, and closure of the small defect following banding procedure. SV = single ventricle; SOC = small outlet chamber; A = aorta; P = pulmonary trunk.

tion of the atrial septum, left AV valve anomalies, small defect between the main chamber and the small outlet chamber, subaortic stenosis, and hypoplasia of the transverse arch with coarctation again emphasizes that this type of single ventricle particularly may be related to altered hemodynamics in intrauterine life. This may occur at the level of the inferior and/or superior vena caval entry into the right atrium or perhaps starting at the placental site which may conceivably disturb the flow pattern across the atrial septum and to the left side of the heart which may indeed alter the shift of the atrial canal to the right and absorption of the bulbus to the left, resulting in single ventricle in some infants.

On the other hand, when single ventricle is seen with a large defect between the main chamber and the small outlet chamber, the embryogenesis of this type of a single ventricle may indeed be somewhat different from those seen in infancy. If altered hemodynamics in intrauterine life can be proven experimentally, it is possible that single ventricle in infancy may be preventible in some. However, one cannot overlook the etiogenesis of single ventricle at the molecular genetic level, and this area should be explored in the future.

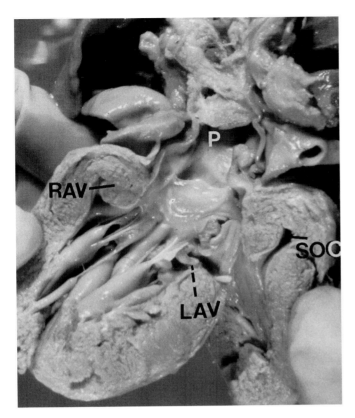

Figure 124: Single ventricle with inverted transposition, pulmonary trunk emerging from the main chamber. RAV = right AV valve; LAV = left AV valve; SOC = small outlet chamber; P = pulmonary trunk.

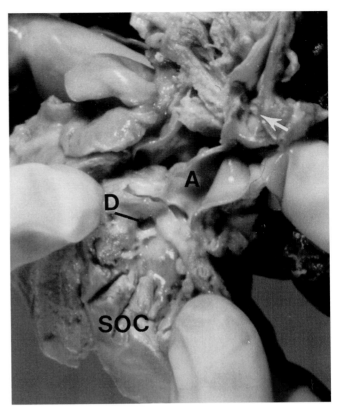

Figure 125: Small outlet chamber showing the spontaneous closure of the defect and coarctation of the aorta. SOC = small outlet chamber; A = aorta; D = spontaneous closure of the defect. Arrow points to coarctation.

The surgical procedures that are being used to correct this lesion in the adult, such as septation procedure and/or Fontan type of a procedure, have to be chosen very carefully after understanding the anatomy. We believe the high incidence of the atrioventricular valve abnormalities and marked hypertrophy of the single ventricular mass are definite contraindications for any type of a surgical procedure. It is again emphasized that the AV valves were "normal" (without obvious anomalies) in only 19 (19%), seven regular and 12 with inverted transposition. In the indeterminate and Holmes hearts, the AV valves were *always* abnormally formed. In 82 (81%), the AV valves were abnormal and in 44 (43.5%) were associated with varying degrees of hypoplasia of the transverse arch and coarctation.

On the other hand, in a selected few cases, perhaps where both AV valves are "more or less normal" with a large defect beneath the aortic valve, a septation procedure may be attempted provided the hypertrophy of the single ventricle has not reached a critical stage.

In some older individuals, perhaps heart or heart and lung transplantation may be considered.

The Conduction System (Fig. 126)

In general, there is an anterior-superior conduction system. The bundle proceeds in the anterior (superior wall of the single ventricle) very close to the pulmonary (in transposition of regular or inverted type) and reaches the defect between the main chamber and the small outlet chamber and gives off the left bundle branch. The right bundle branch proceeds through the defect either subendocardially or intramyocardially to reach the small outlet chamber. In some, the anterior and posterior conduction systems may be well developed and they join together forming a sling. This may give rise to junctional arrhythmias or preexcitation.

Abbreviations:

FC = fetal coarctation; PFO = patent foramen ovale; PDA = patent ductus arteriosus; SOC = small outlet chamber; PPM = posterior papillary muscle; SVC = superior vena cava; TAPVD = total anomolous pumonary venous drainage; PS = pulmonary stenosis; APM = anterior papillary muscle; RAP = right atrial appendage; RAV = right AV valve; LSVC = left superior vena cava; CS = coronary sinus; APM = anterior papillary muscle; PM = papillary muscle; AV valve = atrioventricular valve; Bicuspid AV = bicuspid aortic valve; AA = ascending aorta; LAV = left AV valve; SBE = infective endocarditis; AL = anterior leaflet; RA = right atrium; LA = left atrium; PA = pulmonary atresia.

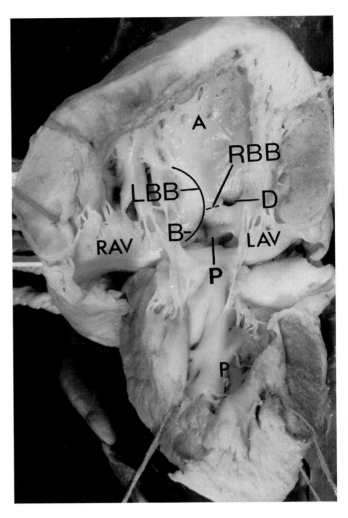

Figure 126: The course of the conduction system in single ventricle with inverted transposition is depicted in the heart specimen. RAV = right AV valve; LAV = left AV valve; P = posterior wall of the single ventricle; A = anterior wall of the single ventricle; B = bundle; LBB = left bundle branch; RBB = right bundle branch proceeding through the defect to the small outlet chamber; D = defect between the single ventricle and the small outlet chamber. (Used with permission from Bharati S, Lev M: The course of the conduction system in single ventricle with inverted (L-) loop and inverted (L-) transposition. *Circulation* 1975. 51:723–730.)

64

Straddling and Displaced Atrioventricular Orifices and Valves (Tricuspid and Mitral)

Definition

Straddling AV Orifice and Valve

In this condition, either one or (rarely) both orifices and valves straddle the ventricular septum to a varying degree over a ventricular septal defect so that some part of the orifice and valve lies in both ventricles.

Complete Straddling AV Orifice and Valve

In this condition, both the anulus and the peripheral connections lie in both ventricular chambers.

Incomplete Straddling AV Orifice and Valve
(a) Basilar or Anular (b) Peripheral

In this condition, either the anulus alone (basilar type) or the peripheral connections (chordae and papillary muscles-peripheral type) lie in both ventricular chambers.

Displaced AV Orifice and Valve

In this condition, either the AV orifice and valve (both the anulus and the peripheral connections) are completely displaced into the discordant (vis-à-vis the valve) morphological ventricular chamber (the opposite ventricular chamber) and have no direct connection with the concordant ventricular chamber.

There was a total of 103 cases. Since most of the cases (83) have already been included in various major entities, the sex and age are not given. However, the subject of straddling AV valve is very important in congenital heart disease and, therefore, all cases (including those already discussed in other categories, and 20 additional hearts) will be dealt with in detail.

Classification of Straddling and Displaced AV Valves

1. Straddling tricuspid orifice and valve—46
   a. Complete—26
   b. Basilar—15
   c. Peripheral—5
2. Straddling mitral orifice and valve—26
   a. Complete—17
   b. Basilar—8
   c. Peripheral—1
3. Straddling of both AV orifices and valves—4
   a. Complete—2
   b. Basilar—1
   c. Peripheral—1
4. Displaced tricuspid orifice and valve—13
5. Displaced tricuspid orifice and valve with straddling mitral orifice and valve—3
6. Displaced mitral orifice and valve with straddling tricuspid orifice and valve—1
7. Straddling and displaced AV orifices and valves in mixed (discordant) levocardia with ventricular inversion—10
   a. Straddling tricuspid valve—6
   b. Straddling mitral valve—1
   c. Displaced tricuspid with straddling mitral valve—1

 d. Straddling right or left AV valve in a criss-cross heart—1
 e. Displaced right (mitral valve) in a criss-cross heart or upstairs-downstairs—1

1a. Straddling Tricuspid Valve, Complete Type (26 cases)

Here a portion of the tricuspid valve, both the anulus and the peripheral connections, pass through a ventricular septal defect which usually is in the form of a common AV canal type of defect (Figs. 1–4). This is a defect situated within the membranous septum and involves the ventricular septal musculature, mostly posteriorly but anteriorly as well, in some cases. In about 12% of the cases, the defect extended into part of the posterior part of the infundibular septum and very often extended apically. Thus, it was usually a large de-

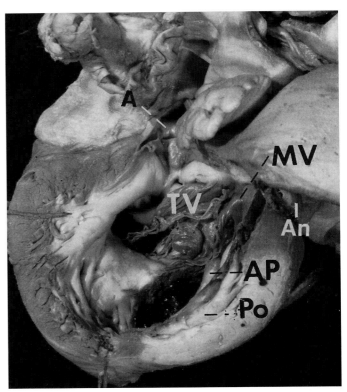

Figure 2: Left ventricular view showing attachment of tricuspid valve to accessory posterior papillary muscle in left ventricle. A = aorta; TV = tricuspid valve; MV = mitral valve; AP = accessory posterior papillary muscle; Po = posterior papillary muscle in left ventricle; An = anterolateral papillary muscle. (Used with permission from Liberthson RR, et al. See Figure 53.)

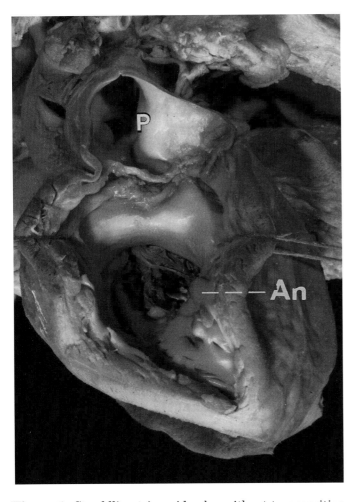

Figure 1: Straddling tricuspid valve without transposition. Right ventricular view showing attachment of tricuspid valve to anterolateral papillary muscle in right ventricle and to rim of VSD. P = pulmonary trunk; An = anterolateral papillary muscle. (Used with permission from Liberthson RR et al. See Figure 53.)

fect. Part of the tricuspid valve, mostly the medial (septal) leaflet, was situated beneath the efferent vessel in the left ventricle and adjacent to the pars membranacea and the central fibrous body, the pulmonic or the aortic-mitral anulus, and the mitral valve (Figs. 1–4).

In some cases, the muscle separated the efferent vessel from part of the anulus. Where there was no efferent vessel in the left ventricle, the anulus lay on the proximal (upstream) wall of the ventricular septal defect, close to the mitral anulus. The septal leaflet and, in some cases, part of the inferior and anterior leaflets, were attached to an accessory posterior papillary muscle (56%) or to the normally formed posterior papillary muscle in the left ventricle (24%). In the remaining 20% of the cases (all with mitral atresia), part of the tricuspid valve was connected to the normal anterior and posterior papillary muscles of the left ventricle.

There was a median ridge, either separately or fused with the accessory posterior papillary muscle of the left ventricle, often extended from the central fibrous body to the apex on the posterior wall. The septal leaflet, in some cases, was attached to this muscle as well. In general, the anterior leaflet of the tricuspid valve was somewhat smaller than normal and the septal leaflet was the largest of the three. The anterior papillary muscle of the right ventricle was usually well developed, but uncommonly it was hypoplastic or even absent. The inferior papillary muscle of the right ventricle was well developed in some cases and absent in others. The tricuspid orifice was smaller than normal in 32%, normal in size in 28%, or larger than normal in 40%. The extent of straddling of the tricuspid valve varied considerably from heart to heart. In some cases it was almost completely connected to the left ventricle, in others, straddling of the valve was moderate to mild.

The atria were situated posteriorly and inferiorly. The atrial septum, in its inferior portion, was moved toward the left so that the right atrium was situated more inferior to the left atrium than normally. The sinus of the right ventricle was smaller than normal in 60% of the cases, normal in size in 12%, and was enlarged in 28%, but a well-developed apical recess and infundibulum were present. The wall of the right ventricle was thicker than normal. The right ventricle was situated anteriorly and to the right of the left ventricle. The left ventricle was enlarged and usually hypertro-

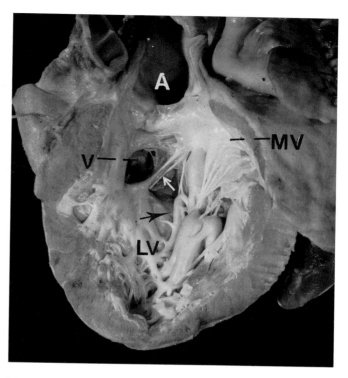

Figure 4: Left ventricular view showing complete straddling tricuspid valve. A = aorta; LV = left ventricle; MV = mitral valve; V = large common AV canal type of ventricular septal defect extending anteriorly and posteriorly. White arrow points to the accessory papillary muscle to which the tricuspid valve is attached. Black arrow points to another accessory posterior papillary muscle to which the tricuspid valve is attached as well.

phied. The mitral orifice and valve were normally placed and formed in 68%, the orifice was stenotic in 12%, and there was mitral atresia in 20% of the cases.

The complexes were:

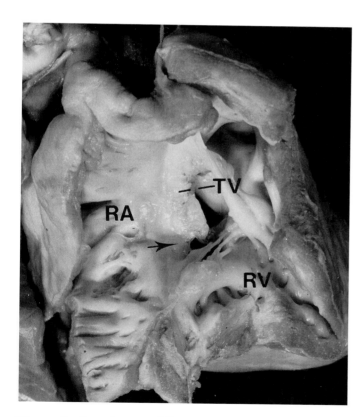

Figure 3: Complete straddling tricuspid valve. Right atrial, right ventricular view. RA = right atrium; RV = right ventricle; TV = tricuspid valve. Arrow points to the septal leaflet of the tricuspid valve passing through a common AV canal type of VSD.

	No. of Cases
Isolated VSD	2
Complete transposition of the great arteries (Figs. 5–8)	8
Complete transposition with tricuspid stenosis	1
Complete transposition with pulmonary stenosis and mitral stenosis	1
Complete transposition with infundibular and valvular pulmonary stenosis (Figs. 9–15)	2
Complete transposition with preductal coarctation of the aorta	3
Complete transposition with pulmonary atresia and mitral stenosis	1
Complete transposition with pulmonary stenosis and mitral atresia (1 with atrial arrhythmias)	1

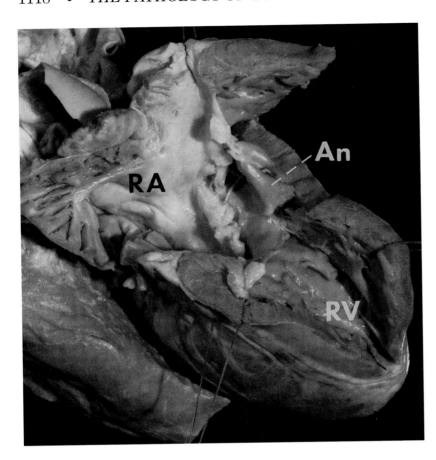

Figure 5: Complete straddling tricuspid valve in complete transposition. Right atrial, right ventricular view. RA = right atrium; RV = right ventricle; An = anterolateral papillary muscle. (Used with permission from Liberthson RR, et al. See Figure 53.)

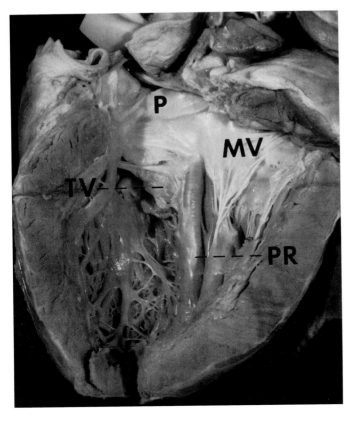

Complete transposition with mitral atresia	2
Double outlet right ventricle with mitral atresia with noncommitted VSD and preductal coarctation	1
Double outlet right ventricle Taussig-Bing, right-sided with preductal coarctation and patent ductus arteriosus	1
Mitral atresia without transposition with preductal coarctation and patent ductus arteriosus	1
Mitral atresia with polyvalvular disease and overriding aorta	1
Tetralogy of Fallot	1

Figure 6: Complete straddling tricuspid valve in complete transposition. Left ventricular view. P = pulmonary trunk; MV = mitral valve; PR = posterior papillary muscle in left ventricle; TV = straddling tricuspid valve. (Used with permission from Liberthson RR, et al. See Figure 53.)

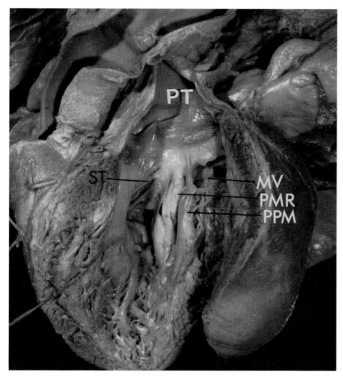

Figure 7: Complete straddling tricuspid valve in complete transposition with common AV canal type of VSD. Left ventricular view. PT = pulmonary trunk; MV = mitral valve; PPM = posterior papillary muscle of left ventricle; PMR = posterior median ridge of left ventricle; ST = straddling tricuspid valve. (Used with permission from Bharati S, Bharati S. See Figure 49.)

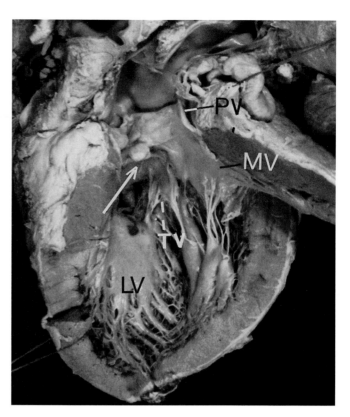

Figure 9: Straddling tricuspid valve in complete transposition with subpulmonary stenosis. Left ventricular view. PV = pulmonary valve; MV = mitral valve; LV = left ventricle; TV = straddling tricuspid valve. Arrow points to the subpulmonary stenosis.

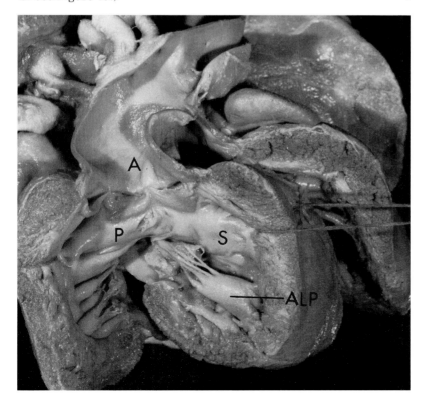

Figure 8: Outflow tract of right ventricle showing the aorta emerging from the right ventricle. A = aorta; P = parietal band; S = septal band; ALP = anterolateral papillary muscle. (Used with permission from Bharati S, Bharati S. See Figure 49.)

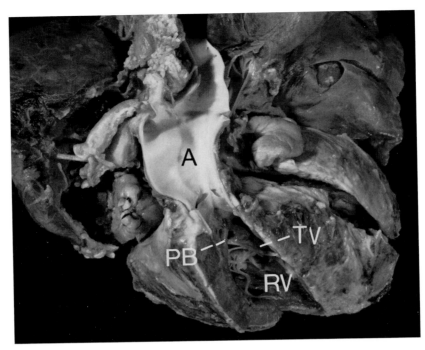

Figure 10: External view of the heart with straddling tricuspid valve in transposition with subpulmonary stenosis. RV = right ventricle; A = aorta; TV = tricuspid valve; PB = parietal band.

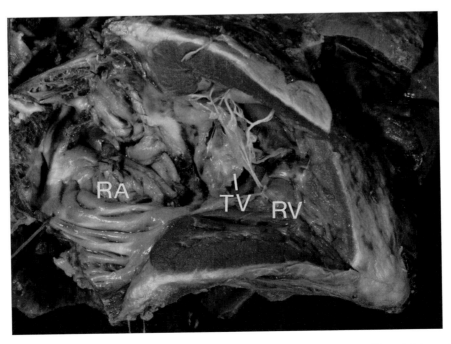

Figure 11: Right atrial, right ventricular view. RA = right atrium; RV = right ventricle; TV = straddling tricuspid valve.

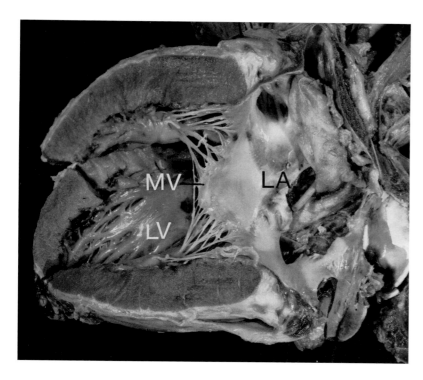

Figure 12: Left atrial, left ventricular view. LA = left atrium; LV = left ventricle; MV = normally formed mitral valve.

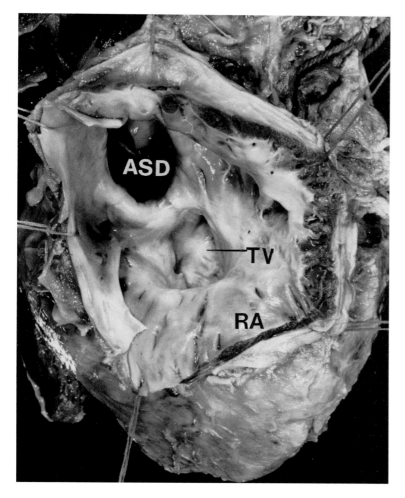

Figure 13: Straddling tricuspid valve in complete transposition with subpulmonary stenosis. Right atrial superior view. ASD = atrial septal defect; TV = straddling tricuspid valve; RA = right atrium.

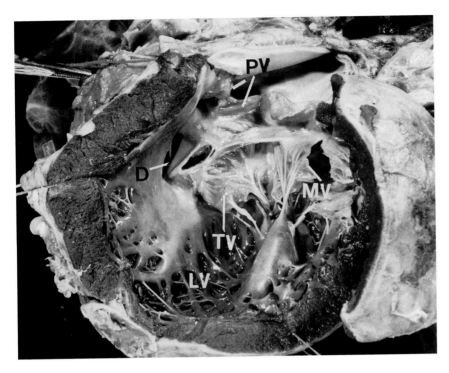

Figure 14: Left ventricular outflow tract view showing the straddling tricuspid valve and subpulmonary stenosis. PV = pulmonary valve; D = defect; MV = mitral valve; LV = left ventricle; TV = straddling tricuspid valve.

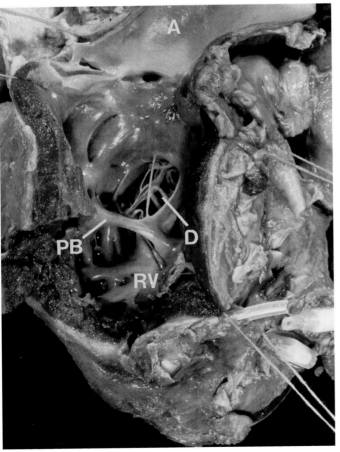

Figure 15: Outflow tract of the right ventricle. A = aorta; D = defect; PB = anomalous parietal band in the right ventricle; RV = right ventricle. Note the connections of the tricuspid valve to the anterolateral papillary muscle situated underneath the anomalous parietal band.

Associated Cardiac Abnormalities

	No. of Cases
Atrial septal defect, fossa ovalis type	8
Bicuspid pulmonic valve	6
Patent ductus arteriosus	7
Double VSD	2

1b. Straddling Tricuspid Valve – Incomplete Form

Basilar or Anular Straddling Tricuspid Valve (15 cases)

In this group, the anulus of the tricuspid valve was prolapsed through a ventricular septal defect, but the peripheral connections of the valve were maintained in the right ventricle as is the case normally. The ventricular septal defect was of the common AV canal type (CAVO) in the majority of the cases, but it involved mostly the membranous septum. The ventricular septal defect was small in 85% of the cases, extending apically in an oblique fashion from the pars membranacea; in 15% of the cases, however, it was very large, extending into the infundibular septum. Thus, part of the anulus of the medial leaflet of the tricuspid valve was situated beneath the efferent vessel in the left ventricle; where there was no efferent vessel in the left ventricle, it was situated on the proximal (upstream) wall of the defect, adjacent to the mitral anulus, as in the complete form.

The atrial septum was markedly deviated in 23%, and in the remainder, the atrial septum and the right atrium were situated more or less in a normal position. The right ventricle was hypertrophied and enlarged in 70% of the cases, and in the remainder it was smaller than normal, but the wall was thickened. The tricuspid orifice was enlarged in 54%, normal in 31%, and small in 15%.

The complexes were:

	No. of Cases
Tetralogy of Fallot with pulmonary atresia and mitral stenosis	1
DORV with subaortic VSD	1
DORV with subpulmonic VSD (Taussig-Bing right ventricular type)	1
DORV with subpulmonic VSD (Taussig-Bing right ventricular type) and pulmonary stenosis	1
Double outlet right ventricle with subpulmonic VSD Taussig-Bing right ventricular type with mild paraductal coarctation	1
Taussig-Bing left-sided with tricuspid stenosis and pulmonary stenosis with common atrium	1
Complete transposition	1
Complete transposition with tricuspid stenosis	1
Premature closure of foramen ovale with preductal coarctation and PDA and overriding aorta	1
Premature narrowing of foramen ovale	1
Transitional coarctation with polyvalvular disease	
ASD and PDA complex with polyvalvular disease and parachute MV	1
ASD, VSD, and PDA with overriding aorta	1
ASD, VSD, PDA with diffuse fibroelastosis of LV and RV	1
VSD, cleft in MV, pulmonary hypertension	1

Major Associated Cardiac Anomalies

	No. of Cases
Patent ductus arteriosus	4
Atrial septal defect, fossa ovalis type	3
Persistent ostium primum	1
Juxtaposed right atrial appendage to the left	2

1c. Peripheral Type of Straddling Tricuspid Valve (five cases)

In this type, the tricuspid anulus, although it was in the normal position, the peripheral connections were mostly in the right ventricle, but a few were in the left ventricle (Figs. 16, 17). This was usually associated with a large common AV canal type of ventricular septal defect that extended anteriorly and/or apically, or the defect was situated in the posterior midseptal region, and the ventricular septal muscle separated the mitral and tricuspid anuli. The septal leaflet of the tricuspid valve at its junction with the anterior or inferior leaflet was attached to well-developed or small accessory posterior papillary muscle in the left ventricle or the attachment was to a normal anterior or posterior papillary muscle in the left ventricle.

The complexes seen in this type of a straddler are:

	No. of Cases
Preductal coarctation with VSD	1
Complete transposition	1
Taussig-Bing, left-sided	1
Complete transposition with pulmonary atresia	1
DORV with isolated truncal inversion with subaortic VSD, pulmonary stenosis, and atypical primum ASD (Figs. 18–23)	1

Major Associated Cardiac Anomalies

	No. of Cases
ASD, fossa ovalis type	2
PDA	2
Isolated cleft in MV	1
Double mitral orifice with MS	1

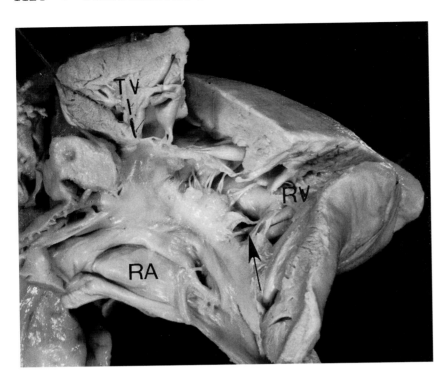

Figure 16: Peripheral straddling tricuspid valve. Right atrial, right ventricular view. RA = right atrium; RV = right ventricle; TV = peripheral straddling tricuspid valve. Arrow points to the chordal extension proceeding through the defect to the opposite chamber.

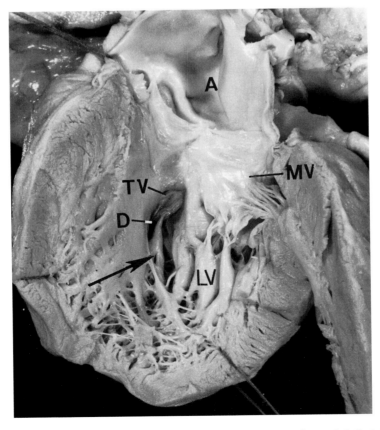

Figure 17: Left ventricular outflow tract showing a large midseptal defect. The straddling tricuspid valve and the peripheral connections are in the left ventricle to an anomalous papillary muscle. A = aorta; MV = mitral valve; LV = left ventricle; TV = straddling tricuspid valve; D = defect, mid septal posterior. Arrow points to the anomalous papillary muscle in the left ventricle.

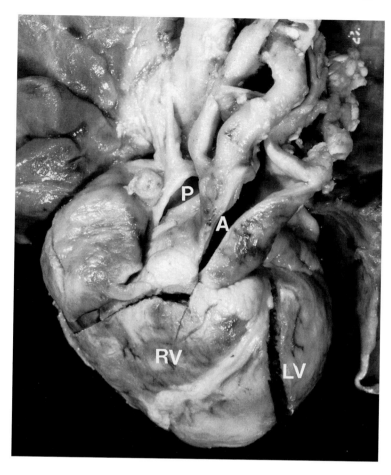

Figure 18: Isolated truncal inversion with atypical ostium primum with peripheral straddling tricuspid valve. A = aorta to the left and anterior; P = pulmonary trunk to the right and posterior; RV = morphologically right ventricle; LV = morphologically left ventricle.

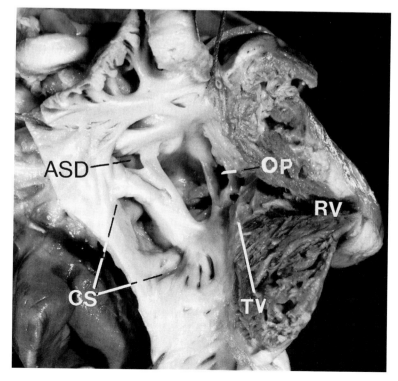

Figure 19: Right atrial, right ventricular view. ASD = atrial septal defect, fossa ovalis type; CS = huge coronary sinus receiving a large left superior vena cava; RV = right ventricle; TV = tricuspid valve; OP = ostium primum defect.

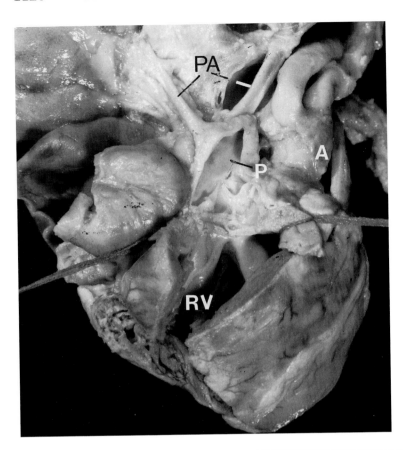

Figure 20: The aorta and the pulmonary trunk emerge from the morphologically right ventricle. The pulmonary trunk is situated to the right and posterior to the aorta – isolated truncal inversion. PA = pulmonary arteries; P = pulmonary trunk; RV = right ventricle; A = aorta.

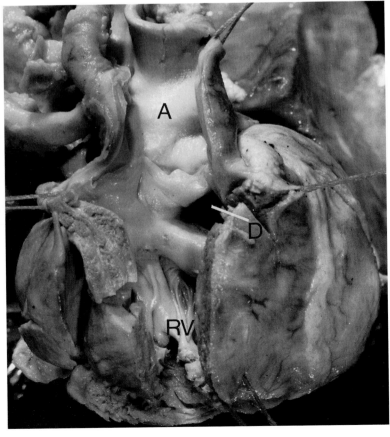

Figure 21: Aorta also emerging from the right ventricle confluent with an anteriorly located ventricular septal defect. A = aorta; D = anteriorly located defect; RV = right ventricle.

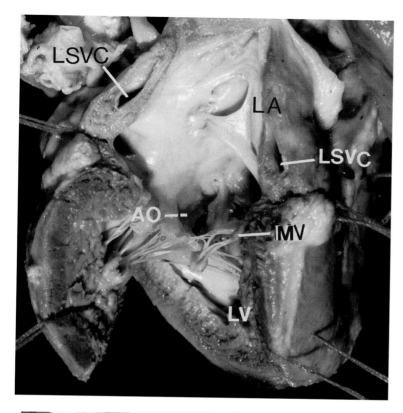

Figure 22: Left-sided view showing the atypical ostium primum with accessory opening in the mitral valve. LA = left atrium; LV = left ventricle; LSVC = large left superior vena cava; MV = mitral valve with no cleft; AO = accessory opening in the mitral valve.

2a. Straddling Mitral Valve, Complete Form (17 cases)

In this entity, the anterior leaflet of the mitral valve was large and incompletely divided into two parts and formed an incomplete cleft-like malformation. At the junction of the two parts, a portion of the leaflet was prolapsed or herniated through a ventricular septal defect (Figs. 24, 25). The valve that herniated was situated either in the center of the proximal (upstream) part of the defect, or distinctly to the right side of the plane of the defect. The peripheral part of the herniated leaflet was connected to the right side of the distal (downstream) wall of the defect in various ways. In 11% of the cases the connections were by way of the chordae, in 78% by way of well-developed single papillary muscle or several papillary muscles, and in 11% by way of small papillary muscles in the right ventricle. In 35% of the hearts the anterior papillary muscle in the left ventricle was absent, or small, or, rarely, the posterior papillary muscle was absent. The papillary muscles of the left ventricle were normal in others.

The defect, in general, was large and was situated in the infundibular septum in its left lateral aspect, with its proximal inferior angle related to the tricuspid anulus or separated from it by a small amount of muscle. Most of the distal portion (downstream) of the defect was unrelated to the tricuspid anulus and lay api-

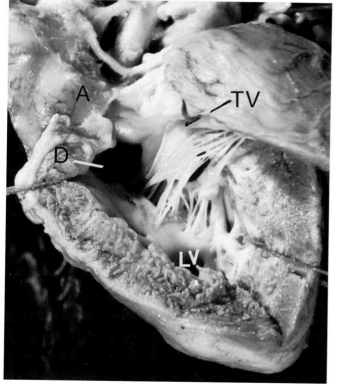

Figure 23: Outflow tract of the left ventricle demonstrating the ventricular septal defect confluent in part with the aorta, with the aorta overriding the defect. LV = left ventricle; A = aorta; D = anteriorly located defect confluent with the aorta; TV = peripheral straddling tricuspid valve.

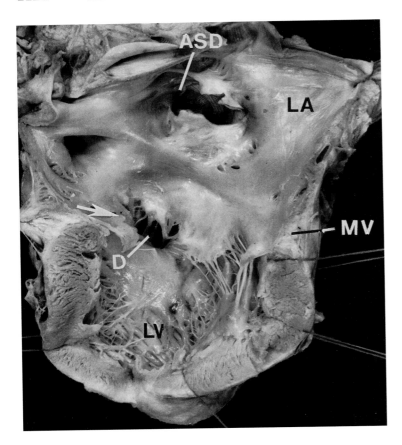

Figure 24: Complete transposition with pulmonary atresia and straddling mitral valve, complete type. Left atrial, left ventricular view. ASD = atrial septal defect; LV = left ventricle; MV = mitral valve; LA = left atrium; D = large defect. Arrow points to the anterior leaflet of the mitral valve with irregular cleft and passing through the defect to right ventricle. Note the absence of anterolateral papillary muscle.

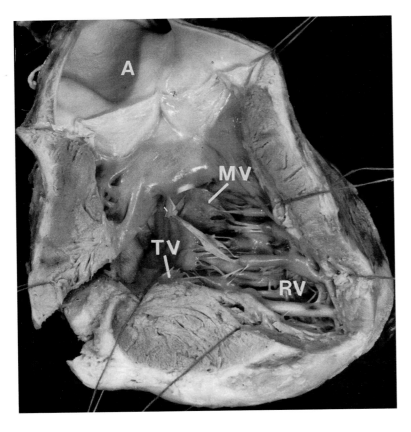

Figure 25: Outflow tract of right ventricle showing the mitral valve attachments. RV = right ventricle; TV = tricuspid valve; MV = complete straddling mitral valve; A = aorta.

cal to the latter. The defect was often confluent with the efferent vessel and often extended posteriorly and involved the membranous septum so that the mitral and tricuspid anuli were contiguous. The defect almost always was related to the pulmonary trunk, although muscle separated it from the pulmonary trunk in some cases. Thus, the herniated portion of the mitral valve, in some cases, obstructed the outflow tract into the pulmonary trunk. Rarely, it obstructed the outflow into the aorta.

Where there was pulmonary atresia with ventricular septal defect (pseudotruncus), the defect was usually separated from the aorta by muscle. There was usually hypertrophy and enlargement of the left atrium, suggesting possible mitral insufficiency. Although, in general, the mitral valve was larger than normal, in four it was smaller than normal. The left ventricle was hypertrophied and enlarged in 41%, normal in size in 35%, and smaller than normal in 34%.

The complexes were:

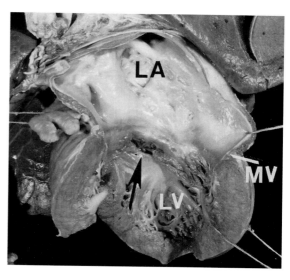

Figure 26: Basilar straddling mitral valve. LA = hypertrophied and enlarged left atrium; MV = mitral valve showing incomplete cleft-like malformation and part of the base of the valve straddling through the defect; LV = left ventricle. Arrow points to the basilar straddling mitral valve.

	No. of Cases
Taussig-Bing, right ventricular type with pulmonary stenosis	6
Taussig-Bing, right ventricular type with fetal coarctation	2
Taussig-Bing, intermediate type with tricuspid stenosis and pulmonary stenosis	1
Taussig-Bing, intermediate type with subpulmonary stenosis	1
Taussig-Bing, left sided	1
Taussig-Bing, left-sided type with tricuspid stenosis	1
Complete transposition with pulmonary atresia	1
Complete transposition with pulmonary stenosis	1
Complete transposition with pulmonary atresia with tricuspid stenosis (large VSD–common ventricle)	1
DORV with subaortic VSD and pulmonary stenosis	1
DORV with noncommitted VSD with common ventricle	1

Major Associated Cardiac Anomalies

	No. of Cases
Atrial septal defect, fossa ovalis type	6
Patent ductus arteriosus	5

2b. Straddling Mitral Valve – Basilar or Anular Type (eight cases)

Here, only the anulus was herniated or prolapsed or straddled through the defect with the anterior leaflet divided into two segments, as seen in the complete form, but the connections of part of the mitral valve were in the left ventricle (Fig. 26). In two hearts, the anterior papillary muscle was absent in the left ventricle, and in others, the papillary muscles were normal. In general, the ventricular septal defect was large, except in one where it was situated in the infundibular septum. This type of a straddler is frequently seen in Taussig-Bing hearts (7), intermediate (3), left-sided (2), right sided (2), and in complete transposition (1).

Associated Cardiac Anomalies

	No. of Cases
Patent ductus arteriosus	2
Bicuspid pulmonic valve with stenosis	1
Coarctation of the aorta	1
Accessory VSD	1
Tricuspid stenosis	2

2c. Straddling Mitral Valve – Peripheral Form (one case)

This was seen in a right-sided Taussig-Bing with tricuspid stenosis and preductal coarctation of the

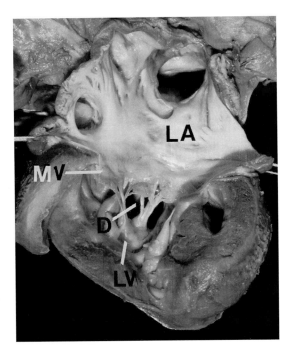

Figure 27: Peripheral straddling mitral valve. Left atrial, left ventricular view. LA = left atrium; LV = left ventricle; D = defect; MV = mitral valve.

aorta (Figs. 27, 28). The mitral valve was not divided into two components. Although the anulus of the mitral valve was in the left ventricle, the peripheral connections of the valve were attached to two papillary muscles through the chordae to the right side of the ventricular septum. There was no distinct anterior papillary muscle in the left ventricle. The defect was similar to what is seen in the basilar type of a straddling mitral valve, but was large.

3. Straddling of Both AV Orifices and Valves (four cases)

Although these cases are very rare, they are important from the standpoint of diagnosis and surgery (Figs. 29, 30). One was a case of complete regular trans-

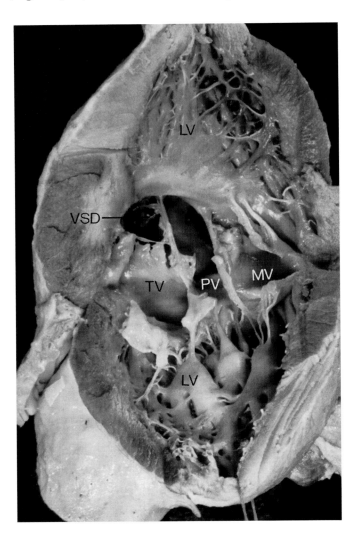

Figure 29: Double straddling AV valve. Left ventricular view showing the large common AV canal type of ventricular septal defect through which both the mitral and tricuspid valves are connected to the left ventricle. LV = left ventricle; MV = mitral valve; TV = tricuspid valve; PV = pulmonary valve; VSD = ventricular septal defect.

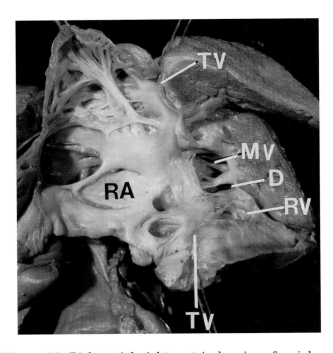

Figure 28: Right atrial, right ventricular view of peripheral straddling mitral valve. RA = right atrium; RV = right ventricle; TV = tricuspid valve; D = large common AV canal type of defect extending more apically; MV = peripheral straddling mitral valve.

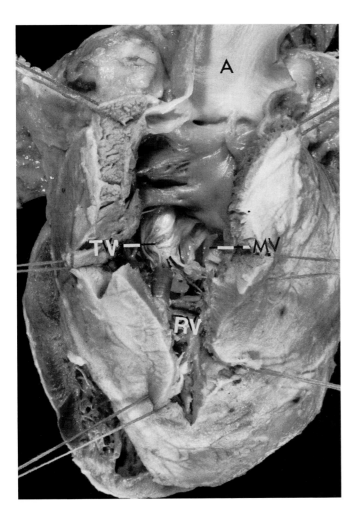

Figure 30: Right ventricle showing connections of both AV valves with aorta emerging from the chamber. RV = right ventricle; MV = straddling mitral valve; TV = straddling tricuspid valve; A = aorta.

position. There was a huge VSD in the base extending both anteriorly and posteriorly. The anterior leaflet of the tricuspid valve straddled through the septum and was connected to a small papillary muscle in the left ventricle. The medial leaflet was connected to both ventricles and the inferior leaflet was connected only to the left ventricle. The anterior leaflet of the mitral valve was attached to an anterior papillary muscle in the right ventricle and also to the regular papillary muscles in the left ventricle. The left ventricle was quite large and the right ventricle was small, consisting mostly of infundibulum with a small part of sinus (Figs. 29, 30).

In a second case of complete regular transposition with tricuspid and pulmonic stenosis, there were two ventricular septal defects, a posterior muscular and an anterior defect separated from the tricuspid valve by

muscle. Part of the peripheral portion of the septal leaflet of the tricuspid valve was connected to an accessory posterior papillary muscle in the left ventricle passing through the posterior ventricular septal defect. The anterior leaflet of the mitral valve was cleft and the anulus of the leaflet herniated or straddled through the large anterior ventricular septal defect and was attached by chordae to the superior part of the right ventricle.

In another case of double ventricular septal defect, one was situated in the posterior part of the anterior septum beneath the arch formed by the septal and parietal bands, related to the tricuspid valve, and the other was a spontaneously closed or closing posterobasal defect. The basilar portion of the tricuspid valve was herniated through the more anterior defect while part of the posterior leaflet of the mitral valve was attached to the closing second defect.

The fourth case was an intermediate type of a Taussig-Bing with tricuspid stenosis. There was a large anterior ventricular septal defect separated from the tricuspid valve by muscle. The septal leaflet of the tricuspid valve straddled through the defect and was connected to accessory papillary muscles in the left ventricle. The anterior leaflet of the mitral valve formed a cleft-like malformation and straddled through the defect and was attached to an accessory papillary muscle in the right ventricle.

4. Displaced Tricuspid Orifice and Valve (13 cases)

In this entity, the tricuspid orifice and valve were completely displaced into the opposite ventricular chamber–left ventricle. There were two types:

(a) resembling single ventricle – 5 cases

(b) with tricuspid stenosis with or without juxtaposed right atrial appendage to the left – 8 cases

In the type resembling single ventricle, both AV valves were connected to a group of anterior and posterior papillary muscles in the left ventricle (Fig. 31). The tricuspid orifice and valvular apparatus were small in two, normal in one, and enlarged in two other cases. The right ventricle consisted of a sinus and an infundibulum, but there was no evidence of tensor apparatus. The ventricular septal defect was in the anterior part of the infundibular septum in three cases, in the posterior part of the septum in one, and in one the anterior defect extended posteriorly as well. The anterior and posterior descending coronary arteries joined together at the apex demarcating the morphologically right from the left ventricle, a finding usually not present in cases of single ventricle.

In the second type with tricuspid stenosis with juxtaposition of the right atrial appendage to the left (six

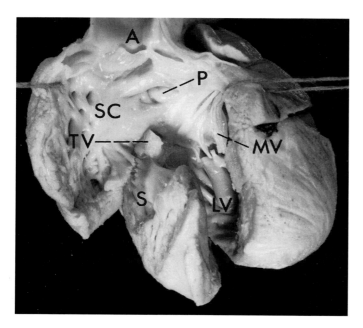

Figure 31: Displaced tricuspid orifice in atypical complete transposition with straddling aorta and pulmonary stenosis. LV = left ventricle; P = pulmonary trunk; S = sinus (apical recess of right ventricle); SC = straddling conus; TV = tricuspid orifice and valve, stenotic; MV = mitral valve; LV = left ventricle; A = aorta. (Used with permission from Liberthson RR, et al. See Figure 53.)

of the eight), there was a minute tricuspid orifice situated beneath the pulmonary orifice in the left ventricle, with small chordal attachments to the wall of that chamber and occasionally to a small papillary muscle (Figs. 32–34). This orifice was close to the VSD in the infundibular septum. The defect was situated below the arch (crista) in some cases, was confluent with the aorta coming from the right ventricle in others with overriding aorta in two (one with straddling parietal band), and in one it involved the membranous septum. In the heart without juxtaposed right atrial appendage to the left, there was an overriding infundibular septum with minute tricuspid orifice entering below this infundibulum. In the six cases with juxtaposed right atrial appendage to the left, the right atrium was displaced posteroinferiorly.

The complexes were:

4a. Type resembling single ventricle

	No. of Cases
DOLV with overriding aorta with preductal coarctation and subaortic stenosis	1
DOLV with overriding aorta with pulmonary stenosis (PS) and mitral stenosis (MS)	1
DOLV with MS, PS, and multiple VSDs (Figs. 35–38)	1
Isolated levocardia, complete transposition with pulmonary atresia	1
Isolated displaced tricuspid valve with tricuspid stenosis (TS), infundibular PS, and subaortic stenosis	1

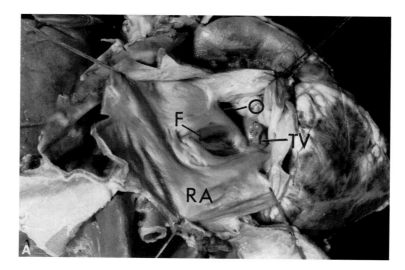

Figure 32: Displaced tricuspid valve with tricuspid stenosis in mesocardia with regular transposition and juxtaposed right atrial appendage to the left. Right atrial view. RA = right atrium; F = fossa ovalis defect; O = opening into right atrial appendage; TV = displaced tricuspid orifice and valve. (Used with permission from Bharati S, et al. See Figure 49.)

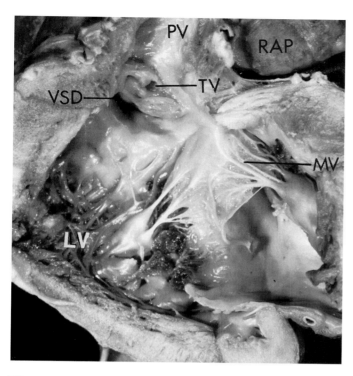

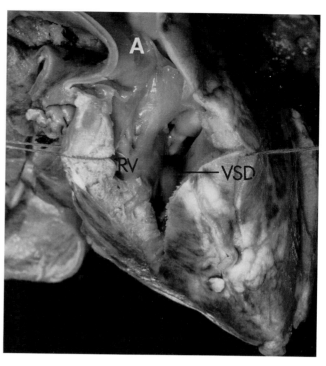

Figure 33: Left ventricular view showing displaced tricuspid valve. MV = mitral valve; RAP = right atrial appendage, juxtaposed to the left; PV = pulmonary valve; TV = displaced tricuspid valve; VSD = ventricular septal defect. (Used with permission from Bharati S, et al. See Figure 49.)

Figure 34: Aorta emerging from the right ventricle. RV = right ventricle; VSD = ventricular septal defect. (Used with permission from Bharati S, et al. See Figure 49.)

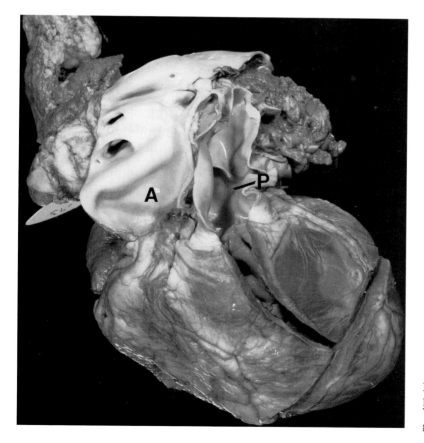

Figure 35: Displaced tricuspid valve with incomplete double outlet left ventricle and multiple VSDs. External view. Note the normally related great arteries. A = aorta; P = pulmonary trunk.

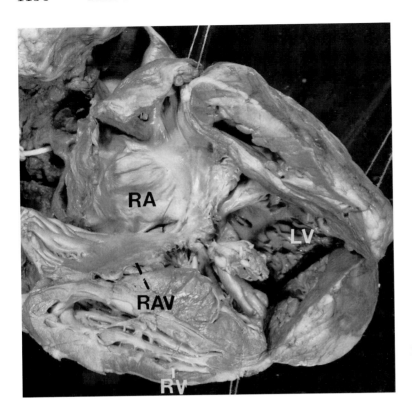

Figure 36: Right-sided view. RA = right atrium; RAV = right AV valve, tricuspid displaced into the morphologically left ventricle; RV = right ventricle; LV = left ventricle.

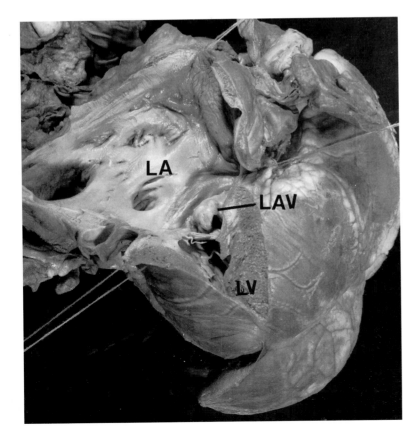

Figure 37: Left atrial, left ventricular view showing mitral stenosis. LA = left atrium; LAV = left AV valve, mitral with stenosis; LV = left ventricle.

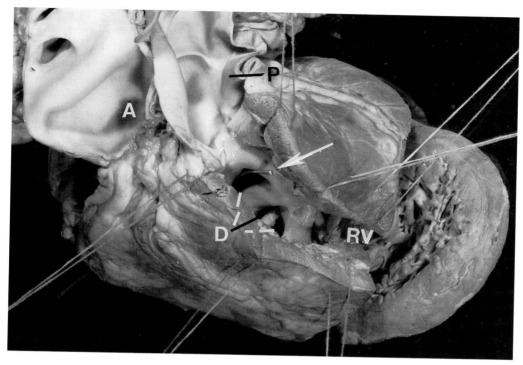

Figure 38: Straddling pulmonary trunk and aorta over the multiple defects. A = aorta; RV = right ventricle; P = pulmonary trunk; D = defects. Arrow points to the straddling pulmonary trunk.

4b. With TS, and superiorly displaced tricuspid valve

	No. of Cases
DOLV with overriding aorta with PS	1
Complete transposition with TS with fetal coarctation, juxtaposed right atrial appendage to the left	1
Mesocardia, complete transposition with TS and subpulmonary stenosis, juxtaposed right atrial appendage to the left	1
Complete transposition with PS, subpulmonary stenosis and TS, juxtaposed right atrial appendage to the left	1
DORV with TS and PS, juxtaposed right atrial appendage to the left	1
Complete transposition with marked TS (functional), atresia, straddling parietal band, double VSD, overriding aorta, juxtaposed atrial appendage to the left	1
Complete transposition with juxtaposed right atrial appendage to the left, VSD, overriding aorta, PS, and small tricuspid valve	1
Complete transposition with TS, VSD, overriding aorta, preductal coarctation	1

Major Associated Cardiac Anomalies

	No. of Cases
ASD, fossa ovalis	3
PDA	3
Juxtaposed right atrial appendage to the left	6
Cor triatriatum sinister	1
Accessory VSD	3
High origin of left coronary	1

5. Combination of Displaced and Straddling Orifices and Valves

Displaced Tricuspid Orifice with Straddling Mitral Orifice (three cases)

One had mitral and pulmonary stenosis with normally related arterial trunks (Figs. 39–41) and the other had complete transposition with pulmonary stenosis. The defect was anteriorly located beneath the arch in the case with normally related vessels, and it was beneath the aorta in the case with transposition. The third case was a case of isolated levocardia with visceral heterotaxy and polysplenia with inverted atria and normal ventricles, and DORV and subpulmonic ventricular septal defect.

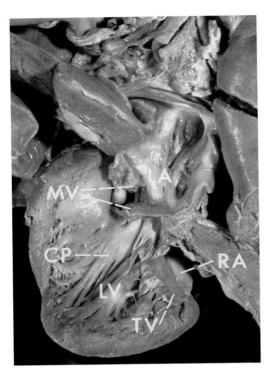

Figure 39: Displaced tricuspid valve with straddling mitral valve. Mitral and pulmonary stenosis without transposition. Bi-atrial and left ventricular view. LA = left atrium; RA = right atrium; TV = tricuspid valve; LV = left ventricle; CP = combined posterior papillary muscle and ridge; MV = straddling mitral valve. Note the tricuspid valve is displaced completely into the left ventricle. (Used with permission from Liberthson RR, et al. See Figure 53.)

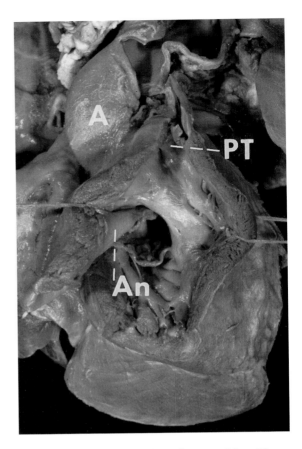

Figure 40: Outflow tract of the right ventricle with normally related great arteries and the straddling mitral valve attached to the anterolateral papillary muscle. A = aorta; PT = pulmonary trunk; An = straddling mitral valve attached to the anterolateral papillary muscle. (Used with permission from Liberthson RR, et al. See Figure 53.)

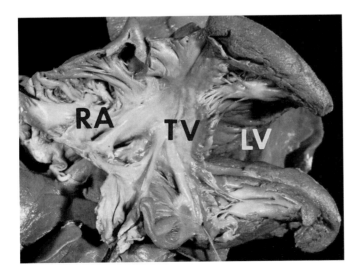

Figure 41: Right atrial, left ventricular view. RA = right atrium; LV = left ventricle; TV = tricuspid valve displaced completely into the morphologically left ventricle. (Used with permission from Liberthson RR, et al. See Figure 53.)

6. Displaced Mitral and Straddling Tricuspid Orifice and Valve (one case)

This was a case of DORV with two ventricular septal defects, one subpulmonic and one common AV canal type. The mitral valve had no connection with the left ventricle, but proceeded through an anterior defect to the right ventricle where it was attached to the papillary muscles, and the tricuspid valve straddled through a common AV canal type of defect and entered both ventricles. The architecture of the right ventricle was typical of a Taussig-Bing heart (Figs. 42–45).

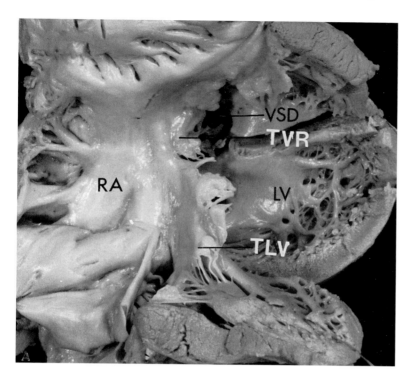

Figure 42: Displaced mitral and straddling tricuspid valve in Taussig-Bing heart. Right atrial, left ventricular view. RA = right atrium; LV = left ventricle; TLV = tricuspid entering left ventricle; VSD = ventricular septal defect; TVR = tricuspid entering right ventricle. (Used with pemission from Bharati S, et al. See Figure 49.)

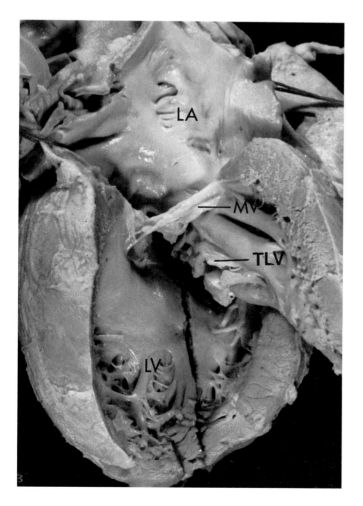

Figure 43: Left atrial, left ventricular view showing displaced mitral valve. LA = left atrium; LV = left ventricle; MV = displaced mitral valve; TLV = straddling tricuspid valve. (Used with permission from Bharati S, et al. See Figure 49.)

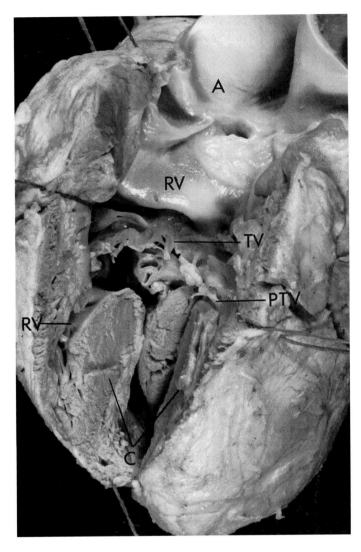

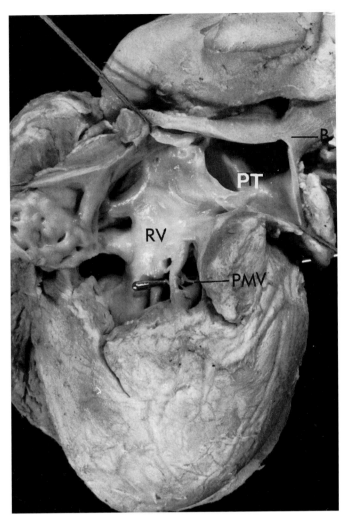

Figure 44: Right ventricular view beneath the aorta. A = aorta; RV = right ventricle; TV = straddling tricuspid valve; PTV = papillary muscle in the right ventricle connected to tricuspid valve; C = cut made by prosector in the ventricular septum. (Used with permission from Bharati S, et al. See Figure 49.)

Figure 45: Right ventricular view beneath the pulmonary trunk. RV = right ventricle; B = banding of pulmonary trunk; PMV = papillary muscle in the right ventricle connected to mitral valve; PT = pulmonary trunk. (Used with permission from Bharati S, et al. See Figure 49.) Note the probe passing through the anterior VSD.

7. Straddling and Displaced AV Valves in Ventricular Inversion (10 cases)

7a. Straddling Tricuspid Valve (6 cases)

Straddling left AV valve (tricuspid valve) was seen in six cases (Figs. 46–49). Five were complete and one was peripheral. In all of these, there was a common AV canal type of ventricular septal defect and in one the defect involved the anterior part of the ventricular septum as well. In one, the defect was restrictive and was situated in the membranous septum. The tricuspid orifice in three cases was quite large and in three it was stenotic. The medial (septal) leaflet of the tricuspid was large and this bridged or crossed over or herniated through the defect and was attached to an accessory posterior papillary muscle in the left ventricle. One had mitral atresia (Figs. 46–49), four had inverted complete transposition (two with subpulmonary stenosis), and two had noninverted double outlet right ventricle, with the aorta to the right and anterior to the pulmonary trunk with no truncal inversion.

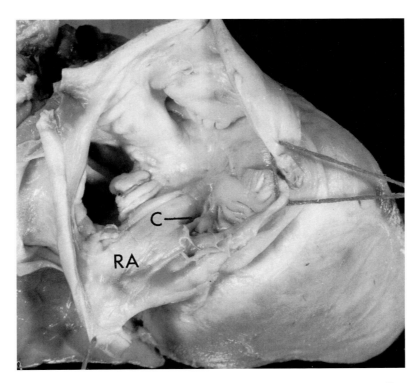

Figure 46: Straddling left AV valve (tricuspid), with right AV valve (mitral) atresia in mixed (discordant) levocardia with ventricular inversion and inverted DORV with pulmonary stenosis. Right atrial view. RA = right atrium; C = coronary sinus. Note the atresia of the mitral valve. (Used with permission from Bharati S, et al. See Figure 49.)

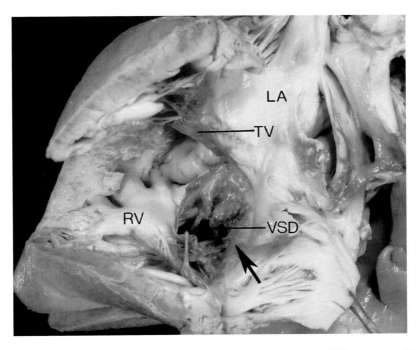

Figure 47: Left atrial, right ventricular view showing the straddling tricuspid valve. LA = left atrium; RV = right ventricle; VSD = ventricular septal defect; TV = straddling tricuspid valve. (Used with permission from Bharati S, et al. See Figure 49.) Note large common AV canal type of defect extending posteriorly. Arrow points to the straddling tricuspid valve.

two cases were inverted DORV with no truncal inver-   ampullary ring remains as the posterior ventricular

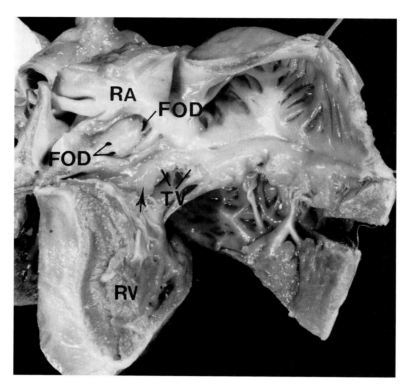

Figure 55: Borderline straddling tricuspid and mitral valves in a common AV canal type of VSD. Right atrial, right ventricular view. RA = right atrium; FOD = fossa ovalis defect; RV = right ventricle; TV = tricuspid valve. Arrow points to the septal leaflet of the tricuspid valve connected to the rim of the common AV canal type of defect.

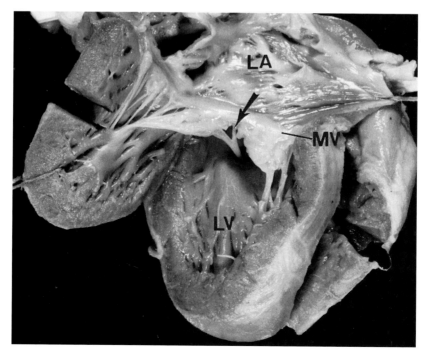

Figure 56: Left atrial, left ventricular view of the same heart as in Figure 54. LA = left atrium; LV = left ventricle; MV = mitral valve. Arrow points to the incomplete cleft-like malformation and accessory chordal extension to the lower margin of the defect.

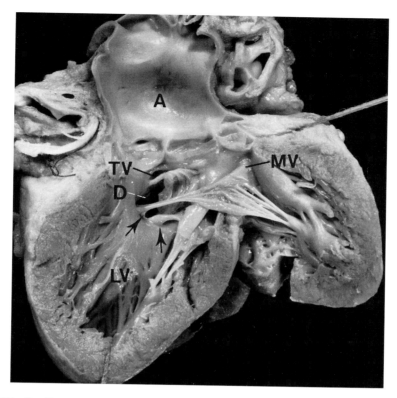

Figure 57: Outflow tract of the left ventricle demonstrating the chordal attachments of the tricuspid and mitral valves to the rim of the CAVO type of defect (same heart as in Figures 55 and 56). A = aorta; MV = mitral valve; TV = chordal extension of the tricuspid valve along the rim of the defect; LV = left ventricle. Two arrows point to chordal extensions from the mitral valve attached to the rim of the defect.

Criss-Cross Hearts and Straddlers

Again, this entity has been described in Chapter 57. Since these hearts are closely related to straddlers and displaced AV valves, we will emphasize some aspects of criss-cross hearts in this discussion.

Fundamentally, in these hearts, the morphological right atrium is connected to the morphological left ventricle, and the morphological left atrium is connected to the morphological right ventricle; yet the chambers, although somewhat altered, were in *relatively* normal position. The type of AV valves corresponded to the distal ventricular chambers.

A true criss-cross heart is one in which both AV orifices are displaced into the oppositely positioned chamber, the opposite chamber being the discordant chamber. The AV valves correspond to the distal chambers. In this view, to be a criss-cross heart, a morphological right ventricle must be anterior and to the right or directly anterior to the left ventricle, or anterior and superior to the left ventricle with the above AV connections (that is, the tricuspid valve entering the morphological right ventricle, and the mitral valve entering the left). Straddling and displaced AV orifices are those in which the valves enter the morphologically discordant (vis-à-vis the valves) chambers, in part or completely. The valves do not correspond to the distal chamber in part or completely. There are hearts in which both AV orifices are displaced as defined above, and the ventricular chambers take on a criss-cross position. A true criss-cross heart may be combined with a straddling AV valve.

Conclusion

In general, straddlers and displaced AV valves are associated with transposition, DORV, the Taussig-Bing group of hearts, mitral atresia, or ventricular inversion. The above data suggest that there might be frequent association of several genes that may be affected together. Or there may also be a tendency for certain groups of genes to be susceptible to alterations in the hemodynamics and/or other factors (such as infections) during the very early stages of the developing embryo that may eventually produce combination of anomalies as described above.

The tendency for certain genes to be associated or grouped together at a certain stage of the developing embryo and the altered hemodynamic effects are to be explored in the future.

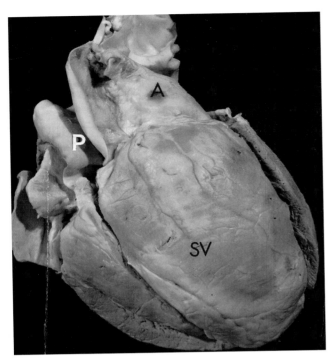

Figure 1: Single ventricle with inverted loop and inverted transposition. Anterior view. A = aorta; P = pulmonary trunk; SV = single ventricle.

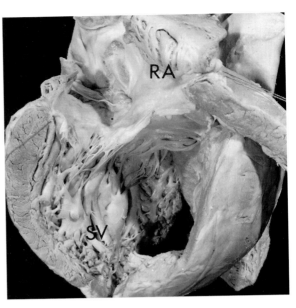

Figure 3: View of the single ventricle from the right side. RA = right atrium; SV = single ventricle.

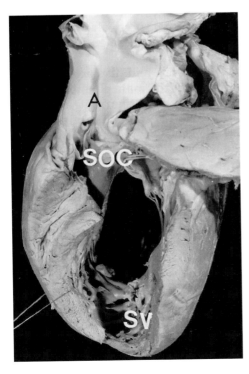

Figure 2: Aorta emerging from the small outlet chamber. SOC = small outlet chamber; A = aorta; SV = single ventricle.

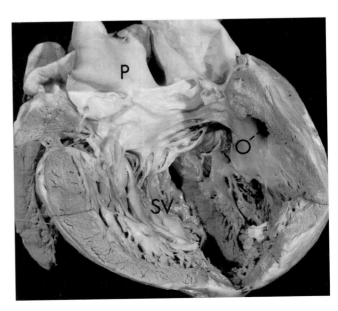

Figure 4: Pulmonary trunk emerging from the main ventricular chamber. P = pulmonary trunk; SV = single ventricle; O = opening between the single ventricle and the small outlet chamber.

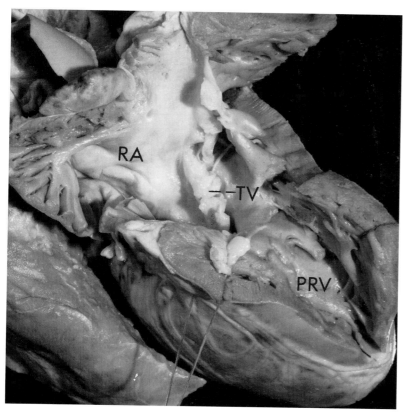

Figure 5: Straddling tricuspid orifice with regular transposition. Right atrial, right ventricular view. RA = right atrium; PRV = primitive right ventricle; TV = straddling tricuspid valve.

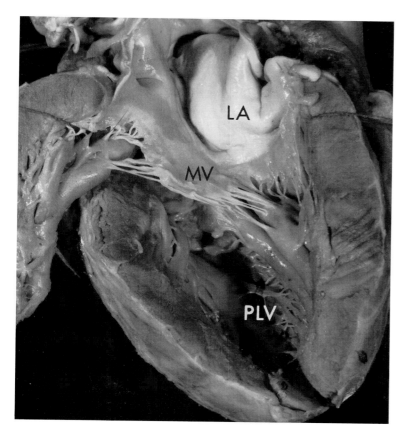

Figure 6: Left atrial, left ventricular view. LA = left atrium; MV = mitral valve; PLV= primitive left ventricle.

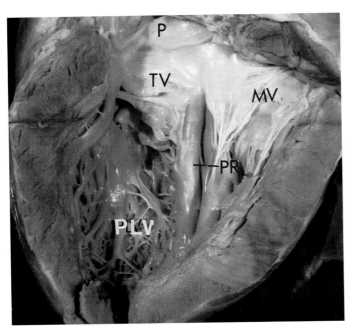

Figure 7: Outflow tract of the left ventricle. PLV = primitive left ventricle; MV = mitral valve; P = pulmonary trunk; TV = straddling tricuspid valve; PR = posterior ridge.

cles. However, the left-sided ventricle contains a portion of sinus that rightfully belongs to the right side, and, therefore, we call the chambers primitive right and left ventricles (Figs. 5–7). It differs from the displaced tricuspid valve in not having any valvular apparatus in the right ventricle.

Possible Embryological Relationship of the Three Entities

In the normal embryological development, the posterior ventricular septum (septum ventriculorum proprium) is made up by a main ventricular septal ridge that extends over the antimesocardial aspect of the ventricle. There is a ventricular counter ridge that is fundamentally the bulboauricular spur which is responsible or concerned mostly with the anterior septum. These ridges extend from the anterior and posterior endocardial cushions to the bulbar cushions.

The main septal ridge cuts across the interampullary ring, thus producing a tricuspid furrow caudally in the proampulla and an aortic groove cranially in the meta-ampulla. During the absorption of the bulbus and its ventral deviation to the left and the shift of

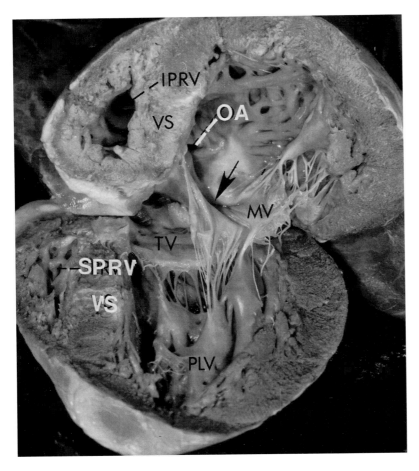

Figure 8: Displaced tricuspid orifice with regular transposition. VS = ventricular septum; MV = mitral valve; TV = tricuspid valve; PLV = primitive left ventricle; SPRV = sinus of primitive right ventricle; OA = opening into aorta; IPRV = infundibulum of primitive right ventricle. Arrow points to where the orifice of the pulmonary trunk is (which is not well seen in the picture).(Used with permission from Bharati S, Lev M. See Figure 9.)

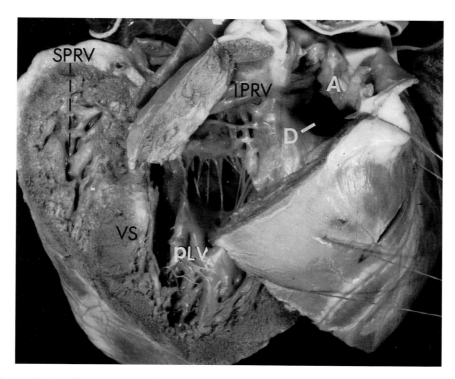

Figure 9: Outflow tract or infundibulum of the right ventricle showing a U-shaped defect confluent with the aortic valve with the aorta overriding the defect. A = aorta; SPRV = sinus of primitive right ventricle; IPRV = infundibulum of primitive right ventricle; VS = ventricular septum; PLV = primitive left ventricle. (Used with permission from Bharati S, Lev M: The relationship between single ventricle and small outlet chamber and straddling and displaced tricuspid orifice and valve. *J Herz* 1979, 4:176–183.)

the atrial canal to the right (or expansion of the atrial canal), the main ventricular ridge swings or moves into a more sagittal plane and the middle portion of the interampullary ring fuses (joins) with the middle portion of the main ventricular ridge. Simultaneously, the tricuspid furrow expands, with its adjacent proampulla, to produce or to form the inflow portion of the right ventricle. Therefore, the developing main posterior ventricular septum consists in part of the interampullary ring. However, its basal part (portion) consists of the main ventricular ridge.

The bulbar septum and meta-ampullary portions of the main ventricular ridge constitute the anterior ventricular septum. To these structures is later fused the bulboauricular spur. The bulbar septum is formed by the fusion of proximal bulbar ridges A (sinistroventral) and B (dextrodorsal). The septum, when formed, lies or is situated obliquely and to the right of the interampullary ring. As the bulbus swings (moves) ventrally and to the left during the process of the absorption of the bulbus, the developing (forming) bulbar septum and the meta-ampullary portion of the main ventricular ridge swing likewise ventrally and to the left, thus giving an abbreviated portion of the bulbus

and meta-ampulla to the definitive left ventricle in a normal heart.

Thus, the posterior (main) muscular ventricular septum consists of two parts: (1) a proampullary portion of the main ventricular ridge, and (2) the central portion of the interampullary ring. The anterior muscular ventricular septum consists of the bulbar septum fused with the bulboauricular spur, and the meta-ampullary portion of the main ventricular ridge. This, therefore, means that the definitive left ventricle consists of proampulla, a small part of meta-ampulla, and a shrunken part of the bulbus. The definitive right ventricle consists of proampulla, meta-ampulla, and a well-developed bulbus.

In single ventricle, straddling tricuspid or displaced tricuspid valve we may hypothesize the following: There may be an abnormality in the formation of the proampullar or meta-ampullar portions of the main ventricular septum and persistence of the interampullary ring, related in some way to lack of movement of the atrial canal to the right. It might be postulated that normally this movement of the atrial canal divides off the interampullary ring. If there is no movement at all of this canal, we have single ventricle and small outlet chamber. Here, the bulbus will be absorbed with a portion of the bulbus going to the main ventricular chamber, but no proampulla is given to the right-sided chamber. Therefore, the right-sided chamber will contain only a shrunken meta-ampulla and bulbus and the opening between the two will be a persistent interampullary ostium.

If, under the same circumstances, the interampullary ring progressed into a sizable posterior septum, even though abnormally formed, and the meta-ampulla remained a sizable structure, it might lead to a displaced tricuspid orifice with primitive right and left ventricles.

If the process of disruption of the interampullary

ring proceeded in part, that is, there is partial movement to the right of the atrial canal, then we might have a straddling tricuspid orifice. Here we would have a primitive right ventricle consisting of a small part of proampulla with the remainder consisting of meta-ampulla and bulbus, and the left ventricle might contain a part of meta-ampulla in addition to a portion of proampulla and shrunken bulbus.

The above speculations are made with the assumption that the bulboventricular loop is normally developed (D-). It is evident that similar speculations could be made with a levo-loop, but the movements of the structures would be in opposite directions.

Anatomic Differences in Ventricular Morphology in Single Ventricle, Straddling Tricuspid and Displaced Tricuspid Valve

	Single Ventricle	*Straddling Tricuspid Valve*	*Displaced Tricuspid Valve*
Left ventricular morphology	Sinuses of both definitive ventricles and infundibulum	Sinus of left ventricle and part of sinus of right ventricle with infundibulum or vestibule	Sinuses of both definitive ventricles and infundibulum
Right ventricular morphology	Infundibulum, in part	Portions of sinus of right ventricle with tricuspid valve apparatus with infundibulum	Portions of sinus of right ventricle without tricuspid apparatus with infundibulum

Basic Philosophy

The fundamental question as to whether single ventricle, straddling tricuspid orifice, or displaced tricuspid orifice should be considered as separate entities or grouped together in one entity depends upon the anatomy as well as the surgical approach.

The Differential Diagnosis Between Single Ventricle, Common Ventricle, Straddling and Displaced AV Valves and Their Significance

Single ventricle must be differentiated from common ventricle, straddling tricuspid orifice, displaced

right or left AV valve, and tricuspid and mitral atresia. In our opinion, these are different anatomic entities and should be dealt with separately, although it is understood that there are hearts where differentiation cannot be made absolutely one from the other because of anatomic indistinguishability in some. However, in most cases, differentiation can be made. We emphasize this factor because of the fact that anatomically the geometry of the hemodynamically altered malformed heart differs considerably from one heart to another, which may indeed be responsible for the mortality and morbidity of the different entities, regardless of the type of surgery.

On the other hand, the genes responsible for all of the above entities are probably closely related and further research at the molecular genetic level is warranted.

66

The Concept of Single Ventricle Complex as Distinct from that of Tricuspid Atresia Complex

In order to understand the concept of single ventricle complex as distinct from that of tricuspid atresia complex, the anatomy of the normal right ventricle should be defined clearly.

Right and Left Ventricles

The normal right ventricle consists of a sinus or inflow tract with a coarsely trabeculated septal surface associated, in many cases if not in most cases, with an apical recess. Above this area is an infundibulum or outflow tract demarcated by a septal and a parietal band that form an arch on the septum beneath the efferent vessel. The infundibulum is sharply demarcated from the sinus or the inlet. The sinus in the normal right ventricle contains the tensor apparatus of the tricuspid valve superimposed on the trabecular surface.

The normal left ventricle consists of inflow and outflow portions, which are not distinctly demarcated from each other. This is related in part to the acuteness of the angle between the two. The normal lower septal surface is finely trabeculated. In the normal heart, the septal portion of the subaortic area (the base) is angulated with the remainder of the septum in such a way as to form a bayonet-like extension of the lower septum. This basal part of the subaortic area in the normal heart may be called a vestibule. This vestibule is usually not sharply demarcated from the remainder of the ventricle.

Ventricular Septum and Anterior and Posterior Descending Coronary Arteries

The ventricular septum is that portion of the ventricular myocardium that separates what we have defined above as right and left ventricles from each other. The architecture of the right and left sides of the septum has already been described. The anterior descending coronary artery normally supplies the anterior two-thirds and the apical portion of the ventricular septum. The posterior descending coronary artery normally supplies the posterior one-third of the septum, excluding its apical portion.

Thus, if these two coronary arteries can be identified, and if they meet in the apical region, we believe it is evidence in favor of the concept that the embryological posterior ventricular septum as well as the embryological anterior septum have formed. These two arteries demarcate the right and left ventricles in our definition of these terms.

It has been convenient in common usage to differentiate between the anterior or infundibular portion of the septum and the more posterior portion of the septum. This has been influenced, in part, by embryological thinking, since the anterior infundibular septum probably arises from the embryonic bulbar septum, and the posterior septum from the embryonic main ventricular septum.

The concept thus has usefulness in anatomy since it is helpful to know whether adequate septation between the chambers is present. There is usually no difficulty in recognizing the anterior septum. We believe that anatomically one can recognize the presence of the posterior septum by the coronary arterial supply.

Tricuspid Atresia

Tricuspid atresia is defined as absence of tricuspid orifice in the presence of a mitral orifice.

Tricuspid Atresia Complex

The term "complex," as we use it, means the presence of a single anomaly or a group of anomalies that have a tendency to occur together, and the reaction of the endocardium, myocardium, valves, epicardium, and the conduction system to the presence of the anomaly or anomalies.

The term "tricuspid atresia complex" refers to that complex which has tricuspid atresia as a base, or any combination of congenital anomalies in which tricuspid atresia is an element.

Single Ventricle Complex

We define single ventricle complex as that in which two AV orifices, or a common AV orifice, enter a single ventricular chamber which gives rise to one of the two efferent vessels. The single ventricular chamber in the majority of the cases communicates with a small outlet chamber that gives rise to the other efferent vessel. Thus, one efferent vessel is related to both AV orifices, or to the common AV orifice, while the other efferent vessel is not related to either AV orifice.

Difference Between Tricuspid Atresia Complex and Single Ventricle Complex

In tricuspid atresia complex, the right ventricle is the right-sided chamber adjacent to the right atrium on the anterior surface of the heart. This chamber consists of an infundibulum, beneath which there is a trabeculated area. The latter area occasionally shows a papillary muscle, although in most cases there is no tricuspid valvular apparatus. We consider this area to be a remnant of sinus. We therefore call this right-sided chamber a *right ventricle morphologically*. The fact that the anterior and posterior descending coronary arteries in most cases demarcate this chamber from the left ventricle (Figs. 1, 2), as in the normal heart, is in favor of this hypothesis.

In single ventricle, the small outlet chamber consists mainly of what we believe to be an *abnormally*

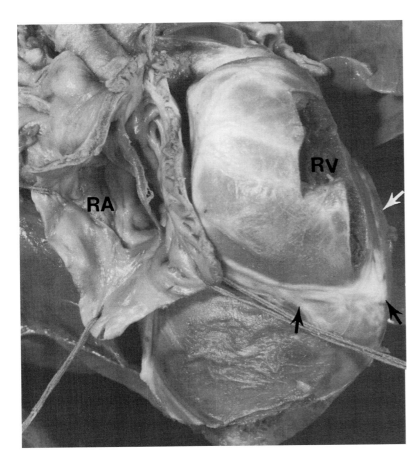

Figure 1: Tricuspid atresia with transposition. Right atrial view. RA = right atrium; RV = right ventricle. Arrows point to anterior and posterior descending coronary arteries joining together at the apex.

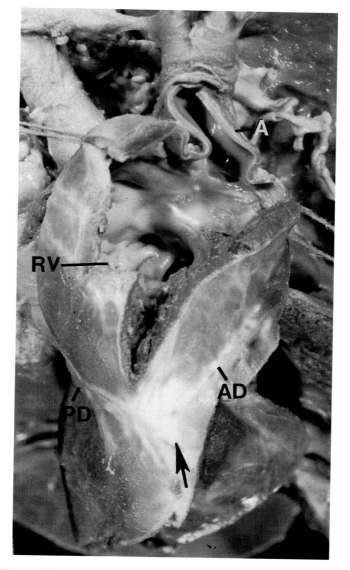

Figure 2: Tricuspid atresia with transposition. Right ventricular view. A = aorta; RV = right ventricle; AD = anterior descending coronary artery; PD = posterior descending coronary artery. Arrow points to the apex formed by the anterior and posterior descending coronary arteries, thereby demarcating the development of the posterior ventricular septum.

developed infundibulum showing abnormally formed septal and parietal bands. At the gross level there may be a small trabeculated area beneath these bands, and on serial sections, we have found trabecular recesses. However, in practically all hearts of what we call single ventricle, there are no distinct anterior and posterior descending coronary arteries meeting at the apex (Fig. 3) as in the normal heart and as in tricuspid atresia. This raises the issue as to the degree to which this chamber corresponds to the normal right ventricle. Thus, in single ventricle complex there is this difference in anatomy from most

cases of tricuspid atresia complex, with or without transposition.

In tricuspid atresia complex, with or without transposition, the left-sided ventricle is clearly identified as a morphologically left ventricle. However, there are abnormalities in the left ventricle in some hearts, such as a muscle bundle proceeding on the posterior wall from the central fibrous body towards the apex. In single ventricle complex, the main ventricular mass has two sinuses and a poorly defined outflow tract. It is questionable whether this should be called a morphologically left ventricle.

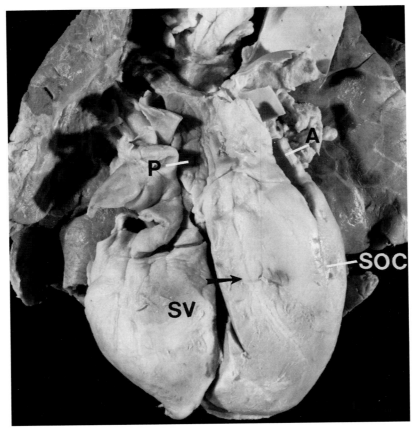

Figure 3: Single ventricle with small outlet chamber with inverted loop (L-) and inverted transposition. A = aorta; P = pulmonary trunk; SOC = small outlet chamber; SV = single ventricle. Arrow points to the right delimiting artery.

Atrioventricular Valves

In tricuspid atresia complex, the mitral valve is clearly identifiable as such, and most often shows little abnormality except hemodynamic change. In single ventricle, on the other hand, the two AV valves resemble each other, and it is difficult to decide which is tricuspid and which is mitral. Furthermore, the peripheral connections of the AV valves are quite different from the normal tricuspid or mitral valves.

Conduction System

In tricuspid atresia, the AV node is found more or less in the area adjacent to the tendon of Todaro and the bundle of His does not pass through the anulus of the efferent vessel but below it (Fig. 4). In single ventricle, on the other hand, there is an anterior conduction system. Here, the AV node is in the roof of the right atrium, unrelated to the tendon of Todaro, and the bundle in this entity passes through or just below the anulus of the efferent vessel anteriorly and superiorly (Fig. 5).

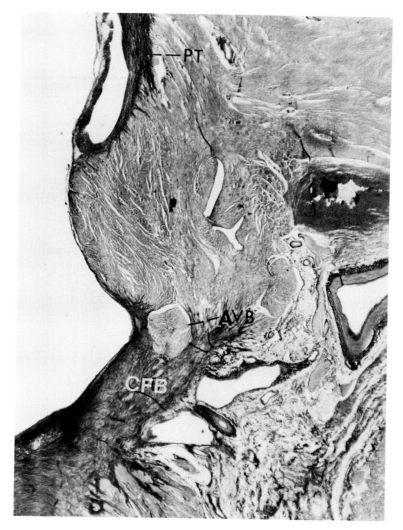

Figure 4: Photomicrograph of AV bundle in tricuspid atresia with regular complete transposition. Weigert-van Geison stain ×15. AVB = AV bundle; CFB = central fibrous body; PT = pulmonary trunk. (Figures 3 and 4 used with permission from Bharati S, Lev M: The concept of tricuspid atresia complex as distinct from that of the single ventricle complex. *Pediatr Cardiol* 1979, 1:57–62).

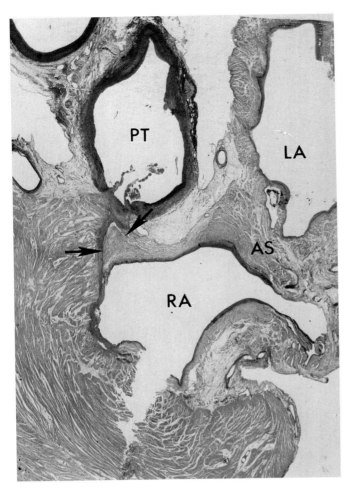

Figure 5: Roof of right atrium and accessory (anterior) AV node forming anterior AV bundle at pulmonic anulus in single ventricle with inverted loop and inverted transposition. Weigert-van Geison stain ×23. AS = atrial septum; LA = left atrium; PT = pulmonary trunk; RA = right atrium. Arrows point to anterior AV node in the roof of the right atrium beginning to form the penetrating AV bundle. (From Bharati S, Lev M: The course of the conduction system in single ventricle with inverted [L-] loop and inverted [L-] transposition. *Circulation* 51:723–730, 1975. By permission of the American Heart Association, Inc.)

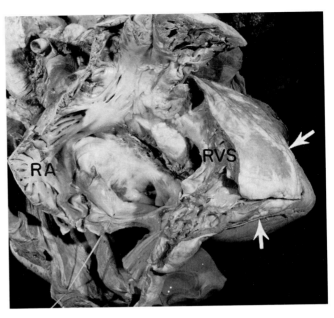

Figure 6: Right side of common AV orifice with common ventricle. RA = right atrium; RVS = right ventricular side of the septum; Arrows point to the anterior and posterior descending coronary arteries joined together at the apex. Note that the inlet as well as the infundibulum is markedly abbreviated.

complete absence of the posterior part of the ventricular septum; nevertheless, the anterior and posterior descending coronary arteries join together at the apex, thereby demarcating development of the posterior ventricular septum (Figs. 6, 7).

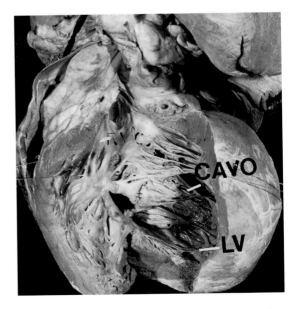

Figure 7: Common AV orifice with common ventricle as seen from the left side. LV = left ventricle; CAVO = common AV orifice. Note the large ventricular component to the common AV orifice.

Because of these morphological coronary arterial, AV valve, and conduction system differences, we consider tricuspid atresia complex and single ventricle complex as two distinct entities.

Common Ventricle Complex

In this entity, two AV orifices, or a common AV orifice, enter a main ventricular chamber, which gives rise to both efferent vessels. One efferent vessel is committed to each AV orifice anatomically, but there is almost

Univentricular Heart

There is, of course, nothing wrong in using the term "univentricular heart" instead of its synonym "single ventricle." However, the concept of univentricular heart should, in our opinion, be restricted to hearts in which two AV orifices open, or a common AV orifice opens into a single or a common ventricular chamber. This would therefore include both what we call single ventricle and what we call common ventricle. We would exclude tricuspid atresia complex from the concept of univentricular heart, single ventricle, or common ventricle.

Basic Philosophy in Congenital Heart Disease

We prefer a descriptive anatomic frame of reference in dealing with congenital heart disease, since the anatomy can be translated into, and is useful in, clinical medicine and surgery. We also prefer the prevailing usage of terms, even when the meaning inferred from derivation may differ from the prevailing meaning. It is important to understand that the meanings of words does evolve with time. Only when the prevailing usage has lost its practical value in communication does that usage need to be changed.

We also prefer to avoid embryology as a frame of reference in terminology. The normal embryogenesis of a part of the heart is often in dispute, and the pathological embryogenesis is in many cases either unknown or only speculative. Therefore, the two main frames of references in discussing the terms and concepts in congenital heart disease are descriptive anatomy and prevailing usage.

Furthermore, the genes responsible for these two entities are most likely unrelated and the answer to this question may be forthcoming through research at the molecular genetic level in the future.

67

Inverted Transposition with Left Atrioventricular Valve Atresia— Mixed Levocardia with Ventricular Inversion and Inverted Transposition with Left Atrioventricular Valve Atresia

In cases of tricuspid atresia with mixed levocardia, ventricular inversion, and inverted transposition, we are not sure as to differentiation between single (primitive) ventricle and mixed levocardia. Of course, if one defines single ventricle as that having two AV orifices, this would exclude tricuspid atresia. If one considered that single ventricle could be present along with tricuspid atresia, then a perusal of the ventricular mass in our cases did not differentiate between the two conditions. Evaluation of the coronary artery circulation, however, showed a long anterior descending coronary artery, an indication that a regular right and left ventricle were present (Fig. 1). We have therefore chosen to discuss this entity as tricuspid atresia with inverted loop and inverted transposition of the great arteries.

The Complex

In general, the aorta emerged anterior and to the left from the small right ventricle (Fig. 2), and the pulmonary trunk was situated to the right side of the aorta and posterior, and there was a long anterior descending coronary artery along the right side of the aorta. The right atrium emptied into a chamber resembling a morphologically left ventricle by means of a mitral valve (Fig. 3). Although architecturally there were anomalous muscle bundles in this chamber, the main ventricular mass in most cases resembled the

morphologically left ventricle, and from this chamber emerged the pulmonary trunk (Fig. 4). The small chamber fundamentally represented an abbreviated outlet or conus or infundibulum and a sinus component as well. Thus, one may consider the ventricular chambers as abnormally developed left and right ventricles. From the right ventricle emerged the aorta over a ventricular septal defect (Fig. 5). The left AV valve was absent (Fig. 6).

Analysis of Our Material

There was a total of 26 cases; 17 were male and 9 were female. The ages ranged from 11 hours to 7 years with a mean age of 7 months, 15 days.

Position of the Great Arteries

The aorta was to the left and anterior (Fig. 7) and the pulmonary trunk to the right and posterior in 17 cases, and in two cases the aorta was directly anterior to the pulmonary trunk (Fig. 8). In four cases they were side by side, the aorta to the left in three, to the right of the pulmonary trunk in one, and in three the aorta was right and posterior and the pulmonary trunk left and anterior (Fig. 9). In 22 cases there was left AV valve (tricuspid) atresia with inverted (L-) transposition. One could make out an altered left ventricular

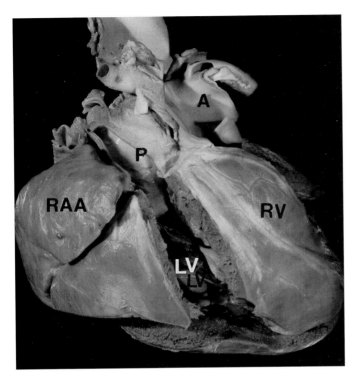

Figure 1: External view of mixed levocardia with left AV valve atresia. RAA = right atrial appendage; P = pulmonary trunk; LV = left ventricle; RV = right ventricle; A = aorta. Note double anterior descending coronary artery. (Used with permission from Lev M, Bharati S. See Figure 14.)

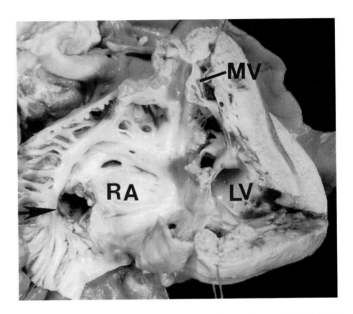

Figure 3: Right atrial, left ventricular view with Blalock-Hanlon procedure resulting in atrial septal defect. RA = right atrium; LV = left ventricle; MV = mitral valve. Arrow points to the defect created by Blalock-Hanlon procedure.

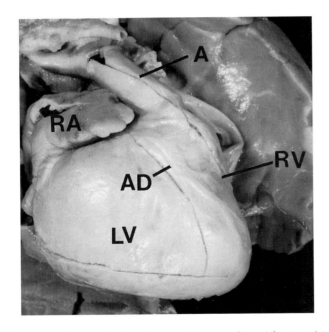

Figure 2: External view of mixed levocardia with ventricular inversion and left AV valve atresia. RA = right atrium; A = aorta, left and anterior; LV = left ventricle; AD = anterior descending coronary artery; RV = right ventricle. Note the pulmonary trunk to the right side of the aorta and posterior hidden by the right atrial appendage.

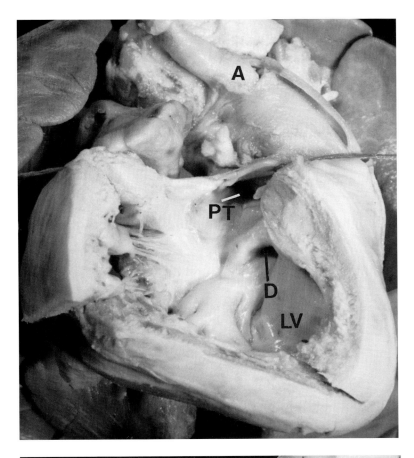

Figure 4: Left ventricular view demonstrating the pulmonary trunk emerging from the morphologically left ventricle. LV = left ventricle; PT = pulmonary trunk; D = defect; A = aorta.

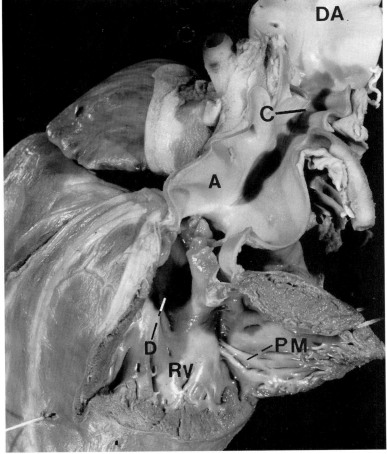

Figure 5: From the morphologically right ventricle emerges the aorta in a somewhat overriding manner over a U-shaped defect. RV = right ventricle; A = aorta; D = U-shaped defect; PM = papillary muscles; C = coarctation; DA = poststenotic dilatation with descending aorta. (Used with permission from Lev M, Bharati S. See Figure 14.)

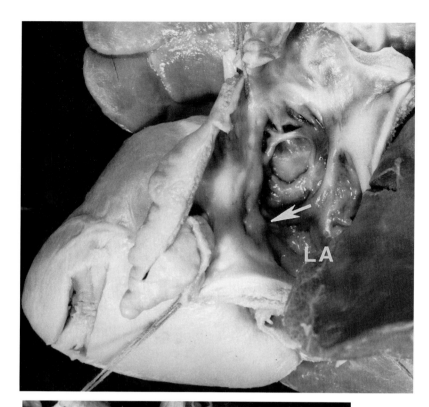

Figure 6: Left atrial view demonstrating the absent left AV valve. LA = left atrium. Arrow points to the atretic left AV valve.

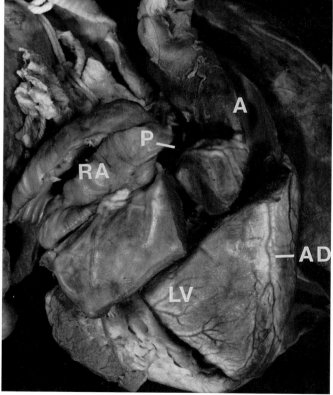

Figure 7: External view of mixed levocardia with ventricular inversion, left AV valve atresia, and pulmonary stenosis. Aorta anterior and to the left. RA = right atrium; LV = left ventricle; AD = anterior descending coronary artery; A = aorta; P = pulmonary trunk.

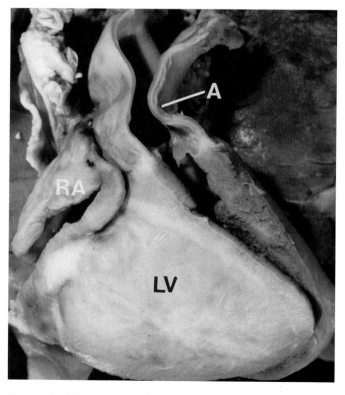

Figure 8: Mixed levocardia with left AV valve atresia and marked pulmonary stenosis with aorta anterior and pulmonary posterior. RA = right atrium; LV = left ventricle; A = aorta.

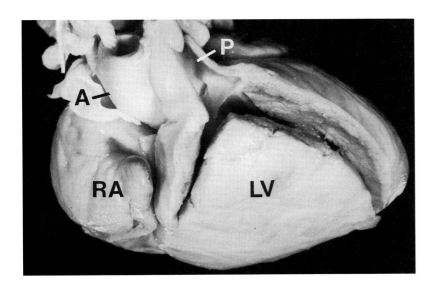

Figure 9: Mixed levocardia with left AV valve atresia with normally related great arteries. A = aorta to the right and posterior; P = pulmonary trunk to the left and anterior; RA = right atrium; LV = left ventricle.

(right-sided) chamber and a small right ventricular (left-sided) conus-like chamber.

The mitral orifice was always enlarged. The pulmonic orifice was atretic in three, was small and stenotic in 11 (markedly stenotic in two), and enlarged in 12. The aortic orifice was smaller than normal in eight cases, and enlarged or normal in size in the remainder. The mitral valve always had two groups of papillary muscles with the usual attachments, and demonstrated normal or increased hemodynamic change in the majority of the cases. In some, the valve presented distinct nodularity and thickening, markedly abbreviated chordae, and widely distributed papillary muscles (Figs. 10–12). The pulmonic valve was unicuspid and thickened in one, bicuspid and thickened in five, and in the remainder the valve was normal. The aortic valve was always normally formed.

The right atrium was hypertrophied and enlarged in all. The atrial septum was abnormally formed in many. The septum primum was redundant with an aneurysm

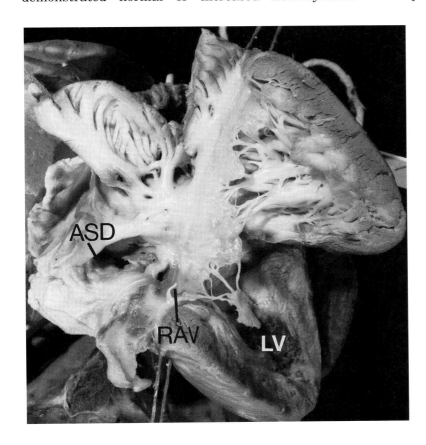

Figure 10: Right atrial, left ventricular view showing the mitral valve. ASD = atrial septal defect; RAV = right AV valve, mitral; LV = left ventricle.

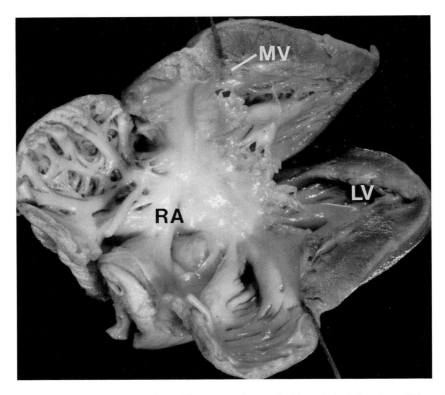

Figure 11: Widely distributed papillary muscles and abbreviated chordae of the mitral valve. Right atrial, left ventricular view. RA = right atrium; LV = left ventricle; MV = mitral valve.

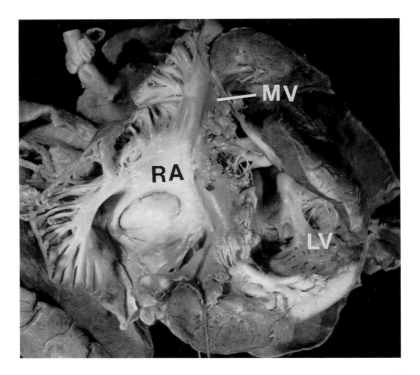

Figure 12: Right atrial, left ventricular view showing the thickening of the mitral valve. RA = right atrium; LV = left ventricle; MV = mitral valve. Note the marked thickening of the mitral valve with abbreviated chordae.

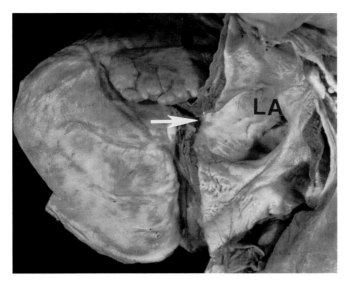

Figure 13: Left atrial hypertrophy in left AV valve atresia. LA = left atrium. Arrow points to the atresia of the left AV valve.

in the region of the fossa ovalis and an oblique foramen ovale, or the foramen ovale was small and patent.

The left atrium was hypertrophied in 50% (Fig. 13), and in the remainder it was normal or hypertrophied and enlarged (Fig. 14) or atrophic (Fig. 15). In general, there was a correlation between the size of the morphology of the left atrium and the morphology of the left and right ventricles when associated with

marked pulmonary stenosis and/or atresia. A small left atrium was associated with a straddling parietal band from the right ventricle which proceeded to the morphologically left ventricle through a small U-shaped ventricular septal defect, and the aorta was overriding to a varying degree. Thus, a small left atrium was associated with a hypoplastic right ventricle and abnormally formed left ventricle (Figs. 15–18).

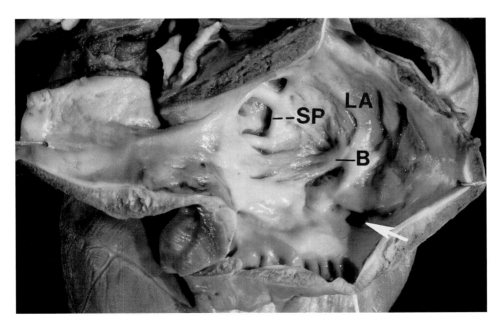

Figure 14: Left atrial hypertrophy and enlargement in atresia of the left AV valve. SP = septum primum; LA = left atrium; B = band in the left atrium. Arrow points to the atretic left AV valve. (Used with permission from Lev M, Bharati S: Transposition of arterial trunks in levocardia. In *Cardiovascular Pathology Decennial 1966–1975*, Ed. SC Sommers, Appleton-Century Crofts, NY, 1975, pp. 1–46.)

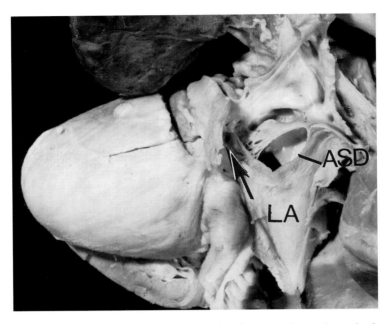

Figure 15: Atrophied left atrium in left AV valve atresia and marked pulmonary stenosis. ASD = atrial septal defect; LA = atrophied left atrium. Arrow points to the atretic left AV valve.

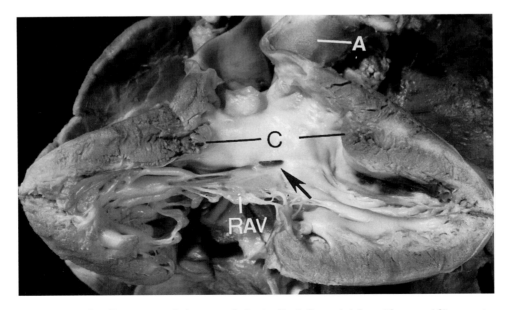

Figure 16: Outflow tract of the morphologically left ventricle with overriding aorta. RAV = right AV valve, mitral; A = aorta; LV = left ventricle. Arrow points to the stenotic pulmonic valve emerging with close relationship to the mitral valve. C demarcates the conus or the small infundibulum for the morphologically right ventricle which has been opened up to demonstrate the aorta emerging from the left and anterior over the infundibulum in an overriding manner.

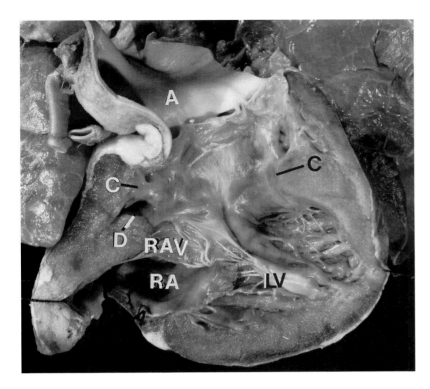

Figure 17: Mixed levocardia with ventricular inversion, left AV valve atresia, and pulmonary atresia and straddling conus. RA = right atrium; RAV = right AV valve, mitral; LV = left ventricle; C = conus or infundibular chamber; D = ventricular septal defect; A = aorta, anterior and to the left. Aorta is distinctly anterior due to pulmonary atresia.

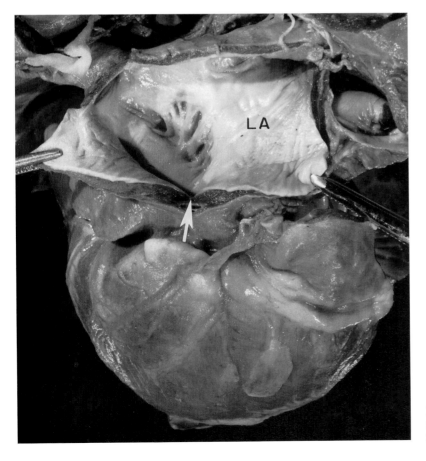

Figure 18: Small left atrium in left AV valve atresia and pulmonary atresia. LA = left atrium. Arrow points to atretic left AV valve.

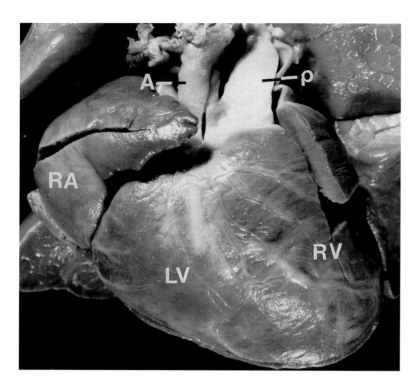

Figure 19: Mixed levocardia with isolated ventricular inversion and left AV valve atresia, and normally related great arteries. RA = right atrium; RV = right ventricle; LV = left ventricle; P = pulmonary trunk; A = aorta.

Isolated Ventricular Inversion and Normally Related Great Arteries

In three cases there was left AV valve atresia and ventricular inversion, but normal relationship of the arterial trunk (isolated ventricular inversion). In two hearts with isolated ventricular inversion and left AV valve atresia, the aorta emerged from the morphologically left ventricle, over a well-developed conus so that there was no aortic mitral continuity, and the pulmonary trunk from the morphologically right ventricle over a typical right ventricular conus (Figs.

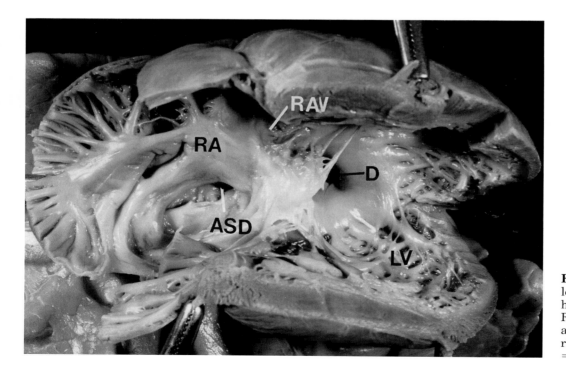

Figure 20: Right atrial, left ventricular view of heart shown in Figure 19. RA = right atrium; ASD = atrial septal defect; RAV = right AV valve, mitral; LV = left ventricle; D = defect.

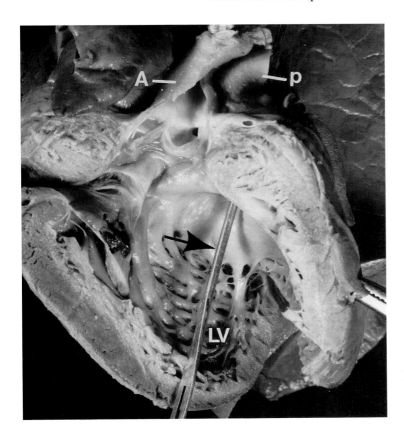

Figure 21: Aorta emerging from the morphologically altered left ventricle. A = aorta; P = pulmonary trunk; LV = left ventricle. Arrow points to the probe passing through the defect.

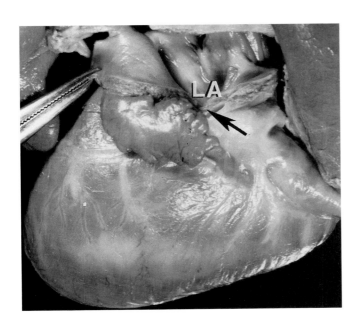

Figure 22: Left atrial view showing the atresia of the left AV valve. LA = left atrium. Arrow points to the atretic left AV valve.

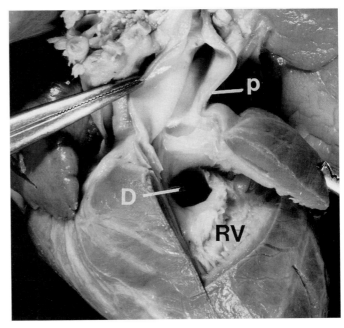

Figure 23: Outflow tract of the right ventricle from which emerges the pulmonary trunk. D = defect; P = pulmonary trunk; RV = right ventricle.

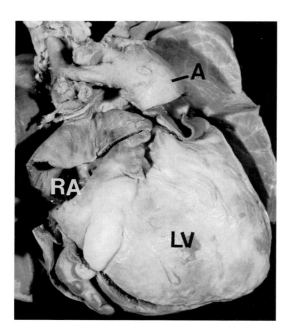

Figure 24: External view of mixed levocardia with ventricular inversion and left AV valve atresia. RA = right atrium; LV = left ventricle; A = aorta.

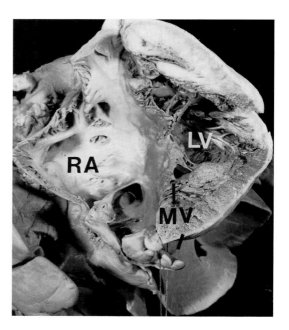

Figure 25: Right atrial, left ventricular view. RA = right atrium; LV = left ventricle; MV = mitral valve. Note the abbreviated chordae and thickening of the mitral valve.

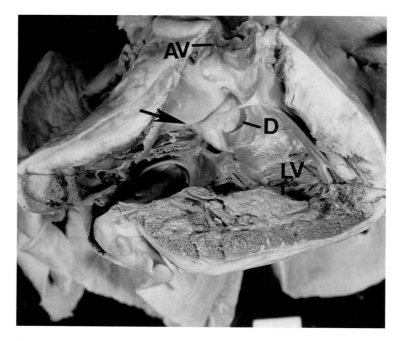

Figure 26: Aorta situated somewhat to the left but emerging from the abnormally formed left ventricle with aortic mitral noncontinuity. AV = aortic valve; LV = left ventricle; D = slit-like defect, as seen from the left ventricle, entering the morphologically right ventricle situated posterosuperiorly. Arrow points to aortic mitral noncontinuity. Note that the architecture of this chamber resembles, in part, the morphologically left ventricle and, in part, the morphologically right ventricle. The inlet is smooth; however, the outlet presents an abnormal conal band or muscle of Lancisi. In addition, there is a straddling muscle band suggesting a straddling conus. Thus, one may say that the inlet or the sinus of this chamber is that of a morphologically left ventricle, and the outlet favors more of that of the outflow tract of the right ventricle. Nevertheless, the aorta emerges from this chamber with aortic mitral noncontinuity.

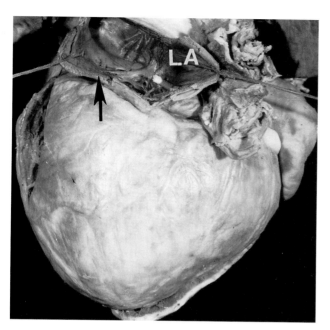

Figure 27: Left atrial view depicting the atresia of the left AV valve. LA = left atrium. Arrow points to the atretic left AV valve.

19–28). In one with isolated ventricular inversion and normally related great arteries, the pulmonary trunk straddled the septum coming from both ventricles (Figs. 29, 30).

In three other cases the aorta, although situated to the left and anterior, straddled over a U-shaped ventricular septal defect, coming from both ventricles. The defect was closing in one, small in five, and slit-like in three. The atrial septum in many presented a patent foramen ovale rather than an atrial septal defect. An abnormal formation of the limbic margin and the septum primum was seen in three.

The coronary circulation was examined in 15 of these cases. The anterior descending coronary artery came off the right-sided coronary artery and joined the vessel coming off the left-sided coronary artery, so that they demarcated off the septum between the two ventricular chambers. The associated cardiac anomalies are given in Table 1. The status of the spleen and extracardial abnormalities are given in Table 2.

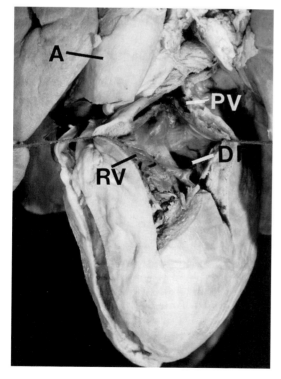

Figure 28: Posterosuperiorly located infundibulum or the outflow tract of the right ventricle. D = defect; RV = right ventricle; PV = thickened, stenotic bicuspid pulmonic valve; A = aorta. This heart may also be interpreted as being a superior-inferior or upstairs-downstairs heart, and despite the fact that the aorta is to the left and anterior, the aorta emerges from the morphologically (although altered) left ventricle, and the pulmonary trunk emerges from the posteriorly located altered right ventricular chamber.

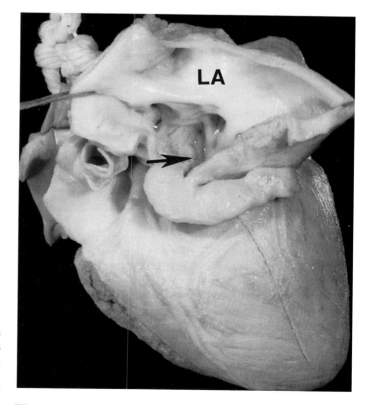

Figure 29: Left AV valve atresia in isolated ventricular inversion. LA = left atrium. Arrow points to the atretic left AV valve.

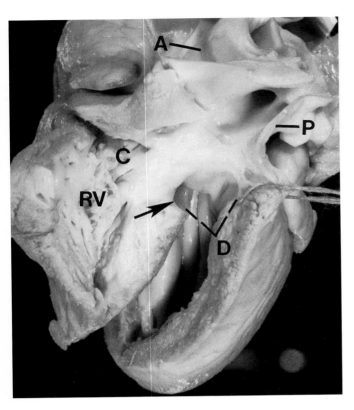

Figure 30: Pulmonary trunk emerging from the right ventricle over a U-shaped defect in an overriding manner. P = pulmonary trunk; A = aorta; C = conus; RV = right ventricle; D = U-shaped defect. Arrow points to the conus-like chamber leading to the aorta

Table 2

Extracardiac Abnormalities and Status of the Spleen in Mixed Levocardia with Left AV Valve Atresia in 18 Cases (Morphological Tricuspid)—all Cases Situs Solitus

Normal spleen with no extracardiac abnormalities—15
Normal spleen with multiple extracardiac abnormalities—1
No data available—2

Table 1

Associated Cardiac Abnormalities in Cases of Mixed Levocardia (Atria in Normal Position, Ventricles Inverted) with Left AV Valve Atresia (Morphological Tricuspid)

Aneurysm of fossa ovalis—5
Remnant of left valve of sinus venosus—1
Abnormal formation of atrial septum with oblique patent foramen ovale—3
Fossa ovalis defect—2 (1 atypical)
Left superior vena cava into coronary sinus—3
Mitral valve insufficiency—1
Mitral valve obstructing the VSD—1
Right aortic arch—2
Fetal coarctation with PDA—3
Adult coarctation—1
Interrupted aortic arch—1
Patent ductus arteriosus—5 (2 tortuous)
Upside down position of left atrium—1
Absent left atrial appendage—1
Double coronary ostia—1
Minute left coronary and large right coronary artery → RV fistula—1
TAPVD (LPV → CS and RPV → right atrium)—1

Comment

Although coarctation of the aorta and interrupted aortic arch occurs in this entity, the aortic valve is normally formed in all cases. It is also of interest that most cases are seen with normal spleen with no extracardiac abnormalities. All of these factors suggest that a palliative procedure such as a modified Fontan or a modified Norwood type of procedure may be entertained in some selected cases. The often encountered abnormal atrial septal morphology suggests abnormal hemodynamics at the atrial level during the second stage of development of the heart.

The genes that are probably involved in the normal development of the cardiac looping might have been affected during the second stage of the development of the heart, resulting in ventricular inversion. Thus, in a way, single ventricle with small outlet chamber with inverted loop and inverted transposition, mixed levocardia with ventricular inversion, and inverted transposition as well as these hearts with ventricular inversion and left AV valve atresia, may be considered as "related hearts genetically." In some, this in turn may affect the developing atrial septa as well.

68

Glycogen Storage Disease

General Statement

Pompe's disease is the infantile form of glycogen storage disease type IIa, in which there is deficient activity of the lysosomal enzyme, acid maltase, or α-1,4 glucosidase transmitted through a single recessive autosomal gene. This is a fatal disease and death is related to cardiac and/or respiratory failure.

In this disease, the heart is enlarged. The myocardium is filled with glycogen. There is usually hypertrophy, and in some cases, enlargement of all the chambers (Fig. 1). The myocardium is very pale. The thickness of the myocardium is relatively greater than the size of the chambers. There may be fibroelastosis in the left ventricle. A localized glycogen tumor was seen only once in this series (Fig. 1).

Analysis of Our Material

There were 12 cases of glycogen storage disease in our series: nine males and three females. The youngest was 1 day old and the oldest was 11 months. The average age was 3 months, 29 days.

The Complex

The apex was formed by the left ventricle in five and by both ventricles in seven. The right atrium was hypertrophied and enlarged in five, hypertrophied in six, and normal in one. The right ventricle was hypertrophied and enlarged in nine and hypertrophied in three. The left atrium was hypertrophied and enlarged in three, hypertrophied in eight, and normal in one. The left ventricle was hypertrophied and enlarged in six and hypertrophied in six.

The Valves

The tricuspid orifice was enlarged in one, normal in size in nine, and smaller than normal in two. The pulmonic orifice was normal in 10 and smaller than normal in two. The mitral orifice was normal in size in 11 and enlarged in one. The aortic orifice was normal in size in nine, smaller than normal in one, and enlarged in two.

The tricuspid valve was normal with normal hemodynamic change for the age of the child in four. It was normal with increased hemodynamic change in five. Mitralization was present in one case. The medial leaflet was connected to several papillary muscles in one case. In another, the medial leaflet was connected to a papillary muscle situated at the junction of the septal and inferior walls of the right ventricle. The pulmonic valve was, in general, normal or occasionally showed increased hemodynamic change. In one case, there was thickening at the base of the valve. The mitral valve was normal in four cases and presented increased hemodynamic change in six. In one case, the hemodynamic change was of the nodular type. In another case, an accessory curtain of tissue extended from the anterior leaflet to the pars membranacea. The aortic valve was normal or presented increased hemodynamic change. In one case, the valve was thickened at the base.

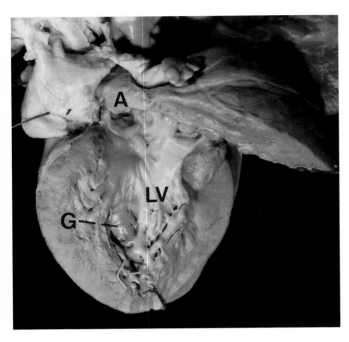

Figure 1: Glycogen storage disease. Left ventricular view. LV = left ventricle; G = glycogenic tumor; A = aorta.

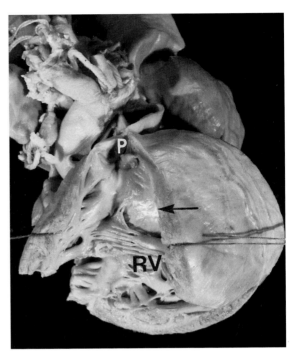

Figure 3: Right ventricular view showing the septal bulge. RV = right ventricle; P = pulmonary trunk. Arrow points to the septal bulge in the infundibulum

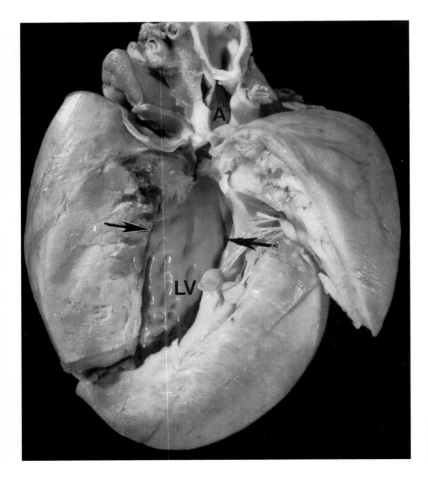

Figure 2: Left ventricular view demonstrating the marked septal hypertrophy. A = aorta; LV = left ventricle. Arrows point to the septal bulge.

The endocardium of all chambers showed either focal or diffuse thickening and whitening in all chambers.

Associated Cardiac Anomalies

Associated cardiac abnormalities were few. Either patent foramen ovale, high origin of coronary ostium, or abnormal architecture of the right and left ventricles were seen. In one case, there was a glycogen tumor-type mass in the left ventricle. In an 11-day-old male, there was tortuous patent ductus arteriosus.

A septal bulge was sometimes see in the left ventricle, either in the outflow tract or in the mid-region, or in both (Fig. 2). It is possible that in some the bulge may extend into the outflow tract of the right ventricle (Fig. 3). This may result in hemodynamically significant obstruction. If hypertrophy of the wall is considerable, this bulge may extend to the base of the anterior group of papillary muscles and may therefore cause abnormal movement of the anterior leaflet of the mitral valve (Fig. 2).

Conduction System

This revealed marked glycogen infiltration in the atria, atrial approaches to the AV node, the AV node, the AV bundle, and the bundle branches. The large cell size associated with glycogen deposition probably causes greater speed of conduction and manifests clinically as short P-R interval in the electrocardiogram in this entity.

Comment

Further research in the next century at the molecular genetic level may indeed provide new avenues in treating the deficient enzyme and thereby this fatal disease may be preventable in some.

69

Gargoylism

Gargoylism or Hurler's disease is a rare heritable disease of mucopolysaccharidoses (MPS-IH) metabolism (deficiency of the enzyme α-L-iduronidase) by way of an autosomal recessive or a sex-linked recessive trait. It affects both males and females with a slight preponderance in the male. The cardiovascular involvement in gargoylism is considered to be thickening of collagen fiber and increase of a MPS-containing large fibroblastic cells. The heart is usually hypertrophied and enlarged. The changes are predominantly seen in the mitral valve in the form of nodular thickening or aneurysmal dilatation of the leaflets with scalloped appearance (floppy) (Fig. 1), less frequently the tricuspid (Fig. 2), the aortic (Fig. 3), and pulmonic valves (Fig. 4) may show such change. The changes in the valve may give rise to mitral stenosis and/or insufficiency clinically. The chordae may also show thickening and may be abbreviated. This may be associated with some focal calcifications. There may be endocardial fibroelastosis of the left atrium and left ventricle. The coronary arteries may show narrowing. Histochemical technique and electron microscopy have differentiated two types of gargoyle cells: (1) classic clear cell containing a pure mucopolysaccharide and (2) a small, less frequently seen cell containing glycolipid. There may be vacuolization of the muscle fibers. Moderate to marked internal and medial thickening of the coronary arteries have been observed. A patent ductus arteriosus has been observed rarely with gargoylism.

Analysis of Our Material

There was a total of six cases: three males and three females. The youngest was 1 year old and the oldest was 13 years old with an average age of 5 years, 4 months, 24 days. The heart was hypertrophied and enlarged from a mild to a moderate degree and the apex was formed by the left ventricle. The right atrium was hypertrophied and enlarged in two and normal in four. The right ventricle was normal in three, hypertrophied and enlarged in two and hypertrophied in one. The left atrium was normal in three, hypertrophied in two, and enlarged in one. The left ventricle was hypertrophied in two, enlarged in two, normal in one, and small in one. The tricuspid and pulmonic orifices were normal in size except in two cases. In these, they were somewhat smaller than normal. The mitral valve was smaller than normal in two, enlarged in two, and somewhat smaller than normal in two. The aortic orifice was smaller than normal in two, enlarged in two, and normal in two.

The Valves

In general, all the valves were markedly thickened, irregular, or cartilaginous. These changes were especially prominent at the line of closure with or without aneurysmal formation. The thickness of the valve extended from the anulus to the edge (Figs. 5–12).

Endocardium

In general, focal or diffuse thickening and whitening were noted in all the chambers.

Associated Cardiac Abnormalities

In general, there were none. However, a 3-year, 11-month-old female had a large ductus arteriosus and she died suddenly. She also had sinus tachycardia and right ventricular hypertrophy. Two months before her death, she also demonstrated first-degree AV block on the electrocardiogram. Two others had patent foramen ovale.

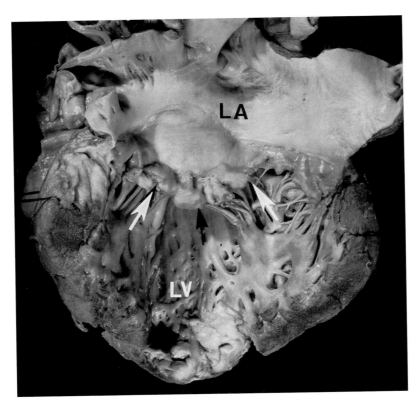

Figure 1: Marked thickening of the mitral valve especially affecting the line of closure to the edge, in the form of scalloping or ballooned-out appearance, with diffuse endocardial thickening of the left atrium and left ventricle. LA = left atrium; LV = left ventricle. Arrows point to the thickened mitral valve. (Used with permission from Okada R, et al. See Figure 5.)

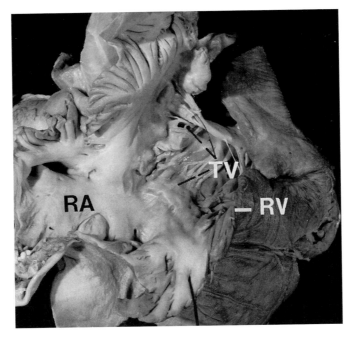

Figure 2: Marked thickening of the tricuspid valve. Right atrial, right ventricular view. RA = right atrium; RV = right ventricle; TV = tricuspid valve.

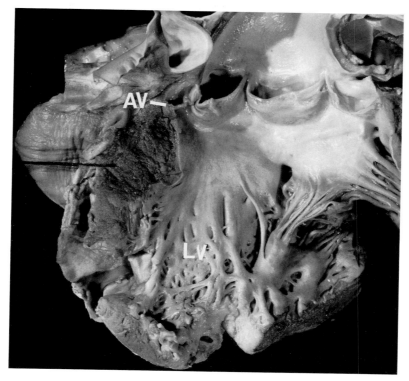

Figure 3: Left ventricular outflow tract showing a thickened aortic valve with fibroelastosis of the left ventricle. LV = left ventricle; AV = aortic valve.

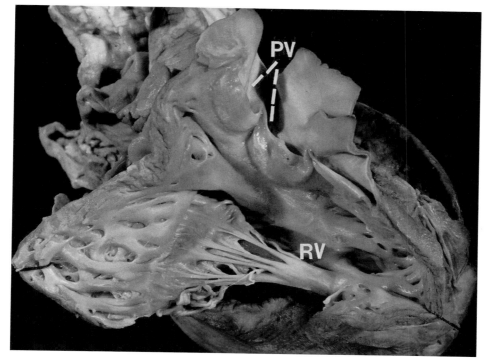

Figure 4: Thickening of the pulmonic valve. RV = right ventricle; PV = pulmonary valve.

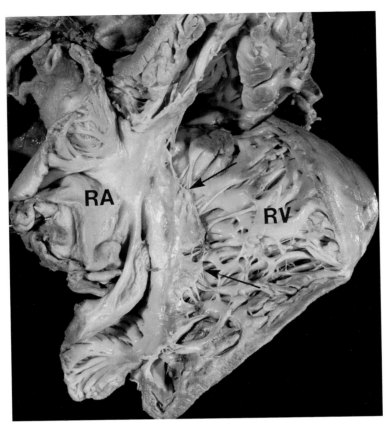

Figure 5: Tremendous enlargement of the right atrium and right ventricle with hypertrophy and diffuse endocardial thickening of the right atrium, right ventricle, and the tricuspid valve. RA = right atrium; RV = right ventricle. Arrows point to the thickened tricuspid valve. (Used with permission from Okada R, Rosenthal IM, Scaravelli G, Lev M. A histopathologic study of the heart in gargoylism. *AMA Arch Pathol* 1967, 84:20–30.)

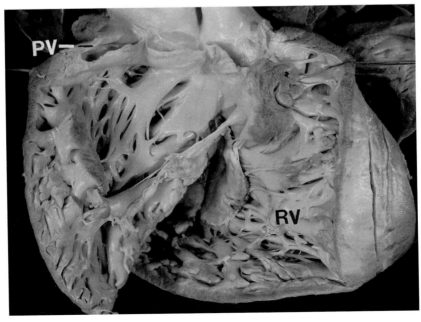

Figure 6: Thickened pulmonic valve with diffuse fibroelastosis of the right ventricle. RV = right ventricle; PV = pulmonary valve.

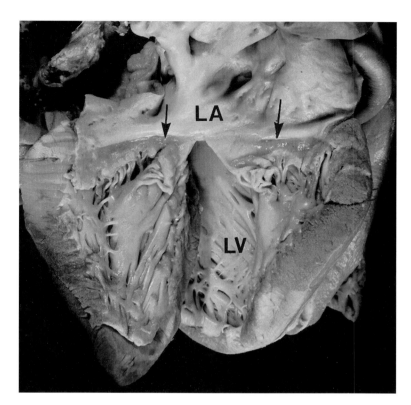

Figure 7: Marked thickening of the endocardium of the left atrium, left ventricle, and the mitral valve. LA = left atrium; LV = left ventricle. Arrows point to the thickened mitral valve.

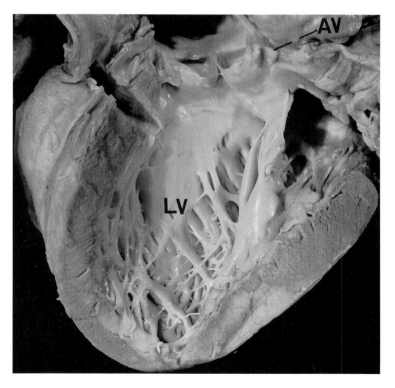

Figure 8: Diffuse fibroelastosis of the left ventricle with thickened aortic valve in the case with patent ductus arteriosus. LV = left ventricle; AV = aortic valve.

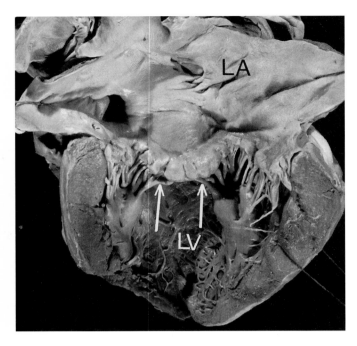

Figure 9: Hypertrophy and enlargement of the left atrium and the left ventricle with a markedly thickened mitral valve from a 13-year-old with gargoylism. LA = left atrium; LV = left ventricle. Arrows point to the markedly thickened mitral valve.

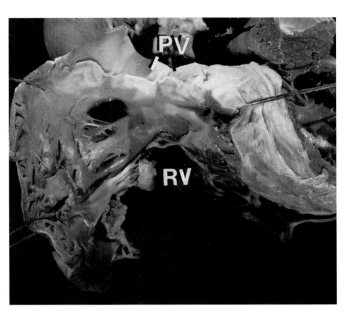

Figure 11: Pulmonic valve, same case as in Figures 9 and 10. Note the markedly thickened pulmonic valve. PV = pulmonary valve; RV = right ventricle.

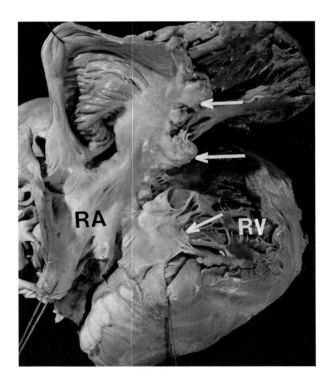

Figure 10: Marked thickening of the tricuspid valve with fibroelastosis of the hypertrophied and enlarged right atrium of the same case as shown in Figure 9. RA = right atrium; RV = right ventricle. Arrows point to the thickened tricuspid valve.

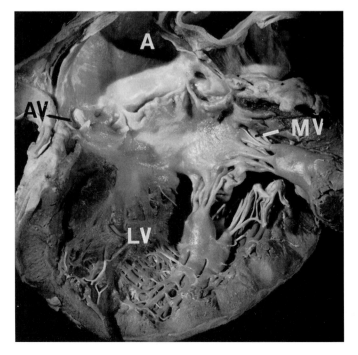

Figure 12: Markedly thickened aortic valve from the case as shown in Figures 9–11. LV = left ventricle; AV = aortic valve; A = aorta; MV = mitral valve. Note the tremendous irregular thickening of the aortic valve.

Conduction System Examination

The conduction system was studied in two cases and both revealed an increase in fibrous tissue in and around the bundle and bundle branches.

Central Fibrous Body and the Valves

The fundamental changes consisted of marked thickening of the valves and the endocardium due to thickening and hyalinization of the collagen fibers. These changes were accompanied by numerous mucopolysaccharide-containing large fibroblasts and an increase in ground substance in the interfibrillary spaces.

Comment

The fundamental pathological change in the heart in gargoylism is thickening of collagenous tissue with little effect on loose connective tissue.

Although there may be a wide range of heterogeneity in phenotypic expression of this disease, it is conceivable that at least in some this disease may be arrested, if not cured, at the genetic level in the future. Further research in the future may be directed toward preventing this disease if at all possible, at least in some.

70

Connective Tissue Dyscrasia– Marfan's Syndrome

Marfan's syndrome is a connective tissue disorder with characteristic features in the cardiac, skeletal, and ocular muscles. The disease is inherited as an autosomal dominant disorder with variable expressivity, causing marked variations in the affected individuals. It is important to emphasize that not all cases are inherited and that there are sporadic cases as well. We therefore include not only the classic cases of Marfan's syndrome diagnosed clinically, but also those cases resembling Marfan's syndrome with many or some of the characteristics, and with distinct involvement of the heart. The major cardiovascular manifestation includes aneurysmal dilatation of the ascending aorta, with aneurysmal dilatation of all the three sinuses of Valsalva to a varying degree, which may lead to rupture of the ascending aorta (Figs. 1–3) and sudden death. This is usually associated with aortic insufficiency (Fig. 4). There may be an association with redundant floppy mitral valve with mitral insufficiency (Fig. 5), aneurysm of the pulmonic sinuses of Valsalva with pulmonary insufficiency (Fig. 6), and in some cases with redundant tricuspid valve and tricuspid insufficiency (Fig. 7). The complex thus produced is one of enlargement of the heart associated with volume hypertrophy of the left atrium and left ventricle. If the tricuspid and pulmonic valves are equally affected, there is global hypertrophy of the heart (Fig. 8).

Analysis of Our Material

There was a total of 26 cases: 14 males and 12 females. The ages ranged from 9 months to 69 years with a mean of 27 years. Fifteen were below 30 years of age and six (23%) were below the age of 16.

The Complex

The heart was hypertrophied and enlarged in all (Figs. 9, 10) with extreme cardiomegaly (huge heart) in two cases. The apex was formed by the left ventricle in 69%, by both ventricles in 23%, and by the right ventricle in 8%. The right atrium was hypertrophied and enlarged in 62%, enlarged in 8%, normal in size in 15%, and hypertrophied in 15%. The huge aneurysm of the ascending aorta usually produced a bulge in the right atrial cavity. (Figs. 11, 12). The right ventricle was hypertrophied and enlarged in 81% (Fig. 13), enlarged in 8%, and normal in size in 11%. Where the aneurysm of the aorta was huge, it not only produced a bulge into the right atrium, but also into the right ventricular outflow tract beneath the pulmonary valve (Fig. 14). The left atrium was hypertrophied and enlarged in 69%, huge (gigantic aneurysm) in 15%, enlarged in 12%, and normal in size in 4%. The left ventricle was hypertrophied and enlarged in 85%, enlarged in 11%, and normal in size in 4% of the cases. The tricuspid orifice was enlarged in 62% and normal in size in 38%. The pulmonic orifice was enlarged in 81% and normal in size in 19%. The mitral orifice was enlarged in 77% and normal in size in 23%. The aortic orifice was enlarged in 77% and normal in size in 23%.

The Valves

Tricuspid Valve

This was normally formed in 30% of the cases. In 70%, the valve showed redundant and nodose leaflets with elongated chordae with numerous connections (Figs. 15–17). The chordae were quite thin and the pap-

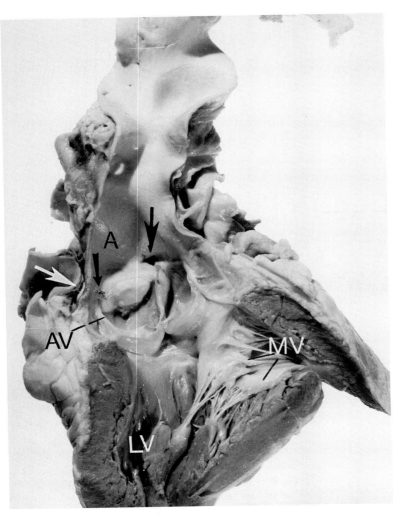

Figure 1: Marfan's syndrome in a young woman with aneurysm of three sinuses of Valsalva, aortic insufficiency, and aneurysm of the ascending aorta with rupture; left ventricular view. LV = left ventricle; MV = mitral valve; A = ascending aorta; AV = aortic sinuses of Valsalva aneurysmally dilated. Arrows point to the rupture. (Used with permission from Novell HA, et al. See Figure 40.)

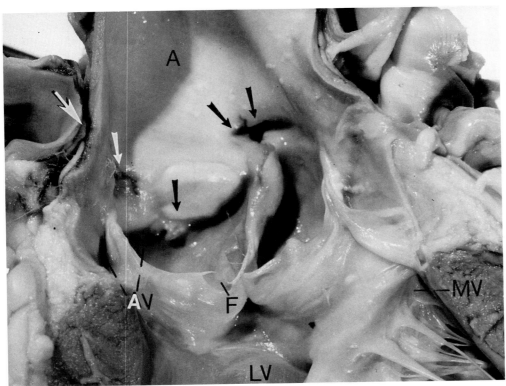

Figure 2: Close-up view of Figure 1 demonstrating the large aneurysm of the three sinuses of Valsalva with fenestration of the aortic valve and rupture. MV = mitral valve; LV = left ventricle; AV = aortic valve aneurysmally dilated; F = fenestration; A = ascending aorta. Arrows point to the rupture. (Used with permission from Novell HA, et al. See Figure 40.)

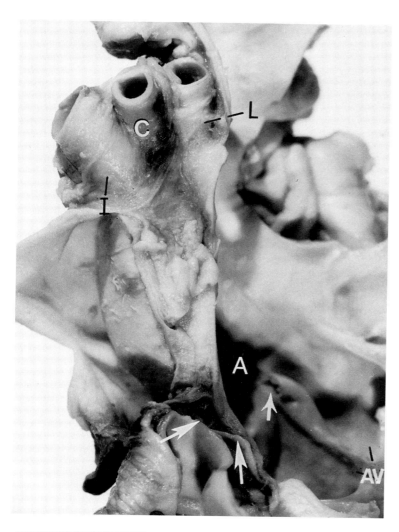

Figure 3: A close-up view of the ascending aorta demonstrating the rupture from Figures 1 and 2. A = ascending aorta; I = innominate; C = common carotid; L = left subclavian; AV = aneurysm of the sinuses of Valsalva distal. Arrows point to the tear in the transverse arch. (Used with permission from Novell HA, et al. See Figure 40.)

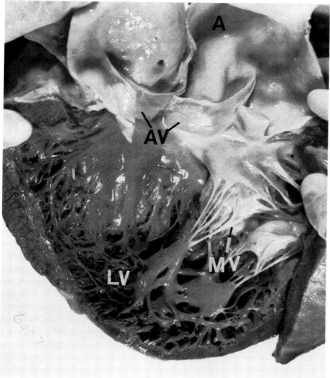

Figure 4: Left ventricular view demonstrating the huge aneurysm of the sinuses of Valsalva of the three aortic cusps with aneurysmal dilation of the ascending aorta, and marked aortic insufficiency. A = aneurysmal dilatation of the ascending aorta; AV = aortic sinuses of Valsalva aneurysmally dilated; LV = markedly enlarged left ventricle; MV = mitral valve.

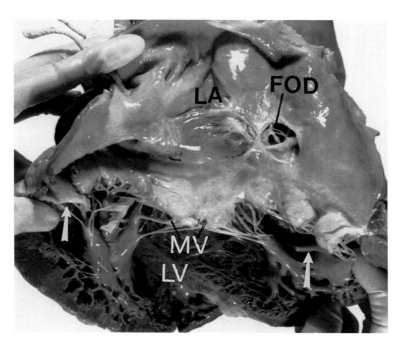

Figure 5: Marked redundancy of the mitral valve with an anular enlargement, and elongated chordae, with a large atrial septal defect; left atrial view. LA = markedly hypertrophied and enlarged left atrium; FOD = fossa ovalis defect somewhat extending posteriorly; MV = markedly redundant and thickened mitral valve; LV = left ventricle. Arrows point to the floppy posterior leaflet. Note the tremendous enlargement of the mitral valve with insufficiency that resulted in a huge left atrium and left ventricle.

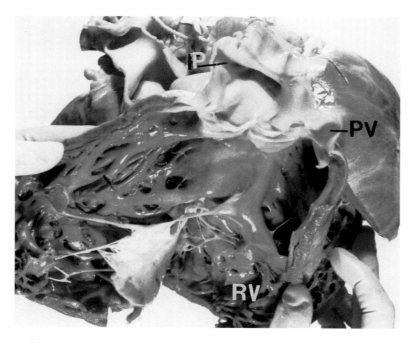

Figure 6: Right ventricular outflow tract demonstrating the aneurysm of the sinuses of Valsalva of the pulmonic valve cusps. RV = right ventricle; P = pulmonary trunk; PV = aneurysm of the sinuses of Valsalva of the pulmonic valve cusps with pulmonary insufficiency.

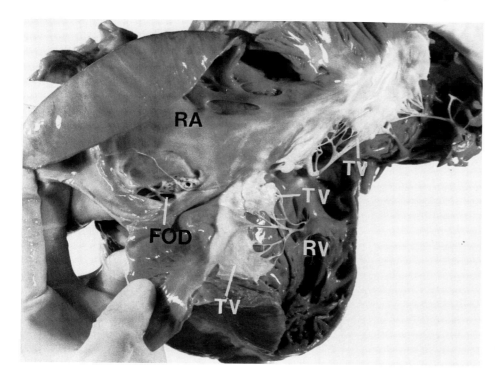

Figure 7: Marked redundancy of the tricuspid valve with tremendous tricuspid insufficiency with atrial septal defect of fossa ovalis type. RA = huge right atrium; FOD = fossa ovalis defect with marked fenestrations in the region of the fossa ovalis; TV = marked thickened redundant tricuspid valve; RV = right ventricle. Note the elongated chordae with considerable thickening.

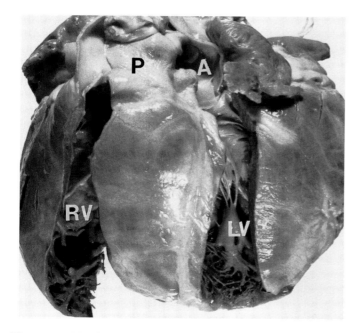

Figure 8: Marfan's syndrome with tremendous enlargement of the heart with aneurysm of the aortic sinus of Valsalva and floppy mitral and tricuspid valves with insufficiency of all the valves; external view of the heart. A = aorta; RV = right ventricle; LV = left ventricle; P = pulmonary trunk.

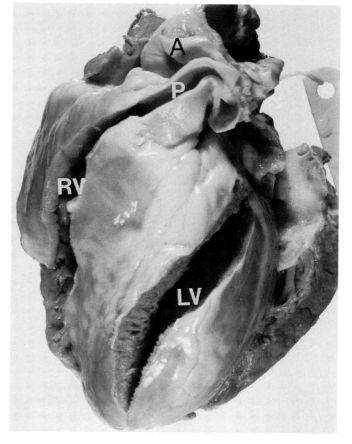

Figure 9: Marfan's syndrome with a hypertrophied and enlarged heart from a 15-year-old boy who died suddenly. A = aorta; P = pulmonary trunk; RV = right ventricle; LV = Left ventricle.

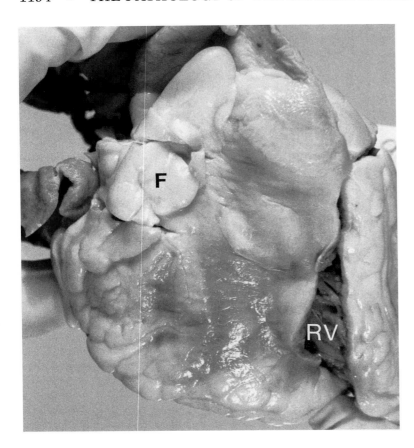

Figure 10: External view of a case of Marfan's syndrome in a 10-year-old boy. RV = right ventricle; F = fat in the right AV sulcus. Note the enlarged heart with marked fatty metamorphosis.

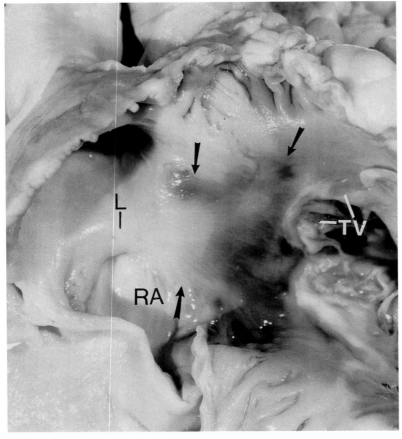

Figure 11: Right atrial view demonstrating the aneurysm of the ascending aorta creating a bulge into the right atrial cavity with hemorrhagic zones in the distal area. RA = right atrium; TV = thickened tricuspid valve; L = limbus fossae ovalis; Arrows point to the bulge with hemorrhagic zones.

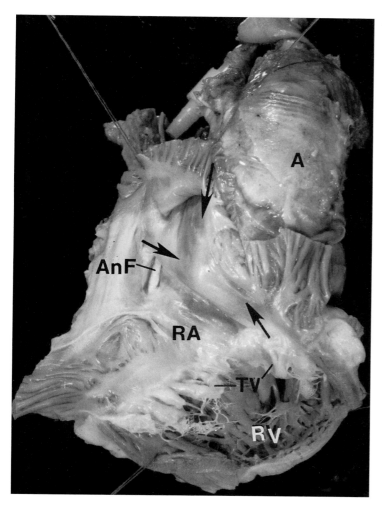

Figure 12: Right atrial, right ventricular view demonstrating the huge aneurysm of the ascending aorta pressing into the right atrial cavity. Note also the redundant tricuspid valve with enlarged orifice, accessory chordal connections and tricuspid insufficiency. RA = right atrium; AnF = aneurysm of the fossa ovalis; A = huge ascending aorta aneurysm; TV = markedly redundant tricuspid valve with anomalous chordae; RV = right ventricle. Arrows point to the bulge created by the aneurysm of the ascending aorta.

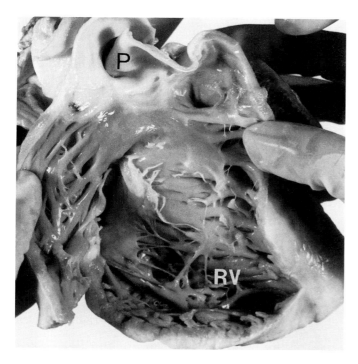

Figure 13: Hypertrophy and enlargement of the right ventricle. RV = right ventricle; P = pulmonary trunk.

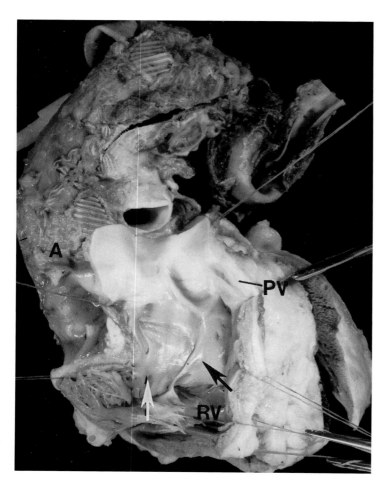

Figure 14: Right ventricular outflow tract demonstrating the ventricular septal bulge created by the aneurysm of the aorta beneath the pulmonary valve. Note also the mild aneurysm of the sinuses of Valsalva of the pulmonic valve cusps. RV = right ventricle; PV = pulmonic valve cusps with mild aneurysms; A = ascending aorta aneurysm with rupture with previous repair, Arrows point to the bulge.

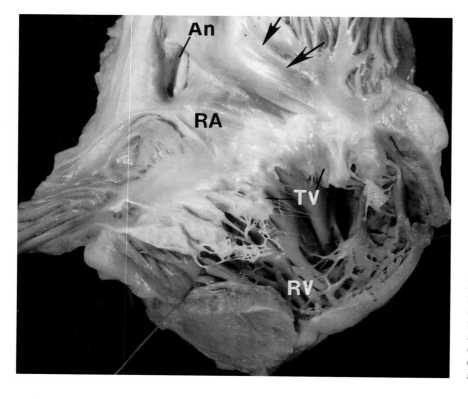

Figure 15: Redundant tricuspid valve with accessory connections as well as the aneurysmal bulge of the ascending aorta into the right atrial cavity. RA = right atrium; RV = right ventricle; TV = redundant tricuspid valve; An = small aneurysm of the fossa ovalis. Arrows point to the aneurysmal bulge of the ascending aorta.

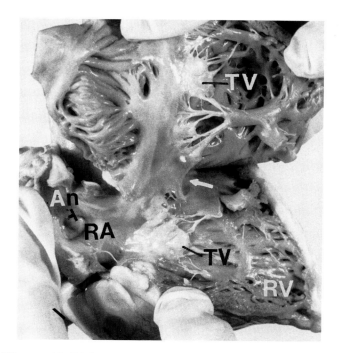

illary muscles were often hypoplastic, poorly developed, and fibrosed. There was a large aneurysm of the leaflets in two and an accessory tricuspid orifice was seen in four (15.3%) (Figs. 18, 19). In one case there were two accessory openings in the tricuspid valve. The papillary muscles revealed fibrosis in approximately 23%. In about 35% of the cases there were numerous, thin, elongated, chordal extensions of the valve. Tricuspid insufficiency was present in 35% of the cases. The intercalated leaflet between the anterior and septal or between the septal and inferior frequently were well developed (Figs. 15–17).

Figure 16: Right atrial, right ventricular view demonstrating redundancy of the tricuspid valve. Note the well-developed leaflet between the septal and anterior leaflets of the tricuspid valve with insufficiency and enlarged right-sided chambers. RA = right atrium; RV = right ventricle; An = small aneurysm of fossa ovalis; TV = tricuspid valve showing the redundant leaflets and thickened chordae. Arrow points to the well-developed intercalated leaflet between the anterior and septal leaflets.

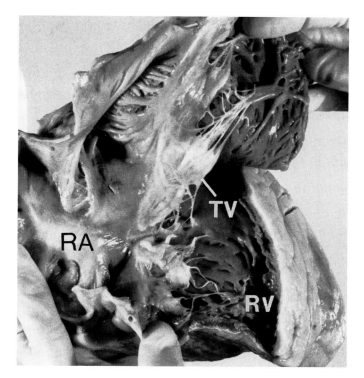

Figure 17: Redundant tricuspid valve and elongated chordae with tricuspid insufficiency. RA = right atrium; TV = tricuspid valve; RV = right ventricle. Note the bulge into the right atrium produced by the aneurysm of the aorta. Note, also, the small aneurysm of the fossa ovalis.

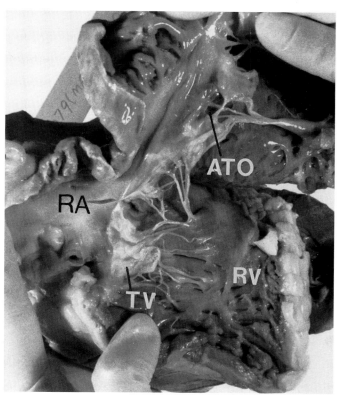

Figure 18: Redundant anterior leaflet of the tricuspid valve with large accessory opening. RA = right atrium; RV = right ventricle; TV = tricuspid valve; ATO = accessory tricuspid orifice.

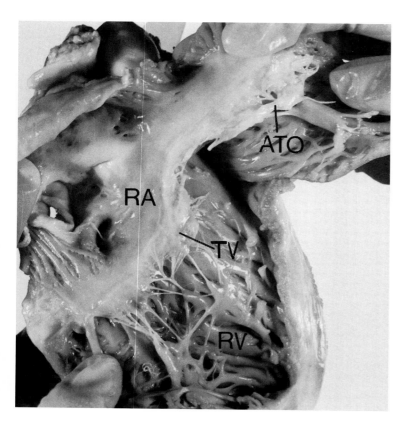

Figure 19: Accessory tricuspid orifice in a case of Marfan's syndrome. RA = right atrium; RV = right ventricle; TV = redundant, enlarged tricuspid valve; ATO = accessory tricuspid orifice. Note the volume enlargement of the right atrium and right ventricle.

Pulmonary Valve

This was normally formed in nine (34.6%). In 50% of the hearts examined, the sinuses of Valsalva of the valve were aneurysmally dilated to a varying degree. The aneurysmal dilatation was mild to moderate and occasionally it was severe. Distinct pulmonary insufficiency with associated aortic insufficiency and/or tricuspid insufficiency was present in five (Figs. 20, 21). Mild to marked fenestrations of the pulmonic valve were present in four (15.3%).

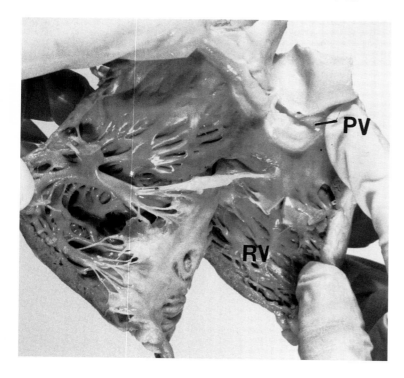

Figure 20: Right ventricular outflow tract demonstrating tremendous enlargement of the right ventricle and pulmonary insufficiency. PV = aneurysmal dilatation of the pulmonic sinuses of Valsalva with fenestration; RV = markedly enlarged right ventricle.

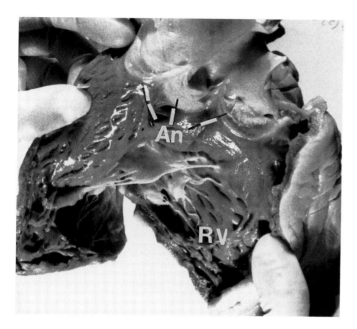

Figure 21: Right ventricular outflow tract demonstrating aneurysm of the sinus of Valsalva with pulmonary insufficiency. An = aneurysmal dilatation of the pulmonic sinus of Valsalva; RV = enlarged right ventricle.

Mitral Valve

This was normally formed in only one case. Thus, practically all of the hearts exhibited redundant leaflets affecting both the anterior and the posterior components to a varying degree. Although both leaflets showed considerable redundancy, ballooning, thickening, and nodularity in 18 (69.2%), either the anterior or the posterior leaflet was more affected (Figs. 22, 23). The ballooning and redundancy of the valve affected mostly the posterior leaflet in seven (Fig. 24). The chordae were usually elongated with numerous chordal extensions for both leaflets in most of the hearts (Figs. 25, 26). Rarely, the chordae were normal or relatively small (Fig. 27). There was significant mitral insufficiency in nine cases (34.6%). This was usually associated with aortic insufficiency and/or tricuspid insufficiency. Infective endocarditis of the mitral valve with significant mitral insufficiency was present in two cases. In one case, in addition, there was marked calcification of the mitral valve. The intercalated leaflets were well developed in many, resulting in quadricuspid mitral valve. In one case there was an accessory orifice (Fig. 28).

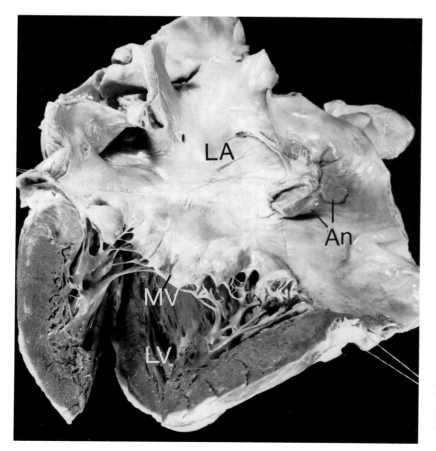

Figure 22: Floppy mitral valve with marked mitral insufficiency and a giant left atrium with aneurysm of the fossa ovalis (aneurysm of the septum primum). LA = giant left atrium; LV = left ventricle; MV = redundant mitral valve; An = aneurysm of septum primum. Note the giant left atrium with a markedly redundant mitral valve with well-developed intercalated leaflets and numerous chordal connections.

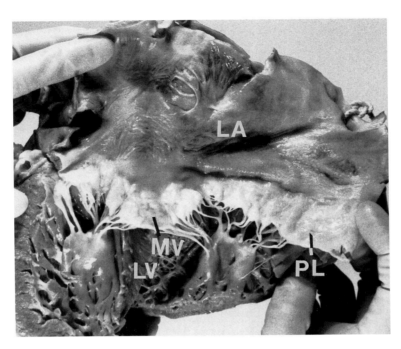

Figure 23: Markedly irregularly thickened and nodose mitral valve (floppy mitral valve) in a 45-year-old male with sudden death. LA = huge left atrium; PL = posterior leaflet; MV = mitral valve; LV = left ventricle. Note the redundant leaflets. Note also the fibrosis of the papillary muscle.

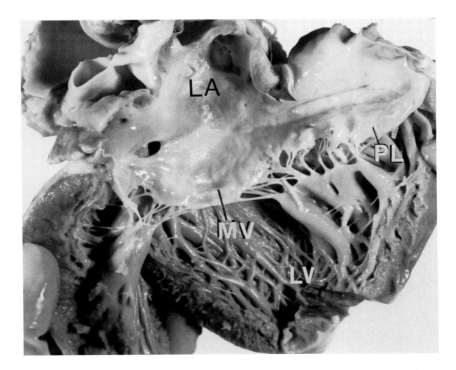

Figure 24: Sudden death in a 15-year-old female with floppy mitral valve affecting the posterior leaflet more than the anterior leaflet; left atrial, left ventricular view. LA = left atrium; LV = left ventricle; MV = mitral valve; PL = markedly redundant posterior leaflet.

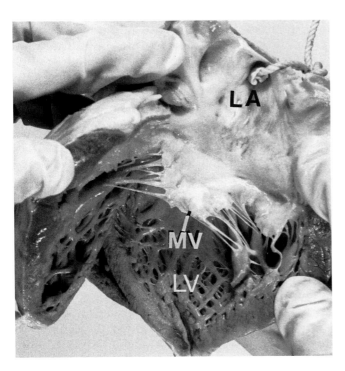

Figure 25: Left atrial, left ventricular view demonstrating a redundant mitral valve with elongated chordae and mitral insufficiency in a 10-year-old female with Marfan's syndrome. LA = hypertrophied and enlarged left atrium; LV = left ventricle; MV = redundant mitral valve with elongated chordae.

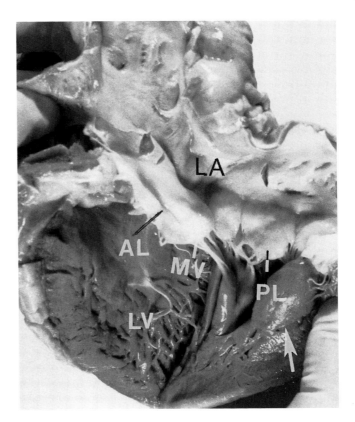

Figure 27: An 8-year-old female with a floppy mitral valve with relatively abbreviated or small chordae but markedly hypertrophied and enlarged papillary muscles; left atrial, left ventricular view. LA = left atrium; LV = left ventricle; MV = mitral valve; AL = anterior leaflet of the mitral valve; PL = posterior leaflet of the mitral valve. Arrow points to the markedly hypertrophied papillary muscle. Note the redundancy of the leaflet throughout the valve.

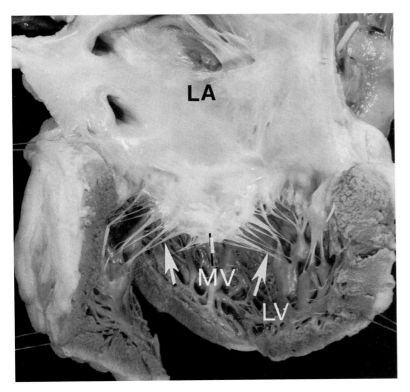

Figure 26: Enlarged mitral orifice with marked thickening and redundancy of the valve with elongated chordae and mitral insufficiency; left atrial, left ventricular view. LA = huge left atrium; MV = mitral valve; LV = left ventricle. Arrows point to the thickened mitral valve and elongated chordae. (Used with permission from Thilenius OG, et al. See Figure 35.)

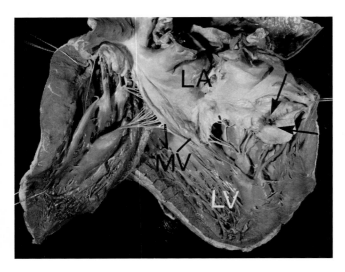

Figure 28: A case of Marfan's syndrome with accessory mitral orifice in the posterior leaflet with marked mitral insufficiency. LA = huge left atrium; LV = markedly hypertrophied and enlarged left ventricle; MV = redundant mitral valve. Arrows point to the accessory opening in the posterior leaflet. Note that the mitral valvular leaflet is markedly enlarged from the anulus to the edge with a huge opening in the posterior leaflet.

Aortic Valve

This was relatively normally formed in three (Fig. 29). However, either the valve was considerably thickened or showed increased hemodynamic change. Aneurysm of all three sinuses of Valsalva to a varying extent was present in 23 (Figs. 30–34). This was associated with aneurysm of the ascending aorta extending to the base of the brachiocephalic vessels to a varying extent (Fig. 35). There was aortic insufficiency clinically of a significant nature in 15 (57.7%). These cases were usually associated with tricuspid insufficiency, pulmonary insufficiency, and/or mitral insufficiency. Fenestrations of the aortic valve were frequently seen. The valve was bicuspid in two cases.

Dissecting aneurysm of the ascending aorta was present in 10. Marfan's syndrome was clinically diagnosed in 15 cases and in 11 others the diagnosis was made as forme fruste Marfan's syndrome.

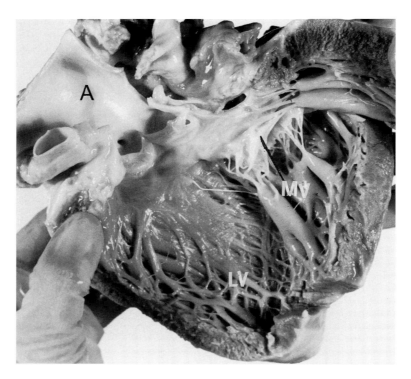

Figure 29: A more or less normally formed aortic valve in a 15-year-old boy. A = aorta; LV = left ventricle; MV = mitral valve.

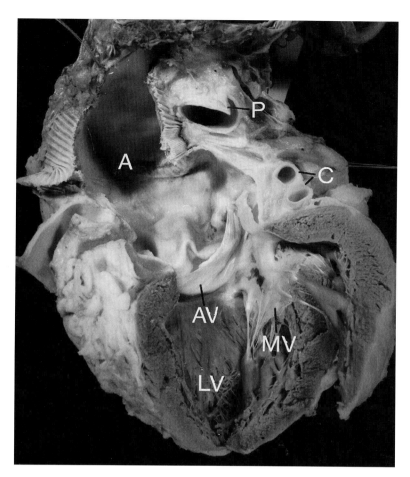

Figure 30: Left ventricular view demonstrating the aneurysm of the sinuses of Valsalva with aneurysmal dilatation of the ascending aorta, old surgery. MV = mitral valve; LV = left ventricle; AV = aneurysmal dilatation of the sinuses of Valsalva; C = aneurysmal dilatation of the coronary arteries; P = pulmonary trunk; A = ascending aorta aneurysm with previous surgery. (Used with permission from Thilenius OG, et al. See Figure 35.)

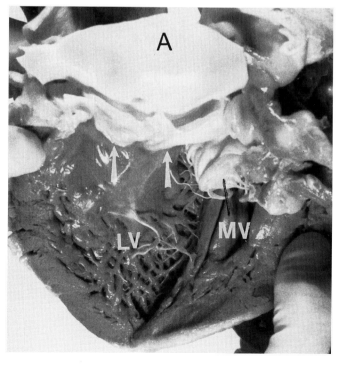

Figure 31: Aneurysm of sinus of Valsalva with floppy mitral valve. A = aorta; LV = left ventricle; MV = floppy mitral valve. Arrows point to the aortic sinus aneurysm.

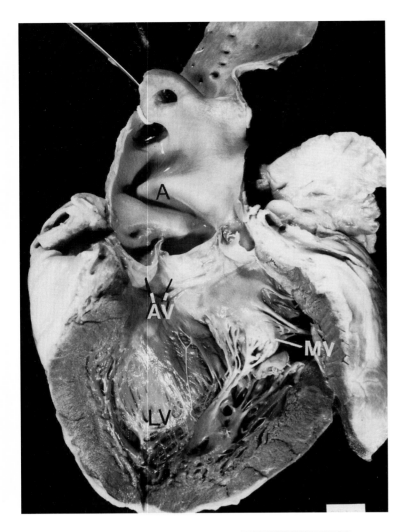

Figure 32: Marfan's syndrome with aneurysm of aortic sinus of Valsalva; left ventricular view. LV = left ventricle; MV = mitral valve; A = aorta; AV = aortic sinus of Valsalva aneurysm.

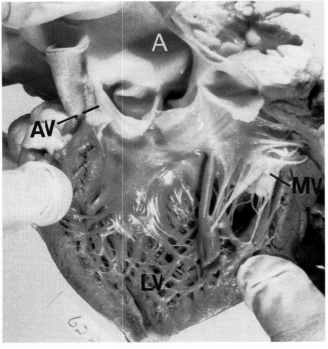

Figure 33: Left ventricular outflow tract demonstrating the aneurysm of the sinuses of Valsalva with aneurysmal dilatation of the ascending aorta. LV = left ventricle; A = ascending aorta; AV = aneurysmal dilatation of the aortic sinuses of Valsalva; MV = mitral valve. Note an accessory muscle proceeding from the inferior group of papillary muscles to the base of the mitral valve. Note the enlarged left ventricle as a result of aortic and mitral insufficiency.

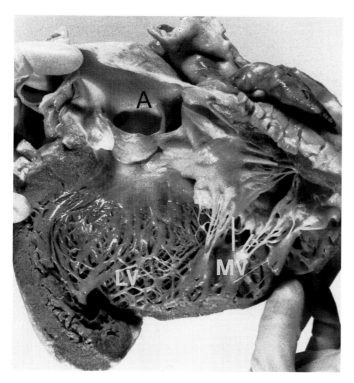

Figure 34: Aneurysm of the aortic sinus of Valsalva with floppy mitral valve. A = aorta; LV = left ventricle; MV = redundant mitral valve.

Coronary Artery Anomalies

	No. of Cases
Dominant left coronary arterial system with small right coronary artery	5
High origin of left coronary ostium	1
High origin of right coronary ostium	1
Right coronary ostium mildly narrowed	1
Right coronary ostium close to the posterior commissure	1
In part intramyocardial course of the anterior descending coronary artery	1
Both coronary arteries relatively small with left main coronary deeply intramuscular at its midportion, with origin of the left circumflex about 3 cm beneath the summit of the ventricular septum, and sudden death	1
Aneurysmal dilatation of all the three coronary arteries	1

Significant Cardiac and Other Anomalies

Coarctation of the aorta	2
Subendocardial infarct of the left ventricle	1
Abnormal band in the right atrium	1

Patent foramen ovale	3
Atrial septal defect, fossa ovalis type	1
Large atypical atrial septal defect extending from coronary sinus area to the inferior vena cava	1
Small left superior vena cava entering the coronary sinus	1
Aneurysm of the fossa ovalis	4

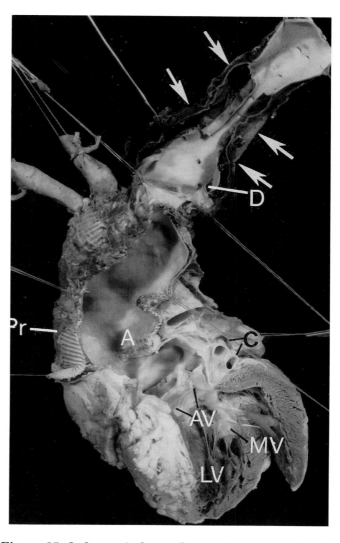

Figure 35: Left ventricular outflow tract demonstrating the huge aneurysm of the ascending aorta with previous rupture and repair, and recent rupture distal with the prosthetic material wrapped around the aorta proceeding up to the base of the brachiocephalic vessels. LV = left ventricle; MV = mitral valve; AV = aneurysm of the aortic sinuses of Valsalva; C = aneurysm of the coronary arteries; A = ascending aorta aneurysm; Pr = prosthetic material used previously for wrapping the ascending aorta up to the transverse arch; D = descending aorta. Arrows point to the rupture. (Used with permission from Thilenius OG, Bharati S, Arcilla RA, Lev M: Cardiac pathology of Marfan's Syndrome: Can dissection and rupture of aortic aneurysms be prevented? *Cardiology* 1980, 65:193–204.)

Fenestrated eustachian valve	2
Strands in the septum primum	1
Marked fatty metamorphosis of the right ventricle	1
Aneurysmal dilatation of the innominate and left common carotid artery	1
Lupus erythematosus (clinically diagnosed)	1
Rupture of the ascending aorta into right atrium with fistulous connection into the right ventricle	1
Thrombosis at the entry at the superior vena cava	1
Surgically induced ventricular septal defect	1
Intractable tachycardia in an identical twin with large membranous septum and sudden death	1
Aneurysm of the membranous septum with sudden death	2
Sudden death	2
Heart block with atypical hypertrophic cardiomyopathy, displaced coronary sinus in central fibrous body, aneurysm of space of His, and cataract with sudden death	1
Sudden death due to recurrent dissection 2 years following wrapping for dissecting aneurysm of the aorta	1
Dissecting aortic aneurysm 11 days postpartum in a young woman with sudden death	1

Types of Valvular Insufficiency

	No. of Cases
Aortic insufficiency	7
Aortic and mitral insufficiency	3
Mitral insufficiency	3
Aortic, mitral, tricuspid and pulmonary insufficiency	2
Mitral and tricuspid insufficiency	1
Aortic, tricuspid and pulmonary insufficiency	3
Tricuspid and pulmonary insufficiency	2

Microscopic Examination

The elastic fibers showed zones of complete disruption with disorganized muscle cells (Fig. 36). There were areas of ground substance that engulfed necrotic muscle cells which were markedly basophilic (Figs. 37–39). The elastic tissue in these areas were not markedly altered.

There was a focal increase in acid mucopolysaccharide. The fibrosa of the mitral valve was elongated and thinned-out with an increase in mucopolysaccharide. The aortic valve cusps were thinned-out and elon-

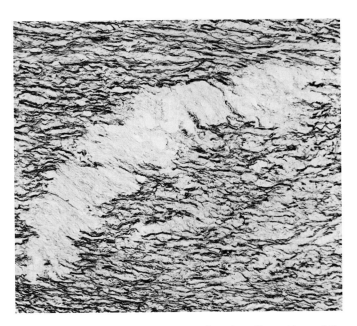

Figure 36: Section of the aorta, showing disruption of the elastic lamella. Weigert-van Gieson stain ×91. (Used with permission from Novell HA, et al. See Figure 40.)

gated, involving the fibrosa as well as the spongiosa. They showed fibrinoid necrosis. There was an increase in spongiosa and fibrosa of the tricuspid valve with disruption of the fibrosa due to increases in mucopolysaccharide and focal fibrinoid necrosis. The chordae showed an increase in mucopolysaccharide. The fibrosa and the anulus of the pulmonic valve revealed loosening of its structures.

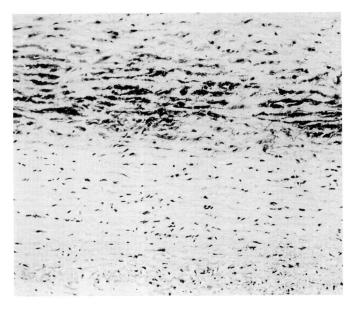

Figure 37: Section of the aorta, showing degenerating muscle cells in the media lying in a sea of ground substance. Hematoxylin-eosin stain ×91. (Used with permission from Novell HA, et al. See Figure 40.)

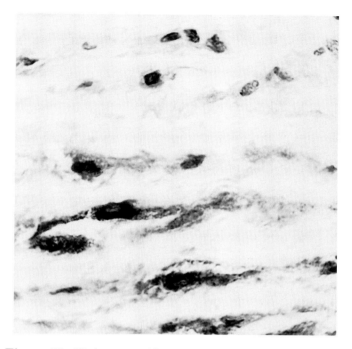

Figure 38: Higher magnification of Figure 37 in the region of the altered muscle cells. Hematoxylin-eosin stain ×520. (Used with permission from Novell HA, et al. See Figure 40.)

Figure 39: Section of the aorta showing markedly increased ground substance in media and to a lesser extent intima, staining positively for acid mucopolysaccharides. Rinehart-Abul Haj stain for mucopolysaccharides ×91. (Used with permission from Novell HA, et al. See Figure 40.)

Comment

Our material presents an increase in the incidence of abnormalities in the aortic mitral, tricuspid, and pulmonic valves in cases of Marfan's syndrome. In addition, we emphasize the variation in morphology of all the valves with significant insufficiency in various combinations (80.7%). Likewise, there is a higher incidence of sudden death in our material (30.7%). On the other hand, coarctation of the aorta (Fig. 40), atrial septal defect (Fig. 7), and bicuspid aortic valve occurred infrequently. It is of interest that both small (hypoplastic)

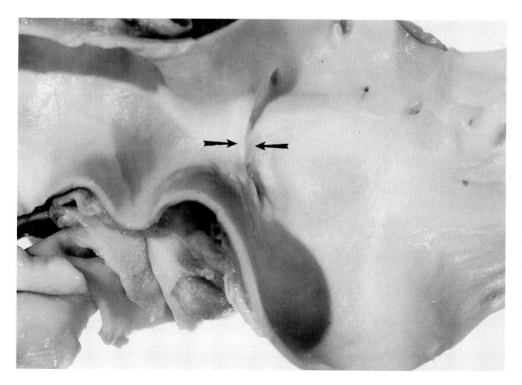

Figure 40: View of the coarctation of the aorta with the dilatation of the aorta distally. Arrows point to the coarctation. Note the poststenotic dilatation of the descending aorta. (Used with permission from Novell HA, Asher LA Jr, Lev M: Marfan's syndrome associated with pregnancy. *Am J Obstet Gynecol* 1958, 75:802–812.)

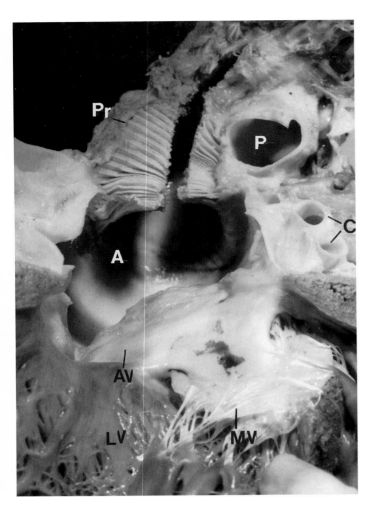

Figure 41: A close-up view of the base of the aortic valve showing the aneurysm of coronary arteries. LV = left ventricle; MV = mitral valve; C = aneurysm of the coronary arteries; AV = aneurysmal dilatation of the aortic sinus of Valsalva; A = aneurysm of the ascending aorta; Pr = prosthetic material wrapped around the aorta for old tear; P = pulmonary trunk.

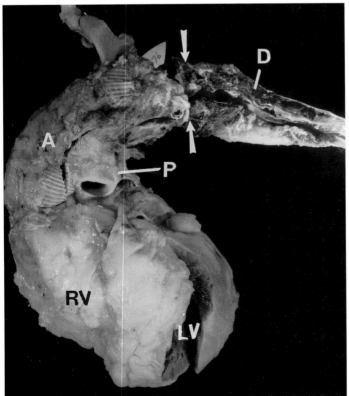

Figure 42: Marfan's syndrome in a 10-year-old boy. Old dissecting aneurysm of the ascending aorta with surgical intervention with recent dissecting aneurysm of the thoracic aorta; external view of the heart. RV = right ventricle; LV = left ventricle; P = pulmonary trunk; A = ascending aorta; D = descending aorta. Arrows point to the ruptured area distal to the previous surgery. Note the hypertrophied and enlarged heart.

coronary arteries and aneurysm of coronary arteries (Fig. 41) were seen in this entity.

The heart was always hypertrophied and enlarged in all cases. This was quite dramatic, especially in the young (Fig. 42). In two, the heart was immense, weighing more than 1,000 grams. In one postoperative heart, where the dissecting aortic aneurysm was wrapped by a Dacron sleeve, there was a recurrence of dissection of the aorta with rupture distal to the sleeve (Fig. 43).

We have included those cases which we consider to be forme fruste Marfan's syndrome where patients exhibited characteristics of Marfan's syndrome but this was not diagnosed clinically. We believe the disease may be quite variable although predominantly affecting the aortic sinuses of Valsalva and the ascending aorta. However, it does affect the entire heart. Although the entire heart is affected to a varying degree pathologically, we are unable to detect the functional abnormality of the valves and the heart clinically due to the limitations in the technologies available today. As technology develops, we will be able to appreciate the abnormal function of the valves and the heart in the future.

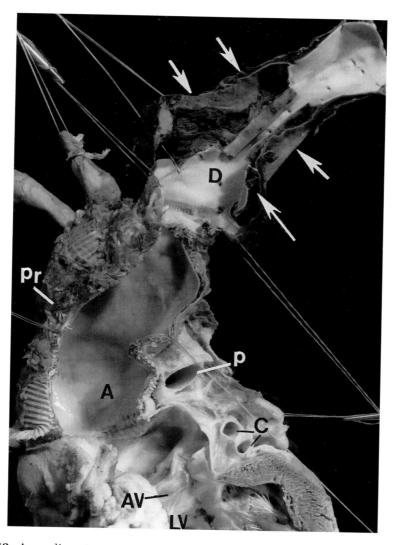

Figure 43: Ascending, transverse, and descending aorta demonstrating the recent tear distal to the previous surgery. LV = left ventricle; C = aneurysmal dilatation of the coronary artery; AV = aneurysmal dilatation of the aortic sinuses of Valsalva; A = ascending aorta aneurysm previously ruptured with old surgery; Pr = prosthetic material wrapped around the ascending aorta up to the transverse arch; D = descending aorta. Arrows indicate the tear in the descending aorta distal to the previous surgery.

Marfan's Syndrome and Its Relationship to the Conduction System

It is not surprising to find various types of arrhythmias, either tachycardias or heart block in this entity, since we are basically dealing with a connective tissue disorder. There is a greater amount of connective tissue throughout the conduction system when compared with the surrounding myocardium. This includes the elastic component which we believe is the most important constituent of the conduction tissue. Likewise, the occurrence of lupus with Marfan's syndrome in our material is not a surprising finding. However, it is emphasized that different types of connective tissue components may be affected in various combinations and may manifest as different disease entities.

Marfan's Syndrome and Fibrillin Genes

Abnormalities in fibrillin metabolism have been identified recently in Marfan's and forme fruste Marfan's syndrome. The gene FBNI, located on chromosome band 15q 21.1, codes for fibrillin, the 350-kd protein which is the main component of extracellular microfibrils. This is considered the locus for mutations that cause variations in connective tissue disorders. Thus, the future will unravel innumerable types of fibrillin disorders expressing innumerable anomalies in all or some of the valves, the aorta, the coronary arteries, the conduction system, and the myocardium to a varying degree (from mild to moderate) in innumerable combinations.

We should also keep in mind that the possibility of one genetic disorder combining with other types of genetic disorders may result in a yet to be created new disorder with its variations!

Research at the molecular-genetic and biochemical level in the next century may unfold the heterogeneous group of fibrillin disorders and their relationship to the clinical manifestation of the disease. Although there may be an intragenetic heterogeneity, future research in this field may shed some light as to the possibility of preventing the fatal types, at least in some.

71

Congenital Polyvalvular Disease

There is a group of hearts that appears to fall into this complex which we call polyvalvular disease. In this disease, the mitral (Fig. 1), the tricuspid (Fig. 2), and the pulmonic valves (Fig. 3), and less frequently the aortic valve (Fig. 4), show remarkably irregular thickening, and redundancy with nodulation involving the base, the anulus, the body of the leaflet, the line of closure, and the edge of the valve. The changes may be marked, moderate, or mild, affecting the various leaflets and cusps. In addition, the chordae and the papillary muscles reveal abnormalities to a varying degree. Thus, in a sense the entire valvular apparatus is affected to a varying degree. This frequently results in mild or moderate-to-severe tricuspid stenosis or insufficiency, pulmonary valvular and infundibular stenosis or insufficiency, mitral insufficiency and/or stenosis, and aortic stenosis or insufficiency. There may also be subaortic obstruction. The aortic and pulmonic valves may be bicuspid. These findings are often associated with atrial septal defect, patent ductus arteriosus, or ventricular septal defect (Figs. 1–4).

Microscopic examination of the valves when compared to normal valves and hemodynamically altered valves of a similar age group reveals that all of the valves are involved in a dysplastic process (Fig. 5). This consists of an increase in spongiosa with vacuolar and lacunar degeneration, and a distinct lack of elastic tissue in the proximalis and in the spongiosa (Figs. 6–9) with an increase in acid mucopolysaccharide content (Fig. 10). The architecture of the valve is thus disrupted with no demarcation between the spongiosa and fibrosa layers. The dysplastic process is similar to but more marked than that seen in a case of single dysplastic valve as in bicuspid aortic valve (Figs. 11, 12). The changes are totally different from that seen in hemodynamic changes (Fig. 13). Clinically, these cases are often associated with trisomy 18 or trisomy 13–15

and multiple extracardiac anomalies, and are called congenital polyvalvular disease. The disease may bear some relationship to connective tissue disorders such as Marfan's syndrome and the isolated cases of floppy mitral or tricuspid valves, or may occur without any relationship to connective tissue disorders or chromosomal abnormalities.

There is usually global hypertrophy of the heart. It is self-evident that the hypertrophy and enlargement of the heart depends on the severity of the functional stenosis and/or insufficiency of the valves as well as the hemodynamics of the shunts at the atrial, ventricular, or ductal level.

Analysis of Our Material

There was a total of 101 cases: 59 females and 42 males. The ages ranged from 24 weeks' gestation stillborn to 42 years, with a mean of 2½ years.

The Complex

The heart was hypertrophied and enlarged in all. The apex was formed by the left ventricle in 40% (Fig. 14), by both ventricles in 32% (Fig. 15), and by the right ventricle in 28%. The right atrium was hypertrophied and enlarged in 91%, was normal in size in 6%, and hypertrophied in 3% of the cases. The right ventricle was hypertrophied and enlarged in 74%, hypertrophied in 25%, and normal in size in 1%. The left atrium was hypertrophied and enlarged in 54%, normal in size in 22%, enlarged in 9%, hypertrophied in 6%, atrophied in 5%, and smaller than normal in 4%. The left ventricle was hypertrophied and enlarged in 52%, hypertrophied in 17%, enlarged in 2%, smaller than normal in 15%, normal in size in 5%, and atrophied in 9% of the cases.

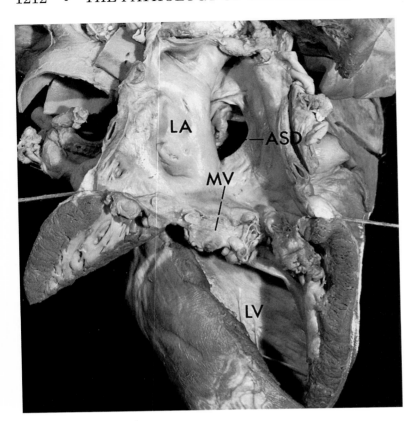

Figure 1: Gross appearance of valves in congenital polyvalvular disease in a case of ASD, VSD, tricuspid, pulmonary, mitral, and aortic stenosis (3 years, 4 months old). Left atrial, left ventricular view showing the redundant mitral valve. LA = left atrium; LV = left ventricle; ASD = atrial septal defect; MV = redundant mitral valve. (Used with permission from Bharati S. See Figure 13.)

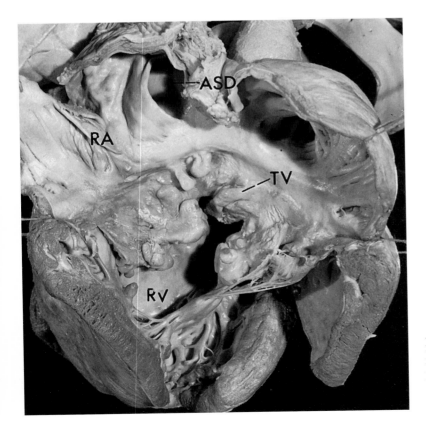

Figure 2: Right atrial, right ventricular view of Figure 1. Note the redundant tricuspid valvular leaflets. ASD = atrial septal defect, fossa ovalis type; RA = right atrium; TV = tricuspid valve; RV = right ventricle. (Used with permission from Bharati S. See Figure 13.)

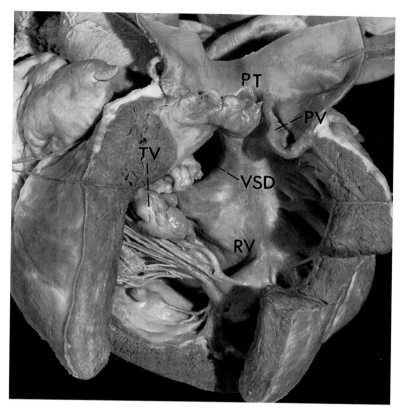

Figure 3: Outflow tract of right ventricle from Figure 2 demonstrating the redundant pulmonary valve. TV = redundant tricuspid valve; RV = right ventricle; VSD = ventricular septal defect; PV = redundant pulmonic valve; PT = pulmonary trunk. (Used with permission from Bharati S. See Figure 13.)

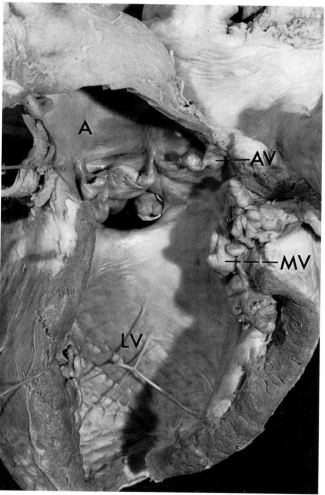

Figure 4: Left ventricular outflow tract view of Figures 1, 2, and 3 demonstrating the U-shaped defect and overriding aorta, with redundant mitral and aortic valves. LV = left ventricle; AV = aortic valve; MV = redundant mitral valve; A = aorta overriding the U-shaped defect. (Used with permission from Bharati S. See Figure 13.)

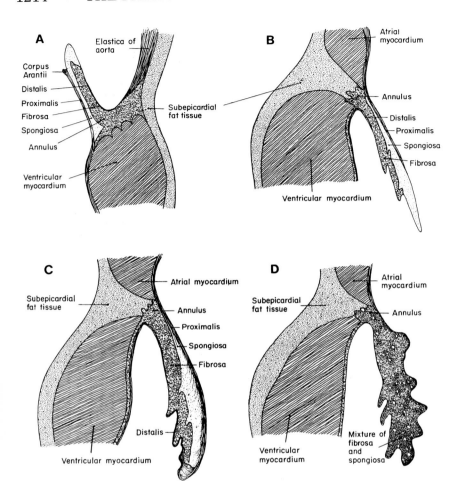

Figure 5: Diagrammatic sketches of (**A**) normal semilunar valve after Gross and Kugel, (**B**) normal atrioventricular valve, (**C**) atrioventricular valve altered by hemodynamic change (increase flow and pressure), (**D**) atrioventricular valve in polyvalvular disease. (Used with permission from Bharati S. See Figure 13.)

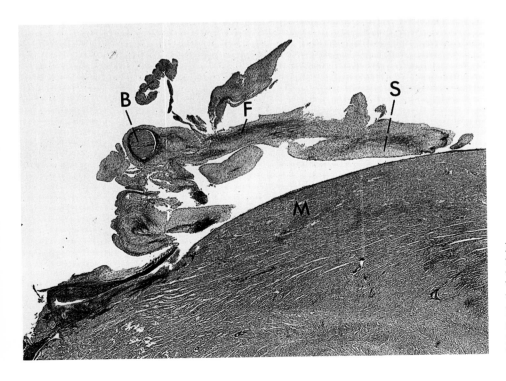

Figure 6: Microscopic appearance of tricuspid valve in congenital polyvalvular disease from a case of ASD, VSD, and PDA complex (41 days old). Weigert-van Gieson stain ×17. F = fibrosa; S = spongiosa; M = myocardium; B = blood cyst. (Used with permission from Bharati S. See Figure 13.)

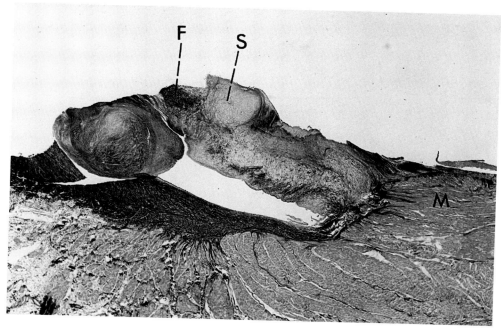

Figure 7: Pulmonic valve in a case of pulmonary, tricuspid, and mitral stenosis, 3 years old. Weigert-van Gieson stain ×15. F = fibrosa; S = spongiosa; M = myocardium. (Used with permission from Bharati S. See Figure 13.)

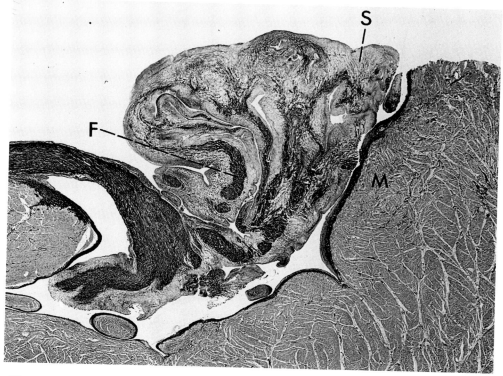

Figure 8: Mitral valve in a case of ASD, VSD, tricuspid, pulmonic, mitral, and aortic stenosis, 3 years, 4 months old. Weigert-van Gieson stain ×15. F = fibrosa; S = spongiosa; M = myocardium. (Used with permission from Bharati S. See Figure 13.)

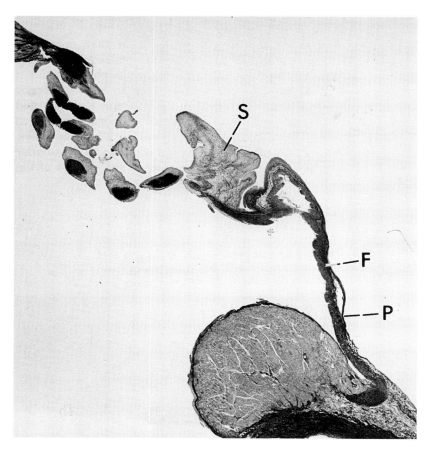

Figure 13: Hemodynamically altered tricuspid valve in a case of VSD and PDA complex, 7 weeks old. Weigert-van Gieson stain ×12. P = proximalis; F = fibrosa; S = spongiosa. (Used with permission from Bharati S, Lev M: Congenital polyvalvular disease. *Circulation* 1973, 47: 575–586.)

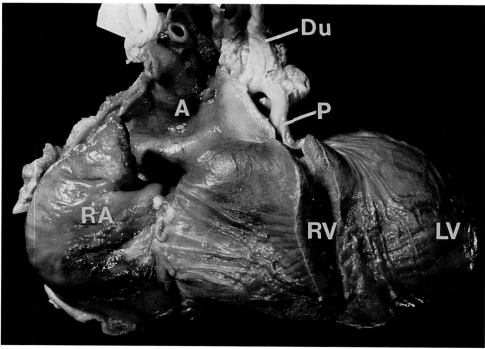

Figure 14: External view of the heart from a case of obstruction and shunt. Note the huge heart with the bifid apex, but nevertheless the apex is formed by the left ventricle, from an 18-day-old infant. RA = tremendously hypertrophied and enlarged right atrium; RV = right ventricle; A = aorta; LV = left ventricle; P = pulmonary trunk; Du = ductus arteriosus.

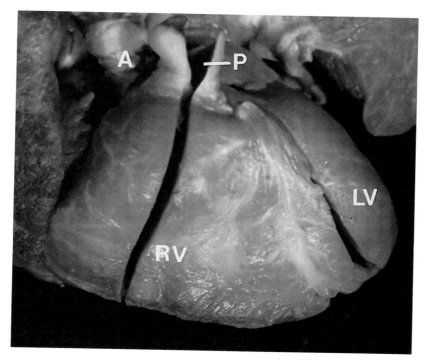

Figure 15: Hypertrophied and enlarged heart in a case of obstruction with shunt, external view. Note that the apex is mildly bifid and formed by both ventricles. RV = right ventricle; LV = left ventricle; P = pulmonary trunk; A = aorta.

Tricuspid Valve

This showed remarkable changes in all hearts to a varying degree. The valvular tissue was considerably redundant, nodose, and thickened in an irregular fashion throughout. The redundancy and nodularity of the valvular substance resulted in the leaflets not being differentiated into three distinct segments (Figs. 16–20). In more than 50% of the hearts examined, the valvular tissue was represented by a sheet or a mass of fleshy tissue with bizarre connections (Fig. 21). In some, the leaflets were quite large, forming aneurysmal dilatation (Fig. 22), which occasionally caused obstruction to the outflow tract into the pulmonary trunk. In approximately 18% of the cases, the chordae were markedly elongated and thinned-out, and the papillary muscles, especially the anterolateral papillary muscle, were poorly developed (Fig. 23). On the other hand, in about 30% of the cases, the chordae were markedly abbreviated (Figs. 17, 19, 24, 25) and thickened, and the papillary muscles were either poorly formed or abbreviated or quite short. Some proceeded directly to the valvular structure and some of them proceeded to the undersurface of the base of the valve. In about 12% of the cases, blood cysts were found. In one, there was an accessory orifice. Rarely, the valve was thickened and irregular from mild to a moderate degree (Fig. 26).

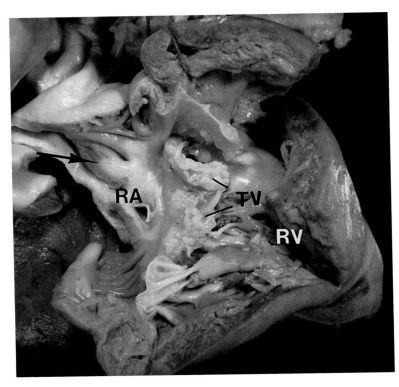

Figure 16: Another example of multiple shunts demonstrating the dysplastic nature of the tricuspid valve. Right atrial, right ventricular view. RA = right atrium; RV = right ventricle; TV = dysplastic thickened tricuspid valve. Arrow points to the aneurysm in the fossa ovalis.

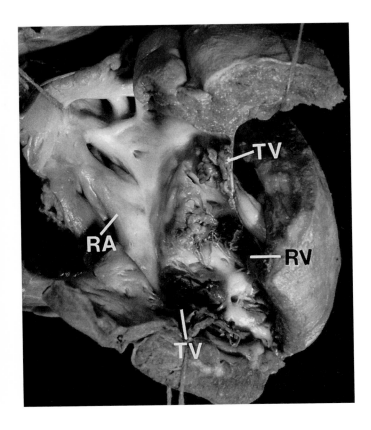

Figure 17: Markedly redundant nodular tricuspid valve with markedly abbreviated chordae. Right atrial, right ventricular view. RA = right atrium; RV = right ventricle; TV = redundant tricuspid valve with abbreviated chordae.

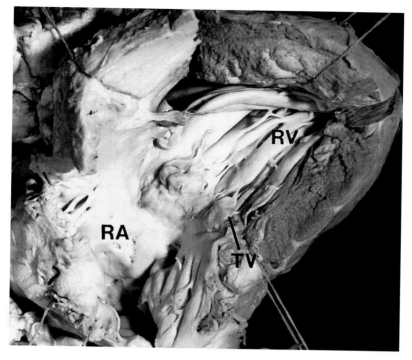

Figure 18: Markedly redundant tricuspid valve with tricuspid stenosis. RA = right atrium; RV = right ventricle; TV = redundant tricuspid valve.

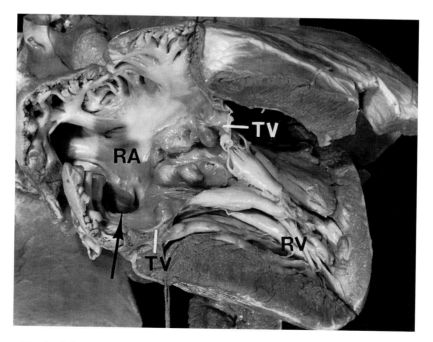

Figure 19: Atrial septal defect at the entry of the inferior vena cava with straddling inferior vena cava – sinus venosus type of atrial septal defect with redundant tricuspid valve with tricuspid stenosis. RA = right atrium; TV = redundant tricuspid valvular tissue with abbreviated chordae; RV = hypertrophied right ventricle. Arrow points to the straddling inferior vena cava through the defect.

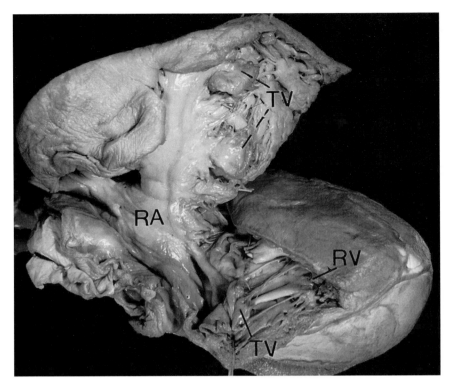

Figure 20: Undifferentiated tricuspid valve ballooned out into several segments. RA = right atrium; RV = right ventricle; TV = tricuspid valve.

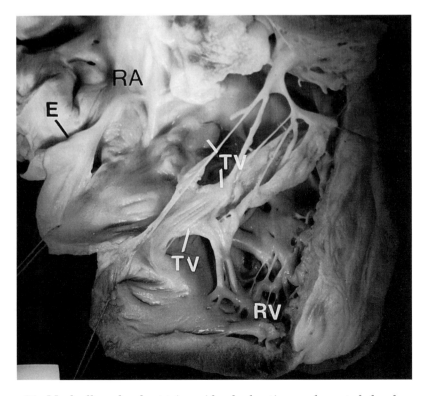

Figure 21: Markedly redundant tricuspid valvular tissue, elongated chordae, and hypoplastic papillary muscles with bizarre connections and tricuspid insufficiency. RA = right atrium; E = hypertrophied and enlarged eustachian valve; TV = redundant tricuspid valve; RV = right ventricle.

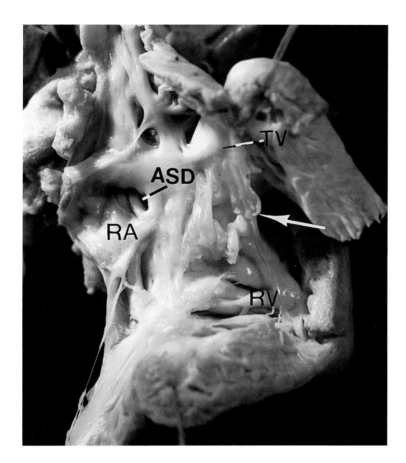

Figure 22: Right atrial, right ventricular view showing the tricuspid valve. RA = right atrium; RV = right ventricle; TV = redundant tricuspid valve; ASD = atrial septal defect of fossa ovalis type. Arrow points to the aneurysm of the tricuspid valvular tissue.

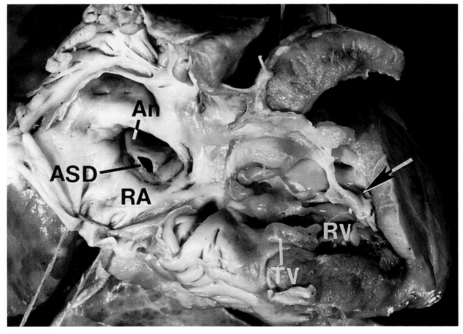

Figure 23: Markedly redundant tricuspid valve with small anulus and hypoplastic papillary muscles with marked tricuspid stenosis and atrial defect. Right atrial, right ventricular view. RA = right atrium; ASD = atrial septal defect of fossa ovalis type; An = aneurysm of the fossa ovalis; TV = redundant tricuspid valve; RV = small right ventricle with thick wall. Arrow points to hypoplastic papillary muscle. Note the small anulus and almost absent chordae and papillary muscles.

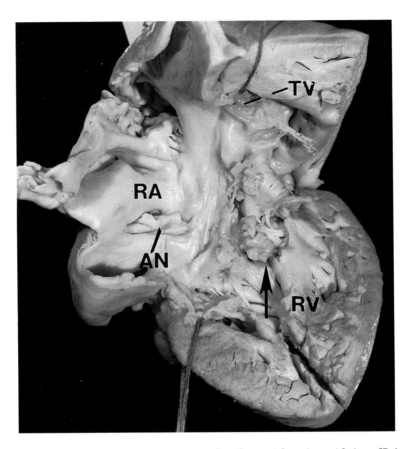

Figure 24: Markedly redundant tricuspid valve with tricuspid insufficiency and aneurysm of fossa ovalis. RA = hypertrophied and enlarged right atrium; An = aneurysm of the fossa ovalis; TV = redundant tricuspid valve; RV = right ventricle. Arrow points to the redundant tricuspid valve.

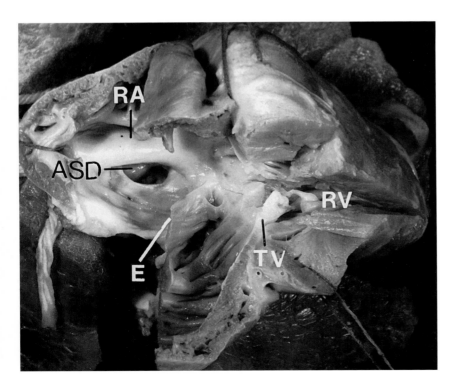

Figure 25: Right atrial, right ventricular view demonstrating marked tricuspid stenosis, redundant leaflets, abbreviated chordae and papillary muscles, large atrial septal defect of the fossa ovalis type, and hypertrophied and enlarged eustachian valve. RA = hypertrophied and enlarged right atrium; ASD = large atrial septal defect, fossa ovalis type; E = enlarged eustachian valve; TV = markedly dysplastic small tricuspid valve; RV = small right ventricle with thick wall.

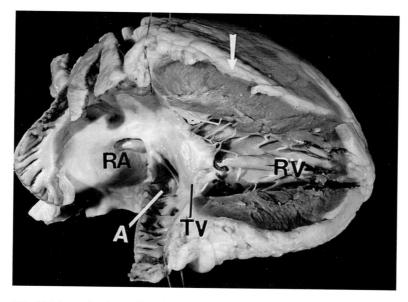

Figure 26: Thickened tricuspid valve with tricuspid stenosis and aneurysm of space of His. RA = right atrium; RV = right ventricle; TV = thickened tricuspid valve; A = aneurysm of space of His. Arrow points to the marked right ventricular hypertrophy.

Semilunar Valves

In addition to the redundancy, nodularity, and irregular thickening of the semilunar valves, the following abnormalities were noted: (Figs. 27–32)

	No. of Cases
Bicuspid aortic valve	21 (20.7%)
Bicuspid pulmonic valve	12 (11.8%)
Bicuspid, aortic, and pulmonic valves	26 (24.7%)
Unicuspid pulmonic valve	3
Unicuspid aortic valve	1
Incompletely divided tricuspid pulmonic valve with low raphé	2
Incompletely divided tricuspid aortic valve with low raphé	1
Quadricuspid aortic valve	1
Quadricuspid pulmonic valve	1
Aneurysm of aortic and pulmonic sinuses of Valsalva	3
Aneurysm of an aortic sinus of Valsalva	9 (8.9%)
Aneurysm of pulmonic sinuses of Valsalva	1
Fenestration of the aortic valve	3
Fenestration of the pulmonic valve	1
Fenestration of the aortic and pulmonic valves	1
Blood cysts in the aortic and/or pulmonic sinuses of Valsalva	3
Widening of commissures of aortic and/or pulmonic sinuses of Valsalva	3
Dome-shaped pulmonic valve with minute opening in the center	1
Pulmonary atresia	2

The semilunar valves were distinctly abnormally formed, in addition to being markedly redundant, nodose, and thickened in approximately 85% of the cases. The valve, although it was tricuspid, showed redundancy and irregular thickening in only about 14%. The aortic and pulmonic valves were more or less normally formed in only one heart but presented increased hemodynamic change. The aortic and/or the pulmonic valve was bicuspid in 58.4%. There was a tendency for increased occurrence of a bicuspid aortic valve in this entity more so than in the pulmonary. Likewise, the aortic valve had a tendency for aneurysmal dilatation, subluxation, and fenestration. Blood cysts in the semilunar valves were infrequently seen.

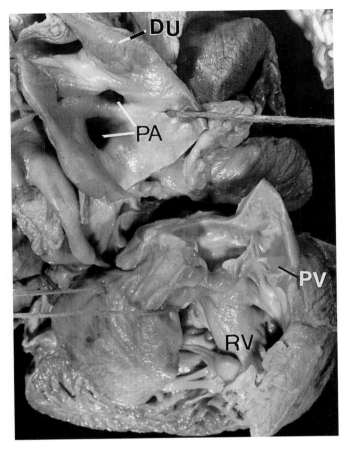

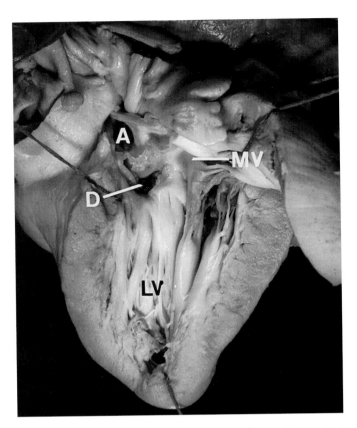

Figure 27: Bicuspid pulmonic valve and huge ductus arteriosus in a case of polyvalvular disease with ventricular septal defect. Outflow tract of the right ventricle. RV = right ventricle; PV = bicuspid dysplastic markedly thickened pulmonic valve; PA = two pulmonary arteries; DU = huge ductus arteriosus.

Figure 28: Another example of multiple shunts demonstrating the ventricular septal defect with nodular thickened aortic valve. LV = left ventricle; D = ventricular septal defect confluent with the aorta; A = aorta; MV = mitral valve. Note the thickened nodular aortic valve.

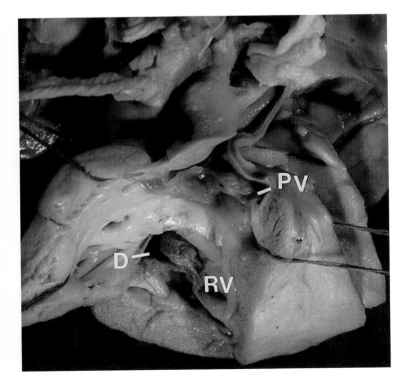

Figure 29: Bicuspid dysplastic pulmonary valve. RV = right ventricle; D = ventricular septal defect; PV = dysplastic thickened pulmonary valve.

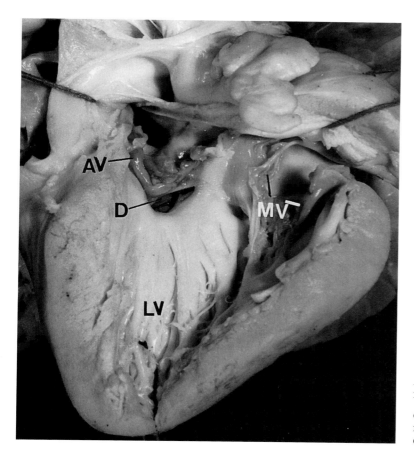

Figure 30: Bicuspid dysplastic aortic valve with a U-shaped ventricular septal defect. LV = left ventricle; MV = thickened mitral valve; AV = redundant nodular bicuspid aortic valve; D = ventricular septal defect; LV = left ventricle.

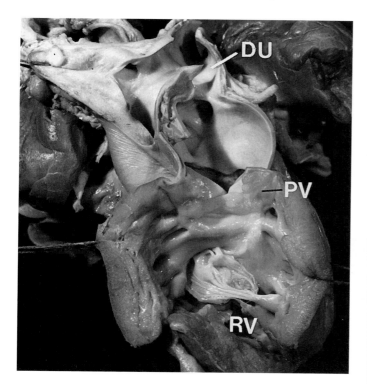

Figure 31: Unicuspid dysplastic pulmonary valve from a case of a multiple shunts, right ventricular outflow tract view. RV = right ventricle; PV = unicuspid dysplastic pulmonary valve; DU = ductus arteriosus.

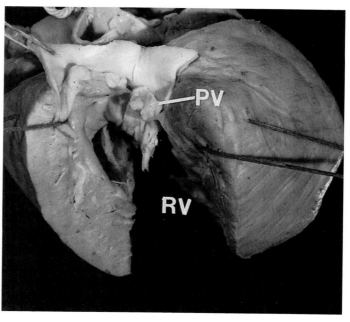

Figure 32: Outflow tract of the right ventricle demonstrating bicuspid thickened pulmonic valve with pulmonary stenosis. RV = right ventricle; PV = pulmonary valve.

Mitral Valve

The mitral valve presented redundancy, nodularity, and irregular thickening affecting both the anterior and the posterior leaflets to a varying extent (Figs. 33–36). In some, the posterior leaflet presented remarkable changes and in others the anterior leaflet showed more changes. In still others, both leaflets presented marked redundancy. These changes may be considered as floppy mitral valve. The chordae were elongated with poorly developed papillary muscles in approximately 22% of the cases. In 25%, the chordae were markedly abbreviated with poorly developed papillary muscles, and the papillary muscles proceeded either to the undersurface of the valve or to the base of the valve to a varying degree. In three, the chordae were completely absent, resulting in the fusion of the papillary muscles with the edge of the leaflet producing arcade-like malformations. Those with markedly abbreviated chordae produced an incomplete formation of an arcade-like mitral valve. One of the papillary muscles was absent, producing a parachute type of deformity in about 11% of the cases. This was present either in the posterior or in the anterior group. Blood cysts were found in five.

We were able to classify congenital polyvalvular disease into six major groups:

	No. of Cases
Group I = with shunts with or without extracardiac obstruction	37
Group II = with intracardiac obstruction with or without extracardiac obstruction	9
Group III = with obstruction and shunts	30
Group IV = without any shunts or obstruction	3
Group V = with major cardiac abnormalities	16
Group VI = with predominant insufficiency of the valves	6
Total	101

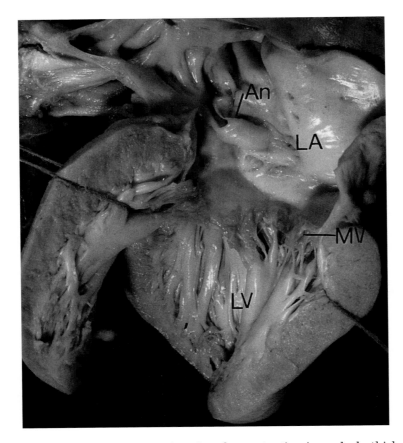

Figure 33: Left atrial, left ventricular view demonstrating irregularly thickened mitral valve, the aneurysm of the fossa ovalis and atrial septal defect. LA = left atrium; MV = irregularly thickened mitral valve; An = aneurysm of the fossa ovalis; LV = left ventricle. Note the trabeculations in the left ventricle.

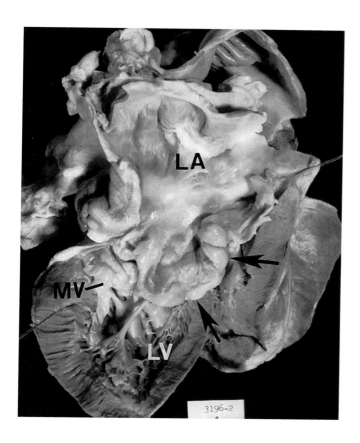

Figure 34: Markedly redundant mitral valve – floppy mitral with mitral insufficiency. Left atrial, left ventricular view. LA = hypertrophied and enlarged left atrium; LV = left ventricle; MV = markedly redundant mitral valve with chordae proceeding to the undersurface. Arrow points to the redundant mitral valve.

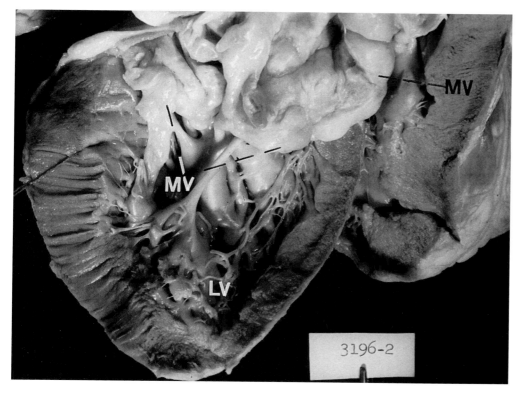

Figure 35: Close-up view of Figure 34 demonstrating the redundant leaflet of the mitral which involves the entire valvular apparatus. MV = mitral valve; LV = left ventricle.

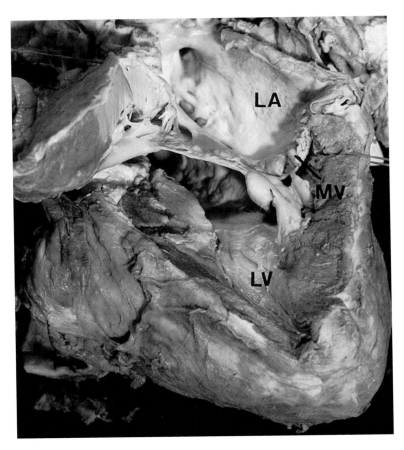

Figure 36: Left atrial, left ventricular view demonstrating irregularly thickened no-dose mitral valve with mitral stenosis and markedly abbreviated chordae. LA = left atrium; MV = thickened mitral valve; LV = left ventricle.

GROUP I

With Shunts with or without Extracardiac Obstructions (Figs. 37, 38)

	No. of Cases
ASD	5
VSD (2 with overriding aorta)	3
ASD and PDA	4
VSD and PDA (2 with overriding aorta)	5
ASD and VSD	2
ASD, VSD, and PDA (2 with overriding aorta)	10
ASD, VSD, and PDA with fetal (preductal) coarctation of the aorta (2 with overriding aorta and straddling TV)	7
ASD, VSD, and PDA with segmental coarctation of the aorta	1

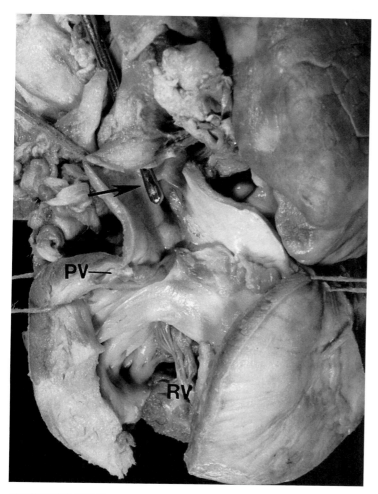

Figure 37: Marked right ventricular hypertrophy, redundant pulmonary valve, and patent ductus arteriosus in congenital polyvalvular disease – group I. RV = right ventricle; PV = pulmonary valve. Arrow points to the probe passing through a large ductus arteriosus.

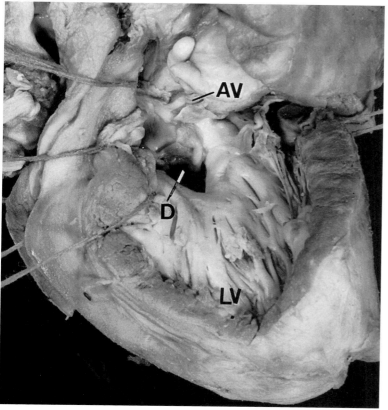

Figure 38: U-shaped subaortic ventricular septal defect with overriding aorta. Note the irregularly thickened aortic valve. LV = left ventricle; D = U-shaped defect; AV = thickened aortic valve.

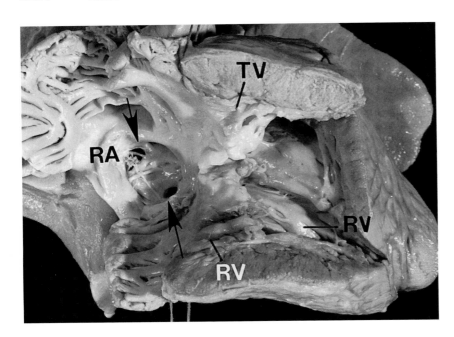

Figure 42: An example of a group III shunt with obstruction, atrial septal defect, and tricuspid stenosis. Right atrial, right ventricular view. RA = right atrium; RV = hypertrophied right ventricle; TV = markedly irregularly thickened tricuspid valve with almost absent chordae and poorly developed papillary muscles. Arrows point to multiple openings in the atrial septum with strands extending across the fossa ovalis.

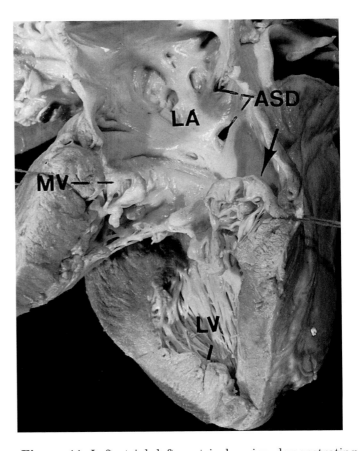

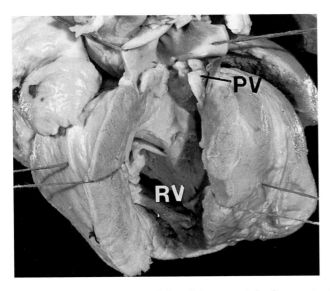

Figure 43: Outflow tract of the right ventricle demonstrating markedly dysplastic bicuspid pulmonary valve with pulmonary stenosis and marked right ventricular hypertrophy. RV = right ventricle; PV = markedly dysplastic bicuspid pulmonic valve.

Figure 44: Left atrial, left ventricular view demonstrating markedly redundant mitral valve with poorly developed papillary muscles, abbreviated chordae, and mitral stenosis. LA = hypertrophied and enlarged left atrium; ASD = atrial septal defect in two different locations; MV = redundant mitral valve; LV = left ventricle. Arrow points to the redundant posterior leaflet.

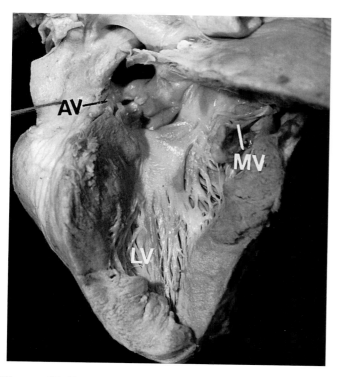

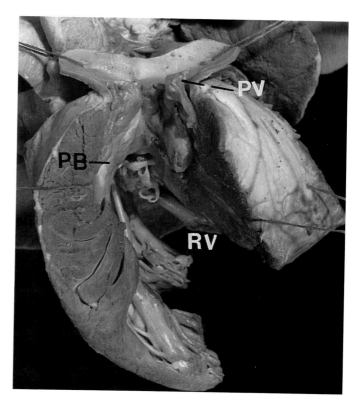

Figure 45: Dysplastic aortic valve with aortic stenosis and left ventricular hypertrophy. AV = aortic valve; MV = mitral valve; LV = left ventricle.

Figure 46: Dysplastic pulmonary valve with marked pulmonary stenosis and poststenotic dilatation of the main pulmonary trunk with tremendous right ventricular hypertrophy. RV = right ventricle; PV = dysplastic pulmonary valve; PB = hypertrophied and deviated parietal band with infundibular pulmonary stenosis.

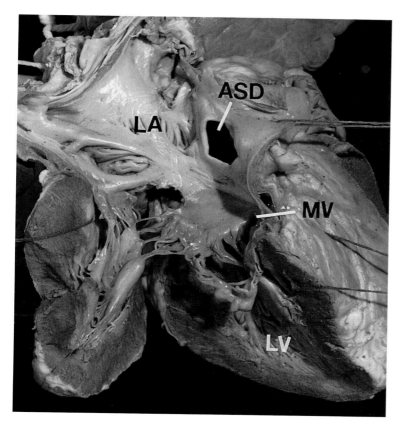

Figure 47: Same heart as in Figure 46. Atypical atrial septal defect of fossa ovalis type close to the entry of the inferior vena cava with straddling inferior vena cava. Left atrial, left ventricular view. LA = hypertrophied and enlarged left atrium; ASD = atrial septal defect in the posterior aspect of the atrial septum; MV = thickened mitral valve with mitral stenosis; LV = left ventricle.

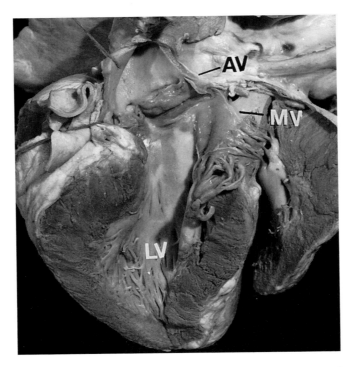

Figure 48: Same heart as in Figure 46. Irregularly thickened aortic valve with aortic stenosis and marked left ventricular hypertrophy. AV = aortic valve; LV = left ventricle; MV = mitral valve.

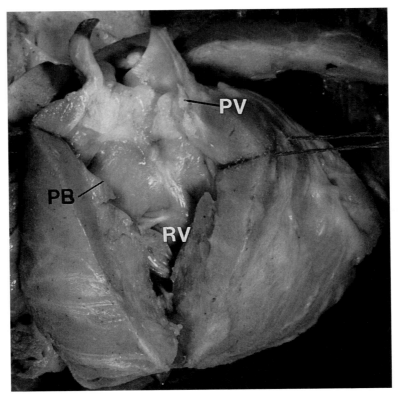

Figure 49: Another example of group III. Bicuspid pulmonary valve and infundibular pulmonary stenosis. RV = right ventricle; PB = deviated parietal band with infundibular stenosis; PV = pulmonic valve.

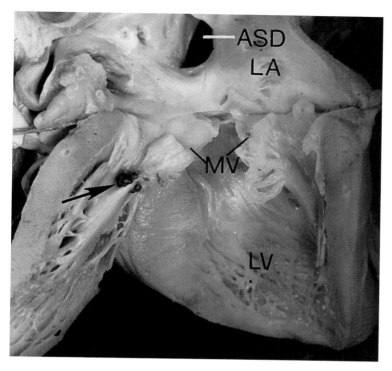

Figure 50: Same heart as in Figure 49. Left atrial, left ventricular view showing the large atrial septal defect and redundant mitral valve with mitral stenosis. LA = left atrium; MV = mitral valve; ASD = atrial septal defect of fossa ovalis type; LV = left ventricle. Arrow points to a huge blood cyst in the chordae between the anterolateral papillary muscle and the valve.

GROUP IV

Without Any Shunts or Obstruction (Figs. 51, 52)

	No. of Cases
Right ventricular hypertrophy	1
All chambers normal	1
Hypertrophy and enlargement of all the chambers	1

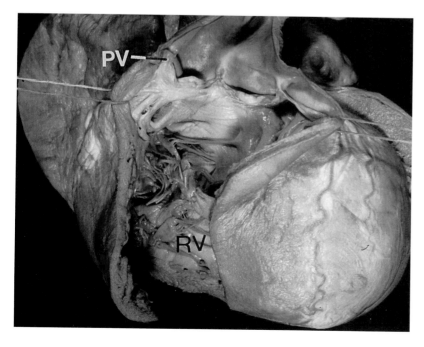

Figure 51: An example of group IV without obstruction and shunt. Irregular thickening of the pulmonic valve with insufficiency. RV = right ventricle; PV = pulmonary valve.

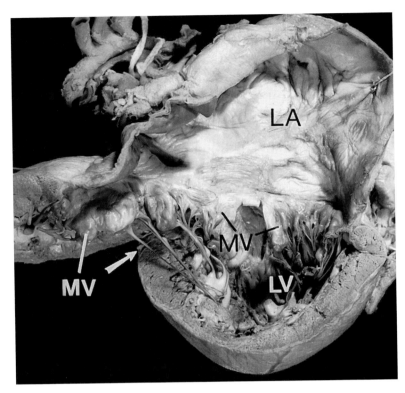

Figure 52: Another example of group IV. Redundant and markedly segmented mitral valve with mitral insufficiency and huge left atrium. LA = tremendously enlarged left atrium; MV = redundant mitral valve; LV = left ventricle. Arrow points to elongated chordae with poorly developed papillary muscles.

GROUP V

With Major Cardiac Abnormalities (Figs. 53–60)

	No. of Cases
DORV, subaortic VSD, and infundibular and valvular pulmonary stenosis	1
DORV, with marked mitral stenosis (almost atresia), ASD, aortic stenosis, and paraductal coarctation	1
DORV with mitral atresia, double VSD coarctation (fetal and adult), and ASD	1
DORV with subaortic VSD, pulmonary and mitral stenosis, and paraductal coarctation	1
DORV with subaortic VSD, and infundibular and valvular pulmonary stenosis	1
Pulmonary atresia with VSD and right aortic arch	1
Tetralogy of Fallot with pulmonary atresia	1
Tetralogy of Fallot with parachute mitral valve with stenosis	1
Tetralogy of Fallot	1
Tetralogy of Fallot – acyanotic	1
Tetralogy of Fallot with ASD (straddling tricuspid valve)	1
Tetralogy of Fallot with ASD and PDA	1
Mitral atresia with double VSD and overriding aorta	1
Premature closure of the foramen ovale with mitral stenosis, VSD, and wide PDA	1
Premature narrowing of the foramen ovale with mitral atresia with fetal coarctation, PDA, and multiple VSDs	1
Noonan's syndrome, aortic, subaortic, and pulmonary stenosis, infundibular pulmonary stenosis, coarctation, ASD, PDA, and restrictive VSD	1

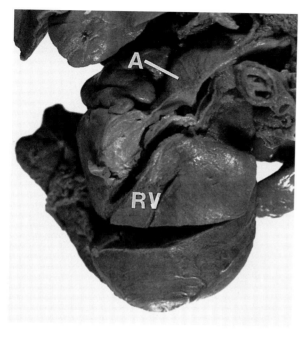

Figure 53: An example of group V. External view of the heart from a stillborn, 39 weeks' gestation with double outlet right ventricle. A = aorta to the right and anterior; RV = right ventricle. Note that the entire heart is practically formed by the right ventricle.

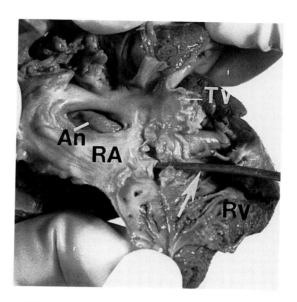

Figure 55: Same heart as in Figure 54, demonstrating the coronary sinus type of atrial septal defect. RA = right atrium; TV = tricuspid valve; RV = right ventricle; An = aneurysm of fossa ovalis. Arrow points to the probe passing through the coronary sinus type of atrial septal defect.

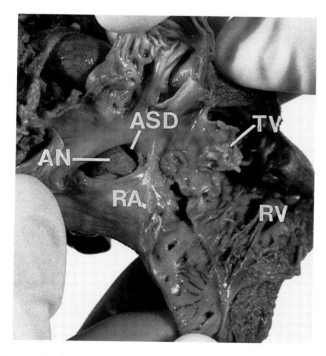

Figure 54: Right atrial, right ventricular view showing the redundant tricuspid valve with almost absent papillary muscles and tricuspid insufficiency. RA = right atrium; TV = tricuspid valve; RV = right ventricle; AN = aneurysm of the fossa ovalis; ASD = atrial septal defect.

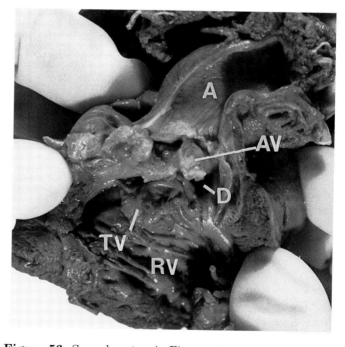

Figure 56: Same heart as in Figures 53–55. Right ventricular outflow tract demonstrating the aorta emerging from the right ventricle over a restrictive small defect. Note the restriction caused by the large irregularly, thickened, nodose aortic valve obstructing the defect. TV = tricuspid valve; RV = right ventricle; A = aorta; AV = markedly redundant aortic valve restricting the defect; D = ventricular septal defect.

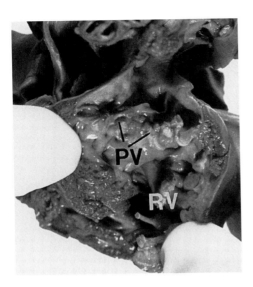

Figure 57: Same heart as in Figures 53–57. Right ventricular outflow tract demonstrating the pulmonary trunk also emerging from the right ventricle. Note the markedly dysplastic bicuspid pulmonic valve. RV = right ventricle; PV = pulmonary valve.

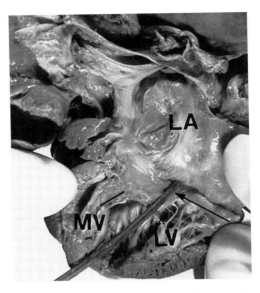

Figure 59: Same heart as in Figure 58. Arrow points to the probe passing through the coronary sinus atrial septal defect at the anulus of the posterior commissure of the mitral valve. LA = left atrium; MV = mitral valve; LV = left ventricle.

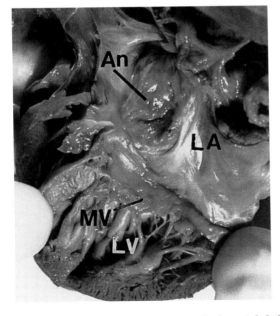

Figure 58: Same heart as in Figure 57. Left atrial, left ventricular view demonstrating the thickened mitral valve and aneurysm of the fossa ovalis. LA = left atrium; LV = left ventricle; MV = mitral valve; An = aneurysm of fossa ovalis.

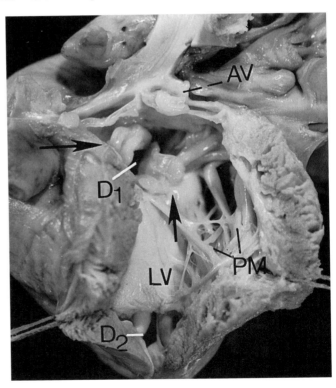

Figure 60: Another example of group V. Mitral atresia with double ventricular septal defects. Left ventricular view demonstrating the hypertrophied and enlarged left ventricle and the two VSDs. AV = bicuspid, thickened, redundant aortic valve; D_1 = common AV canal type of ventricular septal defect extending anteriorly with aneurysm of the tricuspid valve overlying the defect; LV = left ventricle; D_2 = second muscular apical ventricular septal defect; PM = papillary muscles. Arrows point to the redundant tricuspid valve tissue through the first ventricular septal defect.

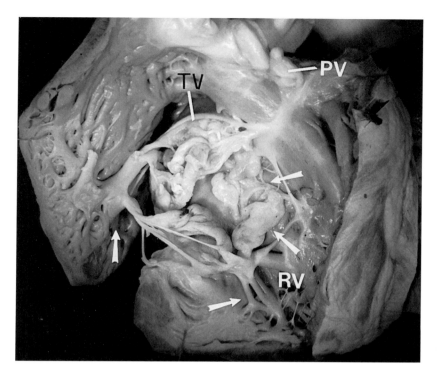

Figure 61: An example of group VI. Right ventricular outflow tract demonstrating the tremendously hypertrophied and enlarged right ventricle as a result of tricuspid and pulmonary insufficiency. TV = tricuspid valve; RV = right ventricle; PV = redundant pulmonary valve. Arrows point to the redundant tricuspid valve with hypoplastic papillary muscles.

GROUP VI

With Predominant Insufficiency of the Valves
(Figs. 61, 62)

	No. of Cases
Tricuspid and mitral insufficiency, with mild pulmonary and aortic insufficiency, and sudden death	2
Probable spontaneous closure of VSD by means of aneurysm of membranous septum with tricuspid and aortic insufficiency	1
Mitral, aortic, and tricuspid insufficiency and coronary artery disease (all valves replaced and coronary artery bypass	1
Mitral and aortic insufficiency, mitral anularplasty, WPW, and sudden death	1
Mitral and tricuspid insufficiency, floppy valves, and sudden death	1

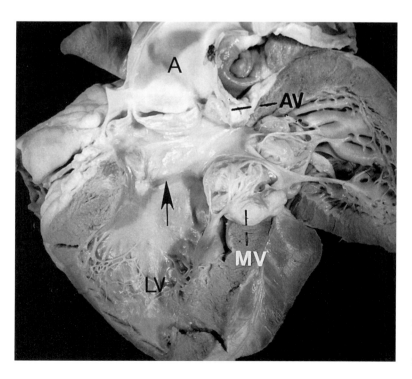

Figure 62: Same heart as in Figure 61. Outflow tract of the left ventricle demonstrating the aneurysm of the membranous septum, thickened aortic valve, and redundant mitral valve with insufficiency. LV = hypertrophied and enlarged left ventricle; MV = redundant mitral valve; A = aorta; AV = aortic valve. Arrow points to the aneurysm of the membranous septum.

Brachiocephalic Vessel Anomalies

	No. of Cases
Origin of right subclavian artery proximal to PDA	1
Retroesophageal right subclavian artery	1
Four brachiocephalic vessels	3
Two subclavian arteries emerging at the junction of ductus with the descending aorta	1
Two brachiocephalic vessels together, and origin of left subclavian artery away from the two vessels	4
Origin of left subclavian artery a considerable distance away from the other two vessels	2
Enlarged intercostals	1

Coronary Artery Anomalies (Fig. 63)

	No. of Cases	
High origin of both coronary ostia (1 close to each other)	5	
High origin of right coronary ostium	4	(12.8%)
High origin of left coronary ostium	4	
Origin of right coronary artery close to posterior commissure (1 with accessory right coronary artery)	3	
Single right coronary artery (1 with narrowing)	2	
Small right coronary artery (1 with high origin)	2	
Large right coronary artery supplying the left anterior descending coronary artery, and small left coronary artery supplying the left circumflex	1	
Hypoplastic anterior descending coronary artery	1	
Right coronary artery giving rise to left circumflex coronary artery	1	
Origin of both coronary ostia emerging from the left sinus of Valsalva	1	

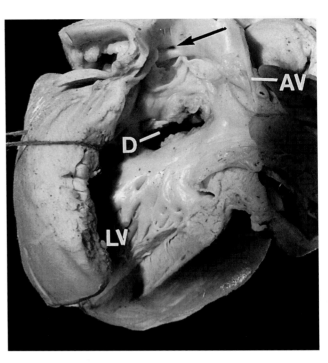

Figure 63: Left ventricular outflow tract demonstrating a somewhat oblique ventricular septal defect with thickened aortic valve and high origin of the right coronary ostium. AV = thickened aortic valve; D = ventricular septal defect; LV = left ventricle. Arrow points to the high origin of the right coronary ostium close to the posterior commissure.

Abnormalities Associated with Ventricles (Fig. 64)

	No. of Cases
Divided right ventricle	1
Anomalous muscle bands in the right ventricle	5
Marked trabeculation of the left ventricular septum	9
Aneurysm of the left ventricular septum	1
Ventricular septal bulge	6
Anomalous muscle bands in the left ventricle	2
Almost absent posterior ventricular septum and abnormal formation of anterior septum	1
Small diverticulum of the right ventricle	2
Fibrosis of the left and the right ventricles	1
Spongy premature ventricular mass	1
Myocardial abscess	1

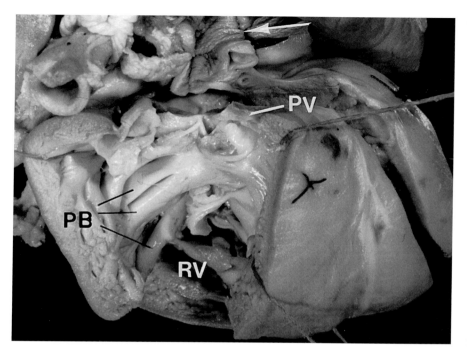

Figure 64: Outflow tract of the right ventricle demonstrating the redundant nodose pulmonary valve, right ventricular hypertrophy, and abnormal orientation of the parietal bands. RV = right ventricle; PV = thickened pulmonary valve; PB = parietal bands. Arrow points to the banding procedure.

In addition to the ventricular septal defect seen with major cardiac abnormalities, the defects varied as follows (Fig. 65):

Double VSD (1 CAVO and the other usual)	1
Double VSD (1 usual and the other midway in the septum)	1
Anterior mid-muscular VSD	1
Small VSD	1
Small restrictive VSD	1
Subaortic obstruction caused by redundant tricuspid valvular tissue	2
CAVO type VSD	2
Aneurysm of membranous septum restricting VSD	2
U-shaped subaortic VSD	3
Redundant tricuspid valve covering the VSD	1

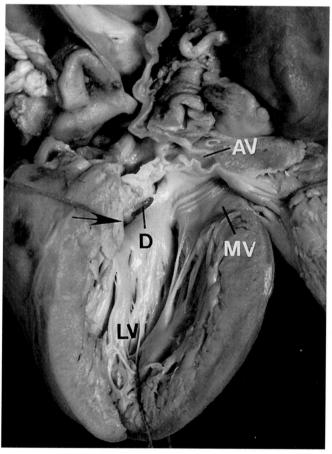

Figure 65: Left ventricular outflow tract demonstrating markedly redundant thickened bicuspid aortic valve prolapsing through a U-shaped defect restricting the defect. LV = left ventricle; MV = mitral valve; AV = irregularly thickened bicuspid aortic valve prolapsing through the ventricular septal defect; D = defect. Arrow points to the defect and the prolapsing aortic valve

Table 1

Extracardiac Abnormalities

	No. of Cases	
Trisomy 18	18 (17.8%)	
Mosaic trisomy 18	1	
Trisomy 13–15	3	(22.7%)
Extra chromosome in 20% of cells with multiple congenital anomalies	1	
Noonan syndrome	1	
Multiple extracardiac abnormalities	21	

Table 2

Other Associated Cardiac Abnormalities in the Atria

	No. of Cases
Oblique patent foramen ovale	6
Aneurysm of fossa ovalis	16
Secondary small ASD posteroinferiorly	2
Accessory coronary sinus type ASD	4
ASD extending to superior vena cava and right pulmonary vein	1
ASD extending to coronary sinus area and inferior vena cava	2
Absent coronary sinus and coronary veins draining into left superior vena cava–to innominate	1
Left superior vena cava entering the coronary sinus	8
Stenosis of the coronary sinus	2
Large fenestrated eustachian and thebesian valves (remnant of sinus venarum component)	8
Aneurysm of space of His	5
Absent right superior vena cava with left superior vena cava entering the coronary sinus	1
Huge rete Chiari	1
Band in the right atrium	2
Band in the left atrium	1
Stenosis of left pulmonary vein	1
Stenosis of right pulmonary artery and peripheral pulmonaries	1

Comment

The Relationship of Polyvalvular Disease to Isolated Dysplastic Valve – Congenital Aortic Stenosis

We want to emphasize that the dysplastic nature of the valve histologically is *different* from a hemodynamically altered valve. However, the dysplastic nature of the valve is somewhat *similar* to an isolated congenitally dysplastic valve such as the valve in aortic stenosis. The amount or quantity of the dysplasticity is greater with a greater amount of disruption of the architecture in polyvalvular disease, when compared to isolated dysplastic valve in aortic stenosis. Thus, the intensity of the dysplasticity and the disruption of the architecture of the valve is greater in polyvalvular disease.

The Relationship of Polyvalvular Disease to Markedly Redundant Common AV Valve Leaflets in Common AV Orifice and Markedly Redundant Quadricuspid or Bicuspid Truncal Valve

Histologically, some of the valves in common AV valve, especially when they are markedly redundant, nodose, and thickened and the redundant quadricuspid or bicuspid truncal valves are almost identical to the valves in polyvalvular disease.

The Relationship of Hemodynamically Altered Valve to Congenital Polyvalvular Disease

The histological manifestation of the hemodynamically altered valve is in the form of elastosis of the proximalis and of the spongiosa with, in some cases, an increase in fibrosa. These changes in the valve may occur either by an increase in pressure or an increase in volume of flow, or the valve may be hemodynamically altered due to normal aging phenomena. However, each individual layer of the valve remains distinct, although altered.

The Relationship of Polyvalvular Disease to Marfan's Syndrome

Although histologically the valves in polyvalvular disease may be similar to those in Marfan's syndrome, the aortas in the cases we studied histologically were normal in polyvalvular disease. There was no evidence of cystic degeneration in the aorta in polyvalvular disease. It is conceivable that congenital polyvalvular disease may be related to forme fruste Marfan's syndrome in which the aorta may not be involved.

The Relationship of Isolated Floppy Mitral and/or Tricuspid Valve to Polyvalvular Disease

The isolated cases of floppy mitral valves that we have studied histologically resemble congenital polyvalvular disease. One may therefore hypothesize that in some isolated floppy valves, without chromosomal and/or extracardiac abnormalities, there may be abnormal formation of the valves related to abnormalities in elastic tissue constituent. This may therefore manifest at varying ages. Therefore, one may consider these as variations in the manifestation of congenital polyvalvular disease.

The Relationship of Polyvalvular Disease to Other Known Diseases of the Valves

Congenital polyvalvular disease is a distinct entity and has no relationship to the valves in Hurler's disease, Ehlers-Danlos syndrome, and serotonism. In Hurler's disease, the fibrosa and anulus of the valve is affected with an infiltration of gargoyle cells. In Ehlers-Danlos syndrome, it is not clear whether the elastic content of the valve is increased or decreased and the architecture of the valve is disturbed or not. In serotonism, on the other hand, the architecture of the valve is not disturbed although there is a fibrous coating of the valve.

The Meaning of Increase in Acid Mucopolysaccharides (AMPs) in the Valve

One may consider the increase in acid mucopolysaccharides in various valvular diseases either congenital or acquired nature as a nonspecific finding.

Therefore, increase in acid mucopolysaccharides as such does not constitute evidence of a congenitally dysplastic valve. However, in addition to an increase in acid mucopolysaccharides, if there is hypoelastification or absence of elastic tissue associated with marked disruption of the architecture of the valve without clear demarcation between the fibrosa and the spongiosa layers (disarray pattern of the valve), one may then call the valve a congenitally dysplastic valve. If this is present in all four valves, the entity may then be called congenital polyvalvular disease. One may then invoke the theory that there has ensued a congenital incomplete differentiation of the valvular apparatus in fetal life. This may indeed be related to abnormal formation of one or several types of elastic tissue constituent at the molecular level.

Relationship of Polyvalvular Disease to Hypertrophic Cardiomyopathy

In addition to valvular abnormalities, the ventricular septum was considerably hypertrophied either in a symmetrical or in an asymmetrical manner in six, and there was one with Noonan syndrome. More recently, we encountered a heart where there was clinically hemodynamically significant left ventricular outflow tract obstruction with mid-septal (asymmetrical) hypertrophy of the ventricular septum associated with abnormalities of all four valves. The above suggests that a combination of chromosomal abnormalities may occur together manifesting in a single heart.

Conclusion

In this disease, we find remarkable changes affecting all of the valves to a varying degree, with a tendency to be associated with abnormal chromosomes, especially trisomy 18 and 13-15. When we first described this entity almost 20 years ago, we had analyzed only 36 hearts. Now we have analyzed 101 cases. When we first described this entity we felt that the aortic valve was the least involved. Now, having analyzed more than 100 hearts of congenital polyvalvular disease, it appears that the abnormalities of the aortic valve also occur quite frequently, perhaps more than the pulmonic valve, such as a bicuspid, unicuspid, quadricuspid, and aneurysm of sinuses of Valsalva of the valve.

In addition, we have now classified congenital polyvalvular disease into six distinct groups. When we originally described this entity, we were able to classify them into four distinct groups. It appears that congenital polyvalvular disease may occur with major cardiac abnormalities especially associated with double outlet right ventricle, tetralogy of Fallot, and mitral valve abnormalities associated with premature narrowing or closure of the foramen ovale. In addition to this group, there is yet another group of hearts where we find that the valvular involvement is dominant, producing insufficiency of the AV valves, particularly the tricuspid and mitral valves, resulting in sudden death.

It is of interest that there is a tendency for overriding of the aorta to occur in this entity. In group III, where there is combined obstruction and shunt, the mitral and/or the aortic valve show significant pathology resulting in either mitral stenosis and/or aortic stenosis. Likewise, coronary artery anomalies are not rare (23.7%). There is a distinct increase in abnormalities in the formation of the atrial and the ventricular septa. This includes aneurysm of the fossa ovalis, and an enlargement or remnant of the sinus venarum valves, with bands in the atrial septum either on the right or the left side. Likewise, abnormal formation of the ventricular septa in the form of anomalous muscle bands or heavy trabeculations or a deviated parietal band (Fig. 64) was not uncommon. The ventricular septal defect showed considerable variation. The defect in some was covered by means of an aneurysm of the membranous septum, or the tricuspid or aortic valve restricting the defect.

Histology of the valve presents distinct characterization of hypoelastification of the valve, with an increase in spongiosa content with an associated increase in acid mucopolysaccharides. The valvular abnormality affected the entire valvular apparatus. Thus, the chordal connections may be abbreviated and papillary muscles poorly developed, and that might result in insufficiency in addition to the stenosis caused by a redundant leaflet. Our histological findings and analysis of the gross heart suggest that we may indeed be dealing with a type of a connective tissue disorder predominantly affecting the elastic tissue and probably the connective tissue as well. Since there is a tendency for this type of valve to occur with abnormal chromosomes and multiple extracardiac abnormalities, the long-term outlook of congenital polyvalvular disease does not appear encouraging. Nevertheless, since there is a minority of patients without chromosomal abnormalities and/or extracardiac abnormalities who may clinically manifest insufficiency of the valves, one may entertain the idea of valvuloplasty rather than prosthetic replacement of the valve. It is also possible that newer techniques using noninvasive methods of analyzing the valvular structures at a very early stage may help in determining the altered hemodynamics of the valves. If minimal to moderate abnormal function of the valves

could be detected by these methods, a partial correction of the valve may be attempted by interventional methods in some selected cases without chromosomal or extracardiac abnormalities.

It is also conceivable that the nature of the abnormality of the elastic tissue and/or the connective tissue may be identified at the molecular and/or the genetic level in the near future. If this can be achieved, one may want to correct this anomaly at a very early stage and/or prevent its occurrence.

However, since the whole heart is affected to a varying degree, especially in those with chromosomal abnormalities and multiple extracardiac anomalies, it is very likely that several types of genes are affected or abnormal, per se, to start with in the very early stages of development of the embryo. From the obvious morphological variations seen within each group of hearts, one may speculate that there probably are many variations in the genes and their mutations, and that in some severe forms of congenital polyvalvular disease, the defect may lie in the earliest or the primary genes responsible for the development of the embryo itself. Some cases of congenital polyvalvular disease may indeed be related to the broad spectrum of manifestations in fibrillin disorders.

72

Congenital Mitral Stenosis

This is a rare entity in which the mitral valve is irregularly thickened with involvement of the chordae (Fig. 1). There is no associated fibroelastosis, fetal coarctation, or hypoplasia of the aortic tract complex. There may be an associated bicuspid aortic valve. There is, of course, biatrial and right ventricular hypertrophy and enlargement (Fig. 2).

Analysis of Our Material

There was a total of eight cases: five females, two males, and one was an animal heart, the youngest being a 2-week-old infant, the oldest 50 years of age, with a mean age of 8½ years. The heart was hypertrophied and enlarged and the apex was formed by the right ventricle in three (Fig. 3), by both ventricles in one, and by the left ventricle in three. The right atrium and the right ventricle were hypertrophied and enlarged in almost all cases except one where it was hypertrophied. The left atrium was hypertrophied and enlarged in five and hypertrophied in two. The left ventricle was hypertrophied and enlarged in two, enlarged in one, normal in two, smaller than normal in one, and atrophied in one. The tricuspid and pulmonic orifices were either normal or somewhat smaller than normal and occasionally enlarged. The mitral orifice was distinctly smaller than normal in all except one where it was very small. The aortic orifice was normal in three and smaller than normal in four.

The Valves

Tricuspid Valve

The tricuspid valve was normally formed but presented increased hemodynamic change in three. In others it showed various abnormalities. The chordae were abbreviated, and anomalous papillary muscles proceeded to the base of the valve, and the valve presented irregular thickening throughout.

Pulmonary Valve

This was normally formed in all, and presented increased hemodynamic change.

Mitral Valve

In general, the valve was markedly irregularly thickened throughout. In one, the thickening of the valve produced fusion at the line of closure along with fused chordae. In one, the irregularly thickened valve produced a very small opening. In addition, there was an accessory orifice. In two, the papillary muscles fused with the edge of the leaflet with hardly any chordal connections in between, presenting an arcade-like malformation (Fig. 1). In one, the anterolateral papillary muscle was hypoplastic and proceeded to the base of the valve. In another, the valve showed irregular thickening throughout, extending from the papillary muscle and chordae, which were fused with the valvular structure in a funnel-shaped fashion.

Aortic Valve

The aortic valve was normally formed in all except one, where it was bicuspid and considerably thickened. A patent ductus arteriosus was seen in two cases below the age of 1 month. In one 3-month-old, there was a small ventricular septal defect associated with a small atrial septal defect, and an overriding aorta with tricuspid stenosis. In the animal heart, there was a suggestion of a spontaneously closed ventricular septal defect. Anomalous muscle bands or chordal extensions were not uncommon in the left ventricle.

We are fundamentally dealing with an abnormally formed valve with a small anulus. The abnormality consists of a marked irregular thickening of the entire valvular apparatus (Fig. 1). The narrowing may occur at the line of closure or at the anulus, or the valve may

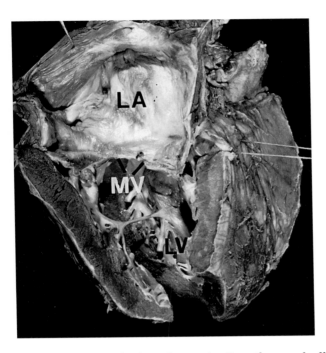

Figure 1: Left atrial view demonstrating the markedly thickened mitral valve with stenosis. LA = left atrium; MV = markedly thickened mitral valve with almost absent chordae; LV = left ventricle. Note the anomalous muscle band stretching across the left ventricular cavity.

taper down into a funnel-shaped opening. The one common denominator in all cases is the markedly abbreviated thickened chordal connections. It is of interest that congenital mitral stenosis is also seen in infancy as well as in adults. This is similar to what we have seen in cases of mitral insufficiency. It should be emphasized that four out of eight, in addition to mitral valve anomaly, also demonstrated distinct abbreviated chordal connections with bizarre papillary muscle attachment to the tricuspid valve in the right ventricle. These findings suggest that the fundamental problem in congenital mitral stenosis may be related to the development of the chordal extensions in both chambers.

Embryology of the Development of Atrioventricular Valves

The atrioventricular valvular apparatus develops from the endocardial cushions, the dextrodorsal bulbar cushion D, and the connections of the endocardial cushions with the muscular trabeculae of the ventricular myocardium. This development occurs in three stages or in three periods. In the first stage, the leaflets are fashioned fundamentally from the endocardial cushions and muscular trabeculae. In the second period, muscle gradually invades and replaces the cushion material. During the third phase, collagen tissue invades

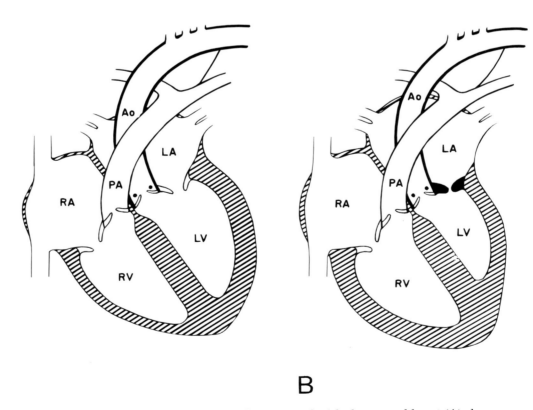

A   B

Figure 2: A diagram of mitral stenosis (B) compared with the normal heart (A) showing the hypertrophied and enlarged left atrium. RA = right atrium; RV = right ventricle; LA = left atrium; LV = left ventricle; AO = aorta; PA = pulmonary artery.

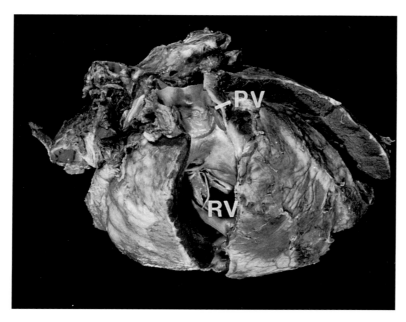

Figure 3: External view of the heart from a case of mitral stenosis where the apex is formed by the right ventricle. RV = right ventricle; PV pulmonary valve. Note the marked right ventricular hypertrophy.

and replaces the muscle tissue. Thus, one may hypothesize that the development of valvular tissue is impeded during the first two stages which may result in markedly abbreviated chordal and anomalous papillary muscle connections. We also would like to emphasize that anatomically the valve is distinctly abnormally formed either in infancy or in the adult heart, thus pointing out the fact that significant stenosis may occur at any age. We theorize that the stenosis may be transient in nature and may affect only part of the valve and not the entire valve. If this can be diagnosed by high technology, one may be able to correct the lesion by means of a nonsurgical technique. It is also emphasized that the tricuspid valve anatomy is well delineated prior to any attempt to correct the mitral valvular stenosis.

We should also keep in mind that the fundamental abnormality may lie in the genes responsible for the normal development of the AV valves. Future research at the molecular-genetic level focusing especially in the formation of the endocardial cushions may indeed help in the understanding the anomalies of the AV valves.

septal leaflet of the tricuspid valve. It is not uncommon to find diffuse fibroelastosis of the left ventricle with previous surgical procedures (Fig. 8).

Since these findings are found in stillborn infants as well as in any age group, we may hypothesize the following. In the stillborn, since the heart is hypertrophied and enlarged, we assume that the arcade mitral valve probably resulted in functional mitral insufficiency in intrauterine life with resultant left atrial and left ventricular enlargement. In addition, in this particular case, it is associated with a small patent ductus arteriosus. The tricuspid valve also presented marked abbreviation of the chordae with considerable thickening with hypertrophy and enlargement of the right-sided chambers. Therefore, one may hypothesize that there was also associated tricuspid insufficiency in intrauterine life, with decreased flow through the ductus, with markedly increased flow across the abnormally formed mitral valve accentuating the mitral insufficiency. On the other hand, when congenital mitral insufficiency is seen in the older age group, one may look upon the situation in a somewhat different manner. The valve, although anatomically abnormally formed, may not hemodynamically cause significant insufficiency for a long time. However, under altered physiological states, it may cause transient insufficiency of the valve affecting only part of the valvular apparatus, thus maintaining a more or less normal physiology, or the function of the valve may be normal to a great extent. With aging changes, the transient insufficiency gradually gets worse, producing significant insufficiency that may eventually become a permanent insufficiency.

We therefore emphasize that insufficiency of the mitral valve may be temporary in nature, affecting only part of the valve (focal) which may get worse with time. Thus, it is clear that newer methods of studying the function of the valves by means of high technology should be developed in the future which may help in early diagnosis and treatment. This is very important because if what we hypothesized can be proven by noninvasive techniques, correcting an insufficient valve at an early stage of its development may prevent the development of volume hypertrophy of the left atrium and the left ventricle.

The marked enlargement of the left atrial appendage also suggests the possibility of preferential abnormal flow patterns directed to one direction. One may therefore postulate that only a part or a component of a valvular apparatus may be affected, both anatomically and functionally, thereby resulting in unequal flow patterns. This may therefore require further innovative nonsurgical methods of correcting that part of the valve.

74

Mitral Atresia with Ventricular Septal Defect Complex

General Statement

In this complex, there is mitral atresia with the aortic orifice patent (Figs. 1, 2). This is associated with one, two or three ventricular septal defects (Figs. 2, 3). The left ventricle, although smaller than normal, is not the miniscule size seen in hypoplasia of the aortic tract complex. Despite the fact that there is absence of mitral orifice and valve, the papillary muscles are usually well developed in the left ventricle (Fig. 3). There is, of course, marked right atrial and right ventricular hypertrophy. There may be coarctation of the aorta or absence of the transverse arch. The foramen ovale, of course, is patent, or there is an atrial septal defect, fossa ovalis type. Occasionally, the aortic orifice is stenotic.

This entity must be differentiated anatomically from premature closure or narrowing of the foramen ovale.

Analysis of Our Material

There were 21 cases of this entity: 11 males and 10 females. The youngest was stillborn and the oldest was 19 years of age, with a median age of 13.4 months.

The Complex

The apex was formed by the right ventricle in nine, mostly by the right ventricle in nine, by both ventricles in two, and by the left ventricle in one.

The right atrium and ventricle were hypertrophied and enlarged in all (Figs. 4, 5). The left atrium was atrophied in 13, small and thick in one, hypertrophied in six (Fig. 1), and hypertrophied and enlarged in one

(Fig. 6). The left ventricle was very small with a thick wall in three, atrophied in nine, small with an average thickness of the wall in eight, and normal in size with average thickness of the wall in one.

The Valves

The tricuspid orifice was enlarged in all (Fig. 4). The pulmonary orifice was enlarged in 19 and normal in size in two. The mitral orifice was atretic in all. The aortic orifice was small in 18 and normal in size in three.

The tricuspid valve showed only marked hemodynamic change in 11. The remainder, in addition, showed other malformations in the anterior leaflet which was divided into two parts with nodulations, irregularities, or thickness. In one case, a straddling tricuspid valve was connected to both ventricles. Mitralization occasionally was noted. In one case, there was a double tricuspid valve.

The pulmonic valve, in general, showed increased hemodynamic change. In one case, it was bicuspid and thick. The aortic valve was either normal or showed increased hemodynamic change in 11. In six it was bicuspid and thick, and in one it was unicuspid and thick. In one case the left anterior cusp was redundant and thick.

The endocardium in all chambers showed focal thickening and whitening. Occasionally, diffuse thickenings were noted.

The types of atrial septal defects are given in Table 1, the types of ventricular septal defects are given in Table 2, the types of abnormalities of the outflow tract of the left ventricle and transverse arch in Table 3, and other associated abnormalities in Table 4.

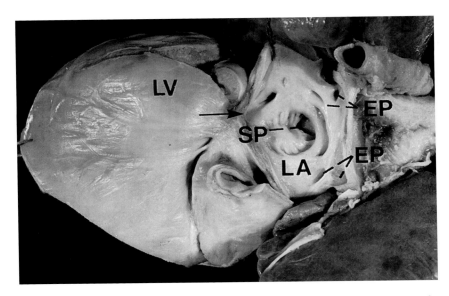

Figure 1: Left atrial and left ventricular view showing atresia of the mitral orifice. LV = left ventricle; LA = left atrium; EP = entry of pulmonary veins; SP = derivative of septum primum. Arrow points to the atretic mitral orifice.

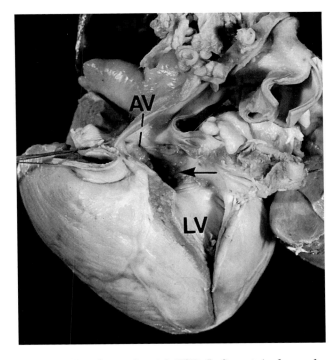

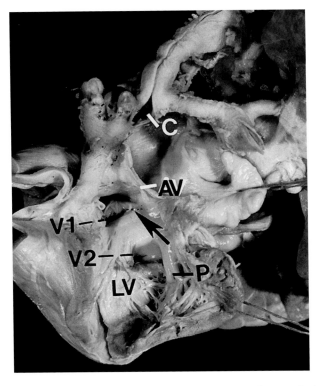

Figure 3: Mitral atresia with double VSD. Left ventricular and aortic view. V1 = first VSD–subaortic U-shaped; V2 = second VSD–posterobasal muscular; LV = left ventricle; AV = aortic valve overriding the defect; C = coarctation of the aorta; P = well-developed posterior papillary muscle. Arrow points to the attachment of the tricuspid valve on the summit of the ventricular septum.

Figure 2: Mitral atresia with VSD. Left ventricular and aortic view. LV = left ventricle; AV = aortic valve. Arrow points to the U-shaped VSD confluent with the overriding aorta.

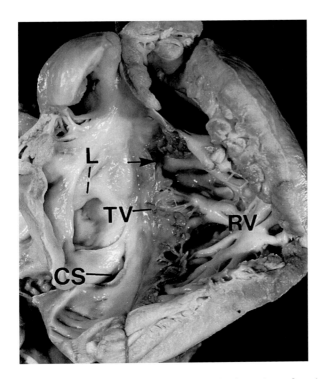

Figure 4: Right atrial and right ventricular view showing the enlargement of both chambers. L = limbus fossae ovalis; TV = enlarged tricuspid valve showing redundancy and thickening; CS = coronary sinus; RV = hypertrophied and enlarged right ventricle. Arrow points to the entry of the VSD beneath the junction of the septal and anterior leaflets of the tricuspid valve. Note also the thickened fossa ovalis with no ASD with an oblique patent foramen ovale not seen in the picture.

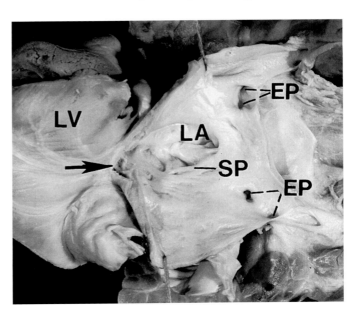

Figure 6: Left atrial view showing the enlarged left atrium. LA = left atrium; EP = entry of pulmonary vein; SP = derivative of septum primum; LV = left ventricle. Arrow points to the atretic mitral orifice.

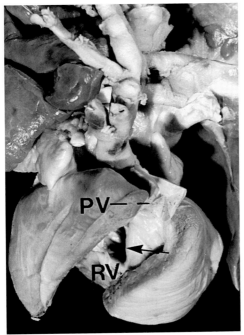

Figure 5: Right ventricular view showing the hypertrophied and enlarged right ventricle. RV = right ventricle; PV = pulmonic valve. Arrow points to the VSD.

Table 1

Types of Atrial Septal Defect

	No. of Cases
Atrial septal defect, fossa ovalis type	2
Large ASD	3
Fossa ovalis defect with aneurysm of the fossa ovalis	1
Large fossa ovalis defect with aneurysm of the fossa ovalis	1
Fossa ovalis defect with proximal ASD	1
Fossa ovalis defect with ostium primum defect	2
Oblique foramen ovale (with aneurysm in 3)	7
Atrial septectomy	2
Atrial septostomy	2

Table 2

Types of Ventricular Septal Defect

	No. of Cases
Small VSD – confluent with aorta	2
VSD, moderate size	2
Usual VSD with overriding aorta	3
Large VSD extending anteriorly with overriding aorta	1
Basal VSD entering the sinus of the right ventricle	1
Large muscular VSD (in the middle) entering the right ventricular sinus	1
Large muscular VSD between the aorta and the posterior part of the ventricular septum	1
Mid-septal VSD	1
CAVO type VSD with straddling tricuspid valve	2
Double defect (basal and apical)	3
Double defect (basal and the other close to the posterior part of the ventricular septum with overriding aorta)	2
Double-defect – both close to base with overriding aorta	1
Double defect (mid-part anterior – a large one at the junction of the sinus and conus and second above the first)	1

Table 3

Abnormalities in the Outflow Tract of the Left Ventricle and the Transverse Arch

	No. of Cases
Aortic stenosis with preductal coarctation and PDA	5
Preductal (fetal) coarctation with probe patent ductus arteriosus	3
Preductal (fetal) coarctation with adult component with wide PDA and probe PDA	2
Preductal (fetal) coarctation with closed ductus	1
Coarctation (clinical surgeon)	1
Paraductal coarctation – almost atresia (with wide PDA)	1
Absence of the transverse arch with PDA	1

Table 4

Other Associated Cardiac and Noncardiac Abnormalities

	No. of Cases
Left superior vena cava entering the coronary sinus	5 (23.8%)
Entry of coronary sinus into both atria	1
High origin of coronary arteries	1
Left pulmonary veins into coronary sinus	1
Aneurysm of the main pulmonary trunk with dissection and rupture	1
Abnormal bands in the right atrium	1
Right subclavian artery from descending aorta	1
Probe PDA in 2-day-old infant with fetal coarctation	1
Circuitous PDA in an 11-day-old infant	1
Small placenta	1

Comment

It is to be noted that the left ventricle is not as small as in hypoplasia of the aortic tract complex, and may thus be used in some cases in the repair as a pumping chamber. At the same time, the frequency of coarctation and the presence of aortic stenosis are important considerations in surgery.

It is of interest that one case lived until 19 years of age. In this case, an atrial septectomy was done in infancy. The left ventricle was smaller than normal and its wall was of average thickness. There was a marked paraductal coarctation with a widely patent ductus arteriosus. Thus, an atrial septectomy may permit survival to adult life.

Although the usual subaortic perimembranous type of ventricular septal defect is common (Fig. 2), it should be noted that the ventricular septal defect may be present anywhere (Figs. 3, 4, 7–9). The defect in many cases is subaortic and U-shaped, confluent with the aortic valve (Figs. 2, 3). The presence of a straddling tricuspid valve in some cases may be expected where there is mitral atresia.

It is to be noted that a large atrial septal defect is uncommon in this entity, and that in seven there was an oblique foramen ovale (Figs. 4, 7) and in three there was an aneurysm in the fossa ovalis (Fig. 9). This raises the question as to whether the basic abnormality embryologically in this entity was in the atrial septum rather than in the mitral valve. One may postulate that there is an impediment to the flow of the blood into the left side in this entity, and, therefore, mitral atresia

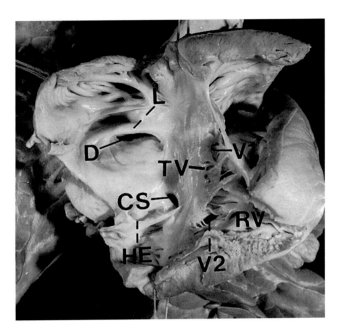

Figure 7: Right atrial and right ventricular view showing the hypertrophied and enlarged right side of the heart and the double VSD. L = limbus fossa ovalis; D = fossa ovalis defect or patent fossa ovalis; CS = coronary sinus; HE = hypertrophied and enlarged eustachian valve; TV = tricuspid valve; RV = right ventricle; V1 = first VSD beneath the junction of the anterior and septal leaflets of the tricuspid valve; V2 = Second VSD beneath the inferior (posterior) leaflet of the tricuspid valve.

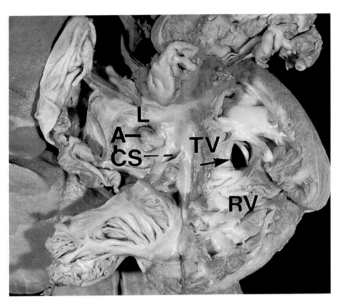

Figure 9: Right atrial and right ventricular view showing the entry of the VSD from Figure 8 in the sinus of the right ventricle. L = limbus fossa ovalis; CS = coronary sinus; TV = tricuspid valve; RV = right ventricle; A = aneurysm of fossa ovalis. Arrow points to the VSD as seen from the right side. Note also the patent foramen ovale

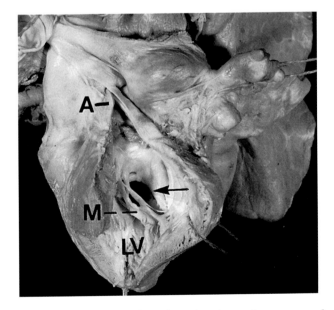

Figure 8: Left ventricular view showing a large muscular VSD. A = aortic valve; LV = left ventricle; M = anomalous muscle bands criss-crossing the defect. Arrow points to the VSD.

with ventricular septal defect is related to the cardiac anomalies premature closure or narrowing of the foramen ovale and hypoplasia of the aortic tract complex in some.

The frequent presence of overriding of the aorta (Figs. 2, 3), and the presence of double outlet right ventricle noted elsewhere (Chapter 13), indicates the general conception that where there is mitral atresia, there is a tendency for the aorta to move to the right to produce double outlet right ventricle. The tendency for the defect to be a U-shaped structure suggests that the basic anomaly is the defective absorption of the bulbus into the left ventricle.

Thus, in some, there may be abnormalities in the genes that are responsible for the normal development of the mitral valve and the proper absorption of the bulbus into the left ventricle. On the other hand, perhaps in some this entity developmentally may fall within the spectrum of hearts with premature narrowing or smallness of the foramen ovale complex.

75

Aortic Atresia with Ventricular Septal Defect

In this anomaly, there is aortic atresia, usually with a large subarterial (anterior or conal) type of ventricular septal defect. Thus, the pulmonary trunk may override the defect (Fig. 1). There is an atrial septal defect of the fossa ovalis type and a widely patent ductus arteriosus. Occasionally, there is absence of the transverse arch. In general, all chambers are hypertrophied and enlarged.

Analysis of Our Material

There was a total of 10 cases: eight males and two females. The youngest was 2 days of age and the oldest 1 year, with an average age of 2 months.

The Complex

The heart was hypertrophied and enlarged. The apex was formed by the left ventricle in four, by the right ventricle in four, and by both ventricles in two. The right atrium and right ventricle were hypertrophied and enlarged in eight and hypertrophied in two. The left atrium was hypertrophied and enlarged in three, normal in three, hypertrophied in two, small in one, and atrophied in one. The left ventricle was hypertrophied and enlarged in five, enlarged in two, normal in one, hypertrophied in one, and small with a thick wall and fibroelastosis in one. The tricuspid orifice was normal in size in five and enlarged in five. The pulmonic orifice was enlarged in nine and normal in size in one. The mitral orifice was normal in three, enlarged in three, small in three, and atretic in one. The aortic orifice was atretic in nine and quite small in one.

The Valves

Tricuspid Valve

The valve was normally formed and showed increased hemodynamic change in three. In three others, there was mitralization of the valve with distinctly increased hemodynamic change. In the remainder, the valve presented varying types of anomalies. The anterolateral and/or the inferior papillary muscle proceeded to the base of the valve, or several irregular papillary muscle connections were seen with a markedly segmented anterior leaflet.

Pulmonic Valve

The pulmonic valve was normally formed, and presented increased hemodynamic change in all but one, where it was bicuspid and markedly thickened.

Mitral Valve

The mitral valve was normally formed and presented increase hemodynamic change in some. It was atretic in one.

Aortic Valve

The aortic valve was atretic in all but one, where it was quite small with marked aortic valvular and subaortic stenosis and overriding aorta.

Endocardium

The endocardium presented either focal or diffuse thickening and whitening, especially in the left atrium and left ventricle.

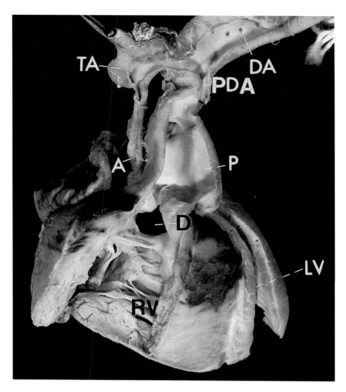

Figure 1: Aortic atresia with ventricular septal defect. A = markedly elongated hypoplastic ascending aorta; TA = transverse arch; P = pulmonary trunk; PDA = ductus arteriosus; DA = descending aorta; RV = right ventricle; LV = left ventricle; D = ventricular septal defect. Note that the pulmonary trunk overrides the defect.

Ventricular Septal Defect

The ventricular septal defect was subarterial (conal, anterior, or infundibular) either of moderate or large size in eight (Fig. 1). Occasionally it was small (Fig. 2). The defect was situated at the junction of the septal and parietal bands in the majority of the cases. It was confluent with the base of the pulmonary valve. The pulmonary trunk overrode the defect in four. The parietal band had a tendency to straddle the defect. In one, the defect was of the usual type, in part membranous and in part muscular type. In one there were two defects, one subarterial and the other submitral.

The associated cardiac anomalies are given in Table 1.

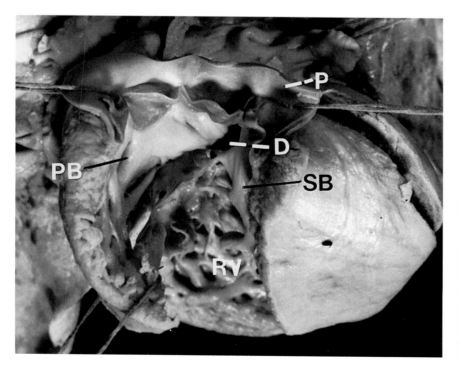

Figure 2: Aortic atresia with ventricular septal defect confluent in part with the base of the pulmonary trunk. Note that the defect extends anterior or distal to the muscle of Lancisi in an oblique angle at the junction of the arch formed by the septal and the parietal bands. Thus, the defect is relatively small but nevertheless confluent with the pulmonic valve. PB = parietal band; SB = septal band; D = defect between the septal and parietal bands; P = pulmonary trunk; RV = right ventricle.

Table 1

	No. of Cases
Atrial septal defect (large or moderate size)	4
Patent foramen ovale	4
Balloon septostomy	1
Aneurysm of fossa ovalis	1
Adult coarctation	1
Absent transverse arch	1
Mitral stenosis	1
Incomplete cor triatriatum dexter	1
Mitral atresia with marked subaortic stenosis with overriding aorta and repair of coarctation in infancy with the distal origin of the left subclavian artery	1

Comment

In this entity there appears to be a tendency for a subarterial defect to be confluent with the base of the pulmonary trunk with overriding of the pulmonary trunk to a varying degree. The pulmonary trunk overrode the septum in four. The ascending aorta was either very small or a minute chord-like structure that proceeded to the base and gave off the two coronary arteries (Fig. 3). As it proceeded towards the transverse arch, it was distinctly larger than the ascending aorta. A wide ductus arteriosus was always present in this entity. It is of interest that there was one case associated with mitral stenosis and one with mitral atresia. Although one could add mitral atresia, in the entity called mitral atresia with ventricular septal defect, we chose not to because of the fact that the ascending aorta was hypoplastic, resembling hypoplasia of aortic tract complex or aortic atresia with VSD. In this remarkable heart there was distinct subaortic stenosis as well as marked aortic stenosis with overriding of the aorta. A coarctation was repaired in infancy and a ductus ligated at that time. There was one with absent transverse arch. Here, the defect was U-shaped confluent with the membranous septum and extended anteriorly and entered the right ventricle at the junction of the anterior and septal leaflets of the tricuspid valve and extended in part to the lower margin of the septal and parietal bands (Figs. 4–6).

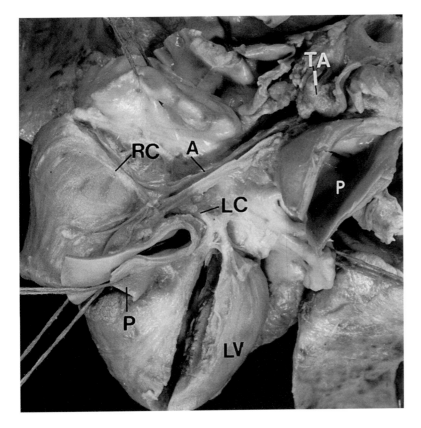

Figure 3: Aortic atresia with VSD, external view of the heart demonstrating the origin of the coronary arteries from the base of the chord-like ascending aorta. P = pulmonary trunk; LV = left ventricle; A = chord-like markedly narrowed hypoplastic ascending aorta; RC = right coronary artery; LC = left coronary artery; TA = transverse arch.

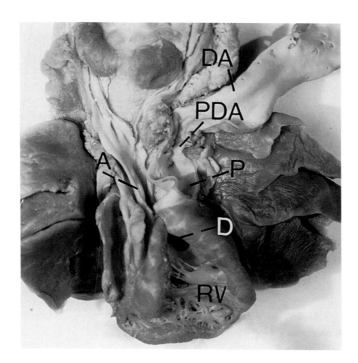

Figure 4: Aortic atresia with absent transverse arch; external view of the heart. RV = large right ventricle; A = very small ascending aorta giving off the brachiocephalic vessels; P = large pulmonary trunk; PDA = patent ductus arteriosus; DA = descending aorta; D = ventricular septal defect. Note the absence of the transverse arch.

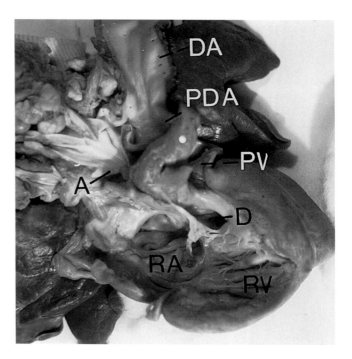

Figure 5: Right ventricular outflow tract view demonstrating the U-shaped defect at the junction of the septal and anterior leaflets of the tricuspid valve involving the lower septal band. A = small ascending aorta; RA = right atrium; RV = right ventricle; D = U-shaped ventricular septal defect; PV = pulmonary valve; PDA = patent ductus arteriosus; DA = descending aorta.

Embryogenesis

Because of the presence of a subarterial defect in almost all hearts, one may hypothesize that the fundamental problem, at least in the majority of the cases, may lie in the formation of the infundibular or bulbar septum without involving the aorticopulmonary septum. Thus, the aorta and pulmonary trunk have distinctly separated, with the coronary arteries emerging from the base of the atretic aortic valve.

The abnormal formation of the infundibular septum may indeed be related to the abnormalities in the genes that are responsible for the development of the septum. Future research at the molecular-genetic level may help in understanding this anomaly.

Since various types of aorticopulmonary anastomosis are being performed today for hypoplasia of aortic tract type of hearts, it is important to delineate the architecture of the outflow tract of the right ventricle as well as the right atrium. Likewise, the tricuspid valvular anatomy should be well delineated. It is also emphasized that since we are dealing with a subarterial defect confluent with the pulmonic trunk, the parietal band may straddle and override the defect and proceed to the opposite chamber to a varying degree which may produce subarterial obstruction at a later date following a Norwood type of procedure.

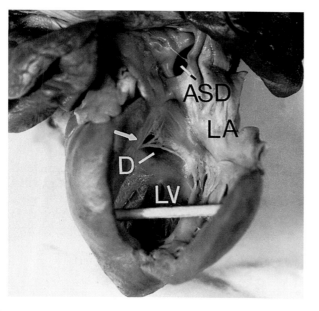

Figure 6: Left atrial, left ventricular view demonstrating a large atrial septal defect of the fossa ovalis type and anomalous attachment of the anterior leaflet of the mitral valve to the lower margin of the defect. LA = left atrium; LV = left ventricle; ASD = atrial septal defect, fossa ovalis type; D = U-shaped ventricular septal defect. Arrow points to the anomalous attachment of the mitral valve to the ventricular septum

76

Pulmonary Atresia with Tricuspid Insufficiency

In this complex, the pulmonary atresia is associated with tremendous enlargement of the tricuspid orifice with considerable thickening and enlargement of the valve. This results in massive tricuspid insufficiency, resulting in tremendous right atrial and right ventricular hypertrophy and enlargement (Figs. 1, 2). The right atrial and right ventricular enlargement may form an aneurysm resulting in paper-thin walls of both chambers. The left ventricle may also be hypertrophied and enlarged. There is, of course, a good-sized atrial septal defect or a patent foramen ovale sometimes associated with an aneurysm of the fossa ovalis. A variation of this complex is complete absence of the tricuspid valve associated with pulmonary atresia (Fig. 3).

Rarely, one sees a pulmonary atresia associated with a normal-sized tricuspid orifice. The right ventricle is then small and thick-walled.

Analysis of Our Material

There was a total of 21 cases: 13 males and eight females. The youngest was a stillborn, the oldest an 18-month-old, with a median age of 1 month. Eighty percent of them were below the age of 48 hours.

The Complex

The heart was greatly enlarged, especially affecting the right side of the heart. The apex was formed by both ventricles in 45%, by the right ventricle in 35%, and by the left ventricle in 20%. The right atrium was hypertrophied and enlarged in all. The right ventricle was hypertrophied and enlarged in all but three, where it was thick-walled with a small chamber. The left atrium was hypertrophied and enlarged in 55%, normal in 30%, and smaller than normal in 15%. The left ventricle was hypertrophied and enlarged in 60%, normal in 20%, enlarged in 10%, and hypertrophied in 10%. The tricuspid orifice was greatly enlarged in 75%, normal in size in 15%, and smaller than normal in 10%. The pulmonic orifice was atretic in all. The mitral orifice was normal in 50% and enlarged in 50%. The aortic orifice was enlarged in 40%, normal in 55%, and smaller than normal in 5%.

The Valves

Tricuspid Valve

The valve was distinctly abnormally formed in all. The valvular tissue was markedly redundant and nodose throughout (Fig. 4). The anterior leaflet was ballooned out in many and formed a sheet of tissue or a sail-like tissue that was inserted close to the base of the pulmonary valve obstructing the outflow tract into the pulmonary trunk (Fig. 5). The anterior leaflet was often greatly enlarged with redundant irregular nodulations with anomalous chordal connections, and frequently with a hypoplastic anterolateral papillary muscle. The valve presented irregular thickening in areas and was thinned out in some. The anterior leaflet was quite frequently attached to the parietal band (Fig. 6), and was occasionally perforated. The septal (medial) leaflet was frequently absent (Fig. 7) or represented by nubbins of irregularly thickened or nodule-like formation of valvular tissue. This was found, in

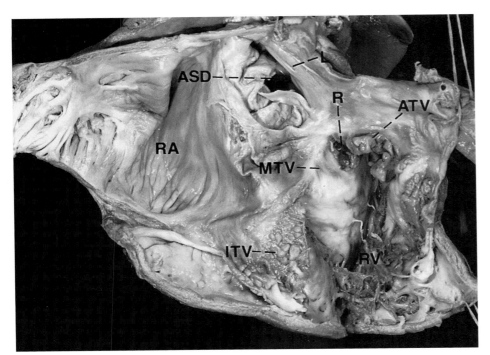

Figure 1: Right atrial, right ventricular view. ASD = atrial septal defect, fossa ovalis type; ATV = anterior leaflet of the tricuspid valve; ITV = inferior tricuspid leaflet with portion of the medial leaflet; L = limbus, fossae ovalis; MTV = medial leaflet of the tricuspid valve; R = red nodule in region of absent medial leaflet; RA = right atrium; RV = right ventricle. Note the tremendously enlarged right atrium and markedly redundant anterior leaflet of the tricuspid valve with partially absent medial leaflet with redundancy of the inferior leaflet. (Used with permission from Bharati S, et al. See Figure 17.)

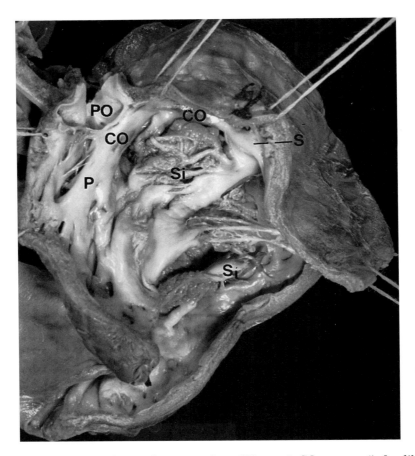

Figure 2: Right ventricular outflow tract view of Figure 1. CO = conus (infundibulum) of right ventricle; P = parietal band; PO = opening in region of the pulmonary atresia produced by valvotomy; S = septal band; SI = sinus of right ventricle. (Used with permission from Bharati S, et al. See Figure 17.)

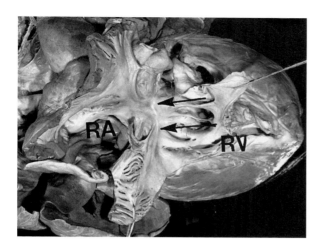

Figure 3: Complete absence of tricuspid valvular tissue. RA = right atrium; RV = right ventricle. Arrows point to the complete absence of the tricuspid valve. Note the anomalous chordal extensions and trabeculations in the small right ventricle with thick wall.

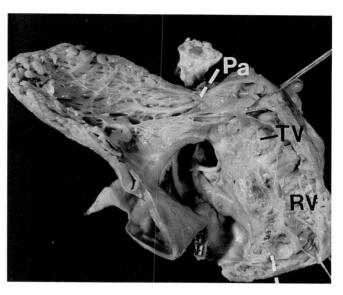

Figure 5: Tricuspid valvular tissue in part redundant and in part thinned out with a huge anulus and tremendously enlarged right ventricle and attachment of the anterior leaflet close to the base of the pulmonic valve. TV = tricuspid valve; RV = right ventricle; Pa = atretic pulmonic orifice.

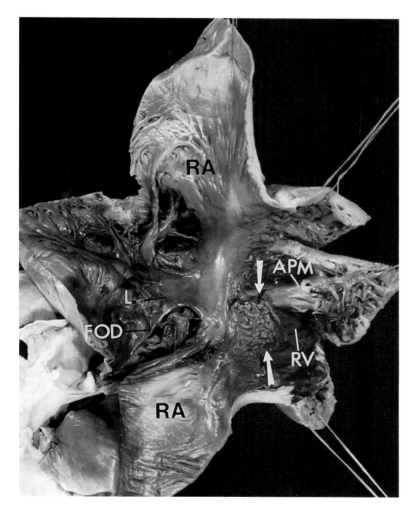

Figure 4: Markedly redundant valvular tissue of all the leaflets with anomalous papillary muscle proceeding to the base of the anterior leaflet. FOD = fossa ovalis defect; L = limbus, fossa ovalis; RA = right atrium; RV = right ventricle; APM = anomalous papillary muscle proceeding to the base of the valve. Arrows point to the markedly redundant nodose valvular tissue.

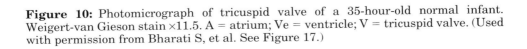

Figure 10: Photomicrograph of tricuspid valve of a 35-hour-old normal infant. Weigert-van Gieson stain ×11.5. A = atrium; Ve = ventricle; V = tricuspid valve. (Used with permission from Bharati S, et al. See Figure 17.)

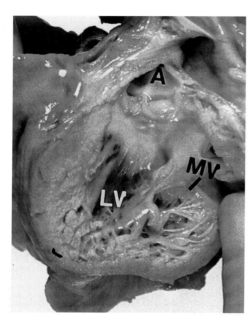

Figure 24: Left ventricular hypertrophy with fibroelastosis and hemorrhage of the endocardium. LV = left ventricle; A = aorta; MV = mitral valve.

Associated Cardiac Anomalies

There were very few associated cardiac abnormalities. There was a single coronary ostium in one, high origin of left coronary ostium in one, blood cysts in the right ventricle in one, and aneurysm of the fossa ovalis in two were noted. The ductus was abnormally small in two newborns.

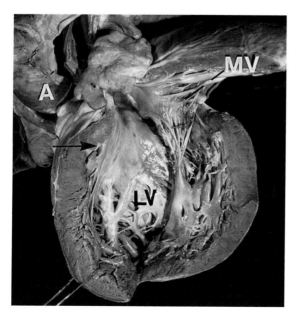

Figure 25: Left ventricular view demonstrating the left ventricular septal bulge. A = aorta; MV = mitral valve; LV = left ventricle. Arrow points to the left ventricular septal bulge.

Comment

Although pulmonary atresia with tricuspid insufficiency is a relatively rare anomaly, this entity should be differentiated from Ebstein's anomaly. In Ebstein's anomaly, there is distinct displacement of the septal and inferior leaflets of the tricuspid valve to a varying degree into the inlet or the sinus of the right ventricle. On the other hand, in this entity we are fundamentally dealing with marked anular enlargement of the tricuspid valve in the majority of the cases with distinctly abnormally formed valvular tissue. Only occasionally is there some suggestion of an incompletely formed valvular tissue slightly displaced into the sinus of the right ventricle. Conventionally, this entity is grouped or classified as *type II pulmonary atresia*, contrasting this with pulmonary atresia with intact ventricular septum which is considered as *type I*. We believe this entity is distinctly different from the entity of pulmonary atresia with intact ventricular septum. Although in both entities we are dealing with intact ventricular septum, the fundamental difference is the size of the tricuspid orifice and the morphology of the tricuspid valve and the right ventricle. In tricuspid stenosis with pulmonary atresia (pulmonary atresia with intact ventricular septum – *type I*), the tricuspid orifice is smaller than normal in the majority of the cases and presents an abbreviated version of a normally formed tricuspid valve. In some there is a tendency for downward displacement of the septal leaflet into the right ventricle. On the other hand, in pulmonary atresia with tricuspid insufficiency, there is tremendous or remarkable valvular abnormality involving the entire valvular apparatus. The right ventricular morphology in these two entities is an exact opposite of the other. In pulmonary atresia with intact ventricular septum, the right ventricle is smaller than normal, with a thick wall and fibroelastosis, in contrast to the right ventricle in this entity where it is enlarged with a thin wall, resembling Uhl's anomaly. Some of the cases of pulmonary atresia with tricuspid insufficiency may be related to Ebstein's malformation of the tricuspid valve.

Embryogenesis

Since the entire valvular apparatus is involved as well as the right ventricular myocardium in this entity, it is conceivable that the fundamental problem may lie in the embryogenesis of the myocardium. Since at the histological level the valve presents in part thinned-out areas and in part thickened areas with hypoelastification, we may in addition invoke the thesis that there may be an associated disturbance in the elastic tissue component of the developing heart involving the specific genes that are responsible for the normal development of the tricuspid and pulmonic valves.

Treatment

If the right atrium and right ventricle are not aneurysmally dilated with paper-thin walls, valvuloplasty may be attempted with plication of the anulus of the tricuspid valve by means of nonsurgical techniques in the newborn period in selected cases and undoing of the pulmonary atresia. Eighty percent of the cases were below the age of 2 days. Thus, the marked enlargement of the heart as a result of tremendous tricuspid insufficiency appears to have occurred during intrauterine life. If the diagnosis is made in intrauterine life, one may think in terms of a balloon valvuloplasty of the pulmonic valve. Efforts should be made to diagnose this entity by means of fetal echocardiography early in fetal life that may help develop methodologies or modalities to prevent the enlargement of the right-sided chambers and the tricuspid valve at an appropriate time as well as aiming toward maintaining the patency of the pulmonic valve.

The genes that are responsible for the normal development of the tricuspid and pulmonic valves may be faulty to start with, and/or a tendency for abnormal development of these valves may be present in some who are genetically predisposed. In some, this anomaly may be related to Ebstein's anomaly of the tricuspid valve.

Future research in these areas at the molecular-genetic level may help in understanding this anomaly.

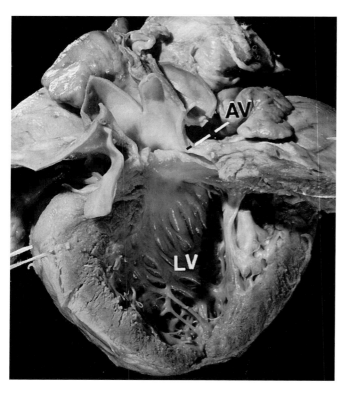

Figure 1: Dysplastic unicuspid aortic valve with aortic and mitral stenosis. AV = irregularly thickened unicuspid aortic valve; LV = hypertrophied left ventricle.

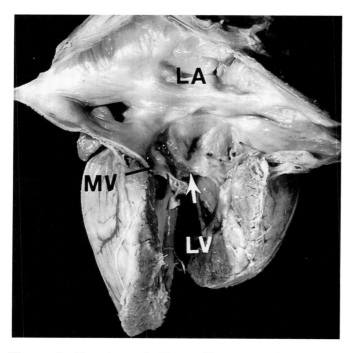

Figure 2: Almost arcade-like malformation of the mitral valve with mitral stenosis and left atrial hypertrophy and enlargement. LA = hypertrophy and enlargement of the left atrium; MV = small mitral with sheet of tissue with practically no chordal connections; LV = left ventricle. Arrow points to the incomplete arcade-like malformation of the mitral valve

Associated Cardiac Abnormalities

	No of Cases
Diffuse fibroelastosis of the left ventricle	10
Focal thickening and fibroelastosis	5
Atrial septal defect of fossa ovalis type, large	1
Fossa ovalis defect	9
Patent foramen ovale	5
Closed foramen ovale in a 6-day-old infant	1
Aneurysm of the fossa ovalis	1
Straddling inferior vena cava	1
Pulmonary hypertension	1
Wide patent ductus arteriosus	10
Probe patent ductus arteriosus	4
Hypoplasia of the transverse arch with coarctation of the aorta	3
Small ascending aorta	7
Ascending aorta, large	4

The coronary arteries were normal in all.

Comment

Although this entity could very well be grouped under the title of aortic stenosis in infancy, we chose to discuss this entity separately. The aortic valve was almost always abnormally formed, similar to aortic stenosis in infancy. However, in contrast to aortic stenosis in infancy, the mitral valve in this entity has markedly abbreviated chordae in all. The mitral valve was smaller than normal in all; the valve presented valvular tissue, abbreviated chordae, and papillary muscles. This we believe is a differentiating factor from aortic stenosis in infancy where the mitral valve may be normally formed. In this entity there is a tendency for the mitral valve to be an incomplete arcade-like formation. The left atrium and left ventricle are either hypertrophied and enlarged or hypertrophied in practically all cases with distinct diffuse fibroelastosis of the left ventricle and the left atrium in 10.

These findings suggest that there probably was hemodynamic alteration in the flow of blood at the atrial septal level during intrauterine life which might have played a role in the abnormal formation of the mitral valve. On the other hand, the presence of fibroelastosis in the left ventricle is tempting to hypothesize a viral etiology during embryogenesis of the heart in the later stages. As we have speculated previously, there are a group of genetically predisposed hearts with left-sided lesions that may be related to altered hemodynamics and/or an infective etiology during the later stages of the development. It is also conceivable that this particular entity may be related to abnormal flow at the superior vena caval and/or at the tricuspid

80

Aneurysm of the Coronary Artery with Fistulous Communications with Cardiac Chambers

In this entity, the right or the left coronary artery communicates with the ventricular or an atrial chamber or a venous structure. It, thereby, becomes cirsoid and aneurysmally dilated. The uninvolved coronary artery is usually normal. The aortic sinuses of Valsalva likewise are normally formed. This produces global hypertrophy and enlargement of the heart.

Analysis of Our Material

There was a total of six cases: three females and three males. The youngest was 15 days of age and the oldest was 67 years, with a median of 20 years. In four, the aneurysm of the coronary artery involved the left coronary, and in two it involved the right. The heart was hypertrophied and enlarged in all.

Right Coronary Artery Aneurysm Entering the Right Ventricle

In a 36-day-old male, the heart was hypertrophied and enlarged. The apex was bifid. The right coronary artery was aneurysmally dilated. The ostium itself was somewhat enlarged and it reached the beginning of the posterior wall of the right ventricle where it communicated with the right ventricular cavity (Fig. 1). The distal portion of the right coronary was normal. The right coronary artery was a dominant vessel supplying the posterior wall of the left ventricle. The left coronary artery gave off the anterior descending coronary artery and a small left circumflex coronary artery.

Right Coronary Artery Aneurysm Communicating with the Right Venous System Proximal to the Coronary Sinus

This was in a 67-year-old female who had aneurysmal enlargement of the right coronary artery which proceeded into the posterior wall of the right ventricle terminating in this wall. Here it communicated with the beginning of the coronary sinus. Distal to this, the venous system was tremendously enlarged in the form of a varix. The left coronary artery and its branches were normal (Figs. 2, 3).

Aneurysm of the Left Main and Left Circumflex Coronaries Entering the Left Atrium

In a 52-year-old male, there was cirsoid aneurysm of the left main coronary and circumflex coronary arteries. The left main coronary artery measured approximately 1.5 cm and gave off a somewhat dilated anterior descending coronary artery. It then proceeded into a cirsoid aneurysmally dilated left circumflex coronary artery and proceeded to the crux on the posterior wall where it opened into the left atrium (Figs. 4–6). In its course, it measured approximately 2 cm in greatest diameter. The right coronary artery was normal. There was marked atherosclerosis of the aorta.

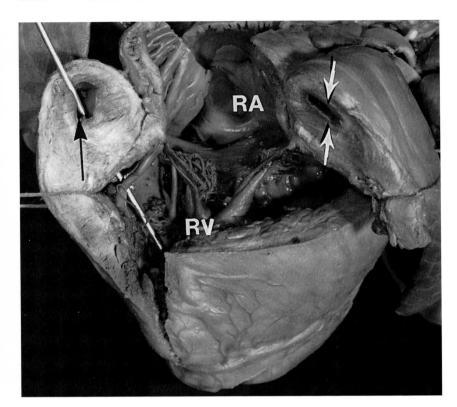

Figure 1: Aneurysmally dilated right coronary artery entering the right ventricle. RA = right atrium; RV = right ventricle. Arrows point to the aneurysmally dilated right coronary artery. Note that the black arrow points to the probe proceeding from the coronary artery into the right ventricle.

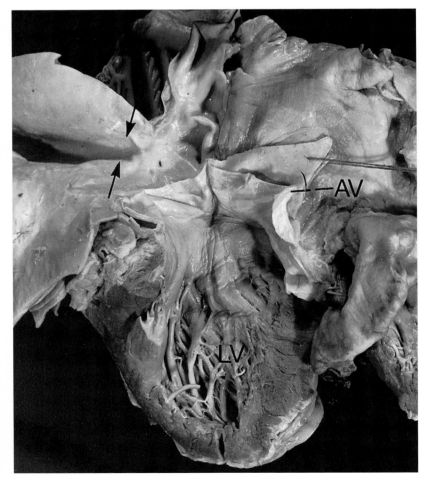

Figure 2: Aneurysmal dilatation of the right coronary artery as seen from the left ventricular and aortic aspect. LV = left ventricle; AV = aortic valve. Arrows point to the aneurysmal dilatation of the right coronary artery.

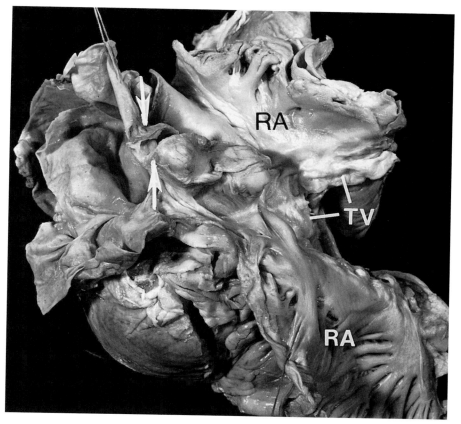

Figure 3: Right atrial view of Figure 2 showing the entry of the aneurysmally dilated right coronary into the coronary sinus. RA = right atrium; TV = tricuspid valve. Arrows point to the entry of the right coronary artery into the coronary sinus.

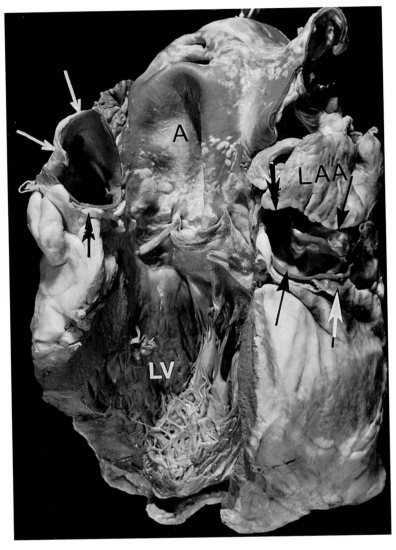

Figure 4: Left ventricular view showing the aneurysm of the left main coronary and the circumflex coronary arteries. A = aorta; LV = left ventricle; LAA = left atrial appendage. Arrows point to the aneurysmally dilated left main coronary artery and the left circumflex coronary artery.

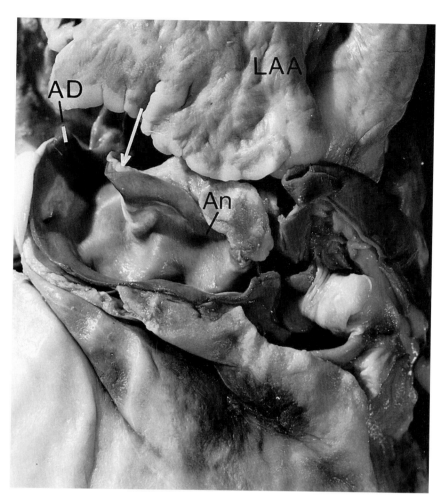

Figure 5: A closer view of the aneurysmal formation of the left main coronary as it proceeds to form the aneurysmal left circumflex coronary artery around the posterior wall. LAA = left atrial appendage; An = aneurysmal dilation of the left circumflex coronary artery; AD = anterior descending coronary artery. Arrow points to the aneurysmal dilatation of the left main coronary artery.

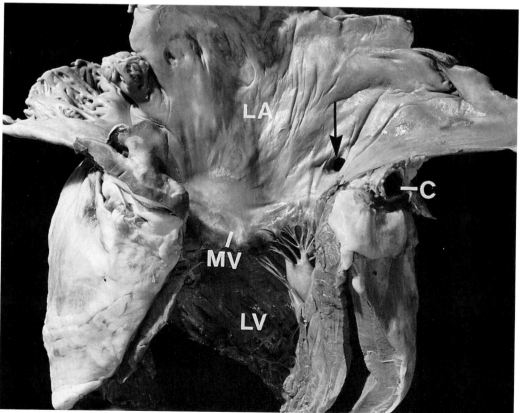

Figure 6: Opening of the left circumflex coronary artery into the left atrium. C = aneurysmally dilated left circumflex; LA = tremendously hypertrophied and enlarged left atrium; MV = mitral valve; LV = left ventricle. Arrow points to the opening of the left circumflex into the left atrium.

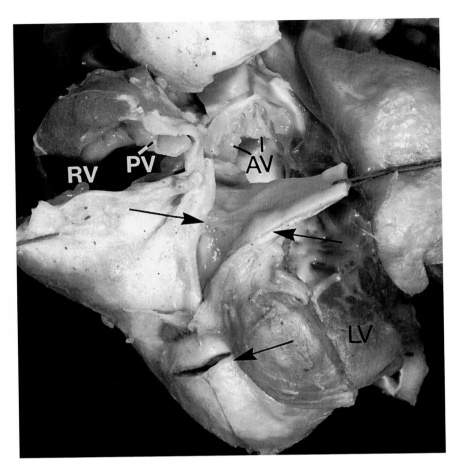

Figure 7: Aneurysmal dilatation of the left main coronary artery and anterior descending coronary artery. AV = aortic valve; PV = pulmonary valve; RV = right ventricle; LV = left ventricle. Arrows point to the aneurysmally dilated left main and anterior descending coronary arteries.

Aneurysm of the Left Main Coronary Artery and Anterior Descending Coronary Artery Entering the Right Ventricle

In a 5-month-old male, the left main coronary artery was huge and led to an aneurysmal dilatation of the anterior descending coronary artery. It proceeded downward into the apex and entered into the lumen of the right ventricle (Figs. 7, 8). The circumflex coronary artery was slightly enlarged and the ascending aorta was somewhat aneurysmally dilated. The left atrium was hypertrophied and the left ventricle was atrophied, with fibroelastosis of the left atrium and left ventricle and marked fibrosis of the myocardium. The associated cardiac abnormality was a widely patent ductus arteriosus.

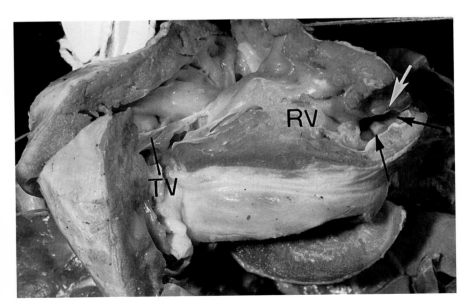

Figure 8: Right ventricular view from the apex demonstrating the opening of the aneurysmal dilatation of the anterior descending coronary artery into the apex of the heart. RV = right ventricle; TV = tricuspid valve. Arrows point to the aneurysmally dilated anterior descending coronary artery entering the right ventricle.

Left Main and Aneurysmally Dilated Left Circumflex Coronary Artery Entering into the Coronary Sinus

This was in a 15-day-old infant who presented with a large left coronary artery and aneurysmally dilated left circumflex coronary artery which entered the coronary sinus. The right-sided chambers were hypertrophied and enlarged and there was atrophy of the left-sided chambers. The associated cardiac abnormalities included hypoplasia of transverse arch with coarctation, patent ductus arteriosus, and an atrial septal defect of fossa ovalis type.

It is, of course, common to have communications between the coronary arterial system and the right ventricular chamber in tricuspid stenosis with pulmonary atresia complex (pulmonary atresia with intact ventricular septum). It is rare, at least, at the gross level, to see such a phenomenon in hypoplasia of the aortic tract complex. One such case is present in this series in which the anterior descending coronary artery communicated with the left ventricle and was thereby aneurysmally dilated.

Aneurysm of Left Main Coronary Artery and Anterior Descending Coronary Artery Communicating with the Left Ventricle

This was in a 5-day-old male infant who died in congestive heart failure. The heart was hypertrophied and enlarged. The limbic margin was displaced close to the superior vena cava proximally. The septum primum was somewhat redundant and formed an aneurysm in the region of the fossa ovalis with a patent foramen ovale (Fig. 9). The tricuspid orifice was greatly enlarged and the septal leaflet was slightly displaced into the right ventricle and was plastered onto the septum (Fig. 9), forming a mild atypical Ebstein-like malformation. The left atrium was hypertrophied with a very small mitral orifice (Fig. 10). The mitral valve was represented by a sheet of tissue with irregular abbrevi-

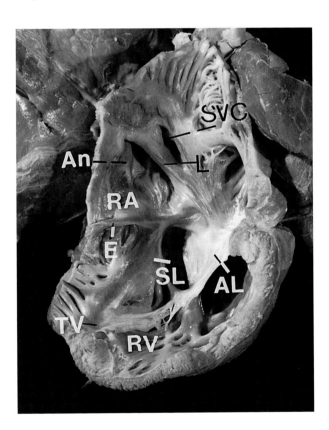

Figure 9: Tremendously hypertrophied right atrium and right ventricle in an infant with hypoplasia of the aortic tract complex and aneurysm of the left main and anterior descending coronary arteries entering into the left ventricle; right atrial, right ventricular view. RA = right atrium; RV = right ventricle; L = limbic margin displaced to the superior vena cava; SVC = superior vena cava; An = aneurysm of the fossa ovalis; E = hypertrophied eustachian valve; TV = tricuspid valve; SL = septal leaflet of the tricuspid valve slightly displaced and is plastered on to the septum; AL = anterior leaflet of the tricuspid valve; RV = markedly hypertrophied and enlarged right ventricle. Note the slight Ebstein-like malformation of the tricuspid valve.

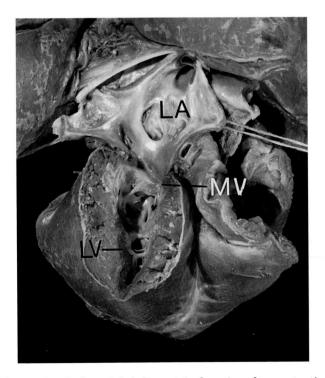

Figure 10: Left atrial, left ventricular view demonstrating the hypoplastic mitral valve with abbreviated chordae and anomalous papillary muscles and small left ventricle and a thick wall with fibroelastosis. LA = left atrium; MV = mitral valve; LV = left ventricle. Note the anomalous chordal and muscle bundles in the left ventricle.

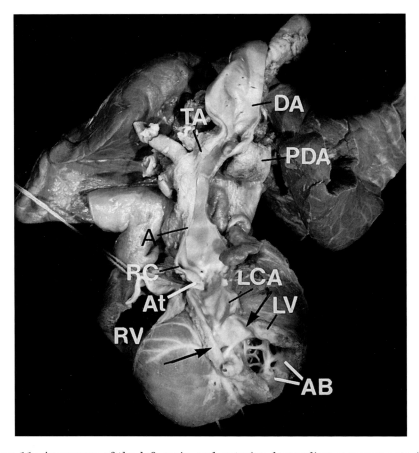

Figure 11: Aneurysm of the left main and anterior descending coronary arteries entering the left ventricle. LV = left ventricle; A = ascending aorta; At = atresia of the aortic valve; RC = ostium of the right coronary artery; LCA = left coronary artery aneurysm; AB = anomalous bands in the left ventricle; RV = right ventricle; DA = descending aorta; PDA = patent ductus arteriosus; TA = transverse arch. Arrows point to the entry of the aneurysm into the left ventricle.

ated chordal connections to anomalous papillary muscles (Fig. 10). The left ventricle was a small chamber, thick walled with fibroelastosis and anomalous chordal extensions throughout. The ascending aorta proceeded to the base of the heart without entering the heart and there was aortic atresia. The right coronary artery was normal. The left main coronary artery formed a large aneurysm and proceeded as an aneurysm of the anterior descending coronary artery which gave off some branches but made direct communication with the left ventricular cavity (Fig. 11). There was no left circumflex coronary artery. There was a wide patent ductus arteriosus.

Comment

The aneurysm of the coronary artery, when it involves the right, may communicate with the coronary sinus or the right ventricle. In both situations, there were no other associated cardiac anomalies and there was

global hypertrophy of the heart. On the other hand, when there is an aneurysm of the left coronary artery, the aneurysm extends either to the left circumflex coronary artery or to the anterior descending coronary artery. When it affected the left circumflex coronary artery, it entered the coronary sinus in one case and the left atrium in the other. In a 52-year-old male, the left circumflex coronary aneurysm had ruptured into the left atrium. On the other hand, in the 15-day-old infant, the left circumflex coronary artery was dilated, tortuous, and entered the coronary sinus. In an infant with hypoplasia of the aortic tract complex (aortic atresia), the aneurysm of the left main and the anterior descending coronary arteries entered the left ventricle with fibroelastosis of the chamber. In one 5-month-old infant, the left coronary artery was larger than normal. The aneurysmal dilatation of the anterior descending coronary artery entered the apex of the right ventricle with marked fibrosis of the myocardium.

It is thus clear that when there is an aneurysm of

the anterior descending or circumflex coronary artery, it may enter the left atrium, coronary sinus, right ventricle, or left ventricle. When the artery communicates with the right ventricle, it produces a tremendous amount of fibrosis in this chamber and in the ventricular septum, and atrophy of the left-sided chambers. When seen in infants, there appears to be a tendency for associated cardiac anomalies such as patent ductus arteriosus, atrial septal defect, and coarctation of the aorta and rarely hypoplasia of aortic tract complex occur to occur. Surgical or nonsurgical methods of closing the communicating fistula should be undertaken before hypertrophy, atrophy, or fibrosis and/or fibroelastosis of the ventricular myocardium occurs. It is also important to delineate the type of coronary artery system before corrective procedures.

81

Abnormal Course or Narrowing of the Pulmonary Trunk and Its Branches

In this anomaly, one pulmonary artery may be dominant. The other may emerge from the dominant vessel behind the trachea, or one vessel may take a long course. This produces hypertrophy and enlargement of the right-sided chambers.

Analysis of Our Material

There was a total of four cases: two males and two females. The ages were 2 days, 1 month 3 days, 6 months 10 days, and 6½ months.

The Complex

The heart was hypertrophied and enlarged in three. The apex was formed by the left ventricle in three and by both ventricles in one. The right atrium and right ventricle were hypertrophied and enlarged in three and hypertrophied in one. The left atrium and left ventricle were hypertrophied and enlarged in two and were of normal size in two. The tricuspid orifice was enlarged in three and normal in one. The pulmonic orifice was enlarged in two and normal in two. The mitral orifice was normal in three and enlarged in one. The aortic orifice was enlarged in three and somewhat smaller than normal in one. The tricuspid valve was normally formed in three. In one the chordae were markedly abbreviated with several accessory small papillary muscles. The mitral and aortic valves were normally formed in all. The endocardium showed focal changes.

Morphology of the Pulmonary Arteries

In one the main pulmonary artery proceeded directly as the left pulmonary artery, and the right lung was supplied by an aberrant pulmonary branch which presumably came from the left. In the second, the main pulmonary trunk proceeded directly as the right pulmonary artery, and the left pulmonary artery emerged from the right pulmonary artery close to its junction with the main pulmonary trunk, took a course between the trachea and esophagus, and proceeded to the left lung. In this case there was a spontaneously closing very small ventricular septal defect and a patent ductus arteriosus. In the third heart, the main pulmonary trunk proceeded as a huge left pulmonary artery. This took a course behind the trachea and behind the tracheal bifurcation and ended in the left lung. Along its course, it gave off a small right pulmonary artery (Figs. 1–4). This was associated with a large left and a very small collapsed right lung and a patent ductus arteriosus. In the fourth case, a 2-day-old infant, the origin of the right pulmonary artery was located posterolaterally on the left side which resulted in a long course of this artery. The right pulmonary artery, as it reached the tracheal bifurcation, divided off into two arteries; one proceeded in front of the bronchi and supplied all the lobes, and the other branch proceeded between the tracheal bifurcation, behind the right side of the bronchus, and supplied the right upper lobe. The ductus arteriosus was widely patent. There was an atrial septal defect, fossa ovalis type, in all four cases.

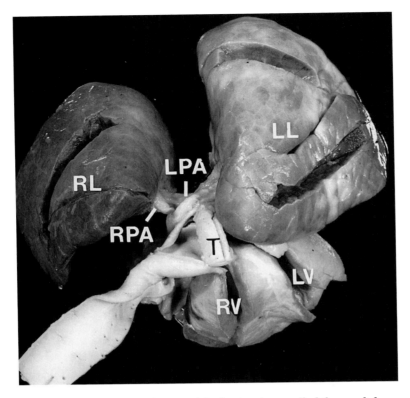

Figure 1: External view of the heart with the trachea pulled forward demonstrating the large left pulmonary artery coursing behind the trachea and a small right pulmonary artery originating from the left. RL = right lung, small collapsed; LL = left lung; RV = right ventricle; LV = left ventricle; T = trachea; LPA = left pulmonary artery, coursing at the tracheal bifurcation proceeding to the left lung; RPA = small right pulmonary artery.

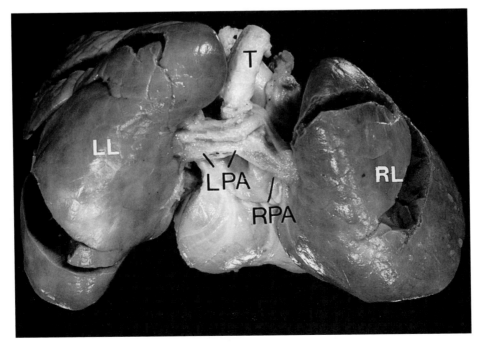

Figure 2: Posterior view of Figure 1 demonstrating the large left pulmonary artery behind the trachea. T = trachea; LL = left lung; RL = small right lung; LPA = large left pulmonary artery; RPA = small right pulmonary artery.

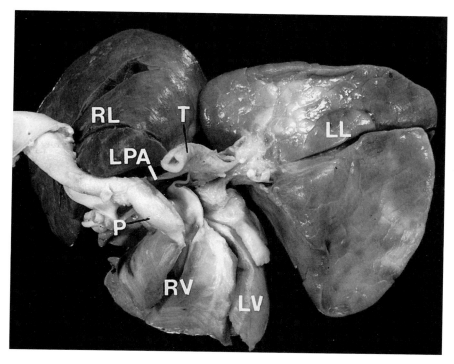

Figure 3: External view of Figures 1 and 2 demonstrating the main pulmonary artery proceeding as the left pulmonary artery. RV = right ventricle; LV = left ventricle; P = main pulmonary trunk; LPA = left pulmonary artery; T = trachea; LL = left lung; RL = right lung. Note the main pulmonary trunk proceeding behind the trachea.

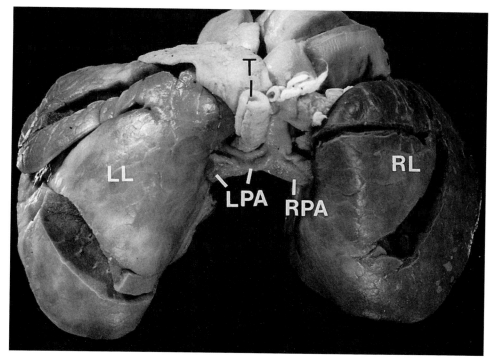

Figure 4: Posterosuperior view of Figures 1–3 demonstrating the pulmonary artery sling created by the large left pulmonary artery as it proceeds behind the tracheal bifurcation to reach the left lung. T = trachea; LL = left lung; RL = right lung; LPA = left pulmonary artery; RPA = right pulmonary artery.

Comment

The size and shape of the pulmonary arteries varied considerably. Likewise, the smaller pulmonary artery was associated with a smaller lung.

It is of interest that in all four cases, there was an atrial septal defect and a patent ductus arteriosus, and in one there was a small spontaneously closing ventricular septal defect. It is evident that the exact anatomy (the size and shape) of the origin and distribution of the two pulmonary arteries and its relationship to the trachea, bronchi, lungs, and esophagus should be well delineated before undertaking any corrective procedures.

82

Origin of a Pulmonary Artery from the Ascending Aorta (Hemitruncus)

In this entity, there is absence of one of the pulmonary arteries (Fig. 1). This artery is given off from the ascending aorta (Fig. 2) or the transverse arch. The artery that usually emerges from the ascending aorta is the right pulmonary artery. When it comes from the arch, it emerges from or close to the base of the innominate artery (Fig. 2). There are two types: those without associated cardiac anomalies and those with.

Isolated Origin of a Pulmonary Artery from the Ascending Aorta

In this type, the ascending aorta usually gives off the right pulmonary artery, while the main pulmonary trunk emerging from the right ventricle proceeds to the left lung. Here, there is a left aortic arch. Because of the left-to-right shunt, there is left atrial and left ventricular hypertrophy. There is also right atrial and ventricular hypertrophy related, probably, to the increased flow into the left lung.

Origin of a Pulmonary Artery from the Ascending Aorta with Associated Cardiac Abnormalities

With Patent Ductus Arteriosus

Here again the ascending aorta gives off the right pulmonary artery with a left aortic arch.

With Tetralogy of Fallot

Unlike the previous types, these are usually with a right aortic arch with the left pulmonary artery arising from the aorta. Rarely, the right pulmonary artery may be absent and the blood supply may come off from the aorta. The hypertrophy and enlargement of the heart resembles that of a classic tetralogy of Fallot despite the fact that there is a built-in left-to-right shunt.

With Double Outlet Right Ventricle with Subaortic Ventricular Septal Defect

Here there will be global hypertrophy of the heart.

Analysis of Our Material

There was a total of 13 cases: eight females and five males. The youngest was a newborn, 11 hours old, and the oldest was 7 years, with an average age of 2 years, 1 month.

Comment

The heart was hypertrophied and enlarged in all. The apex was formed by both ventricles in 38%, by the left ventricle in 31% (Fig. 3), and by the right ventricle in 31%. The right atrium and right ventricle were hypertrophied and enlarged in 70% (Fig. 4), normal in size in 15%, and hypertrophied in 15%. The left atrium was hypertrophied and enlarged in 54% (Fig. 5), normal in size in 23%, smaller than normal in 15% (Fig. 6), and atrophied in 8%. The left ventricle was hypertrophied and enlarged in 46% (Fig. 7), normal in size in 23%, and smaller than normal in 31% (Fig. 8). The tricuspid orifice was enlarged in 46%, smaller than nor-

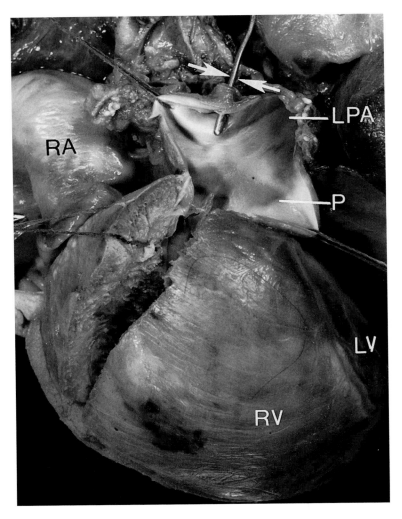

Figure 1: Absent right pulmonary artery, the main pulmonary trunk proceeding directly to the left lung with a small patent ductus arteriosus. RV = right ventricle; LV = left ventricle; P = pulmonary trunk; LPA = left pulmonary artery; RA = right atrium. Arrows point to the probe passing through the small ductus arteriosus. Note the absence of the right pulmonary artery. Note also the tremendous right ventricular hypertrophy and apex formed by the right ventricle.

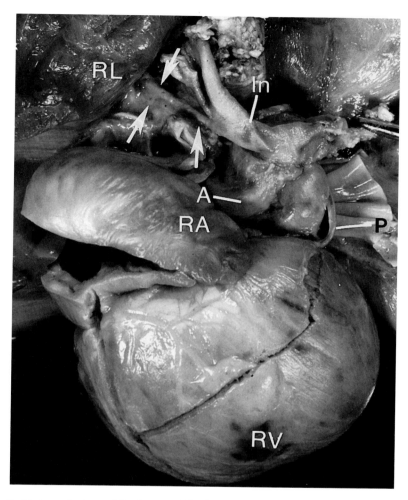

Figure 2: External view of the heart with absent right pulmonary artery and origin of a vessel emerging from the base of the innominate artery proceeding to the right lung. Note the tremendous hypertrophy of the heart with the apex formed by the right ventricle. RA = markedly hypertrophied and enlarged right atrium; RV = right ventricle; P = pulmonary trunk; A = ascending aorta; RL = right lung; In = innominate artery. Arrows point to the vessel emerging from the base of the innominate artery proceeding to the right lung with occlusion.

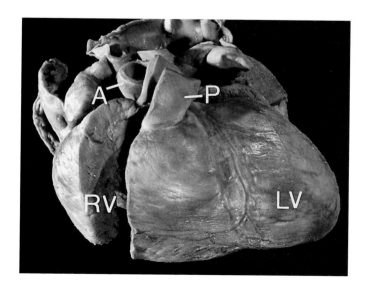

Figure 3: External view of the heart from a case of hemitruncus demonstrating the hypertrophied and enlarged heart with the apex formed by the left ventricle and marked right ventricular hypertrophy. RV = right ventricle; LV = left ventricle; P = pulmonary trunk; A = aorta. (Used with permission from Lev M, Bharati S. See Figure 10.)

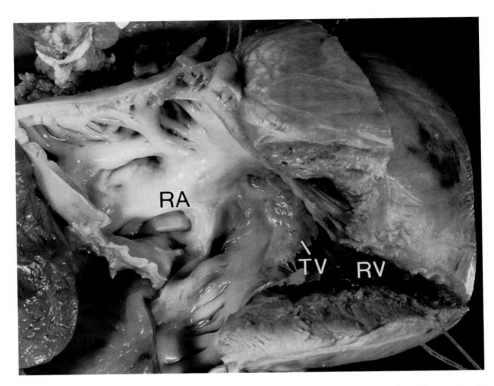

Figure 4: Right atrial, right ventricular view demonstrating tremendous hypertrophy and enlargement of the right-sided chambers. RA = right atrium; RV = right ventricle; TV = tricuspid valve.

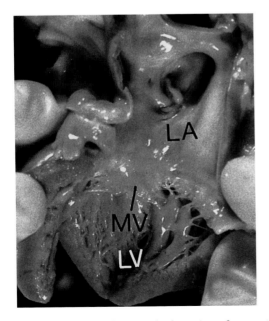

Figure 5: Left atrial, left ventricular view demonstrating the enlarged left side of the heart. LA = left atrium; MV = mitral valve; LV = left ventricle.

mal in 31%, and normal in size in 23%. The pulmonic orifice size was enlarged in 46%, smaller than normal in 38%, normal in size in 8%, and very small in 8%. The mitral orifice was normal in size in 46%, smaller than normal in 31%, and enlarged in 23%. The aortic orifice was normal in size in 54%, enlarged in 31%, and smaller than normal in 15%.

The Valves

Tricuspid Valve

In general, it was normally formed and showed increased hemodynamic change (Fig. 4). The valve was considerably thickened with anomalous papillary muscles which proceeded to the base of the valve in 3.

Pulmonic Valve

In general, the pulmonic valve was normally formed and presented either increased or the usual hemodynamic change. The pulmonic orifice size was very small in one, in one it was bicuspid, markedly

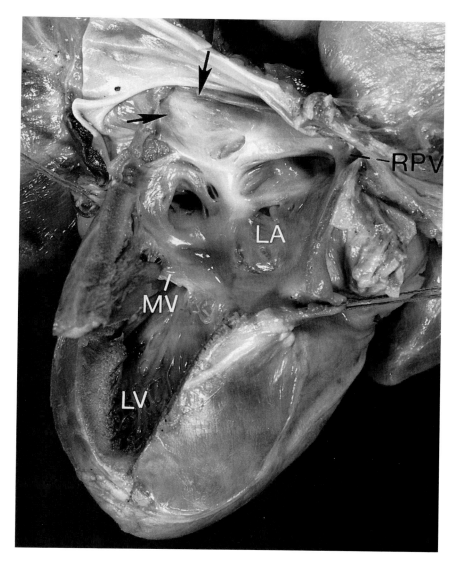

Figure 6: Left atrial, left ventricular view demonstrating the large left pulmonary veins and the small left ventricle. LA = left atrium; MV = mitral valve; LV = left ventricle; RPV = right pulmonary veins entering the left atrium. Arrows point to the large left pulmonary veins.

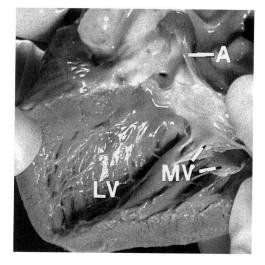

Figure 7: Left ventricular view demonstrating the enlarged left ventricle. LV = left ventricle; MV = mitral valve; A = aorta.

thickened, and irregular, in one the valve was shortened with prominent longitudinal commissures, and the valve was absent in one.

Mitral Valve

The mitral valve was normally formed and presented either increased or normal hemodynamic change. A blood cyst was seen in one.

Aortic Valve

The aortic valve was normally formed and presented either increased or the usual hemodynamic change.

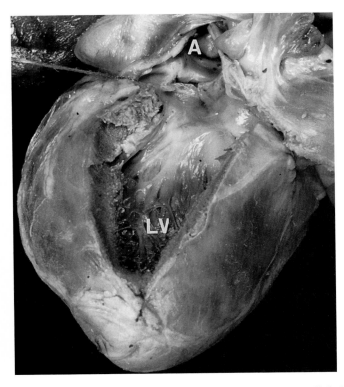

Figure 8: Left ventricular view demonstrating small left ventricle with intact ventricular septum. LV = left ventricle; A = aorta.

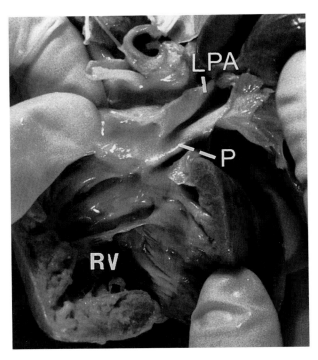

Figure 9: Absent right pulmonary artery in a case of hemitruncus; right ventricular outflow tract view demonstrating the main pulmonary trunk proceeding directly to the left lung. RV = right ventricular hypertrophy and enlargement; P = main pulmonary trunk; LPA = left pulmonary artery.

Isolated Absence of Right Pulmonary Artery (Fig. 9)

There were four cases with the right pulmonary artery emerging from the ascending aorta (Fig. 10) which proceeded directly to the right lung. Their ages were 3 months, 11 hours, 28 days, and 5 months, 21 days. This was associated with a wide patent ductus in one, probe patent ductus arteriosus in two, and markedly elongated and circuitous patent ductus in one.

In one case, a vessel from the base of the innominate artery proceeded to the right lung which was occluded. In another, the patent ductus emerged from the innominate artery and proceeded to the right lung and the left pulmonary artery proceeded upward in an abnormal fashion. In one, the transverse arch gave off two carotid arteries and the two subclavian arteries. From the base of the proximal carotid artery, a tortuous vessel (ductus arteriosus) proceeded to the right lung and the left ductus was closed.

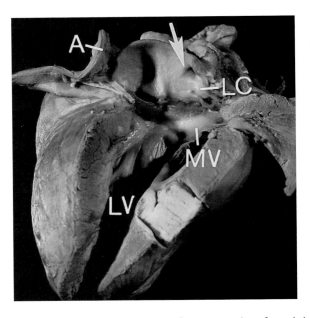

Figure 10: Left ventricular view demonstrating the origin of the anomalous vessel emerging from the ascending aorta. LV = left ventricle; MV = mitral valve; A = ascending aorta; LC = left coronary emerging above the posterior sinus of Valsalva. Arrow points to the origin of the anomalous vessel from the ascending aorta. (Used with permission from Lev M, Bharati S: Transposition of arterial trunks in levocardia. In *Cardiovascular Pathology Decennial 1966–1975*, Ed. SC Sommers, Appleton-Century Crofts, NY, 1975, pp 1–46.)

Right Pulmonary Artery Emerging from the Ascending Aorta with Ventricular Septal Defect and Patent Ductus Arteriosus

In this series, there was one case with isolated ventricular septal defect with patent ductus arteriosus.

Aorticopulmonary Septal Defect with Fetal Coarctation (hypoplasia of transverse arch with coarctation) (Figs. 11–13)

There was one case where the right pulmonary artery was absent and a vessel emerged from the ascending aorta and proceeded to the right lung. In addition, there was a patent ductus arteriosus.

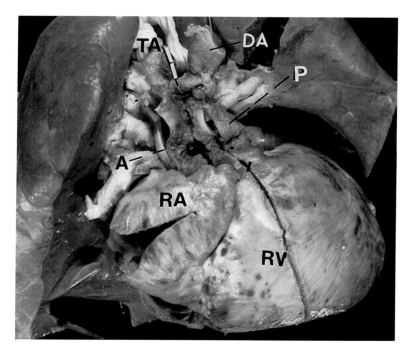

Figure 11: Hemitruncus with aorticopulmonary septal defect and fetal coarctation with surgical repair; external view of the heart. Note the hypertrophied and enlarged heart with the apex formed by both ventricles. RA = right atrium; RV = right ventricle; A = small ascending aorta; P = larger pulmonary trunk; DA = descending aorta; TA = transverse arch.

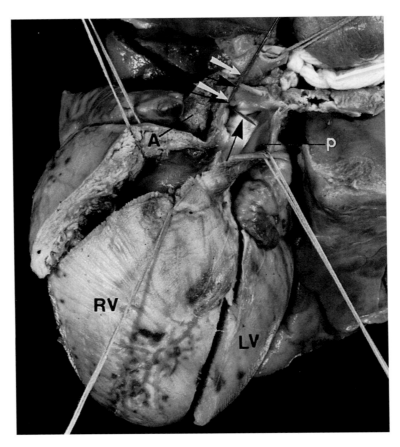

Figure 12: External view of Figure 11 demonstrating the aorticopulmonary septal defect and origin of the right pulmonary artery from the aortic segment. RV = right ventricle; LV = left ventricle; A = aorta; P = pulmonary trunk. The black arrow indicates the probe passing through the aorticopulmonary septal defect. The white arrows indicate the probe passing from the aortic segment to the right pulmonary artery.

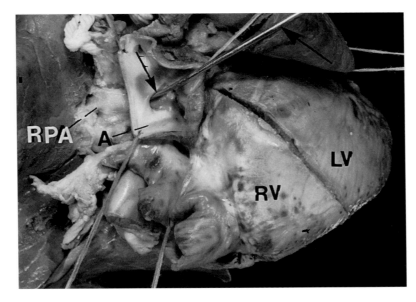

Figure 13: External view of Figures 11 and 12 with an opened aorta demonstrating the origin of the right pulmonary artery from the posterior aspect of the aorta. RV = right ventricle; LV = left ventricle; A = ascending aorta; RPA = right pulmonary artery. Arrow points to the probe passing from the aorta to the right pulmonary artery.

Tetralogy of Fallot with Anomalous Blood Supply from the Ascending Aorta with Absence of One Pulmonary Artery

There were three cases, two with absent left pulmonary artery and one with absent right pulmonary artery. In one, there was a markedly thickened pulmonic valve with absence of the right pulmonary artery. There was a right aortic arch with a vascular ring and the left subclavian artery emerged from the patent ductus arteriosus. A large vessel emerged from the ascending aorta and supplied the right lung (Figs. 14, 15).

In one case with bicuspid pulmonic valve and right aortic arch with absence of left pulmonary artery, an anomalous vessel from the ascending aorta proceeded as the left pulmonary artery. In this case there was also tricuspid stenosis. In the third case of tetralogy of Fallot with absent pulmonic valve, there was absence of the left pulmonary artery with aneurysmal dilatation of the main pulmonary trunk, and the right pulmonary artery and another vessel emerged proximal to the region of the ductus and supplied the left lung.

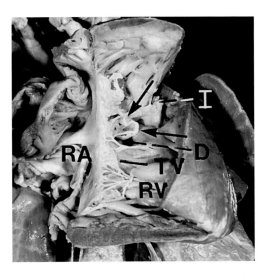

Figure 15: Right atrial, right ventricular view of Figure 14 demonstrating the ventricular septal defect and infundibular narrowing. RA = right atrium; RV = right ventricle; D = ventricular septal defect; TV = tricuspid valve; I = infundibular pulmonary narrowing. Arrows indicate the excess of tricuspid valvular tissue overlying the defect.

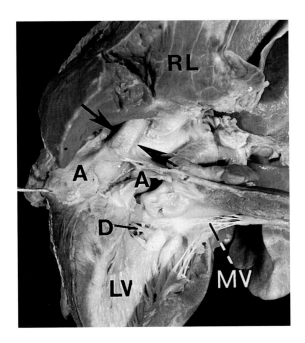

Figure 14: Tetralogy of Fallot with right aortic arch and absent right pulmonary artery and large vessel emerging from the base of the aorta proceeding to the right lung directly; left ventricular view. LV = left ventricle; MV = mitral valve; D = ventricular septal defect; A = aorta pulled forward to demonstrate the large vessel emerging from the base of the aorta; RL = right lung. Arrows point to the vessel proceeding to the right lung. Note the tricuspid valve attached to a varying degree along the rim of the ventricular septal defect.

Double Outlet Right Ventricle with Subaortic Ventricular Septal Defect and Marked Pulmonary Stenosis (Fig. 16)

There was one case with a right aortic arch, with absence of right pulmonary artery. A large vessel emerged from the ascending aorta and proceeded to the right lung, and the left lung was supplied by large bronchial arteries.

Associated Cardiac Abnormalities

In addition to the above-mentioned major cardiac anomalies, four cases had a fossa ovalis atrial septal defect and seven had a patent foramen ovale. In two, there was high origin of the left coronary ostium. In one the coronary ostia emerged above the posterior commissure, and in the other the ostia emerged close to the posterior commissure.

Comment

When there is an anomalous blood supply from the ascending aorta to the lung with absence of one pulmonary artery, it appears that the right pulmonary artery is usually absent. This type of pattern occurs without ventricular septal defect and, in general, without other associated major cardiac anomalies. On the other hand, when absence of a pulmonary artery occurs

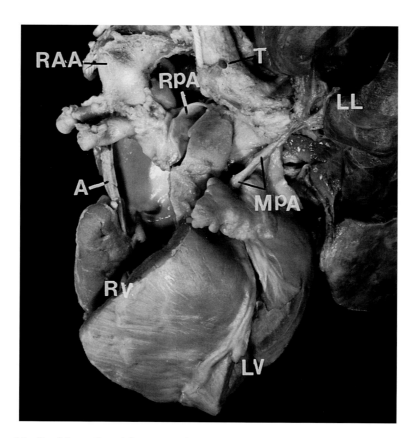

Figure 16: Double outlet right ventricle with marked pulmonary stenosis and absent right pulmonary artery with the main pulmonary trunk proceeding as a cord-like structure to the left lung. A huge vessel emerges from the aorta proceeding to the right lung. RV = right ventricle; LV = left ventricle; T = trachea; RAA = right aortic arch; A = ascending aorta; RPA = right pulmonary artery proceeding from the ascending aorta; MPA = minute main pulmonary trunk proceeding as a left pulmonary artery; LL = left lung.

in tetralogy of Fallot, it appears that the left pulmonary artery seems to be the one that is absent and rarely the right pulmonary artery. It is of interest that hemitruncus may occur in isolated ventricular septal defect, aorticopulmonary septal defect with coarctation of the aorta, and double outlet right ventricle with subaortic ventricular septal defect.

Although the ascending aorta has a tendency to supply the right lung, the size of the vessel that proceeds to the right lung varies considerably. From this material it is clear that the vessel can be large or small or can even be occluded. On the other hand, the vessel may originate from the base of the innominate artery (presumed ductus arteriosus) accompanied or not ac-

companied by a left-sided ductus to the left lung. The ductus arteriosus, likewise, can be small or tortuous, elongated, or sometimes large. It is of interest that in addition to the variation in size and supply of the vessel emerging from the ascending aorta or from the transverse arch of the aorta, one can find bronchial vessels supplying the other lung.

All of the above features suggests that before any surgical correction is contemplated, a very careful analysis of the blood supply to all of the lobes of the lung must be explored thoroughly. It appears that one lobe of the lung could be perfused less and the other more. Thus, there is considerable variation in the blood supply to each lobe of the lung in this entity.

83

Anomalous Blood Supply of a Lung from the Thoracic or Abdominal Aorta

In this entity, the main pulmonary artery and its branches are given off normally. However, there is an abnormal blood supply to the right lung either from the abdominal aorta or the thoracic aorta. This may be accompanied by anomalous pulmonary venous entry to the lung. This group of hearts may be considered as part of a spectrum of scimitar syndrome. The abnormal hemodynamics result in global hypertrophy of the heart.

Analysis of Our Material

There was a total of three cases; all were females. The ages were 3 months, 4 months, and 7 months.

The Complex

The heart was hypertrophied and enlarged. The apex was formed by the left ventricle in two and by both ventricles in one. The valves were normally formed. The endocardium showed focal thickening and whitening.

In a 7-month-old infant, the two right pulmonary veins were absent. An anomalous vessel from the lower abdominal aorta and a vein from the inferior vena cava entered the right lung. Hypertrophy and enlargement of the right-sided chambers with distinct fibroelastosis were present, and a patent foramen ovale was present.

In a 3-month-old infant, atypical branches of the intercostal arteries and the internal mammary artery entered the right lung. This was not accompanied by any veins. Hypertrophy and enlargement of the left-sided chambers and a probe patent foramen ovale were present.

In a 4-month-old infant, the lower right pulmonary veins drained into the inferior vena cava, and an anomalous vessel from the descending aorta supplied the lower right lobe. This was associated with a patent ductus arteriosus. Hypertrophy and enlargement were present in all of the chambers.

Comment

The only common denominator in the above three cases is the involvement of the right lung. In two, the entire right lung was involved. In one, where it was accompanied by an anomalous vein, there was absence of the two right pulmonary veins. In the last case, the right lower pulmonary veins drained into the inferior vena cava. In addition to the normal pulmonary artery supply to the lung, there was a branch from the descending aorta to the right lower lobe.

Embryogenesis

The inferior vena cava develops from a fusion of various parts, the vitellines, the subcardinals, and the supracardinals. One of the sources for the development of pulmonary veins is from a presplanchnic source. This consists of a channel formed from the confluence of the vascular plexus of the lung which extends to the middle part of the sinus venosus. It is therefore conceivable that various types of venous communications can occur in an anomalous manner during the process of development of the various venous channels.

If there is an anomalous pulmonary venous return of more than one vein, this should be corrected. If this is associated with a marked abnormal, huge blood supply to the lung or to one lobe of the lung, it would be wise to ligate the anomalous artery by means of surgical or nonsurgical techniques. Although in all of these cases there is normal pulmonary arterial supply to both lungs, a thorough examination of the arterial and venous supply to both lungs should be undertaken if there is scimitar syndrome. One should rule out sequestration of the lung or a lobe or a part of the lung. The effects of the blood supply, whether it involves only part of the lobe, an entire lobe, or an entire lung, must be studied carefully before undertaking any corrective methods.

84

Double Heart

When two hearts fuse together, the term double heart is used. A double heart is seen in Siamese twins. The fused single heart from the fusion of the Siamese twins is always a complicated heart associated with common atrium, common AV orifice, and complete transposition (Figs. 1–3).

Analysis of Our Material

There were seven pairs of Siamese twins, all females. The heart had a bizarre shape in all. Of the seven double hearts, four hearts will be discussed in some detail.

1. a. single large atrium
   b. three AV orifices
   c. two right ventricles and one left ventricle
   d. abnormal arteries and veins could not be identified.
2. Common atrium for both hearts
   A. Left heart
      a. partially divided atrium
      b. single ventricle small outlet chamber with complete transposition
   B. Right heart, partially divided atrium.
3. This was a case of 36-weeks' gestation stillbirth Siamese twins, female.
   A. Right-sided heart
      a. double outlet right ventricle with common AV canal type of ventricular septal defect and straddling tricuspid orifice and pulmonary stenosis
      b. left superior vena cava entering the coronary sinus
      c. absence of the left side
   B. Left-sided heart
      a. complete transposition, with ventricular septal defect and straddling tricuspid orifice, patent ductus arteriosus, atrial septal defect, fossa ovalis type.

4. Eighteen weeks' gestation Siamese twins (abortion). There was a common atrium, common AV orifice, with truncus arteriosus emerging from the morphological right ventricle, and complete transposition with pulmonary atresia. From the morphological left ventricle no vessel emerged. At the left base of the heart from a small outlet chamber emerged the aorta accompanied by an atretic pulmonary trunk to the right and posterior.

In this case, the Siamese twins were joined together at the midline, and the lungs differentiated into pairs with a distinct trachea of their own. The atrial appendages differentiated into four structures; however, the atria from one heart joined the atria of the other heart by means of a common atrium. The common atrium communicated by means of a common AV orifice with a well-differentiated ventricular mass. From the morphological right ventricle emerged the truncus and from the morphological left ventricle by way of a small outlet chamber emerged an aorta with pulmonary atresia. In other words, ventricular mass did not divide off into two separate hearts, although from the standpoint of atrial appendages, there was an attempt in division of four atrial chambers.

From the above, it is clear that the fused double heart has no distinct four chambers for each heart. In general, one finds a common atrium and either a common AV orifice or a straddling AV valve. The atrioventricular valves, likewise, have not separated off into two sets of tricuspid and two sets of mitral valves. More importantly, the ventricular mass has not separated off into distinct right ventricular and left ventricular morphology for each heart. Although there is a tendency for one ventricular chamber to be predominantly the right ventricle, and the other two ventricular chambers may be consisting of one other right ventricle and one left ventricle, there is no clear evidence for another morphologically left ventricle.

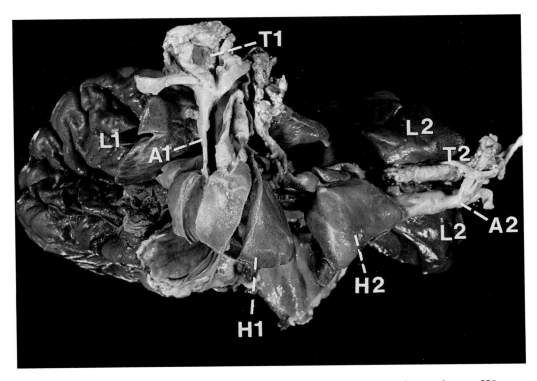

Figure 1: Double heart in Siamese twins—external view. H1 = larger heart; H2 = smaller heart; L1 = lungs for the larger heart; L2 = lungs for the smaller heart; T1 and T2 = trachea 1 and 2; A1 = aorta for the larger heart; A2 = aorta for the smaller heart.

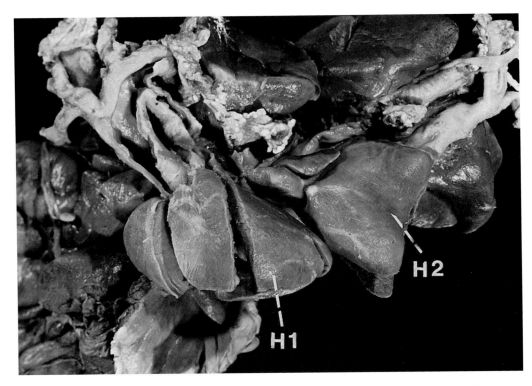

Figure 2: Close-up of Figure 1. H1 = heart #1—larger; H2 = heart #2—smaller.

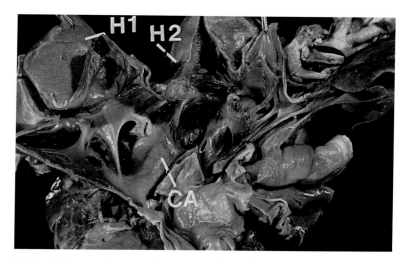

Figure 3: Double heart showing common atrium. CA = common atrium; H1 and H2 = heart #1 and #2.

Comment

Although today there are attempts being made to separate Siamese twins, it would be very difficult to separate one heart from the other. If one of the twins is sacrificed and the other is to retain the fused double heart, it would be almost impossible to create a fourth chambered heart.

85

Primary Pulmonary Hypertension

General Statement

This complex is basically diagnosed clinically. The right atrium and right ventricle are markedly hypertrophied and occasionally enlarged (Fig. 1). The enlargement involves the pulmonary trunk. The left side of the heart is normal or atrophied (Fig. 2) and occasionally the aorta is hypoplastic.

The apex is usually formed by the right ventricle and occasionally by both ventricles. Immense cardiomegaly may be seen occasionally (Fig. 3). The left atrium is usually normal, although it is occasionally small or even enlarged. The tricuspid and pulmonary valves are enlarged. The tricuspid valve, in general, is normally formed and shows increased hemodynamic change. Occasionally, the valve is thickened with accessory papillary muscles. Rarely, there may be an accessory opening with tricuspid insufficiency (Fig. 4). The pulmonic valve usually presents increased hemodynamic change. Rarely, supravalvular stenosis and poststenotic dilatation of the pulmonary trunk, with calcification and thinning of the pulmonary arteries, may be found (Figs. 5, 6). The mitral valve is normally formed but the posterior leaflet may be ballooned-out and thickened in the older age group (Fig. 7). The endocardium of the right atrium and the right ventricle may show focal thickening and whitening, or diffuse fibroelastosis may be present.

Analysis of Our Material

There were 18 cases. All were clinically diagnosed as having primary pulmonary hypertension. There were 11 females and seven males. Eleven were white, four were black, two were Oriental, and one was unknown. The youngest was 4 months of age and the oldest was 32 years of age. Thirteen were beyond the age of 10. The average age was 13 years, 9 months, 7 days.

The heart was always hypertrophied with the apex formed by the right ventricle in 12 and by both ventri-

cles in six. The right atrium and the right ventricle were hypertrophied and enlarged in 14 and hypertrophied in four. The left atrium was normal in eight, small in four, atrophied in two, hypertrophied in two, and hypertrophied and/or enlarged in two. The left ventricle was small in five, atrophied in three, normal in three, enlarged in three, hypertrophied and enlarged in three, and hypertrophied in one.

The Valves

The tricuspid and pulmonic orifices were enlarged in the majority of the cases and occasionally were normal in size. The mitral orifice was normal in 10 and smaller than normal in eight. The aortic orifice was small in eight, normal in eight, and enlarged in two. The tricuspid valve, in general, was normally formed and showed increased hemodynamic change. It was thickened with papillary muscles anchored to the base of the valve in three. In one there was an accessory opening with tricuspid insufficiency. The valve was mitralized in two. The pulmonary valve was normal in all, but showed increased hemodynamic change. In one there was additional supravalvular pulmonary stenosis, poststenotic dilatation of the main pulmonary trunk with calcification, and paper-thin pulmonary arteries.

The mitral valve was normally formed, but was thickened and showed ballooning of the posterior leaflet in the older age group. The aortic valve was normally formed and was fenestrated in one.

Endocardium

In general, the right atrium and right ventricle showed focal or sometimes diffuse thickening and whitening. The marked right ventricular hypertrophy may produce a bulge into the left ventricle cavity in some cases (Fig. 8).

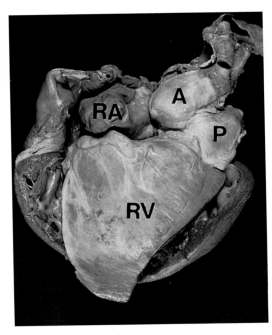

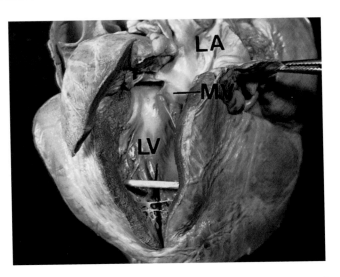

Figure 2: Left side of the heart from Figure 1. Note the small left atrium and small left ventricle with small mitral valve. LA = left atrium; MV = mitral valve; LV = left ventricle.

Figure 1: External view of the heart from a classic case of primary pulmonary hypertension. Note the apex formed by the right ventricle. RV = right ventricle; P = pulmonary trunk; A = aorta; RA = right atrium.

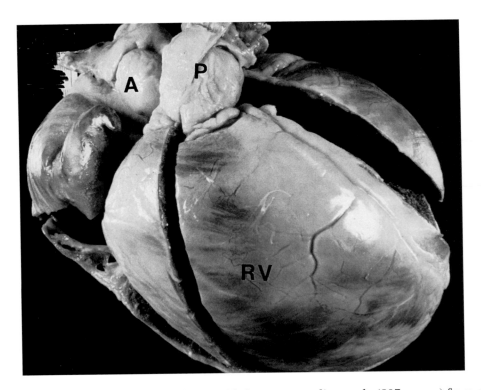

Figure 3: External view of the heart with immense cardiomegaly (807 grams) from a 29-year-old with clinically diagnosed primary pulmonary hypertension. Note the apex is formed by the right ventricle. RV = right ventricle; A = aorta; P = pulmonary trunk.

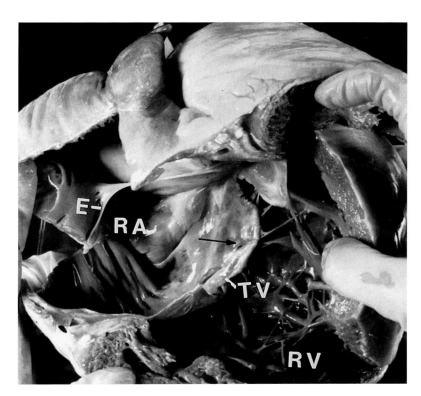

Figure 4: Right atrial, right ventricular view of the heart of Figure 3. RA = right atrium; RV = right ventricle; TV = thickened tricuspid valve; E = eustachian valve. Arrow points to the accessory opening in the septal leaflet.

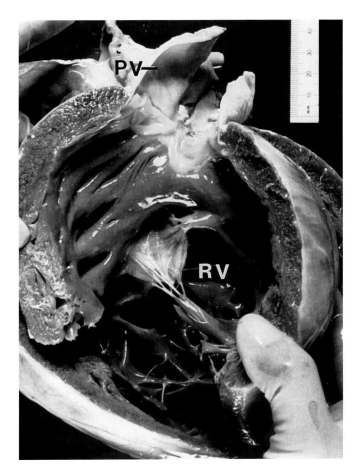

Figure 5: Outflow tract of the right ventricle of Figure 4. RV = right ventricle; PV = pulmonary valve.

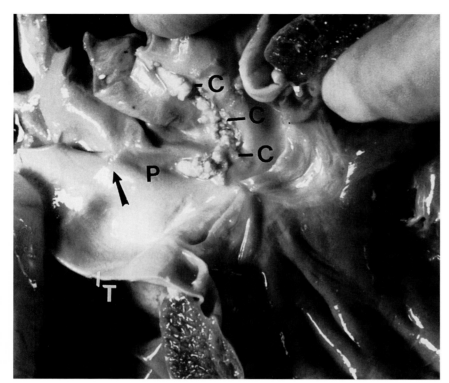

Figure 6: Close-up of the pulmonary valve showing supravalvular stenosis and post-stenotic dilatation with calcification. P = pulmonary trunk; C = calcification; T = thinning of the pulmonary tree. Arrow points to the supravalvular stenosis.

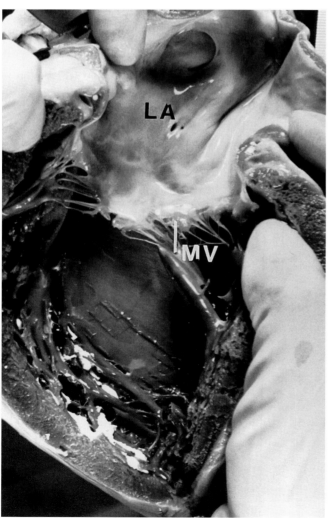

Figure 7: Left side of the above heart showing normal left atrium and thickened mitral valve. LA = left atrium; MV = mitral valve.

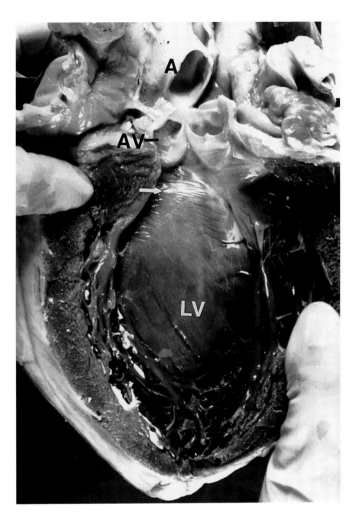

Figure 8: Left ventricular view of the above case. Note the dilated left ventricle with thin wall, thickened aortic valve, and ventricular septal bulge. A = aorta; LV = left ventricle; AV = aortic valve. Arrow points to the left ventricular bulge.

The associated cardiac abnormalities are given in the accompanying table.

Associated Cardiac Abnormalities

	No. of Cases
Rete Chiari	1
Hypertrophied and enlarged eustachian and thebesian valves with fenestrations	2
Oblique patent foramen ovale	2
Atrial septal defect, fossa ovalis type	1
Thrombosis of right atrial appendage	1
Accessory tricuspid orifice with significant tricuspid insufficiency	1
Patent ductus arteriosus ligated in infancy	1
Anomalous parietal bands in right ventricle	2
Marked atherosclerosis of the pulmonary tree	3
Cor pulmonale	3
Supravalvular pulmonary stenosis, post-stenotic dilatation of the pulmonary trunk with calcification and paper-thin pulmonary arteries	1
Right subclavian artery from descending aorta	1
Common brachiocephalic trunk for innominate and left common carotid arteries	1

Comment

Aside from a heart and lung and/or a lung transplantation in selected candidates, this disease remains a challenge. Hopefully, future research at the molecular-genetic level may help in understanding this disease.

86

Premature Closure or Narrowing of the Foramen Ovale

In premature closing (Fig. 1) or narrowing (Fig. 2) of the foramen ovale, either the foramen ovale is closed or markedly narrowed, measuring less than 2 millimeters in the first few days of life. In one type, the fossa ovalis is large, normal, or small in size and is more or less normal in architecture (Fig. 2). In the second type there is no distinct limbus fossa ovalis clearly seen on the right side (Fig. 3), or a defective type of limbus representing the left venous valve component of the septum secundum is present (Fig. 4), whereas the left side shows a pseudolimbus type of formation (Fig. 5). An aneurysm of the fossa ovalis usually accompanies this type of an abnormally formed limbus fossa ovalis (Figs. 2, 3). There is still a third type of an abnormally formed limbus, where the limbus is markedly hypertrophied, quite large (Fig. 5), and the septum primum is almost muscularized with a distinct atrial septal bulge (Figs. 1, 5). In all three types, in general, the limbus fossa ovalis is deviated more proximally close to the entry of the superior vena cava or towards the roof of the atrium (Figs. 1–3, 6).

In the simplest type, there is no mitral or aortic stenosis or atresia and no ventricular septal defect. In this type, there is right atrial and right ventricular hypertrophy and enlargement and hypoplasia of the left atrium and left ventricle. There may be a bicuspid aortic valve or fetal or preductal (hypoplasia of the transverse arch) coarctation of the aorta (Fig. 7).

In the second type, there is a ventricular septal defect. The defect may be of the common AV canal type or the usual subaortic in part perimembranous and in part membranous type. Here the left ventricle is larger than in the previous type (Figs. 8, 9). Again, a bicuspid aortic valve or coarctation is common. Occasionally, there are two ventricular septal defects.

The third type is with aortic atresia without ventricular septal defect. This is associated with a small mitral orifice and a small left ventricle, a thick wall, and fibroelastosis (Figs. 10, 11). The ascending aorta is minute.

The fourth type is with aortic and mitral atresia with practically absent left side of the heart (Fig. 12).

In the fifth type, there is an arcade-like malformation of the mitral valve or a sheet of valvular tissue with a giant or aneurysmally dilated left atrium, left atrial appendage, and a good-sized left ventricle (Fig. 13).

Analysis of Our Material

There was a total of 86 cases: 47 females and 39 males. The youngest was a 28-weeks' gestation fetus and the oldest was 7 weeks of age, with a mean of 4.83 days.

The Complex

The heart was always hypertrophied and enlarged. The apex was formed by the right ventricle in 82% (Fig. 14), by both ventricles in 15%, by left ventricle in 2%, and by a single ventricle in 1%. The right atrium and right ventricle were always hypertrophied and enlarged. The left atrium was atrophied in 38%, small with a thick wall and fibroelastosis in 19%, smaller than normal in 14%, hypertrophied in 10%, very small in 5%, normal in size in 6%, and hypertrophied and enlarged in 8%. The left ventricle was atretic in 50%, very small in 7%, small with a thick wall and fibroelastosis in 10%, smaller than normal in 25%, normal in size in 4%, hypertrophied and enlarged in 4%, and there was hypertrophy and enlargement in a case of single ventricle with small outlet chamber. The tri-

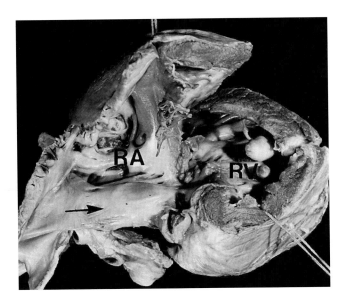

Figure 1: Premature closure of the foramen ovale with marked right atrial septal bulge; right atrial, right ventricular view. RA = markedly hypertrophied and enlarged right atrium; RV = markedly hypertrophied and enlarged right ventricle. Arrow points to the atrial septal bulge. Note the tricuspid valve, markedly redundant and nodose.

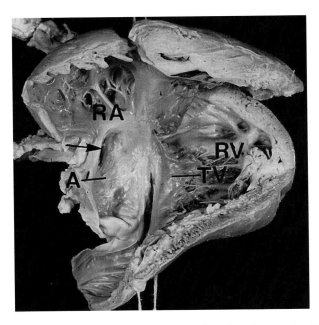

Figure 3: Right atrial, right ventricular view demonstrating the intact atrial septum and the aneurysmal bulge of the atrial septal region. RA = tremendously enlarged right atrium; RV = right ventricle; TV = redundant thickened large tricuspid valve; A = aneurysmal bulge of the atrial septum. Arrow points to the premature narrowing of the foramen ovale.

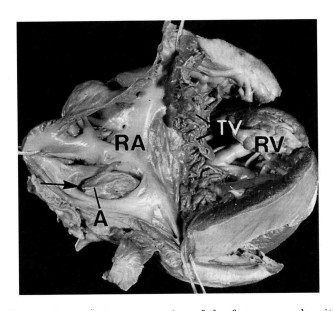

Figure 2: Premature narrowing of the foramen ovale with aneurysm of the fossa ovalis; right atrial, right ventricular view demonstrating the huge right-sided chambers with dysplastic redundant tricuspid valve with probable tricuspid insufficiency. RA = right atrium; A = aneurysm of the fossa ovalis; TV = redundant dysplastic tricuspid valve; RV = right ventricle. Arrow points to the premature narrowing of the foramen ovale.

cuspid orifice was enlarged in 67%, normal in size in 29%, and smaller than normal in 4%. The pulmonic orifice size was enlarged in 74%, normal in 21%, and smaller than normal in 5%. The mitral orifice was atretic in 47%, smaller than normal in 26%, very small (minute) in 20%, and normal in size in 7%. The aortic orifice was atretic in 51%, smaller than normal in 31%, normal in size in 14%, very small in 2%, and enlarged in 2%.

The Valves

Tricuspid Valve (Figs. 1–4, 6)

The valve was normally formed only in 29 (34%) and presented increased hemodynamic change. In the majority of the cases, the valve showed irregular thickening and nodularity with numerous papillary muscles, some of them proceeding to the undersurface of the valve. In some, the chordae were markedly abbreviated. Mitralization of the valve was present in five and blood cysts in five. In one, there was a large accessory tricuspid orifice with insufficiency. In two others, the redundancy of the valvular tissue formed a sheet-like membrane producing tricuspid insufficiency. There was one common atrioventricular orifice of a complete type and another where the tricuspid valve was a complete straddler.

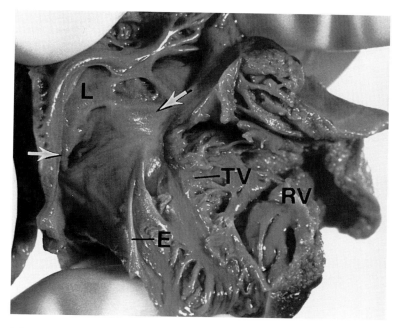

Figure 4: Right atrial, right ventricular view demonstrating the abnormally deviated hypoplastic limbus with premature closure and atrial septal bulge. L = limbic margin; E = enlarged eustachian valve; TV = tricuspid valve; RV = right ventricle. Arrows point to the atrial septal bulge.

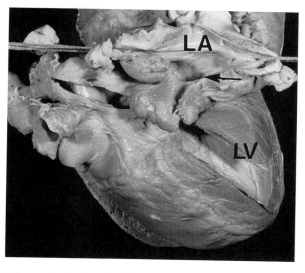

Figure 5: Left atrial, left ventricular view of Figure 1 demonstrating the small left atrium and left ventricle with mitral atresia. LA = small left atrium; LV = small left ventricle. Arrow points to the pseudolimbus type of architecture of the atrial septum and atretic mitral orifice.

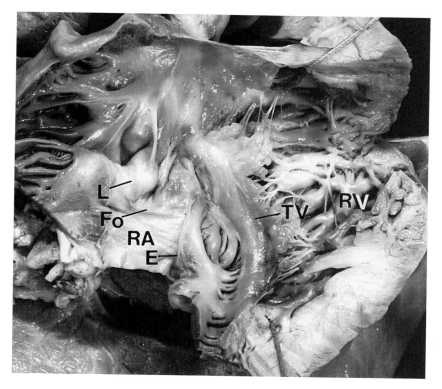

Figure 6: Right atrial, right ventricular view demonstrating the abnormally formed atrial septum. L = markedly hypertrophied and enlarged limbus; Fo = fossa ovalis demonstrating redundancy of the fossa ovalis with some aneurysmal formation; RA = right atrium; E = eustachian valve; TV = enlarged thickened tricuspid valve; RV = markedly hypertrophied right ventricle.

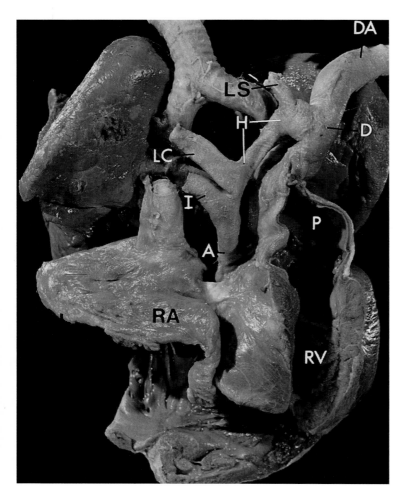

Figure 7: External view demonstrating hypertrophied and enlarged heart with hypoplasia of transverse arch and coarctation of the aorta. RA = huge right atrium; RV = hypertrophied and enlarged right ventricle; A = small aorta; P = large pulmonary trunk; I = innominate artery; LC = left common carotid artery; H = hypoplasia of transverse arch; LS = left subclavian artery emerging distally at the junction of the ductus arteriosus with the descending aorta; DA = descending aorta; D = ductus arteriosus.

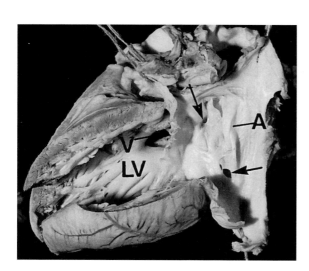

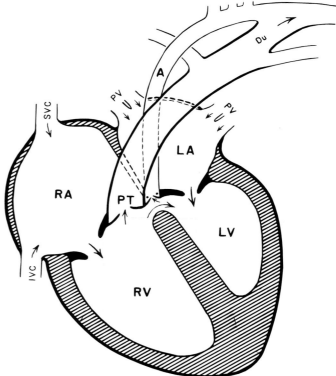

Figure 8: Left atrial, left ventricular view demonstrating the premature narrowing of the foramen ovale and the ventricular septal defect. A = aneurysm of the fossa ovalis; LV = left ventricle; V = U-shaped ventricular septal defect. Arrows point to the small openings in the region of the fossa ovalis.

Figure 9: Diagram depicting the hemodynamics of Figure 8. SVC = superior vena cava; IVC = inferior vena cava; RA = right atrium; RV = right ventricle; LA = left atrium; LV = left ventricle; PV = pulmonary vein; A = aorta; PT = pulmonary trunk; Du = ductus arteriosus.

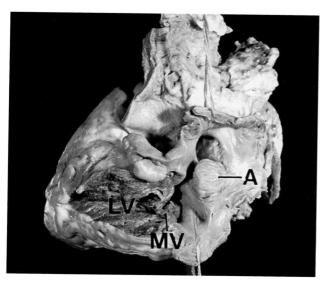

Figure 10: Aortic atresia with small mitral valve, small left ventricle, thick wall, and fibroelastosis; left atrial, left ventricular view demonstrating a huge aneurysm of the fossa ovalis bulging into the left atrial cavity. MV = very small mitral valve; LV = small left ventricle; A = huge aneurysm of the fossa ovalis bulging into the left atrial cavity.

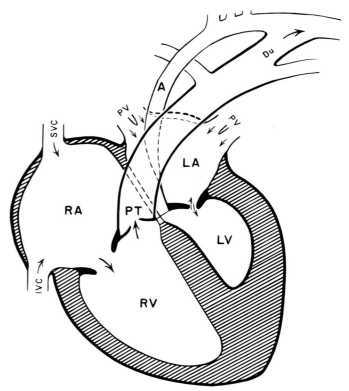

Figure 11: Diagram depicting the hemodynamics of Figure 10. SVC = superior vena cava; IVC = inferior vena cava; RA= right atrium; RV = right ventricle; LA = left atrium; LV = left ventricle; PV = pulmonary vein; A = aorta; PT= pulmonary trunk; Du = ductus arteriosus.

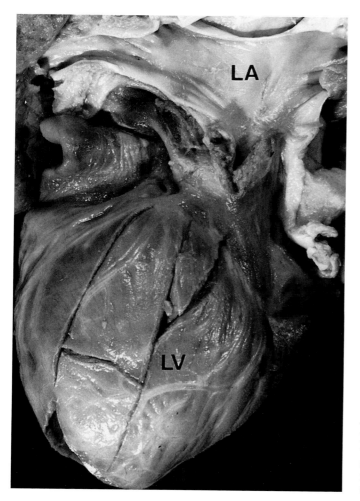

Figure 12: Premature closure of the foramen ovale with aortic and mitral atresia; left atrial, left ventricular view. LA = small left atrium; LV = absent left ventricle. Note the anterior and posterior descending coronary arteries winding around the left ventricle with no cavity.

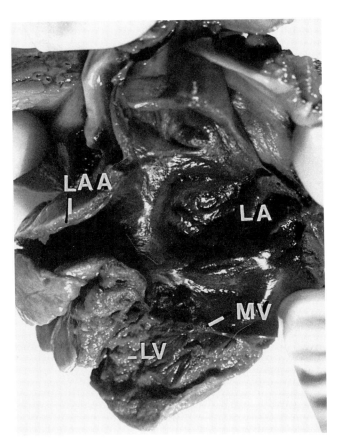

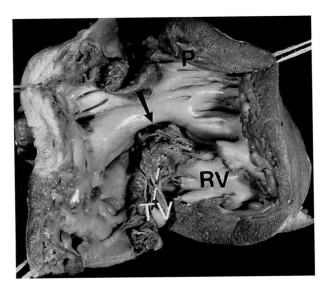

Figure 15: Premature closure of the foramen ovale with a large U-shaped ventricular septal defect and markedly dysplastic tricuspid, pulmonic, mitral, and aortic valves and basilar straddling tricuspid valve; right ventricular outflow tract demonstrating marked right ventricular hypertrophy, a U-shaped defect entering the right ventricle beneath the arch, and absence of the muscle of Lancisi. RV = right ventricle; P = dysplastic pulmonic valve; TV = dysplastic tricuspid valve. Arrow points to the entry of the defect into the right ventricle.

Figure 13: Huge left atrial appendage with premature closure of the foramen ovale and spongy primitive left ventricle. LA = tremendously hypertrophied left atrium; LAA = huge left atrial appendage; MV = minute mitral valve; LV = spongy left ventricle.

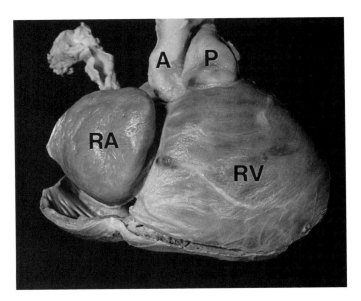

Figure 14: External view of the heart demonstrating the hypertrophied and enlarged heart with a huge right side. RA = tremendously enlarged right atrium; RV = huge right ventricle forming the apex; P = pulmonary trunk; A = aorta.

Pulmonary Valve

In general, the valve was normally formed and presented increased hemodynamic change. The valve was bicuspid in seven, markedly dysplastic in six (Fig. 15), and unicuspid in one. In two, there were aneurysms of the anterior sinuses of Valsalva of the pulmonic valve cusps. There was one case of pulmonary stenosis and another with a blood cyst.

Mitral Valve

The mitral valve was normal in seven. In 25, the valve tissue, when present, was markedly thickened, redundant, attenuated, or shrunken with short thick stubby chordae and papillary muscles (Fig. 16). Some of the papillary muscles proceeded to the base of the valve. In two remarkable cases, the inferior leaflet was distinctly displaced into the septum creating an Ebstein-like malformation of the mitral valve. There was a distinct arcade-like malformation of the mitral valve in three with mitral insufficiency (Fig. 17). Blood cysts were found in two (Fig. 16). In approximately 14% of the cases, there was distinct mitral stenosis.

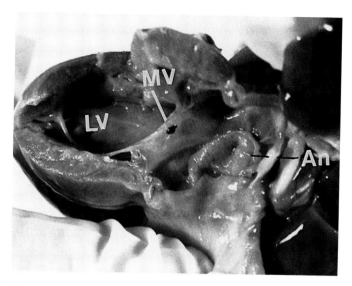

Figure 16: Premature closure of the foramen ovale with a huge left side of the heart demonstrating an aneurysm of the fossa ovalis into the left atrial cavity and the mitral valve. An = huge aneurysm of the fossa ovalis bulging into the left atrial cavity; LV = enlarged left ventricle; MV = mitral valve with a blood cyst.

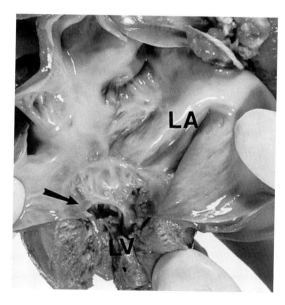

Figure 17: Left atrial view demonstrating arcade mitral valve with mitral stenosis and/or insufficiency in intrauterine life resulting in a giant left atrium. LA = left atrium; LV = left ventricle. Arrow points to the arcade mitral valve with practically no chordae and/or papillary muscles. The mitral valve forms an arch with thickened redundant tissue. Note the enormously hypertrophied and enlarged left atrium with intact atrial septum. (Used with permission from Bharati S, et al. See Figure 25.)

Aortic Valve

The aortic valve was atretic in 47 (55%). The valve was normally formed and presented the usual hemodynamic change in 16 (18.8%). The valve was bicuspid and markedly thickened in 18 (21%), and unicuspid in four (4.7%). In one, the right and left aortic sinuses of Valsalva were aneurysmally dilated and the posterior cusp was quite small.

Endocardium

In general, the endocardium showed focal changes of marked thickening and whitening of the right atrium and the right ventricle. Where there was a mitral orifice, in general, there was diffuse fibroelastosis in many cases of the left-sided chambers.

Atrial Septal Morphology

The foramen ovale was closed completely in 45 (52.3%) (Fig. 18) and the foramen ovale was markedly narrowed (less than 2 mm) in 41 (48%) (Fig. 19). An aneurysm of the fossa ovalis was present in 17 (Fig. 19). The limbus was indistinguishable or hypoplastic and more or less fused with the roof of the atrium and was markedly deviated towards the entry of the superior vena cava in 15. Less frequently, the limbus was very well developed; however, it was oriented close to the superior vena cava proximally with the septum primum markedly thickened (almost muscularized) with a distinct atrial septal bulge into the right atrial cavity (Figs. 18, 19). The majority of them presented with a remnant of the sinus venarum valves, either in the combination of a hypertrophied and enlarged eustachian valve (Fig. 18), or a combined eustachian and thebesian valve, or a Chiari network, or in the form of spatio-intercepto valvulare. Corresponding to the right atrial septal morphology, the left atrial septal morphology likewise revealed considerable variation. The left atrium, when it was smaller than normal, was not infrequently divided into a proximal and a distal segment. The proximal segment consisted of the common pulmonary vein component and the distal segment had the atrial appendage. The aneurysm of the fossa ovalis bulged into the left atrial cavity quite frequently (Figs. 8, 10, 16, 20). In six, there were anomalous bands in the left atrium. In two the left atrial appendage was absent and in four it was gigantic (Figs. 13, 21).

Wherever there was associated anomalous pulmonary venous return, there was a tendency for the atrial septum to be markedly hypertrophied and bulge into the right atrial cavity. The left superior vena cava entered the coronary sinus in 12, and the left superior vena cava entered the left atrium in one, and a distinct double-chambered left atrial type of morphology was present in six.

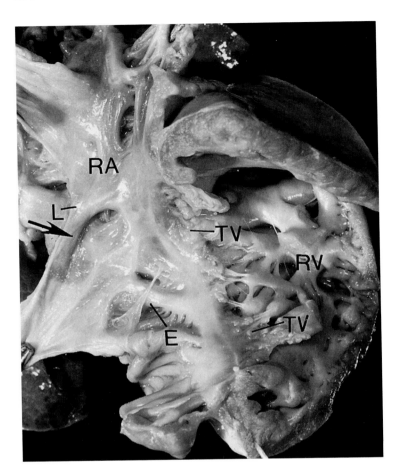

Figure 18: Premature closure of the foramen ovale; right atrial, right ventricular view demonstrating huge right-sided chambers. RA = right atrium; E = combined eustachian and thebesian valve; TV = tricuspid valve; L = limbus fossae ovalis; RV = hypertrophied and enlarged right ventricle. Arrow points to the premature closure of the foramen ovale. (Used with permission from Lev M, Arcilla R, Rimoldi HJA, Licata RH, Gasul BM: Premature narrowing or closure of the foramen ovale. *Am Heart J* 1963, 65:638–647.)

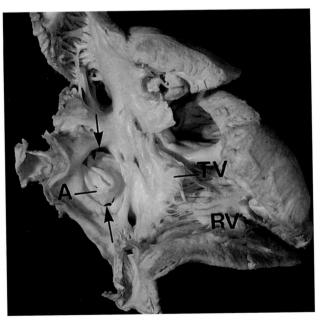

Figure 19: Premature narrowing of the foramen ovale with ventricular septal defect; right atrial, right ventricular view demonstrating huge right-sided chambers. A = aneurysm of the fossa ovalis; TV = tricuspid valve; RV = right ventricle. Arrows point to the premature narrowing of the foramen ovale.

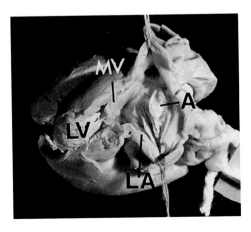

Figure 20: Premature closure of the foramen ovale with aneurysm of the fossa ovalis bulging into the left atrium; left atrial, left ventricular view. LA = left atrium; LV = very small left ventricle; MV = small mitral valve; A = aneurysm of the fossa ovalis bulging into the left atrial cavity.

Ventricular Septal Morphology

In approximately 39% of the cases, there was an associated defect in the ventricular septum. In premature closure of foramen ovale, 18 were associated with ventricular septal defects and 14 of the premature narrowing of the foramen ovale cases had ventricular septal defect. In general, the ventricular septal defect was a U-shaped deficiency in the summit of the ventricular septum and in the majority of the cases was confluent in part with the aortic valve involving the membranous part of the ventricular septum and extending anteriorly to it. This was associated with overriding aorta and the tricuspid valve was either a straddler or attached to the septum to a varying degree (Figs. 22, 23). Rarely were there two defects (Fig. 24). The variations in ventricular septal defects were as follows:

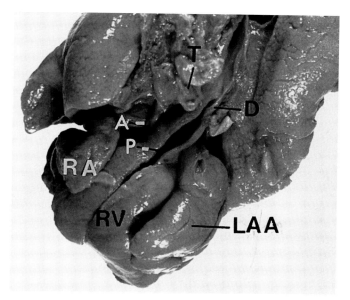

Figure 21: Premature closure of the foremen ovale with a huge left atrial appendage; external view of the heart. RA = right atrium; T = trachea; RV = right ventricle; A = small aorta; P = larger pulmonary trunk; D = ductus arteriosus; LAA = huge left atrial appendage.

	No. of Cases
Large posterobasal ventricular septal defect	2
Common AV canal type of ventricular septal defect	2
Double ventricular septal defect (one defect closed spontaneously)	2
Small ventricular septal defect	2
Minute ventricular septal defect	1
Associated overriding of the aorta	10
Pars membranacea type of a ventricular septal defect	1
Common atrioventricular orifice of a dominant right form	1

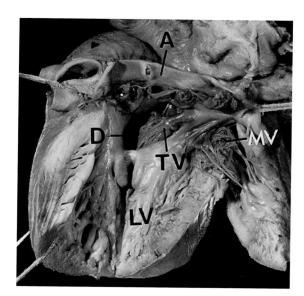

Figure 22: Left ventricular view of Figure 21 demonstrating the U-shaped ventricular septal defect confluent with the base of the aortic valve and straddling tricuspid valve. Note the dysplastic tricuspid mitral and aortic valves. A = aorta; D = U-shaped defect; LV = left ventricle; MV = mitral valve; TV = tricuspid valve attached to the ventricular septal defect and the base of the aortic valve to a varying degree.

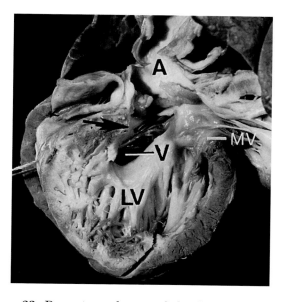

Figure 23: Premature closure of the foramen ovale with straddling tricuspid valve and overriding aorta. LV = left ventricular hypertrophy and enlargement; MV = mitral valve; V = U-shaped ventricular septal defect; A = overriding aorta. Arrow points to the straddling tricuspid valve.

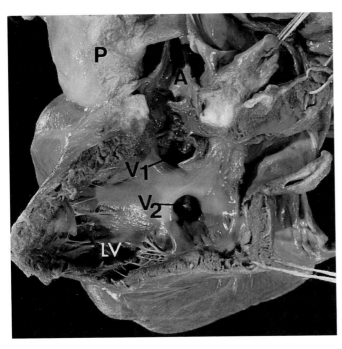

Figure 24: Double ventricular septal defect in a case of premature closure of the foramen ovale with overriding aorta; left ventricular view. LV = left ventricle; V_1 = defect beneath the aorta; V_2 = second muscular defect midway between the base of the mitral valve and the apex of the heart; A = aorta; P = pulmonary trunk. Note the mild overriding of the aorta with redundant tricuspid valvular tissue confluent with the base of the aortic valve.

Double Outlet Right Ventricle with Premature Narrowing of Foramen Ovale

There appears to be a tendency for double outlet right ventricle to occur with this anomaly. When there was double outlet right ventricle, it was usually associated with ventricular septal defect. However, rarely in this entity double outlet right ventricle was seen without a ventricular septal defect. When there was double outlet right ventricle with ventricular septal defect, the defect may be a subaortic type, or a doubly committed type, or a noncommitted type. The types of double outlets were as follows:

No. of Cases

Premature narrowing of the foramen ovale with double outlet right ventricle without ventricular septal defect with fetal coarctation, patent ductus arteriosus with very small coronary sinus, atrial septal defect and the origin of both coronary ostia close to each other with the anterior descending coronary artery proceeding in front of the pulmonary trunk   1

Premature closure of the foramen ovale with double outlet right ventricle of subaortic ventricular septal defect with subaortic stenosis, aortic stenosis, fetal coarctation, and marked mitral stenosis with PDA   1

Double outlet right ventricle with subaortic ventricular septal defect with circuitous PDA, mitral stenosis, and pulmonary stenosis with normal drainage of all the pulmonary veins into the left atrium with a large vein from the right lobe entering the azygos draining into the superior vena cava   1

Premature narrowing of the foramen ovale with double outlet right ventricle and subaortic ventricular septal defect with mitral stenosis and high origin of the right coronary ostium and patent ductus arteriosus   1

Premature closure of the foramen ovale with double outlet right ventricle, subaortic ventricular septal defect with levoatrio cardinal vein draining the left atrium into the innominate vein and into the superior vena cava with fetal coarctation   1

Double outlet right ventricle with doubly committed ventricular septal defect with subaortic stenosis, coarctation of the aorta and high origin of the left coronary ostium   1

Double outlet right ventricle with noncommitted ventricular septal defect with infundibular and pulmonary stenosis and straddling tricuspid valve, CAVO type of VSD with right coronary artery proceeding from the left in front of the pulmonary valve anteriorly with a probe patent ductus arteriosus in a newborn   1

Total or Partial Anomalous Pulmonary Venous Return with or without Stenosis of the Pulmonary Veins

In addition to double outlet right ventricle, there appears to be a tendency for stenosis or atresia of the pulmonary veins with or without total or partial anomalous pulmonary venous return. The anomalous pulmonary venous drainage, either total or partial, showed marked variations. The variations are as follows:

No. of Cases

Right upper pulmonary vein into the right atrium   1

	No. of Cases
Right two pulmonary veins into the left superior vena cava	1
Right upper pulmonary vein into the right superior vena cava	1
Right pulmonary veins draining into the right superior vena cava with coarctation and aneurysmal dilatation of the innominate and left common carotid arteries with small left subclavian artery with the posterobasal VSD	1
Total anomalous pulmonary venous drainage with stenosis at the junction of the left superior vena cava with the coronary sinus	1
Partial anomalous pulmonary venous drainage with pulmonary hypertension (right upper pulmonary veins into right superior vena cava) and stenosis of the pulmonary vein at its entry into the left atrium	1
Total anomalous pulmonary venous return with stenosis (common pulmonary veins entering azygos and azygos entering the superior vena cava with stenosis and second set of common pulmonary veins atretic at the junction with the left atrium and left pulmonary veins entering the left superior vena cava with *no left atrial appendage* and left subclavian artery emerging from left common carotid artery	1
Stenosis of the pulmonary veins with fetal coarctation, aortic stenosis, tricuspid insufficiency and patent ductus arteriosus	1
Total anomalous pulmonary venous drainage into the right atrium close to the entry of the inferior vena cava with elongated tortuous cirsoid closing ductus arteriosus in a newborn	1
Stenosis of the pulmonary vein with coarctation of the aorta	1

Morphology of the Ascending Aorta, Transverse Arch, and Descending Aorta

Where there was aortic and mitral atresia without a ventricular septal defect, the ascending aorta was usually a minute cord-like structure and the transverse arch usually was somewhat larger than the ascending aorta. This was associated with a prominent crista reunion which may be considered a coarctation of the aorta. As stated previously, where the mitral orifice was opened, there was associated mitral stenosis and/or aortic stenosis.

	No. of Cases
Hypoplasia of the transverse arch with coarctation and a widely patent ductus arteriosus	12
Common brachiocephalic vessels	1
Distal origin of the left subclavian artery	3
Absent transverse arch	1
Right subclavian artery from distal part of the transverse arch	1

Coronary Artery Anomalies

These were frequently found when associated with double outlet right ventricle. In addition to those anomalies previously stated, the following were present:

	No. of Cases
High origin of the left coronary ostium	1
High origin of both coronary ostia	2
Double coronary ostia	1

Premature Closure of Foramen Ovale with a Giant Left Atrium

There were three remarkable hearts with a giant left atrium: two with premature closure (Figs. 17, 25)

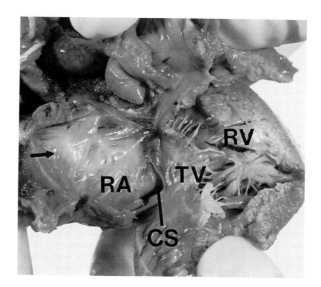

Figure 25: Premature closure of the foramen ovale with arcade mitral valve and insufficiency (intrauterine) and a huge left atrium; right atrial, right ventricular view. RA = tremendously enlarged right atrium; CS = coronary sinus; TV = tricuspid valve; RV = right ventricle. Arrow points to the atrial septal bulge produced by the huge left atrium. (Used with permission from Bharati S, Patel AG, Varga P, Husain AN, Lev M: In utero echocardiographic diagnosis of a unique case of premature closure of foramen ovale with mitral insufficiency and large left atrium. *Am Heart J* 1991, 122:597–600.)

and one with premature narrowing of foramen ovale. One was a 31-weeks' gestation stillborn infant with premature closure of the foramen ovale. In all three, the mitral valve was an arcade-like malformation with a markedly thickened valvular leaflet that obviously produced tremendous mitral insufficiency in intrauterine life resulting in a giant left atrium. All were associated with coarctation of the aorta. The stillborn presented with spongy premature ventricles and small pulmonary veins.

Morphology of the Right and Left Ventricle

Uncommonly, the right and left ventricles presented anomalous muscle bundles. In the left ventricle, the anomalous muscles were usually in the posteroseptal wall. These were frequently seen with ventricular septal defects (Figs. 26, 27). Uncommonly, there was a distinct left ventricular septal bulge (Fig. 28).

Patent Ductus Arteriosus

In a 30 weeks' gestation infant, a very small ductus was closing with a small coronary sinus. A probe patent ductus was present in two stillborn infants. A very small ductus was present in five other newborn infants.

There was one case of trisomy 13–15 born to a mother who was 17 years of age and had used cocaine during pregnancy. This infant was born with multiple congenital anomalies, coarctation, common AV canal type of a huge ventricular septal defect, and the tricuspid valve covered the defect to a considerable extent.

Other Rare Features

A very small coronary sinus type of atrial septal defect was seen in three. These measured less than 2 mm in greatest dimension and the defects were usually present with double outlet right ventricle. In one, it was large.

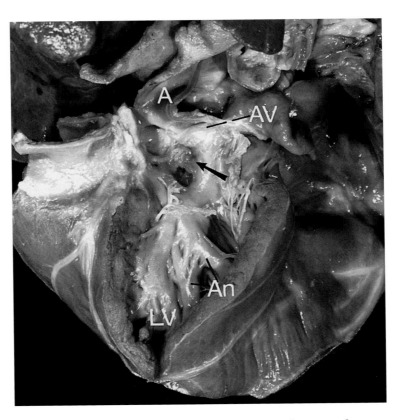

Figure 26: Left ventricular outflow tract demonstrating the anomalous muscle bundles and a U-shaped deficiency (defect) confluent with the aortic valve with redundant endocardial tissue probably restricting the defect. LV = left ventricle; An = anomalous muscle bundles; A = ascending aorta; AV = aortic valve. Arrow points to the endocardial tissue beneath the aortic valve restricting the defect.

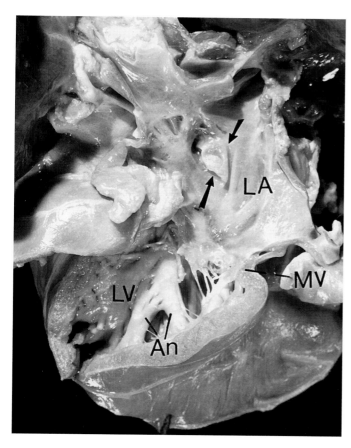

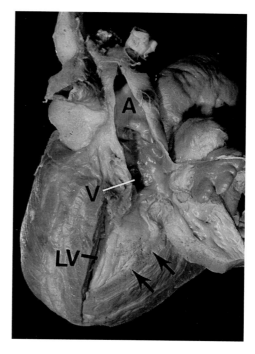

Figure 28: Left ventricular view demonstrating a small ventricular septal defect confluent with the base of the aortic valve and a small left ventricle. LV = left ventricle; V = ventricular septal defect confluent with the base of the aorta; A = ascending aorta. Arrows point to the ventricular septal bulge.

Figure 27: Left atrial, left ventricular view demonstrating the aneurysm of the fossa ovalis and the anomalous architecture of the left ventricle. LA = left atrium; MV = mitral valve; An = anomalous muscle bundles in the left ventricle; LV = left ventricle. Arrows point to the aneurysm of the fossa ovalis.

Single Ventricle with Small Outlet Chamber

This was a Holmes heart with total anomalous pulmonary venous return to the right atrium (right pulmonary veins to coronary sinus and left veins into the right atrium) with marked pulmonary valvular and infundibular stenosis and absent left AV valve. There were two small defects between the main ventricular chamber and the small outlet chamber. There was also a distal origin of the left subclavian artery.

Comment

It is evident that premature closure of foramen ovale may broadly be grouped into those salvageable cases and those difficult or almost impossible to salvage (Fig. 29). As seen from the material, in a little less than 40% of the cases, there is an associated large or

good-sized ventricular septal defect resulting in a sizable (enlarged, Fig. 30) normal, or somewhat smaller than normal) left ventricle in approximately 30% of the cases. Therefore, at least some selected cases may be looked upon as salvageable.

It is important to rule out stenosis and/or total or partial anomalous pulmonary venous drainage. Likewise, corrective procedures by means of surgical or nonsurgical techniques for coarctation of the aorta may be considered judiciously in some selected cases provided the pulmonary venous return is adequate and appropriate without any pulmonary hypertension.

With recent advances made in fetal echocardiography, it is possible that this entity may be picked up early in fetal life in the future and either pharmacological or interventional procedures may be attempted in some selected cases to enlarge the atrial septum (enlarge the narrowed foramen ovale) which may permit the growth of the left side of the heart and may prevent the associated abnormalities such as mitral valve anomalies with stenosis or insufficiency, subaortic stenosis, aortic stenosis, and varying types of coarctation of the aorta to develop in intrauterine life.

The entity of premature closure of the foramen ovale associated with a large left atrium merits some

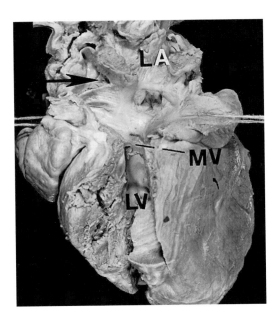

Figure 29: Premature closure of the foramen ovale with marked mitral stenosis and small left ventricle, left side of the heart. LA = left atrium; MV = very small mitral valve; LV = very small left ventricle with thick wall. Arrow points to the premature closure of the foramen ovale.

discussion. It is obvious that significant mitral stenosis and/or insufficiency had occurred in intrauterine life in these infants. The fact that the heart has formed normally suggests that originally the foramen ovale was smaller than normal in intrauterine life with possible anatomic abnormalities in the mitral and/or the aortic valve. At a later date in intrauterine life, there probably was development of significant mitral insufficiency that elevated the left atrial pressure and had closed the abnormally formed atrial septum. This, therefore, had resulted in a huge left atrium with a good-sized left ventricle at birth. We, therefore, hypothesize that to start with there might have been some abnormal hemodynamics at the placental level or at the inferior or superior vena caval level or at the narrowed foramen ovale level, or the abnormal hemodynamics might be at the tricuspid valvular and/or pulmonic valve level. It is also of interest that there were a few cases with a very small or closed ductus associated with this lesion. This suggests that there could have been some abnormal hemodynamics occurring at the ductus level as well in intrauterine life.

Attempts should be made through innovative techniques to diagnose the abnormal hemodynamics occurring at the placental level, inferior vena caval level, su-

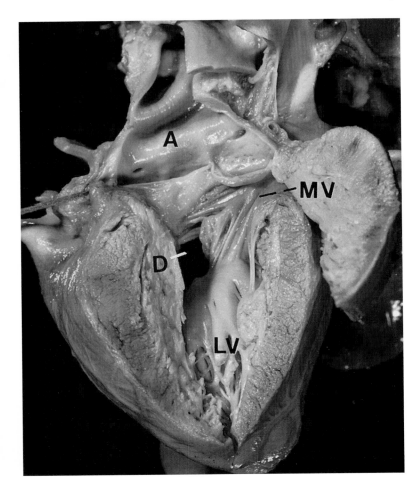

Figure 30: Premature closure of the foramen ovale with large VSD and sizable left ventricle. A = aorta; LV = left ventricle; MV = mitral valve; D = huge subaortic ventricular septal defect.

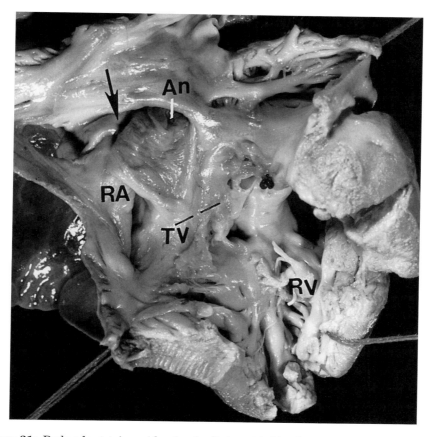

Figure 31: Redundant tricuspid valve leaflets, with blood cysts and greatly enlarged right atrium, right atrial, right ventricular view. RA = right atrium; RV = right ventricle; An = aneurysm of the fossa ovalis; TV = redundant tricuspid valve with blood cysts. Arrow points to the premature closure of the foramen ovale.

perior vena caval level, tricuspid valve, pulmonic valve, ductus arteriosus level, and at the atrial septal level in intrauterine life, which in return may help discover new methods of correcting the abnormal hemodynamics in intrauterine life by pharmacological and/or biochemical methods.

The heart with single ventricle had two small defects between the main chamber and the small outlet chamber with atresia of the left AV valve. The tendency for mitral atresia or marked mitral stenosis to occur in double outlet right ventricle and the association of anomalous pulmonary venous drainage in this entity strongly suggest an abnormal hemodynamic flow pattern to the left side of the heart in intrauterine life. We have previously demonstrated that the aorta has a tendency to rotate to the right to a varying degree resulting in double outlet right ventricle whenever there is an abnormality of the mitral valve in the form of atresia or stenosis.

The frequent association of tricuspid valve abnormalities, such as redundancy of the leaflets, blood cysts, and abnormal peripheral connections (Figs. 31, 32) with enlargement of the right atrium strongly sug-

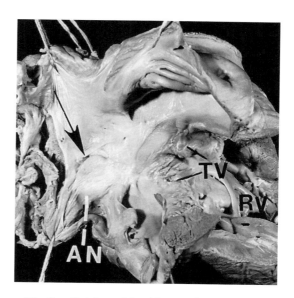

Figure 32: Small tricuspid orifice, redundant leaflets, and huge right atrium in premature closure of the foramen ovale, right atrial, right ventricular view. An = aneurysm of the fossa ovalis; TV = tricuspid valve, small anulus and redundant leaflets RV = right ventricle. Arrow points to the premature closure of the foramen ovale.

gests tricuspid insufficiency and/or stenosis in intrauterine life. Although there probably are multiple factors that might have played a role in the production of premature narrowing or closure of the foramen ovale complex, the forces that are responsible for tricuspid insufficiency should be carefully evaluated in the future.

The fundamental causes, such as abnormalities in the genes that are responsible for the appropriate development of the limbus fossae ovalis, including the septum secundum, the septum primum, and the sinus venarum components, are to be explored at the molecular-genetic level in the future. On the other hand, the frequent association of a U-shaped ventricular septal defect as well as double outlet right ventricle suggests the possibility that the genes that are responsible for the proper absorption of the bulbus into the left ventricle might be affected in some.

87

Absence of Transverse Arch (Interrupted Aortic Arch) with Ventricular Septal Defect

In this complex, the transverse arch between the left common carotid artery and the left subclavian artery (Fig. 1) or distal to the left subclavian is absent. Then, the pulmonary trunk forms the descending aorta, usually through a widely patent ductus arteriosus.

General Statement

The heart presents global hypertrophy, in general, with enlargement of all of the chambers, with a subaortic ventricular septal defect that may enter the right ventricle beneath the arch formed by the septal and the parietal bands (Fig. 2), or it may enter the right ventricle at the region of the arch (intracristal) confluent with the base of the pulmonic valve. In these instances, there may be overriding of the pulmonary trunk (Fig. 3) and/or overriding of the aorta. The parietal band from the right ventricle has a tendency to straddle through the septal defect confluent with the base of the pulmonary valve and proceed to the opposite ventricle, and may produce subaortic stenosis with or without fibroelastic ridges beneath the aortic valve (Fig. 4). In the majority of the cases, there is a bicuspid aortic valve with a small anulus. There is a greater tendency for atrial septal defect of the fossa ovalis type to be associated with this entity. Rarely interrupted aortic arch is seen with aorticopulmonary septal defect and an intact ventricular septum.

Analysis of Our Material

There was a total of 67 cases: 32 males, 34 females, and one animal heart. The youngest was a stillborn and another 34 weeks' gestation newborn and the oldest 5 years of age, with a median age of 2½ months. The heart was hypertrophied and enlarged in all with the apex formed by the left ventricle in 49% (Fig. 1) by both ventricles in 42%, and by the right ventricle in 9% (Fig. 5).

The Complex

The right atrium was hypertrophied and enlarged in 91%, normal in size in 3%, and enlarged in 6%. The right ventricle was hypertrophied and enlarged in 92% (Fig. 6) hypertrophied in 3%, normal in size in 3%, and enlarged in 2%. The left atrium was hypertrophied and enlarged in 73%, enlarged in 6%, hypertrophied in 7%, normal in size in 11%, and atrophied in 3%. There was one case of common atrium that was hypertrophied and enlarged. The left ventricle was hypertrophied and enlarged in 65%, hypertrophied in 4%, enlarged in 14%, normal in size in 8%, smaller than normal in 3%, (Fig. 6), and atrophied in 6%. The tricuspid orifice size was normal in 43%, enlarged in 25%, and smaller than normal in 32%. The pulmonic orifice size was enlarged in 75%, normal in size in 19%, and smaller than normal in 6%. The mitral orifice was normal in size in 36%, smaller than normal in 36%, and enlarged in 28%. The aortic orifice size was smaller than normal in 83% and normal in size in 17%.

The Valves

Tricuspid Valve

This was, in general, normally formed and showed increased hemodynamic change. The valve was redun-

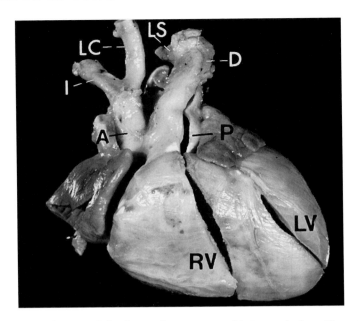

Figure 1: External view of the heart from a case of interrupted aortic arch. Interruption is occurring distal to the left common carotid artery. RV = right ventricle; LV = left ventricle; P = pulmonary trunk; A = small ascending aorta; I = innominate artery; LC = left common carotid artery; D = ductus arteriosus forming the descending aorta; LS = left subclavian artery emerging at the junction of the ductus with the descending aorta.

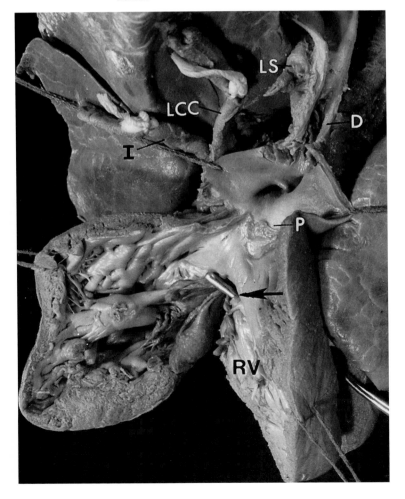

Figure 2: Right ventricular outflow tract demonstrating the defect entering beneath the arch formed by the septal and parietal bands (subcristal defect) with straddling parietal band. RV = right ventricle; P = pulmonary trunk; I = innominate artery; LCC = left common carotid artery; D = closing ductus arteriosus; LS = left subclavian artery. Arrow points to the probe emerging from the left ventricle at the junction of the anterior and septal leaflets of the tricuspid valve and the straddling parietal band.

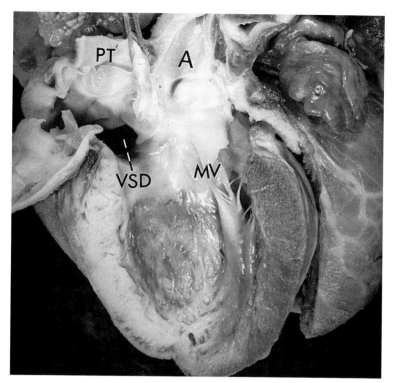

Figure 3: U-shaped ventricular septal defect in the anterior part of the ventricular septum away from the membranous septum with overriding pulmonary trunk; left ventricular view. MV = mitral valve; VSD = U-shaped ventricular septal defect in the anterior septum confluent with the pulmonary trunk; PT = pulmonary trunk overriding the defect; A = aorta.

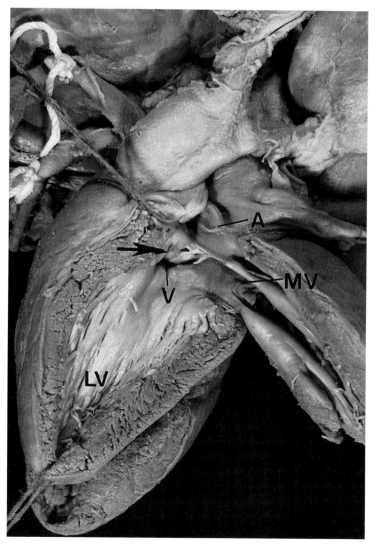

Figure 4: Left ventricular outflow tract demonstrating straddling conal muscle through the defect as well as narrowing of the outflow tract of the left ventricle into the aorta. LV = left ventricle; V = small (restrictive) ventricular septal defect; A = small aortic valve; MV = mitral valve. Note the anomalous anterior papillary muscle of the mitral valve proceeding to the base of the valve. Arrow points to subaortic obstruction.

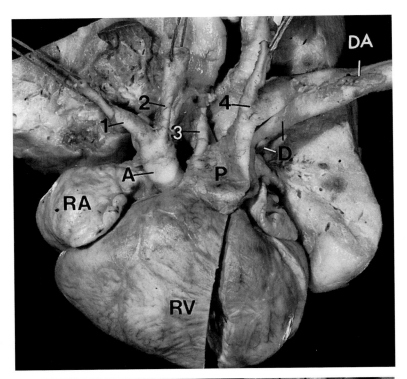

Figure 5: Interruption of the aortic arch (absent transverse arch distal to the two carotid arteries and the right subclavian artery emerging from the pulmonary trunk (3) and the left subclavian artery emerging from the junction of the ductus with the descending aorta (4). RA = right atrium; RV = right ventricle; A = small ascending aorta; 1 = left common carotid artery; 2 = right common carotid artery; 3 = right subclavian emerging from the main pulmonary trunk; 4 = left subclavian artery emerging from the junction of the ductus with the descending aorta; P = large pulmonary trunk; D = ductus arteriosus; DA = descending aorta. Note the apex is formed by the right ventricle.

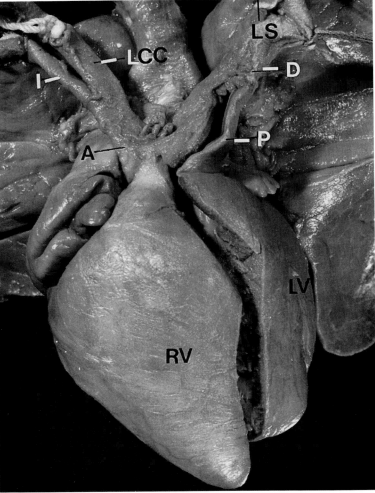

Figure 6: Interrupted aortic arch with small left ventricle, apex formed by the right ventricle and interruption distal to the left common carotid artery, and left subclavian emerging from the descending aorta. RV = huge right ventricle; LV = very small left ventricle; A = small ascending aorta; I = innominate artery; P = pulmonary trunk; LCC = left common carotid artery; D = closing ductus arteriosus; LS = left subclavian emerging from the descending aorta.

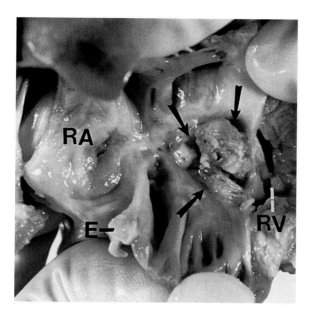

Figure 7: Candida albicans infective endocarditis of the tricuspid valve occluding the tricuspid valve with marked tricuspid stenosis in a postoperative case of absence transverse arch. RA = right atrium; RV = right ventricle; E = hypertrophied and enlarged eustachian valve. Arrows point to the infective endocarditis almost occluding the tricuspid valve.

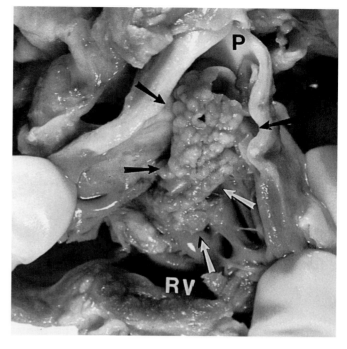

Figure 8: Outflow tract of the right ventricle demonstrating the huge irregular vegetation proceeding into the main pulmonary trunk and occluding the two pulmonary arteries. RV = right ventricle; P = pulmonary trunk. Arrows point to the irregular huge Candida infective endocarditis occluding the outflow tract of the right ventricle into the pulmonary trunk.

dant with tricuspid stenosis in two, blood cysts in two, and the valve was mitralized in five. In seven, the chordae were markedly abbreviated with bizarre connections with the papillary muscles. In three, the valve was markedly thickened and in six, either the papillary muscle from the anterior or posterior group proceeded to the base of the valve. There was one remarkable heart with candida thrombosis occluding the tricuspid valve proceeding to the main pulmonary trunk (Figs. 7, and 8).

Pulmonary Valve

The pulmonic valve was usually normally formed and presented increased hemodynamic change. Blood cysts were present in one. Infective endocarditis (candida thrombosis) was occluding the valve producing pulmonary stenosis in another (Fig. 8). Aneurysm of sinus of Valsalva was present in two. The valve cusps presented thickening throughout in one. The main pulmonary trunk was aneurysmally dilated in three. In four, the right pulmonary artery emerged very close to the base of the pulmonic valve and in two the left pulmonary artery emerged much higher than the right. In one, the cusps were separated with pulmonary insufficiency.

Mitral Valve

In general, the valve was normally formed and presented increased hemodynamic change. Blood cysts were found in four, and the valve was markedly thickened with abbreviated chordae (Fig. 9) or it presented a sheet of tissue with bizarre connections and abbreviated chordae in five. In four, the papillary muscles either from the anterior or the posterior group proceeded to the base or the edge of the valve (Fig. 10). In one there was mitral atresia and there was another with common atrioventricular orifice of the intermediate type.

Aortic Valve

In 35 (52%) the valve was bicuspid and in two it was unicuspid. Many of the bicuspid and tricuspid valves presented considerable thickening. In the remainder, the valve was normally formed but presented some increased hemodynamic change. In one bicuspid valve, one cusp was considerably larger than the other. The valve was markedly thickened in five and in a couple of cases the sinus of Valsalva was quite outpouched.

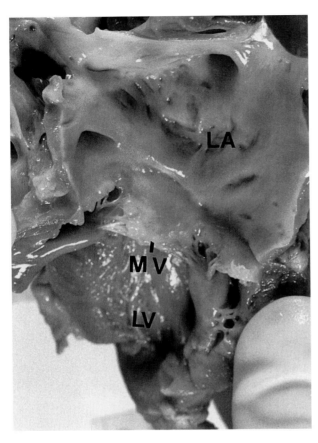

Figure 9: Left atrial, left ventricular view demonstrating the hypertrophy and enlargement of the left atrium with markedly abbreviated chordae. LA = left atrium; MV = mitral valve; LV = left ventricle. Note the hypertrophied papillary muscles with abbreviated chordae.

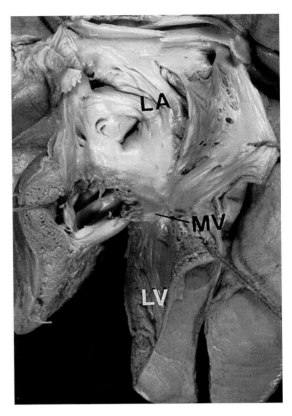

Figure 10: Left atrial, left ventricular view demonstrating the small mitral valve, and the anomalous papillary muscle connections with mitral stenosis. LA = enlarged left atrium; LV = left ventricle; MV = small mitral valve. Note the abbreviated chordae and papillary muscles proceeding directly to the valve leaflets or to the undersurface of the leaflet causing mitral stenosis. Note also the redundant mitral valve tissue.

Morphology of Ventricular Septal Defect

In general, in this entity, the defect had a tendency to be situated beneath the aortic valve in part in the membranous septum and either extended in an oblique manner towards the apex or extended further anteriorly. However, there were many variations in the location and size of the defect in more than 50% of the cases. The VSD variations were as follows:

	No. of Cases
Large anterior (subarterial or intracristal) VSD (1 with overriding pulmonary trunk and aorta)	8
Anterior ventricular septal defect entering the right ventricle beneath the arch	2
Oblique ventricular septal defect	2
In part intracristal and in part subcristal VSD	1
Double ventricular septal defect (the second defect mid-muscular anterior, or anterior muscular)	4
Spontaneously closing ventricular septal defect	2
Anteroapical ventricular septal defect	1
U-Shaped deficiency confluent with the base of the aortic valve but entering the right ventricle beneath the arch or crista	1
U-shaped deficiency of the anterior septum with overriding pulmonary trunk	1
Intermediate type of common atrioventricular orifice with common atrium	1
CAVO type of ventricular septal defect with overriding aorta and infundibular pulmonary stenosis	1
Mid-muscular ventricular septal defect	1
Posterior ventricular septal defect	2
Slit-like ventricular septal defect (1 below the arch and 1 between the sinus and conus)	2

	No. of Cases
Large ventricular septal defect	1
Tricuspid valve attached to the crest of the septum	1

Interrupted (Absent) Transverse Arch with Aorticopulmonary Septal Defect

There was a total of six hearts (8.9%): five males and one female. The ages were stillborn, 4 days, 10 days, 17 days, 1 month, and 1 month, 20 days. In all, the ventricular septum was intact with interruption distal to the left subclavian artery with a patent ductus forming the descending aorta. The type of interruption varied, although in all it occurred distal to the left subclavian artery. The various types of interruptions in these six hearts are as follows:

	No. of Cases
Interruption distal to the left subclavian artery	3
Interruption distal to the left subclavian artery with right descending aorta	1
Interruption distal to the left subclavian artery with right pulmonary artery emerging from the posterior aspect of the aorticopulmonary septum	1
Interruption or marked narrowing (complete obliteration) of the transverse arch distal to the left subclavian artery with aorticopulmonary defect 2 cm above the pulmonary valve and close to two pulmonary arteries with a closing ductus arteriosus	1

Although there is a common denominator of interruption occurring distal to the left subclavian artery in interrupted aortic arch with aorticopulmonary septal defect, there are some variations. The important variation is the origin of the right pulmonary artery emerging from the aortic segment of the aorticopulmonary septal defect.

Patterns of Interruption of the Arch with Ventricular Septal Defect

	No. of Cases
Interruption distal to left common carotid artery	34 (75.5%)
Interruption distal to left subclavian	11 (24.5%)

In three, there was distinct tissue connecting the ascending and the descending aorta; however, the lumen was completely obliterated. In others, a distinct statement as to the type of interruption could not be made. The origin of the brachiocephalic vessels in those where a statement could be made definitely is as follows:

	No. of Cases
Left subclavian artery originating from descending aorta	9
Both subclavian arteries originating from descending aorta	3
Right subclavian artery from descending aorta	2
Left subclavian artery from patent ductus arteriosus	1
Left subclavian artery from junction of the main pulmonary trunk and left pulmonary artery and right subclavian artery from ascending aorta	1
One subclavian artery from the main pulmonary trunk and the other from patent ductus arteriosus	1
Left subclavian artery from descending aorta and right subclavian artery from right pulmonary artery	1
Left subclavian artery at the junction of patent ductus and descending aorta	2

It is evident that interruption of the aortic arch occurs quite frequently distal to the left common carotid artery and less frequently distal to the left subclavian artery. The origin of the left subclavian artery originating from the descending aorta appears to be the most common form of pattern regardless of the fact whether the interruption occurs distal to the left subclavian artery or distal to the left common carotid artery. However, there appears to be a tendency for abnormal origin of the right subclavian artery when interruption occurred distal to the left subclavian artery.

Subaortic Area

In general, the subaortic area was distinctly smaller than normal with a small aortic valve and a small anulus in approximately 85% of the cases. The anatomic variations seen in the subaortic area are as follows:

	No. of Cases
Subaortic stenosis (3 with aortic stenosis and 1 supravalvular aortic stenosis)	20 (29.8%)
Straddling conus (parietal band) (2 with overriding pulmonary trunk)	12 (17.9%)

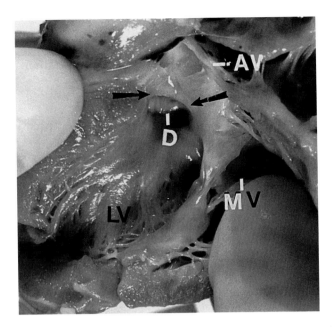

Figure 11: Left ventricular view demonstrating the bicuspid aortic valve and the prominent endocardial ridge immediately beneath the aortic valve proceeding in a circumferential fashion producing subaortic obstruction distal to the surgically closed ventricular septal defect. AV = bicuspid aortic valve, small anulus; MV = mitral valve; LV = left ventricle; D = ventricular septal defect closed surgically. Arrows point to the fibroelastic ridge immediately beneath the aortic valve.

Straddling conus with subaortic stenosis (1 with aortic stenosis and 1 with
overriding pulmonary trunk)   2 (2.9%)
Fibroelastic ridge beneath the aortic
valve   2

Frequently, the subaortic area immediately beneath the aortic valve presented fibroelastic ridge in a circumferential manner (Fig. 11). However, these ridges were not quite prominent.

Comment

Interrupted aortic arch (absent transverse arch) is an uncommon entity. Although it is usually associated with a ventricular septal defect, it may occur with an intact ventricular septum. The origin and course of the pulmonary arteries should be well delineated prior to total surgical correction.

When there is a defect, it is usually of a subarterial type and there is a tendency for the parietal band from the right ventricle to straddle through the defect with the pulmonary trunk and/or the aorta to override the septum to a varying degree. It is noteworthy that the ventricular septal defect varied in size, shape, and location in more than 50% of the cases. The location and size of the defect and its relationship to the great ar-

Table 1

Associated Cardiac Abnormalities

	No. of Cases
Atrial septal defect, fossa ovalis type	41 (61%)
Large atrial septal defect, fossa ovalis type	8
Patent foramen ovale	10
Premature narrowing of foramen ovale	1
Large fossa ovalis defect extending to the proximal region	3
Aneurysm of fossa ovalis	2
Aneurysm of space of His	2
Left superior vena cava entering coronary sinus	3
Absent coronary sinus with coronary veins entering a small left superior vena cava	1
Remnant of sinus venosus valves	1
Tricuspid stenosis	1
Tricuspid stenosis and aortic stenosis	1
Tricuspid stenosis with aortic stenosis and insufficiency	1
Aneurysm of the membranous septum	1
Anomalous muscles in the left ventricle	2
Deviated parietal band in the right ventricle	1
Left pulmonary artery smaller than the right	1
Closing patent ductus arteriosus	8
Stenosis of the ductus arteriosus (catheter proven)	1
High origin of both coronary ostia	6
High origin of right coronary ostium	1
Origin of one coronary ostium above the other	1
Single right coronary ostium	1
Two coronary ostia from anterior sinus of Valsalva	1
Mitral atresia	1
Common AV orifice intermediate type with common atrium	1
Small mitral valve	1
Mitral stenosis (1 with severe coarctation or atresia)	3
Extensive collateral anastomosis	1
Overriding aorta	2

Table 2

Associated Extracardiac Abnormalities

	No. of Cases
Trisomy 18	1
Multiple extracardiac abnormalities (3 abnormal spleens)	16
Accessory spleen	2

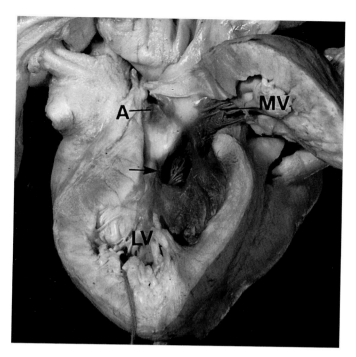

Figure 12: Left ventricular outflow tract view demonstrating the ventricular septal defect that extends from the membranous part of the ventricular septum somewhat posterior and extending anteriorly in an oblique angle with the tricuspid valve attached to the crest of the septum. A = aortic valve; MV = mitral valve; LV = left ventricle. Arrow points to the tricuspid valve attachment to the defect. Note the muscle separating the aorta from the defect. Note also the bicuspid thickened small aortic valve.

teries should be understood before surgical correction. Uncommonly, small defects (Fig. 4) occur in this entity or the defect has a tendency to close or the tricuspid valve may plug the defect (Fig. 12).

Today, interrupted aortic arch is being operated on with some success. The following factors may be related to the high mortality and/or the morbidity in this entity. As indicated above, a straddling parietal band may produce subaortic obstruction sooner or later. It is important to realize that the subaortic area is inherently smaller than normal in this entity. Associated with this narrowing of the subaortic area is a small aortic valve that has a tendency to be bicuspid in many. It appears that the aortic stenosis in this entity may not be manifest adequately prior to surgery due to the presence of a ventricular septal defect. Following surgery, the aortic stenosis may be mild to start with but may become marked over time. The bicuspid aortic valve may be susceptible to infective endocarditis. The presence of fibroelastic ridges immediately adjacent to the base of the aortic valve may promote the growth of subaortic stenosis postoperatively in some cases. In postoperative cases at the junction of the anastomotic site, there may be prominent circumferential ridge that

may cause significant obstruction at a later date (Fig. 13).

It should be noted that in less than 10% of the cases the left ventricle was small or even atrophied. These cases may present a picture of hypoplastic left heart syndromes. A careful morphological examination of the left atrium, the mitral valve, and the left ventricle should be undertaken in all cases of interrupted aortic arch before any total surgical correction is contemplated. The extremely small left ventricle and mitral valve abnormalities may not permit total surgical correction in some. The mitral valve, in one-third of the cases, was smaller than normal with or without stenosis. It was not uncommon to find thickening of the mitral valve with abbreviated chordae and anomalous papillary muscle connections. It is important to carefully analyze the function of the mitral valve prior to surgery. In the presence of a ventricular septal defect and a sizable atrial septal defect, the function of the mitral valve may not be ascertained or may not be determined accurately before surgery.

In some, the overriding pulmonary trunk may be quite dominant and may give a clinical picture of double outlet left ventricle especially when it is associated with a U-shaped deficiency in the summit of the ventricular septum, anterior to the membranous septum,

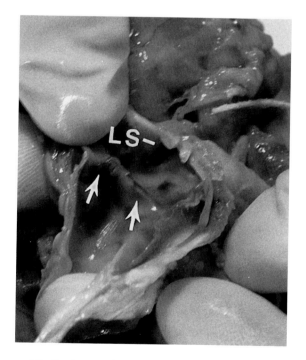

Figure 13: Postoperative anastomotic site of the transverse arch demonstrating a distinct circumferential ridge. Distal to the anastomosis emerges the left subclavian artery. LS = left subclavian artery. Arrows point to the circumferential ridge at the level of the surgically anastomosed area between the ascending and descending aorta.

and confluent with the pulmonic valve. It is of interest to note that an atrial septal defect of the fossa ovalis type is quite frequently noted in this entity. However, an occasional case of premature narrowing of the foramen ovale is also seen.

Ductus Arteriosus

Although the ductus arteriosus forms the descending aorta, it has a tendency to close spontaneously sooner or later. The closure of the ductus or closing ductus arteriosus was seen in nine infants.

Interrupted aortic arch seen with other major cardiac abnormalities such as tricuspid atresia with transposition, Taussig-Bing group of hearts, single ventricle, and truncus will be discussed along with those entities.

Embryogenesis

Here we are usually dealing with an abnormality related to the fourth arch derivative and to some extent the sixth arch derivative as well. The fact that we find in many cases a straddling parietal band, U-shaped ventricular septal defect overriding of the pulmonary trunk and/or of the aorta with smallness of the subaortic area suggests that there is abnormal formation and absorption of the bulbus into the left ventricle to a varying degree. Thus, if the abnormality primarily involves the bulbar septum alone and/or in combination with the membranous septum and the main ventricular septum, the defect occurs in varying locations and shapes. If, on the other hand, the bulbar septum had normally formed but the defect fundamentally occurs distally, in a localized manner affecting the fourth and the sixth arches, there may be an aorticopulmonary septal defect with interrupted aortic arch.

Further, the multiple extracardiac malformations, including DiGeorge's syndrome, in a sizable number of cases (28%) suggest the possibility that abnormalities may fundamentally be present in several genes at several levels that may alter the developing embryo. In addition, alterations in hemodynamics, as such, during these stages may further complicate the developing heart. Research in these areas should be explored in the future.

88

Stenosis or Atresia of the Pulmonary Veins

Stenosis or atresia of the pulmonary veins may be seen in several forms. A common pulmonary vein may be stenotic or the common pulmonary vein may join an accessory chamber that may in return be atretic and have no connection with the left atrium. The stenosis of the pulmonary veins may affect all of the veins individually with marked thickening and diffuse narrowing of the veins (Fig. 1). On the other hand, the narrowing and thickening may affect only the right or the left veins. There is usually hypertrophy and enlargement or hypertrophy of the right-sided chambers with smallness or atrophy of the left-sided chambers.

Analysis of Our Material

There was a total of eight cases: four males and four females. The youngest was a newborn, 23 hours old, and the oldest was 9½ months old, with a mean age of 3 months.

The Complex

The heart was hypertrophied and somewhat enlarged. The apex was formed by both ventricles in five, by the right ventricle in two, and by the left ventricle in one (Fig. 2). The right atrium and right ventricle were hypertrophied and enlarged in the majority of the cases and hypertrophied in the remainder. The left atrium was atrophied in four, small with a thick wall in two, and normal size in one. There was one case with a common atrium where there was hypertrophy of this chamber. The left ventricle was atrophied in five, small in one, normal in one, and enlarged in one. The tricuspid orifice was enlarged in two, normal in three, and smaller than normal in three. The pulmonic orifice was

enlarged in six and normal in two. The mitral orifice was smaller than normal in four (in one it was very small), normal in size in three, and there was one case with mitral atresia. The aortic orifice was smaller than normal in four, normal in three, and atretic in one.

The Valves

Tricuspid Valve

In general, the tricuspid valve was normally formed and presented increased hemodynamic change. There was mitralization of the leaflet in two, and accessory papillary muscles in the inferoseptal wall in two. In the remaining hearts, there was considerable thickening of the valvular structure with some anomalous papillary muscles.

Pulmonary Valve

This was always normally formed and presented increased hemodynamic change.

Mitral Valve

In five, the valve was normally formed and presented the usual hemodynamic change. In one, the valve was atretic, in another the valve was very small, and in one it was markedly thickened.

Aortic Valve

The aortic valve was normally formed. It showed the usual hemodynamic change in six, a bicuspid markedly thickened valve with aortic stenosis in one, and it was atretic in one.

1371

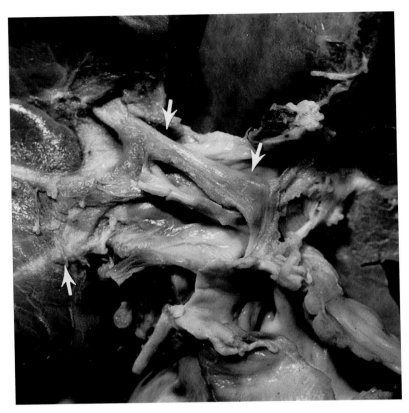

Figure 1: Posterior view of the heart showing marked thickening and narrowing of the pulmonary veins. Arrows point to the pulmonary veins.

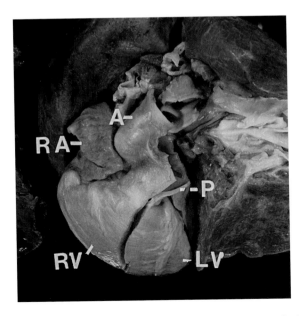

Figure 2: External view of the heart which is relatively small, with an apex formed by the left ventricle. RA = right atrium; RV = right ventricle; LV = left ventricle; A = aorta; P = pulmonary trunk.

Endocardium

The endocardium presented distinctly increased focal thickening and whitening in all of the chambers.

There was considerable variation in stenosis of the veins. Therefore, we are enumerating each case separately as follows.

1. Stenosis of the common pulmonary vein with fossa ovalis type atrial septal defect and patent ductus arteriosus.
2. Stenosis of the common pulmonary vein with aortic and mitral atresia, absence of the atrial septum, wide patent ductus arteriosus and a left superior vena cava entering the left-sided appendage.
3. Stenosis of the right pulmonary veins (Fig. 3) and stenosis of the left lower pulmonary veins with patent ductus arteriosus and probe patent foramen ovale.
4. Atresia of the left pulmonary veins (Fig. 4) with fossa ovalis type atrial septal defect and atrophy of left pulmonary artery.
5. Stenosis of the pulmonary veins with fossa ovalis type atrial septal defect.
6. Stenosis of the pulmonary veins with oblique patent foramen ovale.

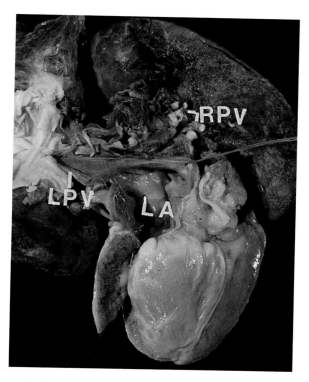

Figure 3: Stenosis of the right pulmonary veins. LA = left atrium; RPV = stenosis of the right pulmonary vein; LPV = left upper pulmonary veins entering the left atrium normally.

7. Stenosis of the pulmonary veins with atrial septal defect, ventricular septal defect, and oblique patent foramen ovale.
8. Stenosis of the pulmonary veins (right more than the left) with fetal coarctation (hypoplasia or transverse arch), distal origin of two subclavian arteries, right pulmonary artery smaller than the left, wide patent ductus arteriosus, and the right atrial appendage resembling that of the left, and the left atrial appendage was minute, with hypoplastic monolobate both lungs.

Comment

It is obvious that there are tremendous variations associated with this entity. The pulmonary artery on the affected side is usually smaller than normal. The stenotic pulmonary veins may be markedly abbreviated and short or elongated. Stenosis of the pulmonary veins is often associated with tremendous proliferation of the connective tissue surrounding the veins up to their entry into the left atrium, or at its junction with the latter. This, therefore, suggests that we may be dealing fundamentally with some type of a connective tissue disorder related to the veins and/or an injury or some other external stimuli that could have resulted in

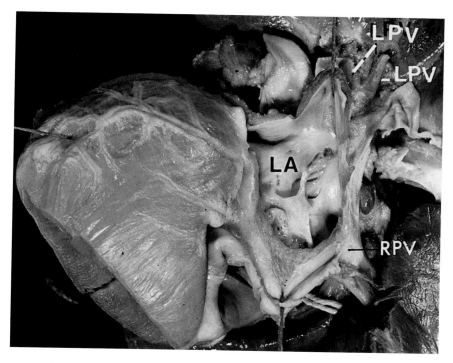

Figure 4: Atresia of the left pulmonary veins as seen from the left atrial view. LA = left atrium; RPV = right pulmonary veins entering the left atrium normally; LPV = markedly thickened small and atretic left pulmonary veins.

1374 • *THE PATHOLOGY OF CONGENITAL HEART DISEASE*

the proliferation of the exuberant amount of connective tissue surrounding the veins. In none of the cases was a true levo-atrial cardinal vein found except in one, where a left superior vena cava entered the left-sided atrial appendage. This may be considered a variant of the levo-atrial cardinal vein. However, in this case there was a common atrium and a coronary sinus.

Thus, the excessive connective tissue proliferation around the pulmonary veins, both before and after surgery, may be one of the reasons for high mortality and morbidity. The relationship of the specific connective tissue proliferation associated with this entity deserves further research at the molecular-genetic level in the next decade.

It is evident that a thorough examination of the pulmonary arterial system and the lung parenchyma is mandatory before any type of correction of the stenotic veins is contemplated. It is wise to undertake any type of correction before atrophy of the left atrium and left ventricle set in.

89

Other Complexes

The following unusual complexes were present in this series. There was a total of 152 cases; 85 were male subjects, 62 were female subjects, four were unknown and one was an animal.

Miscellaneous Mitral Valve Anomalies

10-month-old male
  Mitral anular enlargement with some redundancy of the valve and aneurysm of the left atrium

69-year-old female
  Aneurysm of the pars membranacea
  Calcific mitral valve and redundant, segmented anterior leaflet with mitral insufficiency (Figs. 1, 2)

35-hour-old female infant
  Infective endocarditis in the mitral and the tricuspid valves, patent foramen ovale, tricuspid stenosis with PDA, and hemorrhagic myocardium

48-year-old
  Mitral stenosis and insufficiency and prosthetic valve replacement, etiology unknown

39-year-old male
  Irregularly thickened bicuspid or unicuspid pulmonic valve with fenestrations and pulmonary insufficiency (Fig. 3)
  Irregularly thickened mitral valve

14-year, 9-month-old male
  Thalassemia, clinical, and hemochromatosis of the myocardium and the mitral valve

47-year-old male
  Possible Marfan's syndrome with dissecting aneurysm, and slight dilatation of the aortic sinus of Valsalva
  Aneurysmal dilatation of the anterior leaflet of the mitral valve, and mitral insufficiency

2-day-old male
  Left-sided Ebstein's anomaly of the mitral valve (in atrioventricular concordant heart) with stenosis and insufficiency, giant left atrium, divided left ventricle, fossa ovalis atrial septal defect, and patent ductus arteriosus
  Redundant tricuspid and mitral valves with abbreviated chordae, tricuspid and mitral insufficiency. (Figs. 4–7)

28-year-old male
  Bicuspid aortic valve, infective endocarditis extending to mitral valve, and aneurysm of aortic leaflet of the mitral valve

2-month-old male (35-weeks' gestation – triplet)
  Dysplastic pulmonary valve with marked pulmonary stenosis and infundibular stenosis
  Thickened pulmonic, tricuspid, and mitral valves, mitral stenosis, hypertrophic cardiomyopathy, spontaneous closure of ventricular septal defect, and immense cardiomegaly

Infant male
  Atypical mitral stenosis and probable insufficiency, possible subaortic stenosis, and aneurysm of left atrium and left ventricle (Figs. 8–10)

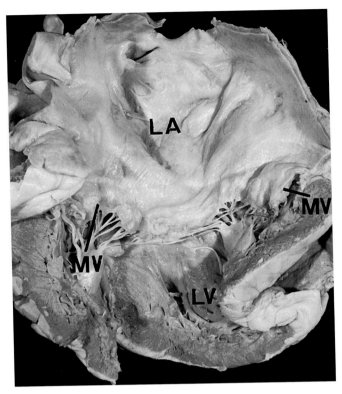

Figure 1: Floppy mitral valve and aneurysm of the membranous septum in a 69-year-old female. Left atrial, left ventricular view. LA = left atrium; LV = left ventricle; MV = enlarged mitral valve with redundant anterior and posterior leaflets. Note the huge left atrium and left ventricle.

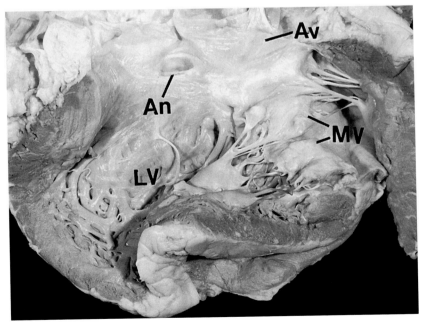

Figure 2: Left ventricular outflow tract demonstrating aneurysm of the membranous septum. MV = mitral valve; AV = aortic valve; LV = left ventricle; An = aneurysm of the membranous septum. Note the huge left ventricle.

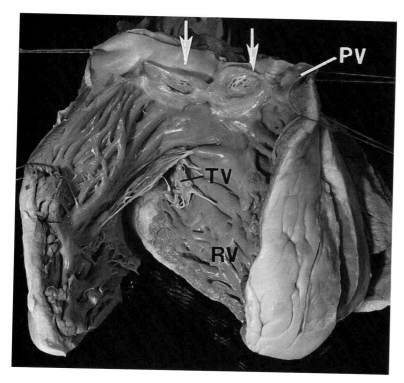

Figure 3: Thickening of the pulmonic valve cusps with fenestrations and pulmonary insufficiency. RV = right ventricle; TV = tricuspid valve; PV = pulmonary valve. Arrows point to the thickened pulmonic valve with fenestrations.

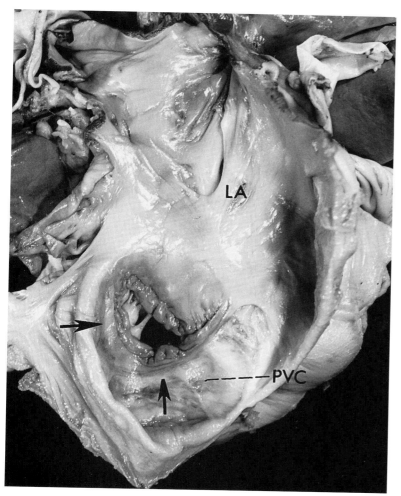

Figure 4: Ebstein-like malformation of the mitral valve with mitral stenosis. Left atrial view. LA = left atrium, hypertrophied and enlarged; PVC = proximal ventricular chamber. Arrows point to the displaced inferior leaflet into the proximal ventricular chamber. (Used with permission from Ruschhaupt DG, et al. See Figure 7.)

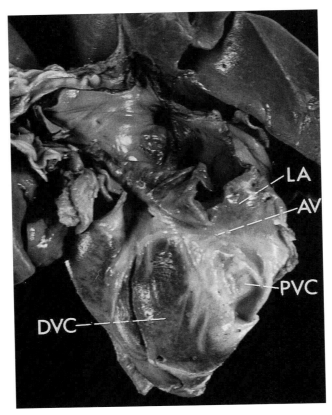

Figure 5: The proximal and distal ventricular chambers as seen from the posterior view. LA = left atrium; AV = atrioventricular sulcus; PVC = thinned-out proximal ventricular chamber; DVC = distal ventricular chamber.

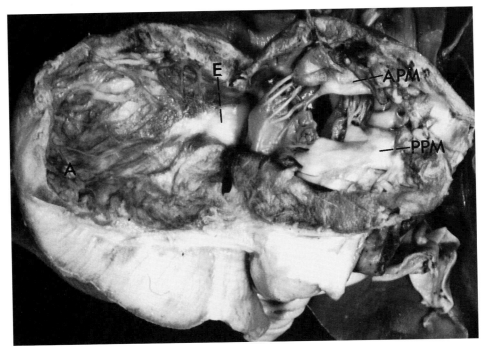

Figure 6: Endocardial fibroelastosis of the left ventricle. E = endocardial fibroelastosis; APM = anterior papillary muscle; PPM = posterior papillary muscle. (Used with permission from Ruschhaupt DG, et al. See Figure 7.)

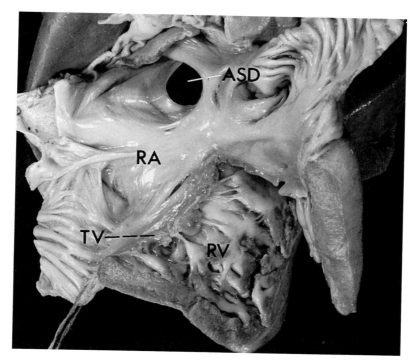

Figure 7: Atrial septal defect, fossa ovalis type in Ebstein's anomaly of the mitral valve. Right atrial, right ventricular view. RA = right atrium; RV = right ventricle; TV = tricuspid valve, ASD = atrial septal defect, fossa ovalis type. (Used with permission from Ruschhaupt DG, Bharati S, Lev M: Mitral valve malformation of Ebstein type in absence of corrected transposition. *Am J Cardiol* 1976, 38:109–112.)

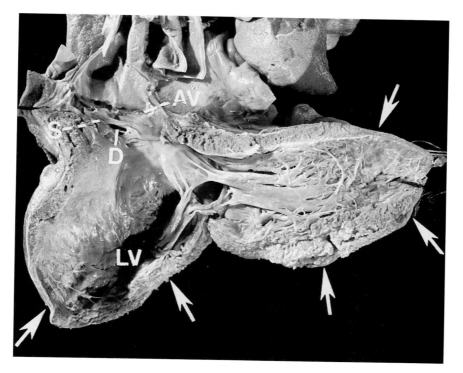

Figure 8: Congenital aneurysm of the left ventricle in a newborn infant. Left ventricular view demonstrating a large left ventricle. LV = huge left ventricle; AV = aortic valve; S = subaortic ridge and a small ventricular septal defect; D = ventricular septal defect. Arrows point to the aneurysmally dilated thin wall of the left ventricle.

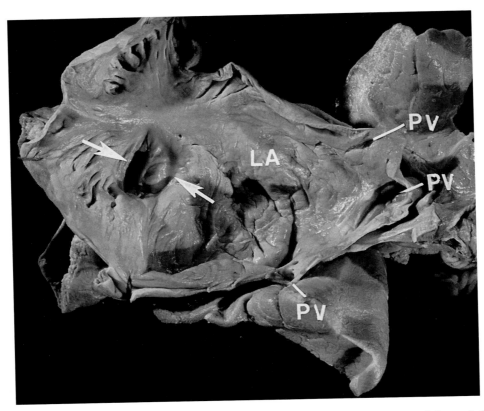

Figure 9: Redundant mitral valve with stenosis and insufficiency, and huge left atrium. PV = pulmonary veins entering the left atrium; LA = left atrium aneurysmally dilated. Arrows point to the redundant mitral valve with stenosis and insufficiency.

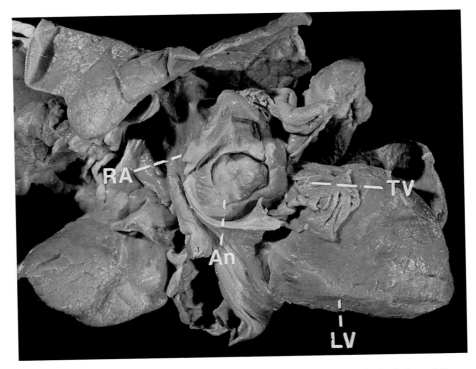

Figure 10: Same heart as seen from the right atrial view. Note the bulging of the septum primum into the right atrial cavity forming an aneurysm. RA = right atrium; An = aneurysm of the septum primum; LV = left ventricle; TV = tricuspid valve.

Tumors

10-month-old male

Fibroma of interventricular septum, obstruction to left ventricular outflow tract and right ventricular outflow tract with surgery

1-month-old male

Rhabdomyoma of the ventricular septum, outflow tract of the left ventricle and the mitral valve (Figs. 11, 12)

10-day-old male

Rhabdomyoma of the ventricular septum

5-month-old female

Multiple rhabdomyoma of myocardium obstructing the tricuspid and mitral orifices, and obstruction to the left ventricular outflow tract, and right ventricular outflow tract (Figs. 13–15)

7-month-old female

Multiple rhabdomyomatosis

8-year-old male

Lipoma of the myocardium in the anterior wall of the left ventricle (2.3 cm)

Redundant tricuspid valve

Tuberous sclerosis

66-year-old female

Lipoma of atrial septum

16-year-old female

Large tumor mass in the anterior leaflet of the mitral valve with subaortic stenosis and systemic hypertension

1½-month-old male

Tumors in the right ventricle

9-day-old male

Cysts in the right atrial wall with thrombus, and multiple tumors of the myocardium

Atrial septal defect, fossa ovalis type, preductal coarctation, and bicuspid aortic valve (Figs. 16–18)

1-month-old male

Tumor of the atrial septum (Fig. 19), supravalvular ridge in the mitral and aortic valves

8-year-old female

Tumor metastasis of the tricuspid valve (Fig. 20) occluding the right pulmonary artery and infiltration of tumor masses in both lungs (osteogenic sarcoma)

Primary tumor sacrococcygeal malignant teratoma, resected at 2 years and followed by radiotherapy, at age 6 diagnosed as osteogenic sarcoma of the left ileum and hip replacement, tumor extension into inferior vena cava and the heart

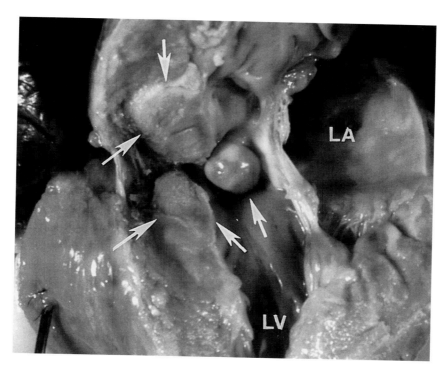

Figure 11: Rhabdomyoma of the left ventricle obstructing the outflow tract into the aorta. LA = left atrium; LV = left ventricle. Arrows point to the rhabdomyoma obstructing the outflow tract of the left ventricle.

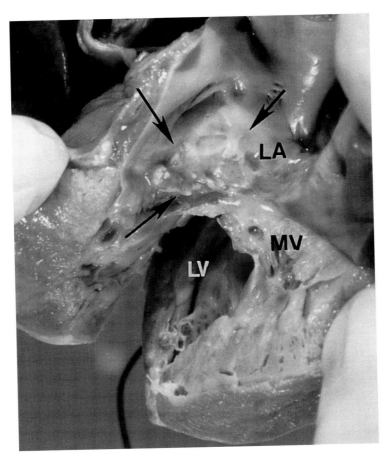

Figure 12: Left atrial, left ventricular view showing the area of rhabdomyoma that was surgically removed from the left atrium. LA = left atrium; LV = left ventricle; MV = mitral valve. Arrows point to the surgical removal of rhabdomyoma.

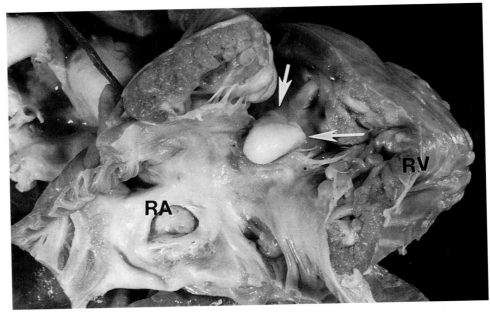

Figure 13: Multiple rhabdomyomas of the heart. Right atrial, right ventricular view. Arrows point to the large tumor at the junction of anterior and septal leaflets of the tricuspid valve. RA = right atrium; RV = right ventricle.

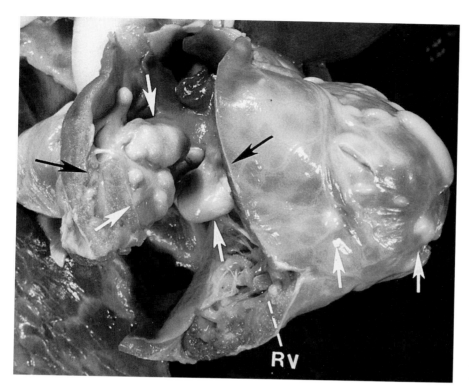

Figure 14: View of the right ventricular outflow tract. Arrows point to some of the tumors. RV = right ventricle.

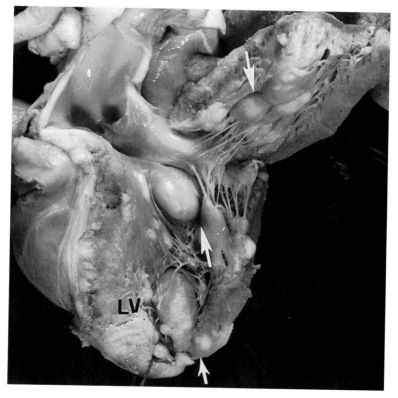

Figure 15: Left ventricular view. LV = left ventricle. Arrows point to some of the tumors. (Used with permission from Bharati S, et al. See Figure 23.)

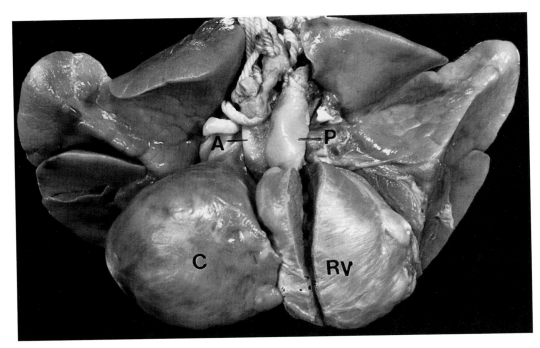

Figure 16: Cyst in the right atrium, external view of the heart. RV = right ventricle; C = cyst; A = aorta; P = pulmonary trunk.

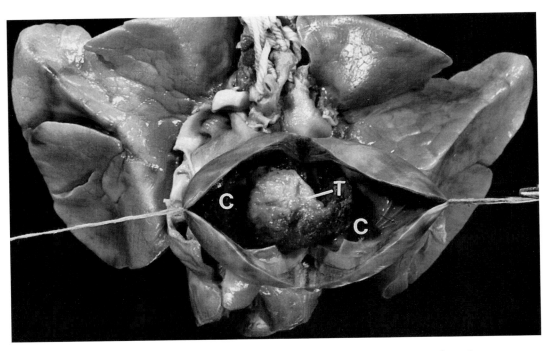

Figure 17: Cyst in the right atrium, with thrombus. C = cyst; T = thrombus.

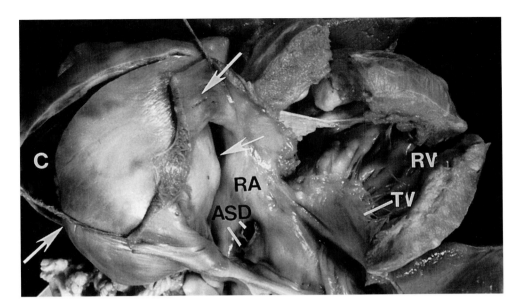

Figure 18: Right atrial, right ventricular view showing the relationship of the cyst to the right atrium. RA = right atrium; RV = right ventricle; TV = tricuspid valve; C = cyst; ASD = atrial septal defect, fossa ovalis type. Arrows point to the cyst.

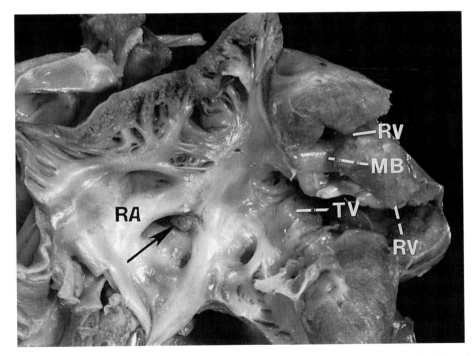

Figure 19: Small tumor in the atrial septum and anomalous muscle band dividing the right ventricle into an inlet and an outlet. RA = right atrium; RV = right ventricle; TV = tricuspid valve; MB = anomalous muscle band stretching from the parietal wall to the undersurface of the anterior leaflet of the tricuspid valve dividing the right ventricle into two segments. Arrow points to the cyst.

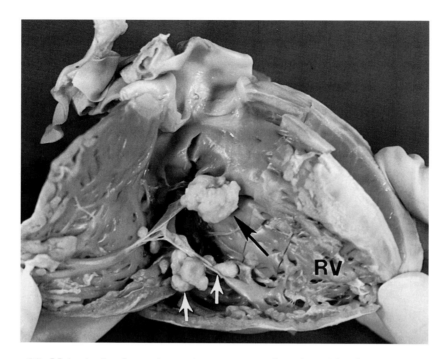

Figure 20: Metastasis of an osteogenic sarcoma to the tricuspid valve in a 16-year-old girl. RV = right ventricle. Arrows point to the tumor on the tricuspid valve. (Used with permission from Bharati S, Lev M. See Figure 23.)

27-weeks' gestation female
  Tumor mass in Bachmann's bundle with intractable supraventricular arrhythmia in utero, and cardiomegaly

Young male
  Myxoma – surgical specimen (Figs. 21, 22)

Middle-aged female
  Sarcoma – frozen section (Fig. 23)

Miscellaneous Aortic Valve Problems

5-week-old female
  Patent ductus arteriosus, bicuspid aortic valve, and aortic stenosis complex

7 years, 7-month-old male
  Double mitral orifice with mitral insufficiency and fenestration of the aortic valve

44-year-old male
  Irregularly thickened fenestrated aortic valve, aortic insufficiency, and subaortic ridges with stenosis

4-day-old male
  Bicuspid aortic valve with aortic stenosis, pulmonary stenosis, and patent ductus arteriosus

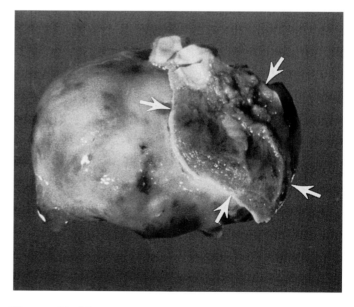

Figure 21: Myxoma in a young male – surgical specimen, gross appearance. Arrows point to the region of attachment of the tumor to the atrial septum. (Used with permission from Bharati S, Lev M. See Figure 23.)

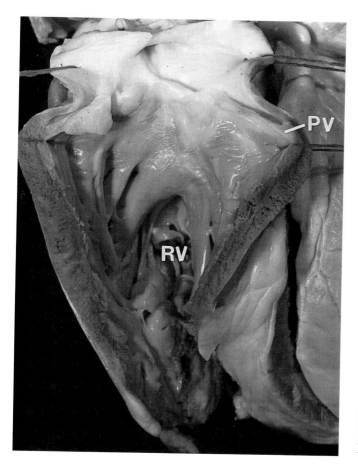

Figure 28: Congenital aortic and pulmonary stenosis in an 18-year-old male. Outflow tract of the right ventricle demonstrating unequal size and diffuse thickening of the pulmonic valve. RV = right ventricle; PV = pulmonary valve.

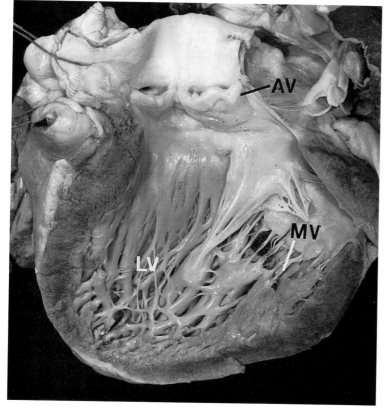

Figure 29: Incompletely divided tricuspid, thickened aortic valve with stenosis and possible insufficiency. AV = aortic valve; MV = mitral valve; LV = left ventricle.

Newborn male
    Huge atypical atrial septal defect, fossa ovalis and proximal type, with paraductal coarctation, and polyvalvular disease

4½-year-old female
    Atrial septal defect, ventricular septal defect (common AV canal type), pulmonary infundibular stenosis, and cleft in the anterior leaflet of the mitral and tricuspid valves

4-month-old male
    Atrial septal defect, ventricular septal defect, mitral stenosis, overriding aorta, redundant tricuspid valve, and left superior vena cava entering the coronary sinus

9-day-old male
    Atrial septal defect, fossa ovalis type, tricuspid insufficiency, patent ductus arteriosus, diffuse fibroelastosis, and origin of the left coronary artery from the noncoronary cusp

54-year-old male
    Atrial septal defect, fossa ovalis type, multiple accessory tricuspid orifices, thickened shortened chordae, tricuspid insufficiency, and pulmonary stenosis

4-day-old male
    Persistence of fetal circulation, clinical, atrial septal defect, patent ductus arteriosus, and thickening of all the valves

2-year, 9-month-old male
    Atrial septal defect, ventricular septal defect, tricuspid stenosis, tricuspid insufficiency and surgery, pulmonary stenosis, diffuse fibroelastosis of all chambers, and sudden death

3-hour-old male
    Cardiomegaly, etiology unknown, atrial septal defect, fossa ovalis type, aneurysmally dilated patent ductus, and high origin of right coronary ostium

8½-year-old female (Figs. 30–34)
    Isovaleric acidemia, clinical atypical Uhl's?, primitive ventricular mass with formation of diverticula of right and left ventricles

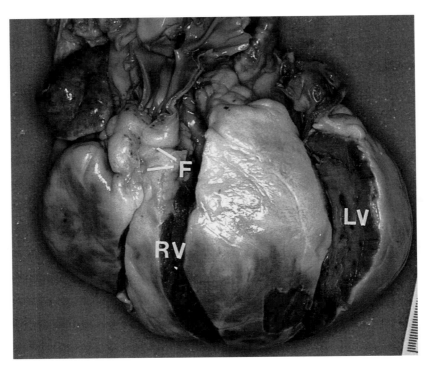

Figure 30: Atypical Uhl's anomaly. External view of the heart. Note the huge heart. LV = left ventricle; RV = right ventricle; F = fat.

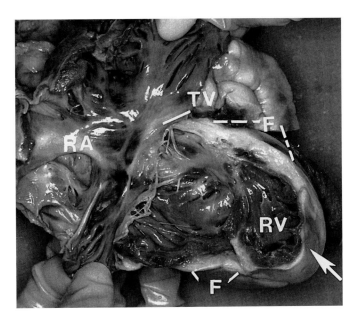

Figure 31: Right atrial, right ventricular view demonstrating the marked fatty infiltration in the anterior wall of the right ventricle and thinned out right ventricle apically. RA = right atrium; RV = right ventricle; TV = tricuspid valve; F = fat in anterior and inferior walls of the right ventricle. Arrow points to thinned out right ventricle.

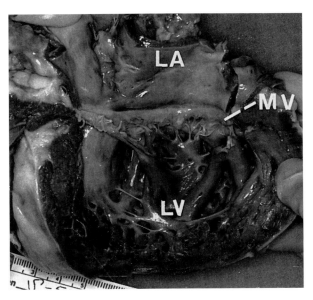

Figure 33: Left atrial, left ventricular view demonstrating some redundancy of the mitral valve. LA = left atrium; LV = left ventricle; MV = mitral valve.

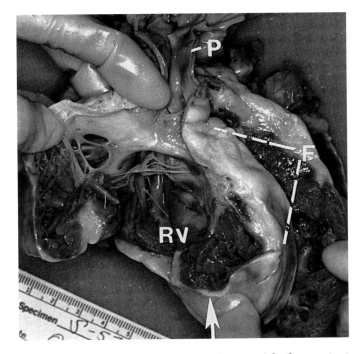

Figure 32: Outflow tract of the right ventricle demonstrating the fatty infiltration replacing the anterior wall of the right ventricle from the base to the apex. F = fat in anterior wall of the right ventricle; RV = right ventricle; P = pulmonary trunk. Arrow points to the paper-thin right ventricle.

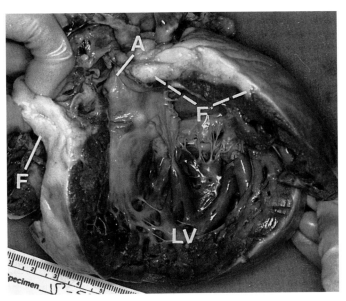

Figure 34: Outflow tract of the left ventricle demonstrating the marked fatty infiltration in the anterior wall of the ventricular septum. LV = left ventricle; A = aorta; F = fat in anterior wall of the left ventricle.

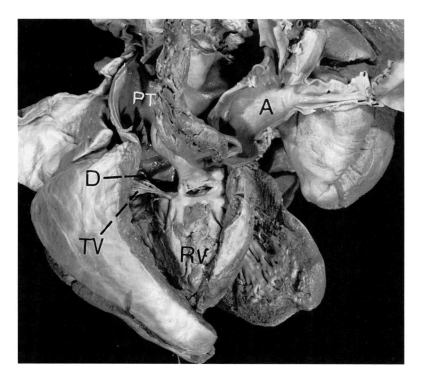

Figure 35: Trunco-conal inversion with Taussig-Bing anomaly. RV = right ventricle; TV = tricuspid valve; D = U-shaped defect confluent with the pulmonary trunk; PT = pulmonary trunk; A = aorta. Note that the aorta is to the left and anterior, and the pulmonary trunk is to the right and anterior.

Hypoplasia of the right ventricle with possible tricuspid stenosis and absence of myocardium in the anterior wall of the right ventricle, mesoposition of heart, atrial septal defect, fossa ovalis type, accessory tricuspid orifice with tricuspid insufficiency, distinct inflow and outflow of the left ventricle

3½-month-old female
Inverted Taussig-Bing (truncoconal inversion) (Figs. 35–38), subpulmonary ventricular septal defect, preductal coarctation, and patent ductus arteriosus complex

6-week-old male
Muscular ventricular septal defect, subaortic stenosis, and anomalous muscle bands in the left ventricle
Right aortic arch and right descending aorta

12-year-old female
Ventricular septal defect and divided right ventricle
Straddling tricuspid valve with insufficiency
Infundibular pulmonary stenosis and aortic stenosis

2-day-old male
Aortic and mitral atresia with ventricular septal defect, and remnants of sinus venarum valves

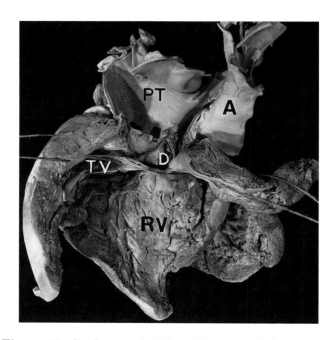

Figure 36: Outflow tract of the right ventricle demonstrating the pulmonary trunk emerging to the right of the aorta confluent with the defect. TV = tricuspid valve; RV = right ventricle; PT = pulmonary trunk; D = defect; A = aorta. (Used with permission from Shaffer AB, et al. See Figure 38.)

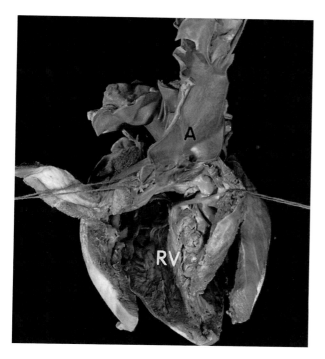

Figure 37: Aorta emerging from the right ventricle unrelated to the defect. A = aorta; RV = right ventricle. (Used with permission from Shaffer AB, et al. See Figure 38.) Note that the aorta is to the left and anterior.

8-year-old male (30-weeks' gestation)
  Redundant tricuspid valve with tricuspid insufficiency, aneurysm of the membranous septum, probable closure of ventricular septal defect, and cardiomegaly
  Mental retardation

Stillborn female
  Patent foramen ovale, aneurysm of the fossa ovalis, and small patent ductus arteriosus
  Subpulmonary stenosis, and subaortic stenosis

6-day-old female
  Fossa ovalis defect, tricuspid stenosis, pulmonary stenosis, mitral stenosis, and aortic and subaortic stenosis
  Uni- or bicuspid valve, bizarre left ventricle with fibroelastosis, mural thrombus, and coronary arteries thickened

10-day-old female
  Redundant tricuspid and pulmonic valves with tricuspid and infundibular pulmonary stenosis and subaortic stenosis, and anomalous bands in the right atrium

28-hour-old male
  Small ventricular septal defect, aneurysm of the sinus of Valsalva, and subluxation of the aortic cusp
  Aneurysm of the fossa ovalis, bicuspid pulmonic valve, small right pulmonary artery, and right pulmonary vein
  Anomalous muscle bands in the left ventricle, and origin of the coronary ostia above the sinus

6-month, 21-day-old female
  Ventricular septal defect, and paraductal coarctation of the aorta
  Right pulmonary artery emerging close to the base of the pulmonic valve, and single coronary artery

26-year-old male
  Common ventricle, huge ventricular septal defect with truncoconal inversion and straddling conus

1-month, 26-day-old female
  ASD and multiple ventricular septal defects, mitral stenosis, and aortic stenosis

5-day-old female
  Double aortic arch with interrupted transverse arch, and atrial and ventricular septal defects
  Bicuspid aortic and pulmonic valves

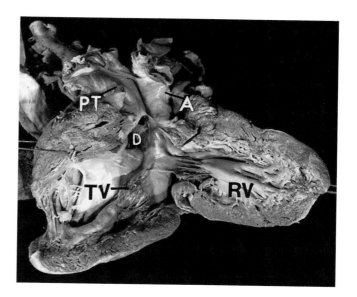

Figure 38: Outflow tract of the right ventricle demonstrating both vessels emerging side by side. TV = tricuspid valve; A = aorta to the left and anterior; PT = pulmonary trunk to the right; D = defect confluent with the pulmonary trunk; RV = right ventricle. (Used with permission from Shaffer AB, Kline IK, Lev M: Truncal inversion with biventricular pulmonary trunk and aorta from right ventricle (variant of Taussig-Bing complex). *Circulation* 1967, 36:783–788.)

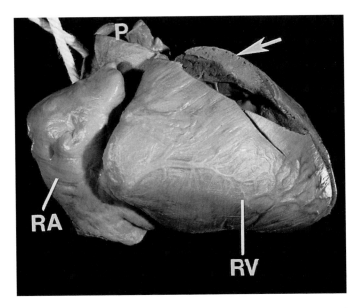

Figure 41: Marked hypertrophy of the heart, apex formed by the right ventricle in an infant with a patent foramen ovale, pulmonary stenosis, and aortic stenosis. RA = right atrium; RV = right ventricle; P = pulmonary valve. Arrow points to right ventricular hypertrophy.

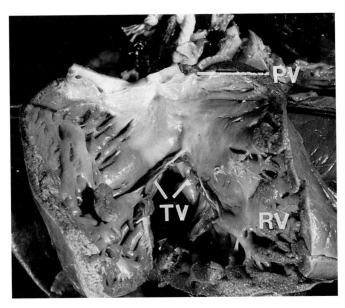

Figure 43: Outflow tract of the right ventricle demonstrating a large right ventricle and a thickened tricuspid valve. RV = right ventricle; TV = thickened tricuspid valve; PV = pulmonary valve.

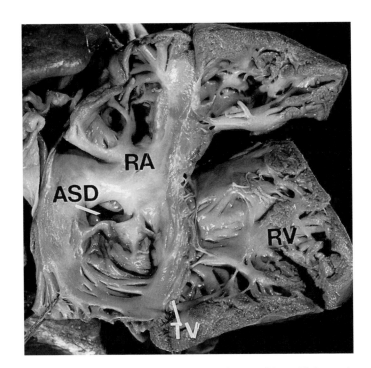

Figure 42: Congenital tricuspid and mitral insufficiency in an infant. Right atrial view. Huge right side. RA = right atrium; RV = right ventricle; ASD = atrial septal defect, fossa ovalis type; TV = tricuspid valve. Note that the tricuspid valve is enlarged with abbreviated chordae and a somewhat thickened valve.

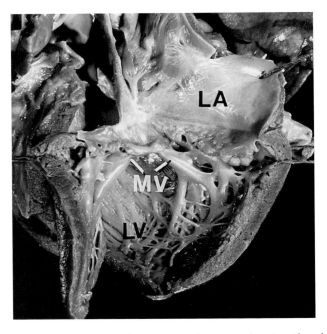

Figure 44: Left atrial, left ventricular view showing the abnormal mitral valve with mitral insufficiency. LV = left ventricle; LA = left atrium; MV = irregularly thickened mitral valve with papillary muscles more or less fusing with the leaflet with hardly any chordal extensions and mitral insufficiency.

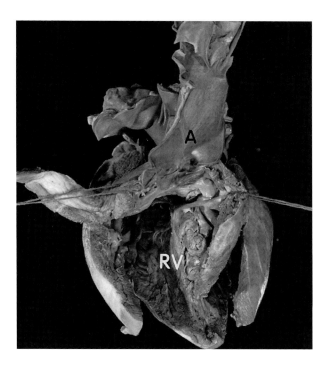

Figure 37: Aorta emerging from the right ventricle unrelated to the defect. A = aorta; RV = right ventricle. (Used with permission from Shaffer AB, et al. See Figure 38.) Note that the aorta is to the left and anterior.

8-year-old male (30-weeks' gestation)
  Redundant tricuspid valve with tricuspid insufficiency, aneurysm of the membranous septum, probable closure of ventricular septal defect, and cardiomegaly
  Mental retardation

Stillborn female
  Patent foramen ovale, aneurysm of the fossa ovalis, and small patent ductus arteriosus
  Subpulmonary stenosis, and subaortic stenosis

6-day-old female
  Fossa ovalis defect, tricuspid stenosis, pulmonary stenosis, mitral stenosis, and aortic and subaortic stenosis
  Uni- or bicuspid valve, bizarre left ventricle with fibroelastosis, mural thrombus, and coronary arteries thickened

10-day-old female
  Redundant tricuspid and pulmonic valves with tricuspid and infundibular pulmonary stenosis and subaortic stenosis, and anomalous bands in the right atrium

28-hour-old male
  Small ventricular septal defect, aneurysm of the sinus of Valsalva, and subluxation of the aortic cusp
  Aneurysm of the fossa ovalis, bicuspid pulmonic valve, small right pulmonary artery, and right pulmonary vein
  Anomalous muscle bands in the left ventricle, and origin of the coronary ostia above the sinus

6-month, 21-day-old female
  Ventricular septal defect, and paraductal coarctation of the aorta
  Right pulmonary artery emerging close to the base of the pulmonic valve, and single coronary artery

26-year-old male
  Common ventricle, huge ventricular septal defect with truncoconal inversion and straddling conus

1-month, 26-day-old female
  ASD and multiple ventricular septal defects, mitral stenosis, and aortic stenosis

5-day-old female
  Double aortic arch with interrupted transverse arch, and atrial and ventricular septal defects
  Bicuspid aortic and pulmonic valves

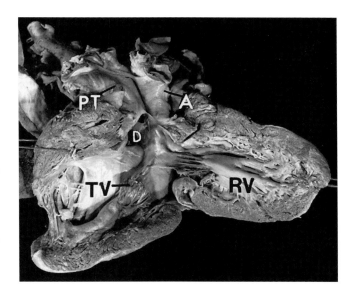

Figure 38: Outflow tract of the right ventricle demonstrating both vessels emerging side by side. TV = tricuspid valve; A = aorta to the left and anterior; PT = pulmonary trunk to the right; D = defect confluent with the pulmonary trunk; RV = right ventricle. (Used with permission from Shaffer AB, Kline IK, Lev M: Truncal inversion with biventricular pulmonary trunk and aorta from right ventricle (variant of Taussig-Bing complex). *Circulation* 1967, 36:783–788.)

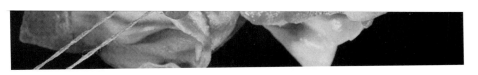

Figure 40: Outflow tract of the right ventricle demonstrating the normal pulmonary valve. RV = right ventricle; PV = pulmonary valve.

Muscular Dystrophy, Friedreich's   3-month-old female

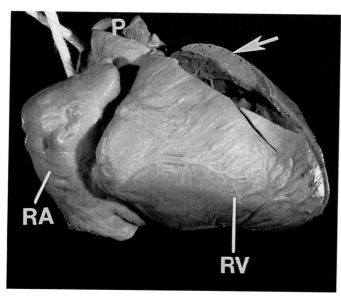

Figure 41: Marked hypertrophy of the heart, apex formed by the right ventricle in an infant with a patent foramen ovale, pulmonary stenosis, and aortic stenosis. RA = right atrium; RV = right ventricle; P = pulmonary valve. Arrow points to right ventricular hypertrophy.

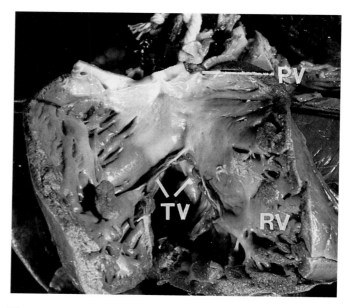

Figure 43: Outflow tract of the right ventricle demonstrating a large right ventricle and a thickened tricuspid valve. RV = right ventricle; TV = thickened tricuspid valve; PV = pulmonary valve.

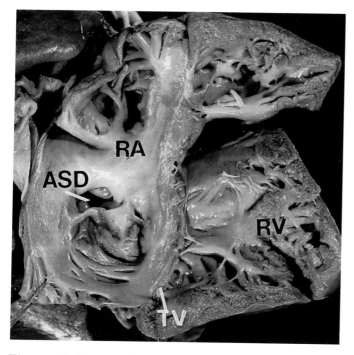

Figure 42: Congenital tricuspid and mitral insufficiency in an infant. Right atrial view. Huge right side. RA = right atrium; RV = right ventricle; ASD = atrial septal defect, fossa ovalis type; TV = tricuspid valve. Note that the tricuspid valve is enlarged with abbreviated chordae and a somewhat thickened valve.

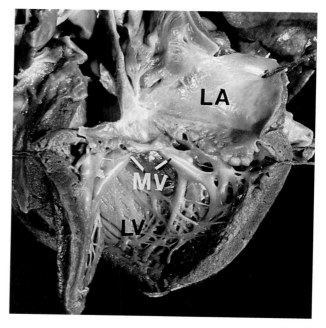

Figure 44: Left atrial, left ventricular view showing the abnormal mitral valve with mitral insufficiency. LV = left ventricle; LA = left atrium; MV = irregularly thickened mitral valve with papillary muscles more or less fusing with the leaflet with hardly any chordal extensions and mitral insufficiency.

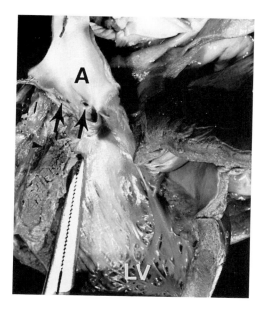

Figure 45: Outflow tract of the left ventricle demonstrating hypertrophy and enlargement of the left side and high origin of both coronary ostia. A = aorta; LV = left ventricle. Arrows point to the high origin of both coronary ostia.

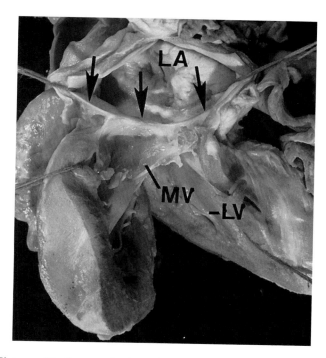

Figure 47: Supravalvular mitral stenosis in a 1-month-old female. LA = left atrium; MV = mitral valve; LV = left ventricle. Arrows point to the supravalvular membrane proximal to the mitral valve but distal to the left atrial appendage. Note the small mitral valve.

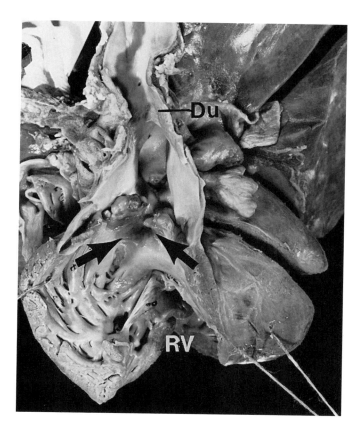

Figure 46: Marked redundancy of the pulmonic valve, pulmonary insufficiency, and huge ductus arteriosus in an infant. RV = right ventricle; Du = huge ductus arteriosus. Arrows point to the markedly thickened pulmonic valve. Note the large right ventricle.

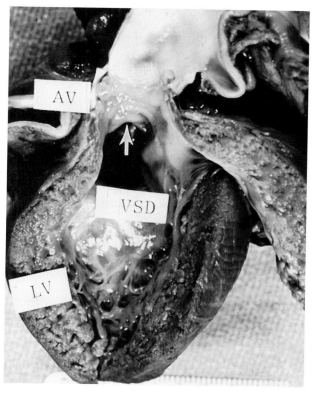

Figure 48: Partial absence of the aortic valve in an infant with a large ventricular septal defect. LV = left ventricle; AV = aortic valve; VSD = ventricular septal defect. (Used with permission from Issenberg HJ, Mathew R, Kim ES, Bharati S: Congenital absence of the noncoronary aortic cusp. *Am Heart J* 1987, 113(2):1;400–402.) Arrow points to the absent noncoronary aortic valve cusp.

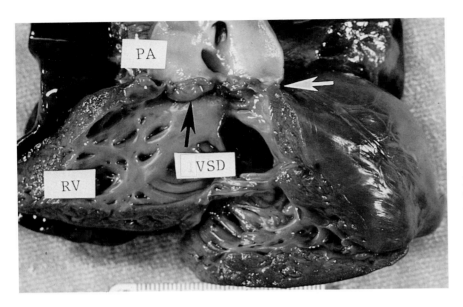

Figure 49: Outflow tract of the right ventricle in absent noncoronary aortic cusp demonstrating the ventricular septal defect extending in part to the base of the pulmonary trunk with dysplastic pulmonary valve. RV = right ventricle; VSD = ventricular septal defect; PA = pulmonary artery. Arrows point to the dysplastic pulmonary valve.

9-month-old male

Infective endocarditis of the pulmonary valve and outflow tract with obstruction

1-month-old female

Infective endocarditis of the tricuspid valve, right atrium, and thrombus of the pulmonary trunk

Hypertrophied and enlarged right atrium and right ventricle

Other – Miscellaneous

2½-year-old female

Cutis laxa, acquired type (Figs. 50–52)

Chronic aortitis with aneurysm of the ascending aorta and destruction and complete occlusion of right coronary with stenosis of left coronary ostium

Chronic arteritis of main pulmonary trunk

Hypertrophy and enlargement of all the chambers

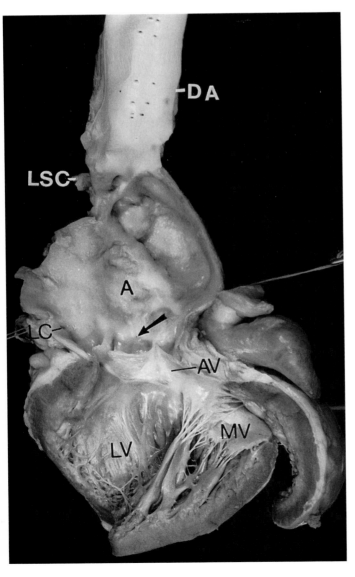

Figure 50: Aneurysm of the ascending aorta, aortitis in a 2½-year-old child with fatal cardiovascular disease and cutis laxa following acute febrile neutorphilic dermatosis. A = aneurysm of the ascending aorta; LV = left ventricle; AV = aortic valve; DA = descending aorta; LC = left coronary artery, high origin; LSC = left subclavian artery; MV = mitral valve. (Used with permission from Muster AJ, Bharati S, Herman JJ, Easterly NB, Crussi FG, Holbrook KA: Fatal cardiovascular disease and cutis laxa following acute febrile neutrophilic dermatosis. *J Pediatr* 1983, 102(2):243–248.) Arrow points to the occluded right coronary ostium. Note that the ascending aorta is markedly dilated showing mucoid, thickened flabby wall resembling syphilitic aortitis.

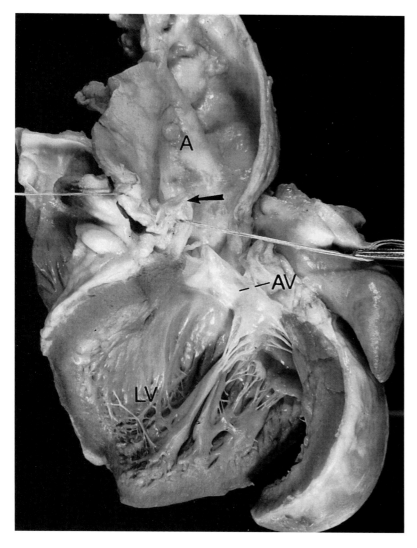

Figure 51: Aorta showing evidence of mucosal thickening destructive changes with marked narrowing of the left coronary artery. LV = left ventricle; AV = aortic valve; A = aorta. Arrow points to narrowing of the left coronary artery.

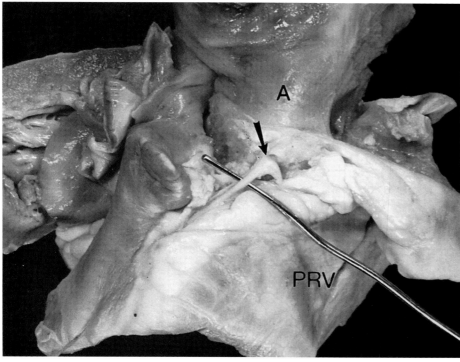

Figure 52: Cutis laxa, acquired type, with stenotic small right coronary artery. A = aorta; PRV = parietal wall of right ventricle. Arrow points to the right coronary artery, and the probe lifts the small right coronary artery.

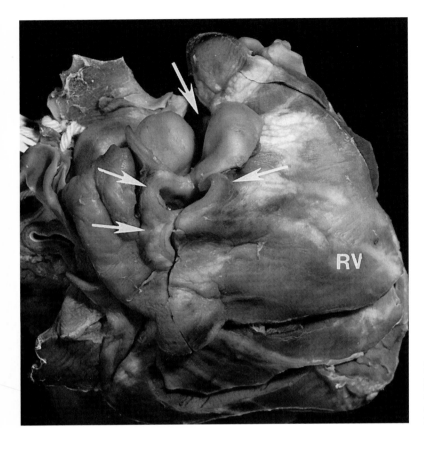

Figure 53: Infantile arteriosclerosis and aneurysm of the coronary arteries in a newborn. External view of the heart. RV = right ventricle. Arrows point to the opened aneurysmally dilated right coronary artery.

4½-month-old female
    Infantile arteriosclerosis, aneurysm formation of coronary arteries and calcification (Figs. 53–56)

30-minute-old female
    Agenesis of the left lung, and hypoplasia of the left pulmonary artery and left pulmonary veins

4-month-old male
    Absence of the right pulmonary artery, bilateral ductus, and right ductus from innominate artery and occlusion

35-week gestation, 34-hour-old male
    Origin of the right coronary artery from right side of the left sinus of Valsalva and proceeding between the pulmonary artery and aorta to the right AV groove with possible compression

11-week-old female
    Small accessory coronary artery from the pulmonary trunk
    Hypertrophy and enlargement of the heart

2-day-old female
    Aortic and mitral atresia, total anomalous pulmonary venous return into the right atrium, hepatic vein into the right atrium, and absent coronary sinus

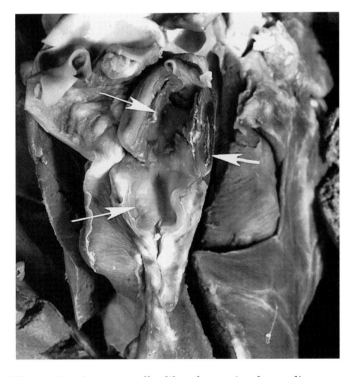

Figure 54: Aneurysmally dilated anterior descending coronary artery. Arrows point to the open anterior descending coronary artery. External view of the heart.

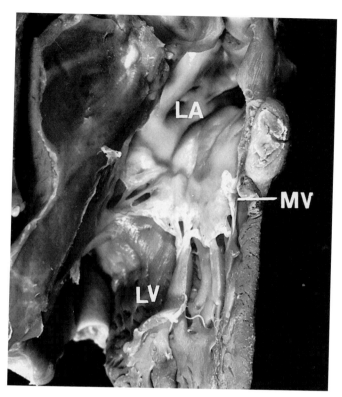

Figure 55: Small mitral valve with thickening in infantile arteriosclerosis. LA = left atrium; LV = left ventricle; MV = thickened mitral valve.

Superior vena cava entering the left atrium, and anomalous right subclavian artery from the descending aorta

3-month-old female
Osteogenesis imperfecta and pulmonary hypertension, clinical, thickened tricuspid valve, and papillary muscle proceeding to the base

6-day-old female
Common ventricle with aortic atresia with normally related vessels

2-day-old male
Persistence of fetal circulation, clinical, dysplastic tricuspid valve, and high origin of both coronary ostia

33-year-old male
Familial cardiomyopathy, etiology unknown

25-year-old male
Familial cardiomyopathy, etiology unknown
Diffuse fibroelastosis of the left ventricle

1-month-old male
Atrophy of the left ventricle due to starvation and relative hypertrophy of right ventricle may be related to reversed ductus

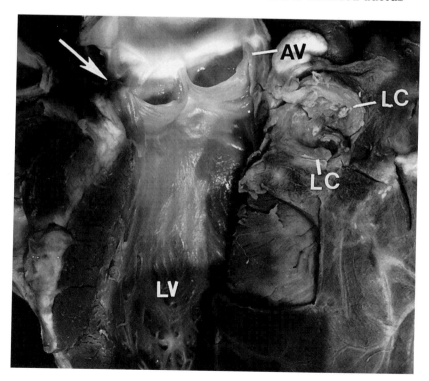

Figure 56: Left ventricular outflow tract demonstrating a normally formed aortic valve. LV = left ventricle; AV = aortic valve; LC = aneurysmally dilated left circumflex, calcific. Arrow points to the aneurysmally dilated right coronary ostium emerging above the sinus of Valsalva.

High origin of both coronary ostia, and patent ductus arteriosus

18-month-old male
  Cystic hygroma
  Hypertrophy and enlargement of the heart, small cyst in anterior wall of the aorta, mild aneurysmal dilatation of the ascending aorta, and ventricular septal bulge

49-year-old male
  Cardiomyopathy
  Focal fibrotic scars in the left ventricle, old myocarditis?

4-day-old male
  Absent ventricular septum with aortic and mitral atresia complex

47-year-old female
  Primary disease of the myocardium
  Thrombus formation in the right ventricle
  Anomalous muscle band from the ventricular septum on the left side to the anterior wall

2-month, 17-day-old male
  Global hypertrophy of the heart

3½-hour-old male
  Aneurysm of the left ventricle

6-day-old male
  Recent anteroseptal infarction of the left ventricle and hypertrophy of the heart

18-day-old male
  Aneurysm of the left ventricle and necrosis of the left ventricle

13-year, 6-month, 14-day-old female
  Narrowing of the left anterior descending coronary artery with massive infarct of the left ventricle and aneurysm formation, global hypertrophy, and fibroelastosis of the left ventricle (Figs. 57–60)

Animal
  Fatty infiltration of the anulus of the medial leaflet of the tricuspid valve, and tachycardia

79-year-old male
  Fibrous diverticulum in posterior wall at the junction of the left atrium and left ventricle and left AV groove with calcification and thrombus formation and mitral insufficiency, mitral valve surgery

2-month-old female
  Huge diverticulum of the right ventricle with VSD (Figs. 61–64)

18-day-old male
  Bizarre-shaped heart
  Abnormal formation of all the valves and tricuspid stenosis (Fig. 65)

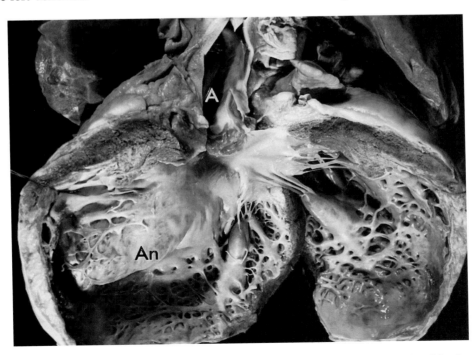

Figure 57: Aneurysm of the left ventricle in a 13½-year-old child who died suddenly. A = aorta; An = aneurysm in left ventricle. (Used with permission from Bharati S, et al. See Figure 60.)

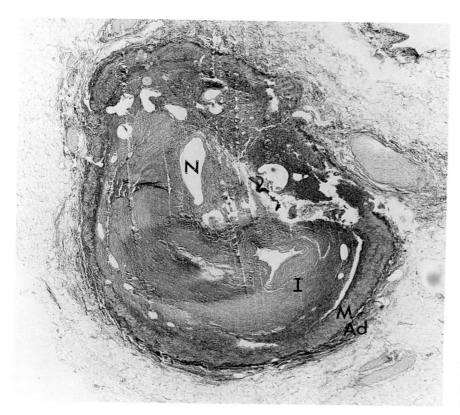

Figure 58: Histologic examination of the coronary artery showing thrombus almost occluding the lumen with marked narrowing. Ad = adventitia; M = media; I = intima; N = narrowing of the coronary artery. (Used with permission from Bharati S, et al. See Figure 60.)

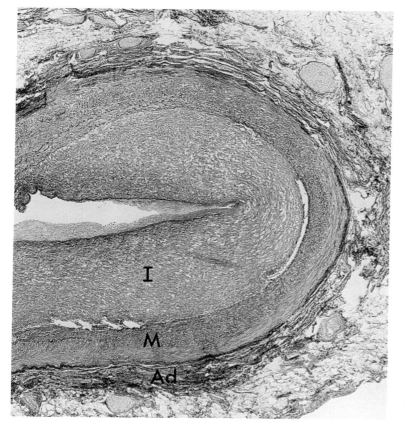

Figure 59: Marked narrowing of the left circumflex coronary artery. Ad = Adventitia; M = media; I = intima. (Used with permission from Bharati S, et al. See Figure 60.)

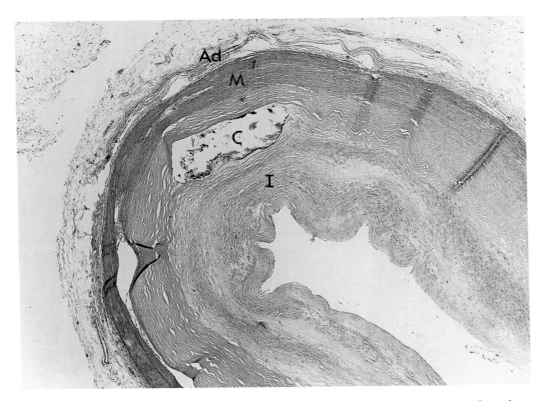

Figure 60: Marked narrowing of the right coronary artery with calcification. Ad = adventitia; M = media; I = intima; C = calcium in the medial wall. (Used with permission from Bharati S, Fisher EA, Yaniz RA, Hastreiter AR, Lev M: Infarct of the myocardium with aneurysm in a 13-year-old girl. *Chest* 1975, 67:369–373.)

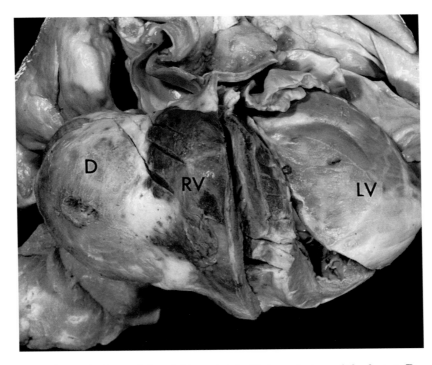

Figure 61: Diverticulum of the right ventricle. External view of the heart. D = diverticulum; RV = right ventricle; LV = left ventricle. (Used with permission from Bharati S, et al. See Figure 64.)

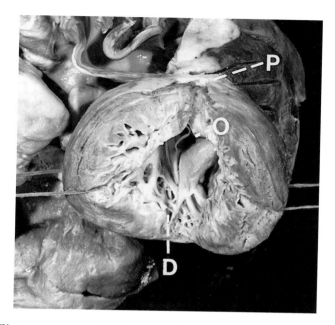

Figure 62: Diverticulum opened up. P = pulmonary trunk; D = diverticulum; O = opening in the diverticulum is divided by the parietal band into two chambers. (Used with permission from Bharati S, et al. See Figure 64.)

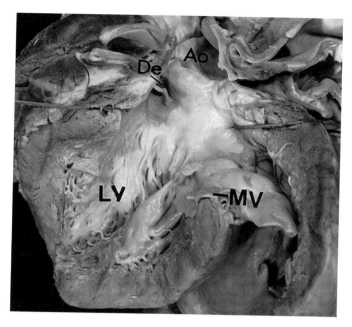

Figure 64: Outflow tract of the left ventricle. LV = left ventricle; MV = mitral valve; De = defect; Ao = aorta. (Used with permission from Bharati S, Rowen M, Camarata SJ, Ostermiller Jr WE, Singer M, Lev M: Diverticulum of the right ventricle. *Arch Pathol* 1975, 99:383–386.)

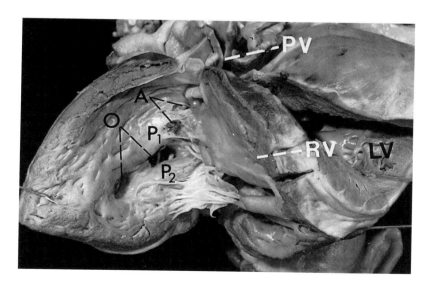

Figure 63: Outflow tract of the right ventricle. RV = right ventricle; P$_1$ = parietal band 1; P$_2$ = parietal band 2; O = two openings in the right ventricle; PV = pulmonary valve; LV = left ventricle.

2-month-old male
  Large left superior vena cava entering the coronary sinus, large eustachian valve, incomplete cor triatriatum dexter, VSD, and PDA (Fig. 69)

45-year-old male
  Eustachian valve close to the AV nodal area (Fig. 70)

1-month-old male
  Three-chambered heart with DORV, straddling right AV valve, and displaced mitral valve into the accessory chamber, accessory right ventricle? (Figs. 71–76)

6-month-old male (30–32 weeks' gestation)
  Calcification of the right ventricle and ventricular septum
  Severe hyaline membrane disease, anemia, severe bronchopulmonary dysplasia and cor pulmonale, and congestive heart failure (Fig. 77)

16-day-old female
  Huge left superior vena cava entering the coronary sinus, small right pulmonary artery, large PDA, right ventricular hypertrophy (Figs. 78, 79)

8½-month old female
  Huge atria, small ventricles with possible mitral and tricuspid stenosis (Figs. 80, 81)

19-year-old male
  Pulmonary hypertension, congestive heart failure
  Leontiasis ossei
  Scoliosis
  Right atrium hypertrophied and enlarged
  Bicuspid pulmonary valve
  Both coronary arteries from right cusp and anterior descending artery in front of the pulmonary trunk)

54-year-old female
  Hypertrophied and enlarged left ventricle
  Hypertrophied and enlarged right ventricle
  Left pulmonic sinus extending down into the conus with fenestration

Unknown
  Rete Chiari (Fig. 82)

Unknown
  Aneurysm of the fossa ovalis (Fig. 83)

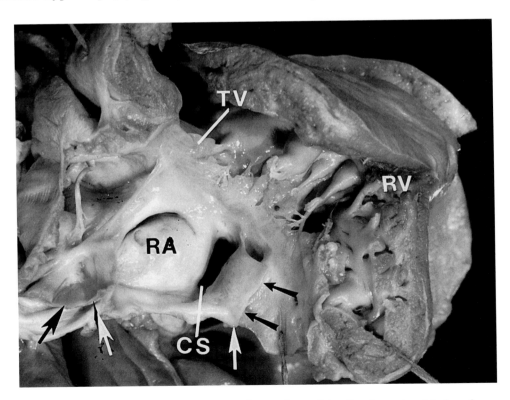

Figure 69: Incomplete cor triatriatum dexter formed by the hypertrophied and enlarged combined eustachian and thebesian valves. RA = right atrium; RV = right ventricle; TV = tricuspid valve; CS = large coronary sinus receiving a left superior vena cava. Three arrows (together) indicate the cut end of the eustachian valve, and the two arrows (away from each other) indicate the other half of the eustachian valve close to the superior vena cava.

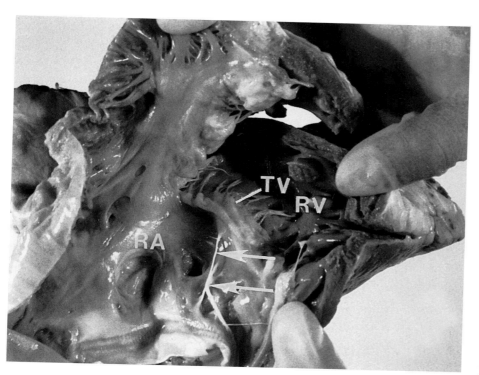

Figure 70: Eustachian valve inserted very close to the septal leaflet of the tricuspid valve near the region of the AV node and His bundle with mild displacement of the thebesian valve and septal hypertrophy in a 45-year-old male. RV = right ventricle; TV = tricuspid valve – note the redundant leaflets; RA = right atrium. Arrows point to the eustachian valve insertion close to the AV node and its approaches.

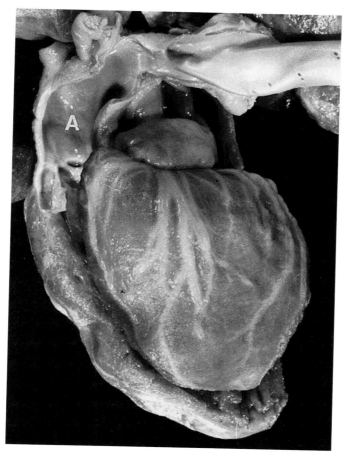

Figure 71: Three-chambered or tri-ventricular heart, DORV complex. External view of the heart. Aorta emerging anteriorly and somewhat to the left. A = aorta.

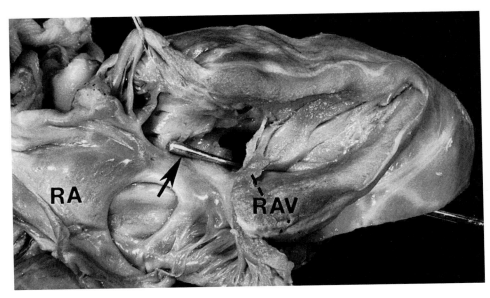

Figure 72: Right atrial, right ventricular view demonstrating right AV valve straddling through a defect to the posteriorly located sinus-like chamber. RA = right atrium; RAV = right atrioventricular valve. Arrow points to the probe and the straddling right atrioventricular valve.

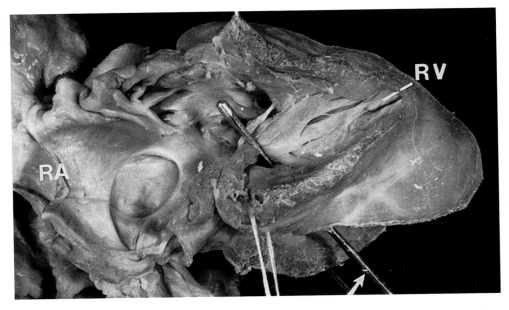

Figure 73: Right atrial, right ventricular view demonstrating the communication between the right ventricle and another chamber situated posteroinferiorly. RA = right atrium; RV = right ventricle. Arrow points to the probe passing through the accessory sinus-like chamber and emerging into the right ventricle at its base

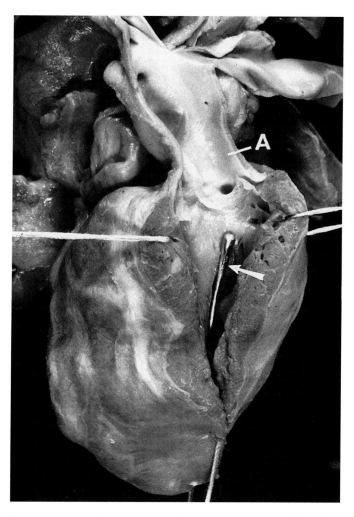

Figure 74: Aorta emerging from the right ventricle. A = aorta. Arrow points to the probe passing through the right ventricle to the accessory chamber.

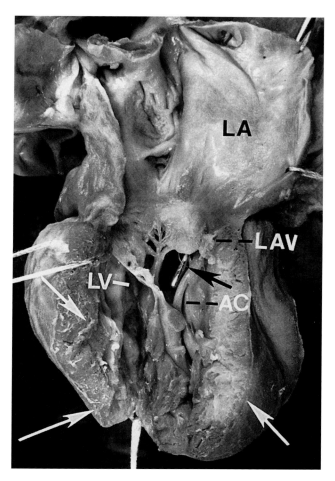

Figure 75: Left atrial view demonstrating the left AV valve entering a small sinus-like chamber. LA = left atrium; LAV = left AV valve; LV = left ventricle; AC = accessory chamber. Black arrow points to the right AV valve entering the accessory chamber. White arrows point to the walls of the accessory chamber.

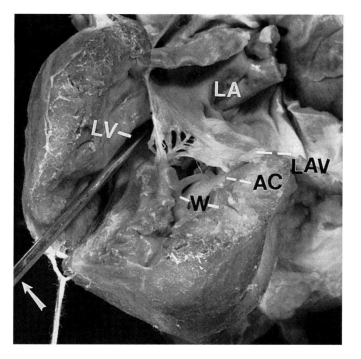

Figure 76: Left-sided view demonstrating the left atrium communicating with the accessory sinus-like chamber demarcated by ventricular septal walls and the left ventricle. LA = left atrium; LAV = left AV valve; AC = accessory chamber; W = distinct septal walls for the accessory chamber; LV = left ventricle. Arrow indicates probe passing through the left ventricle.

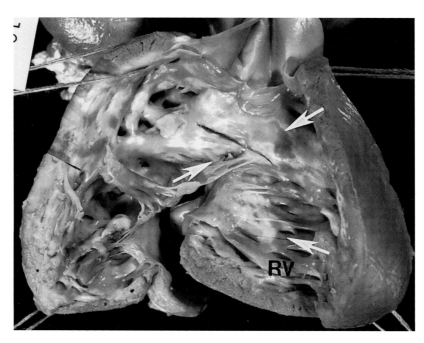

Figure 77: Calcification of the right ventricle in a 6-month-old boy with cor pulmonale and congestive heart failure. RV = right ventricle. Arrows point to calcification.

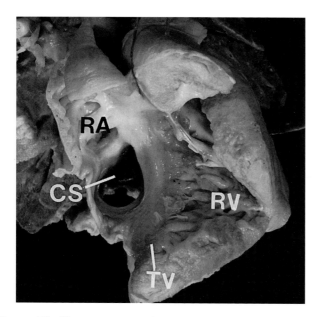

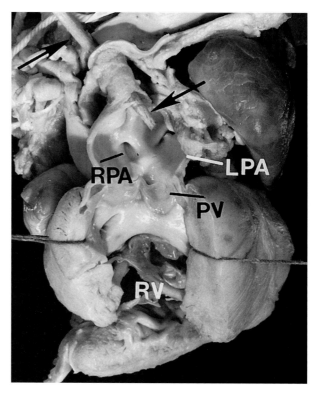

Figure 78: Huge coronary sinus receiving a large left superior vena cava with a small right pulmonary artery. Right atrial, right ventricular view demonstrating the huge coronary sinus. RA = right atrium; RV = right ventricle; TV = tricuspid valve; CS = coronary sinus.

Figure 79: Outflow tract of the right ventricle demonstrating a small right pulmonary artery. RV = right ventricle; PV = pulmonary valve; RPA = right pulmonary artery, small; LPA = left pulmonary artery. Arrows point to the probe passing through the ductus arteriosus.

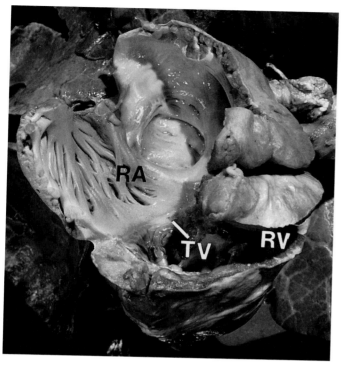

Figure 80: Huge atria and small ventricles with possible tricuspid and mitral stenosis in a 8½-month old female. Right atrial view. RA = huge right atrium; TV = small tricuspid valve; RV = small right ventricle.

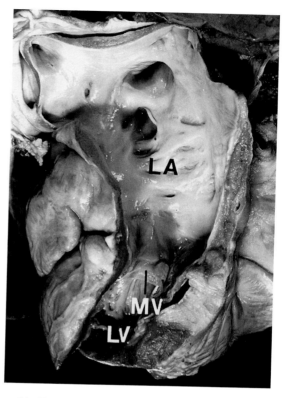

Figure 81: Left atrial, left ventricular view. LA = huge left atrium; MV = small mitral valve with possible stenosis; LV = small left ventricle. (Used with permission from Lev M. See Figure 82.)

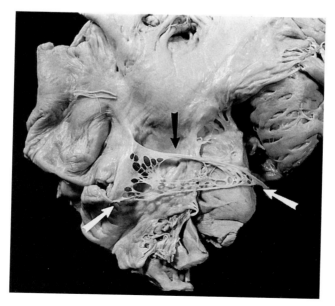

Figure 82: Rete Chiari. Arrows point to Chiari network. (Used with permission from Lev M: *Autopsy Diagnosis of Congenitally Malformed Hearts.* Charles C. Thomas, Springfield, Illinois, 1953.)

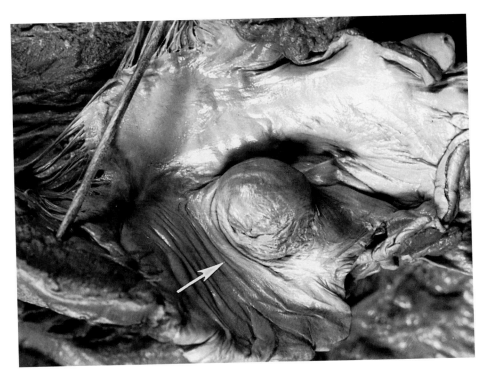

Figure 83: Aneurysm of fossa ovalis, left atrial view. Arrow points to aneurysm.

Newborn male
    Aneursym of fossa ovalis with oblique patent fora-
    men ovale, closing PDA
    Redundant tricuspid valve with tricuspid insuffi-
    ciency, multiple extracardiac anomalies, displaced
    coronary sinus close to the tricuspid valve

Newborn male, second of twins
    Aortico-right ventricular tunnel (Figs. 84–91)

Female, 14 days
Gamete in vitro fertilized transfer (Gift)
    Fertilized ovum (not the biological ovum) trans-
    planted. The infant had interrupted aortic arch
    and probably DiGeorge syndrome.

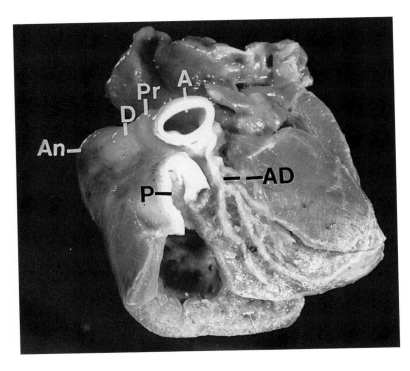

Figure 84: Aortico-right ventricular tunnel. Anteroseptal view. AD = Anterior descending coronary
artery; P = pulmonary trunk; A = aorta; Pr = outpouching of the aorta (proximal chamber of tunnel);
D = membranous structure beneath the aorta (distal
chamber of tunnel); An = aneurysmal dilation of
right ventricle. (Used with permission from Bharati
S, et al. See Figure 91.)

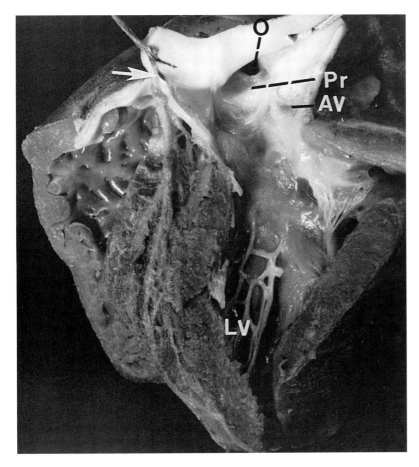

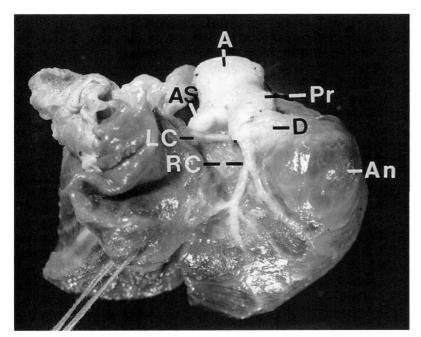

Figure 85: Same as Figure 84, right lateral view. A = posterior surface of aorta Pr = outpouching of aorta (proximal chamber of tunnel); D = membranous structure beneath the aorta (distal chamber of tunnel); An = aneurysm of right ventricle; RC = right coronary artery; LC = left circumflex coronary artery; AS = aneurysmal dilatation of the posterior aortic sinus of Valsalva (outpouching on the posterior side of the aorta). (Used with permission from Bharati S, et al. See Figure 91.)

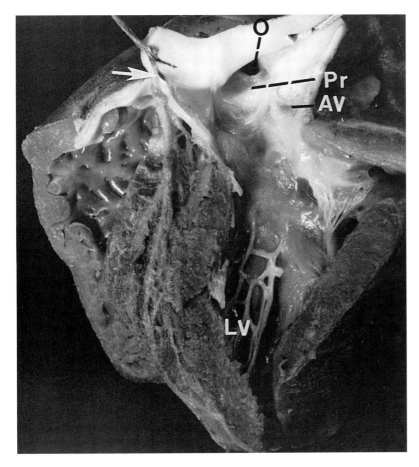

Figure 86: Same as Figure 84, left ventricular view and view of base of aorta. Pr = proximal chamber of tunnel; O = opening from the proximal chamber into the distal chamber of the tunnel; AV = aortic valve; LV = left ventricle. Arrow points to the left coronary ostium. (Used with permission from Bharati S, et al. See Figure 91.)

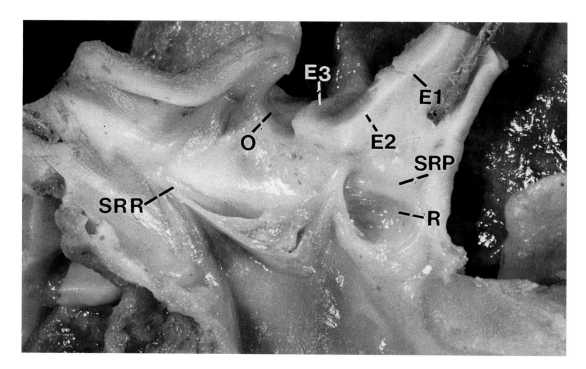

Figure 87: Same as Figure 84, close-up view of the aortic sinuses of Valsalva. A section has been taken out from the aortico-right ventricular tunnel. SRR = supravalvular ridge of right sinus of Valsalva; SRP = supravalvular ridge of posterior sinus of Valsalva; E1 = edge of cut surface of aorta; E2 = edge of cut surface of proximal chamber of tunnel; E3 = edge of cut surface of distal chamber of tunnel; O = opening of proximal to distal chamber of tunnel; R = ridge demarcating aneurysm of posterior sinus of Valsalva.

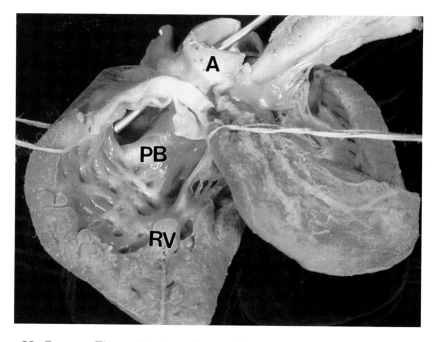

Figure 88: Same as Figure 84, view of tunnel from aorta to right ventricle. Rod is in the tunnel and it enters into the aorta and right ventricle. PB = parietal band; RV= right ventricle; A = aorta. (Used with permission from Bharati S, et al. See Figure 91.)

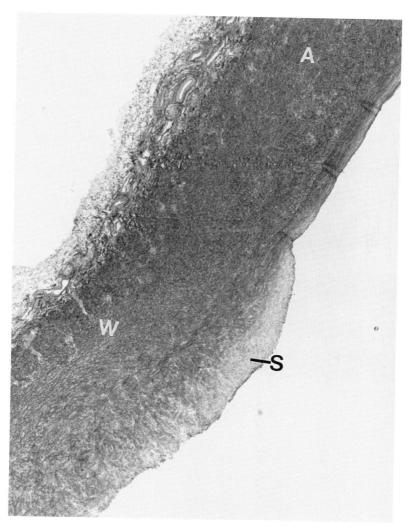

Figure 89: Histology of aortic wall and wall of adjacent pouch (proximal chamber of tunnel). Weigert-van Gieson stain; ×39. A = aorta; W = wall of adjacent pouch; S = spongiosa. (Used with permission from Bharati S, et al. See Figure 91.)

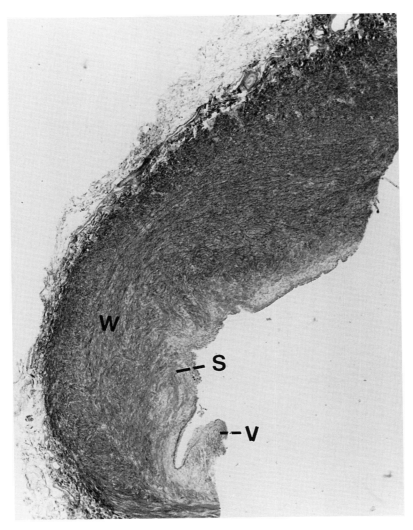

Figure 90: Same as Figure 84, wall of pouch adjacent to aorta (proximal chamber of tunnel). Weigert-van Gieson stain; ×39. W = wall of pouch; S = spongiosa-like tissue; V = valve-like structure.

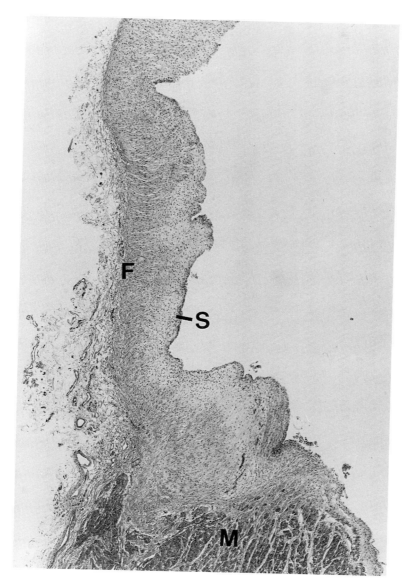

Figure 91: Same as Figure 84, wall of pouch adjacent to myocardium of right ventricle (distal chamber of tunnel). Hematoxylin-eosin stain; ×39. S = spongiosa; F = dense fibrous tissue; M = myocardium. (Used with permission from Bharati S, Lev M, Cassels DE: Aortico-right ventricular tunnel. *Chest* 1973, 63:198–202.)

90

Incidental Anomalies

In these cases, incidental findings were found in otherwise normally formed hearts. In some there were acquired heart diseases such as coronary artery disease, myocardial infarction, hypertensive heart disease, myocarditis, or carcinoma of the lung. In still others there were aging changes in the heart. There was a total of 114 cases, and they are grouped as follows:

	No. of Cases
Coronary artery anomalies	23
Bicuspid aortic valve	19
Quadricuspid aortic valve	3
Left superior vena cava entering the coronary sinus	14
Quadricuspid pulmonic valve	12
Aneurysm of the membranous septum	8
Aberrant right subclavian artery	5
Diverticulum of the left ventricle	3
Chordae and bands in the left ventricle	3
Double mitral orifice	3
Irregular thickening of mitral valve, cleft	3
Anomalies of all valves	3
Double tricuspid valve	3
Anomalies in the right atrium	5
Muscle band in the left atrium	1
Aneurysm of the pulmonic valve	1
Origin of the right pulmonary artery close to the pulmonary trunk	1
Miscellaneous	4

Coronary Artery Anomalies

There was a total of 23 cases. The ages ranged from a 22-weeks' gestation fetus to an 88-year-old male. Fourteen were males, six were females, and three were animals.

Single Coronary Artery

A single coronary ostium was present in five: four males and one female (82 years, 6 months, 83 years, 59 years, and 77 years). These were five cases as incidental findings in otherwise normal hearts. These arose from the left anterior sinus of Valsalva in four and one from the right aortic sinus (Fig. 1). In three cases the single coronary artery divided off into right and left coronary arteries. In one, the left coronary artery gave off the entire circulation terminating in the AV groove as the ramus ostii cavae superioris. The 6-month-old female also had an associated small patent ductus arteriosus, right aortic arch, and bicuspid aortic and pulmonic valves.

Single Coronary with Small Accessory Coronary Ostium from the Pulmonary Trunk

In an 83-year-old female there was a single right coronary artery which gave off the right and left coronary arteries with an accessory coronary ostium from the pulmonary trunk and was associated with acquired heart disease and Mönckeberg's sclerosis of the aortic valve.

Left Circumflex from the Right Sinus of Valsalva

There was a total of three cases: two males, 59 years and 51 years old, and one female, 69 years old. There was coronary artery disease in one male.

There were two coronary ostia in the right anterior sinus of Valsalva. The larger ostium led into the right main coronary artery. This gave off two small branches to the conus, then continued as the right circumflex coronary artery. The smaller ostium ran behind the

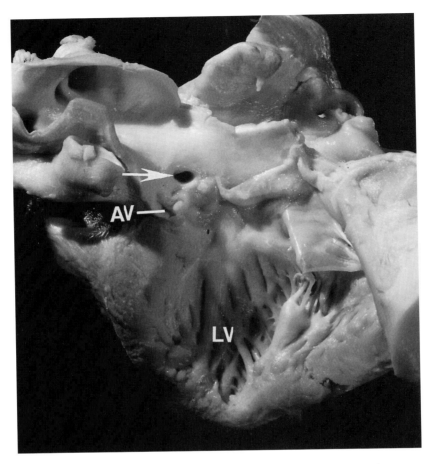

Figure 1: Single coronary ostium emerging above the right cusp. Note the unequal size and irregularly thickened valve. Note the large noncoronary cusp and the two small left and right cusps. LV = left ventricle; AV = aortic valve. Arrow points to the single coronary ostium.

aorta to reach the anterior aspect of the heart between the left margin of the pulmonary trunk and the left atrial appendage. This formed the left circumflex coronary artery. The coronary artery originating in the left sinus of Valsalva formed the anterior descending coronary artery.

In the 59-year-old, the anterior descending coronary artery originated from the left coronary ostium. The left circumflex coronary artery, however, emerged from the right coronary ostium. The right had its usual course. The right and the anterior descending arteries were considerably narrowed.

Both Coronary Ostia from the Right

In one 57-year-old male, both coronary ostia emerged from the right sinus of Valsalva. The left coronary ostium proceeded through the septum onto the anterior wall of the septum where it divided into the anterior descending and the left circumflex arteries and stopped at the obtuse margin. The right coronary artery was normal and formed the posterior descending

artery and proceeded over the posterior wall of the left ventricle and gave off branches to the latter.

High Origin of Coronary Ostium

There was a total of three cases. In one 59-year-old male this was associated with severe three-vessel disease, old and recent infarction, and mitral valve calcification. In a 1-year, 7 day-old female, the right coronary artery emerged high. In the other, a 6-month, 12-day-old male child, the right coronary artery arose from the posterior portion of the right sinus of Valsalva and the left ostium arose about 0.7 cm above the left cusp (Fig. 2).

High Origin of Both Coronary Ostia

This was a 63-year-old where both coronary ostia were facing each other adjacent to but considerably above the commissure between the right and the left cusps (approximately 0.5 cm above the commissure) (Fig. 3).

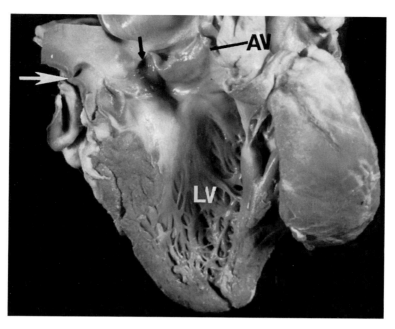

Figure 2: High origin of the left coronary ostium approximately 7 mm above the supravalvular ridge and emerging close to its junction with the right cusp, right coronary emerging close to the posterior cusp. LV = left ventricle; AV = aortic valve. White arrow points to the high origin of the left coronary ostium; small black arrow indicates the origin of the right coronary ostium.

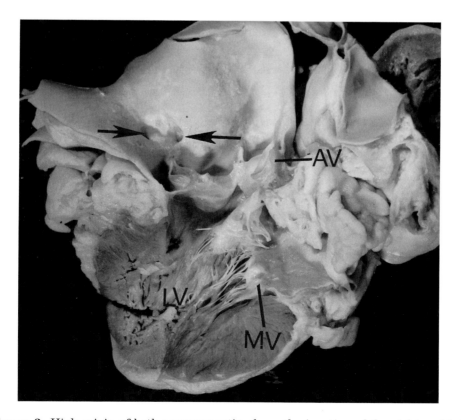

Figure 3: High origin of both coronary ostia above the junction of the right and left cusps in a 63-year-old asymptomatic man. LV = left ventricle; AV = aortic valve; MV = mitral valve. The two arrows point to the right and left coronary ostia emerging above the junction of the right and left cusps.

Double Left and Double Right Coronary Arteries

This was seen in an 88-year-old male. The anterior right gave off the conal branch and the larger ostium situated posteriorly was the main right coronary artery. The more anterior ostium from the left gave rise to the anterior descending coronary artery and the more posterior gave rise to the left circumflex artery.

Minute Left Coronary Artery and Dominant Right Coronary Artery

This was seen in a 44-year-old female. The left coronary artery was a minute vessel and formed a short anterior descending coronary artery. The right coronary artery supplied most of the circulation. It had two ostia. One ostium gave rise to a remarkable vessel that proceeded downward into the substance of the septum. The other coronary artery had the typical distribution of the right main coronary artery.

Origin of the Left Coronary Artery from the Right and Coursing Through the Infundibulum of the Right Ventricle with Old and Recent Infarctions

This was seen in two, a 49-year-old and a 54-year-old, both males. In one the left proceeded intramyocardially through the infundibulum after originating from the right sinus and surfaced into the interventricular sulcus as a small vessel and gave off the left circumflex coronary artery. There was occlusion and marked narrowing of the right and the left circumflex arteries. In the other the left again was a small vessel with a dominant right circulation.

Origin of Left Coronary Artery from the Right with an Oblique Course Between the Main Pulmonary Trunk and the Aorta

This was seen in a 47-year-old female associated with a left superior vena cava entering the coronary sinus and pulmonary emboli to pulmonaries bilaterally.

Origin of the Left Coronary Ostium from the Posterior Sinus of Valsalva

In a 22-weeks' gestation male fetus, the above pattern of coronary artery was seen.

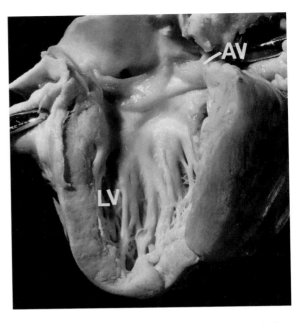

Figure 4: Bicuspid aortic valve in a child. LV = left ventricle; AV = bicuspid aortic valve.

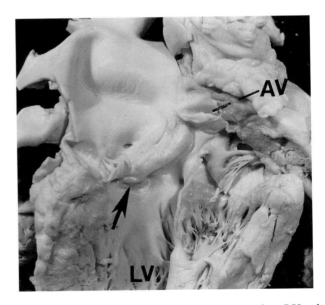

Figure 5: Bicuspid aortic valve. AV = aortic valve; LV = left ventricle. Arrow points to the bicuspid valve. (Used with permission from Lev M. See Figure 17.)

Small Right Coronary Artery and Double Ostia

This was seen in three animals.

Bicuspid Aortic Valve

There were 19 cases of bicuspid aortic valve unassociated with aortic stenosis or insufficiency in most cases. Twelve were males, six were females, and one was an animal heart.

In all cases in this series, two of the normal three cusps were represented by one cusp with a raphé in its midst. Most frequent was lack of subdivision between the right and the left cusps. Less frequent was lack of subdivision between the right and posterior (Figs. 4, 5). There were no cases of lack of subdivision between the left and posterior.

When seen in the younger age group, there was associated recent or healed bacterial endocarditis with calcification (4). When seen in the older age group, these valves showed marked hemodynamic change (Figs. 6, 7), frequently with calcification, extending to the mitral valve and rarely insufficiency of the aortic valve was present. In one there was aneurysm of the sinus of Valsalva adjacent to the ascending aorta and rupture. In two there was a high origin of the left coronary artery with a small right coronary artery. In one there was fenestration of the septum primum and pulmonic valve and blood cysts in the mitral valve.

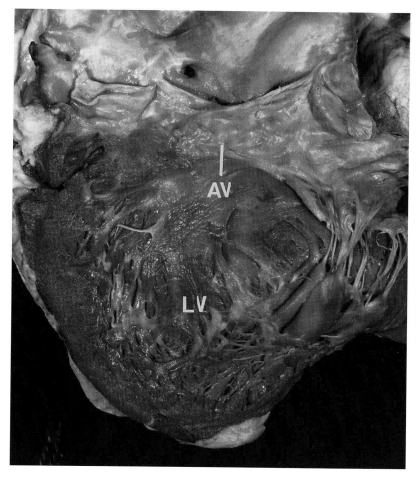

Figure 6: Bicuspid aortic valve, bicuspidality formed by the right and posterior cusps. Bicuspid valve in a 63-year-old male, asymptomatic. LV = left ventricle; AV = bicuspid aortic valve.

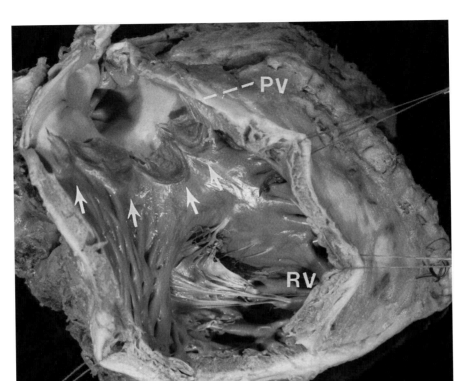

Figure 10: Quadricuspid pulmonary valve. RV = right ventricle; PV = pulmonary valve, quadricuspid. Arrows point to quadricuspid pulmonic valve.

sufficiency, and the small left superior vena cava entered the coronary sinus. Two others had acquired heart diseases and fenestrations in the tricuspid and/or the mitral valve. In one, the aging was quite marked in the aortic and mitral valves with calcification and aortic valve fenestration. The 20-year-old female had recurrent ventricular tachycardia, partial Uhl's anomaly, and died suddenly. There was one who had aging changes with calcification of the aortic valve, infective endocarditis in the tricuspid valve, left superior vena cava entering the coronary sinus and aneurysm of the fossa ovalis, and a small fossa ovalis defect. One 80-year-old female had classic aging changes with calcification of the aortic and mitral valves. It is noteworthy that in addition to the above, quadricuspid pulmonic valves were seen in otherwise normal hearts of two teenagers who died suddenly.

Aneurysm of the Pars Membranacea

There were several cases in which an aneurysm of the pars membranacea was present without a ventricular septal defect and several in which a ventricular septal defect was associated. In some of these cases we found it difficult to distinguish an aneurysm of the pars membranacea from a defect of the ventricular septum which was closed by the tricuspid valve.

These aneurysms bulged into the medial part of the anterior tricuspid leaflet or at the junction between the anterior part of the medial leaflet and medial part of the anterior leaflet. Sometimes the parietal band was somewhat deviated or architecturally abnormal.

Aneurysm of the Membranous Septum Associated with Ventricular Septal Defect

There was a total of four cases; three were males and one was female. The ages ranged from 1 year to 87 years. In two the ventricular septal defect was closed in the region of the membranous septum and there was outpouching of the septal leaflet of the tricuspid valve. In two others there was an associated small ventricular septal defect (Fig. 11). In one there was associated anomalous trabeculations in the left ventricle and a fenestrated pulmonic valve and a thickened aortic valve (Fig. 12).

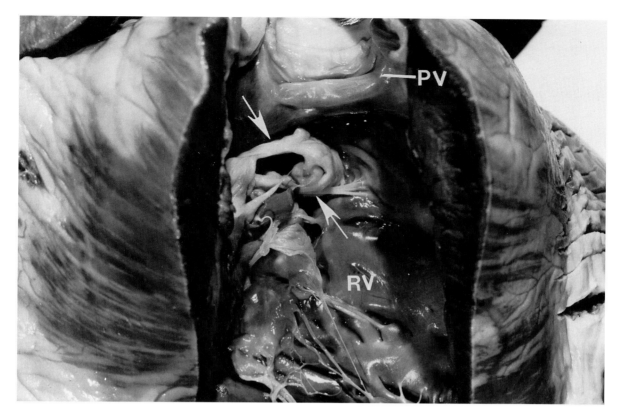

Figure 11: Aneurysm of the membranous septum and closing ventricular septal defect as seen from the right side. RV = right ventricle; PV = pulmonary valve. Arrows point to the aneurysm with irregular ridges.

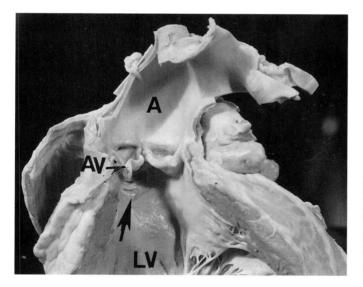

Figure 12: Aneurysm of the membranous septum beneath the thickened aortic valve with closure of the ventricular septal defect. A = aorta; AV = aortic valve, thickened; LV = left ventricle. Arrow points to the closed ventricular septal defect. (Used with permission from Lev M, See Figure 17.)

Aneurysm of the Membranous Septum

There was a total of four cases; three were males and one was female. The ages ranged from 4 months to 60 years. In all, the junction of the medial and anterior leaflets formed outpouching or ballooning with marked hemodynamic change and thickening of the tricuspid valve. In one, there was an associated aneurysm of the fossa ovalis and a fossa ovalis defect (Figs. 13–15). In one, there was a high origin of the left coronary ostium and an anomalous parietal band.

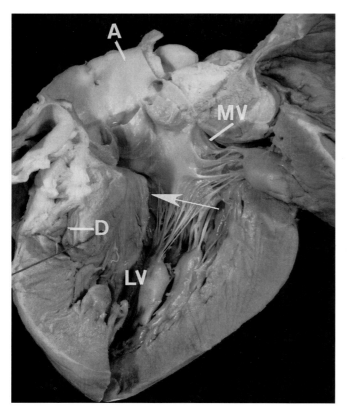

Figure 18: A small diverticulum in the anterior ventricular septum in a 17-year-old boy. LV = left ventricle; MV = mitral valve; A = ascending aorta; D = small diverticulum. Arrow points to the fibroelastic ridge on the summit of the septum.

Chordae and Bands in the Left Ventricle

There were three cases: two males and one female (newborn, 16 years, and 26 years, 8 months). Aberrant chordae of the left ventricle was seen in one. Atypical muscle bands were found in two (one with thrombosis in the bifurcating pulmonary arteries). A group of bands with chordae bridged the cavity of the left ventricle close to the apex. They had their origin at the base of the anterior papillary muscle.

Double Mitral Orifice

There were three cases of this anomaly: one in a 7-year-old, one in an 8-year-old, and another in a 64-year-old. All were male subjects. In one case, the posterior (inferior) leaflet had an opening in it close to the posterior commissure (Fig. 19). The leaflet tissue of this opening was connected to the normal papillary muscles by chordae. In the other two cases, the aortic leaflet of the mitral valve close to the anterior commissure presented a second opening. The surrounding valve tissue was connected by chordae to the usual papillary muscles (Figs. 20, 21).

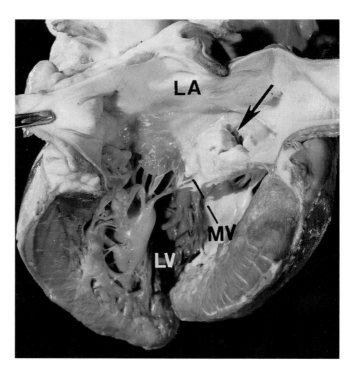

Figure 19: Accessory mitral orifice in the mitral leaflet close to the posterior commissure in an 8-year-old male. LV = left ventricle; LA = left atrium; MV = mitral valve. Arrow points to the accessory mitral orifice.

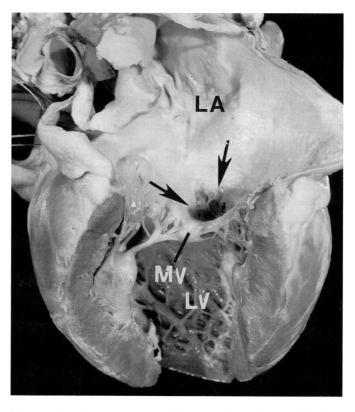

Figure 20: Double mitral orifice. LA = left atrium; LV = left ventricle; MV = mitral valve. Arrows point to the large opening within the substance of the anterior leaflet.

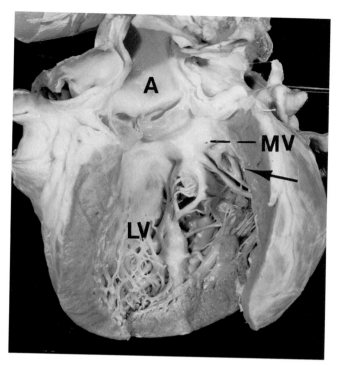

Other Anomalies in the Mitral Valve

There was a total of three cases: two females and one male (19½ months, 22 years, and 78 years). In a 19-month-old child, there were unusual thickenings of the mitral valve that were more extensive and different than the ordinary aging changes seen in this valve. Again, this was not associated with mitral insufficiency or stenosis (Fig. 22). Anomalous muscle bands in the left atrium and thickening of the mitral valve and chordae of the anterior leaflet forming a cleft-like malformation was seen in a 22-year-old female (Fig. 23). In a 78-year-old male with rheumatic heart disease, there was irregular thickening of the mitral valve, and fibrosis of the papillary muscle was present (Fig. 24). These changes are not similar either to aging or to the usual rheumatic mitral valve disease.

Figure 21: Left ventricular outflow tract demonstrating the connections of the accessory orifice. A = aorta; LV = left ventricle; MV = mitral valve. Arrow points to accessory mitral valve with accessory chorda proceeding to the papillary muscle.

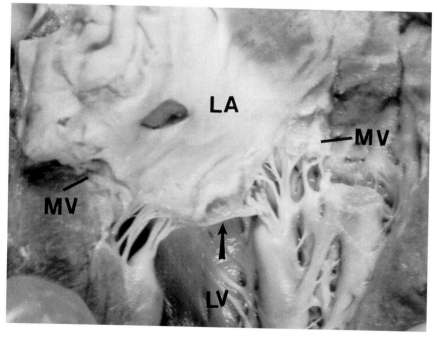

Figure 22: Irregularly thickened grayish nodules in the mitral valve in a 19-month-old female. LA = left atrium; LV = left ventricle; MV = mitral valve. Arrow points to thickening.

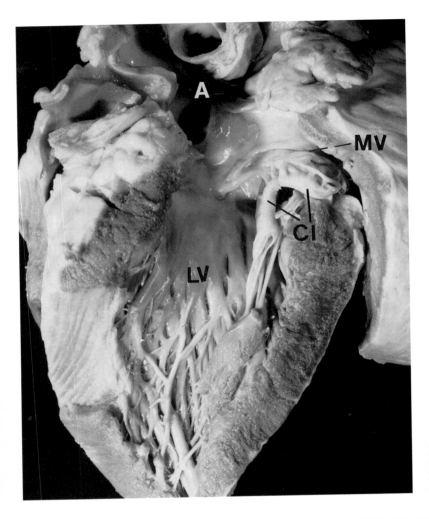

Figure 23: Cleft in the anterior leaflet of the mitral valve in a 22-year-old female. A = aorta; LV = left ventricle; MV = mitral valve; Cl = cleft in the anterior leaflet with thickened edges.

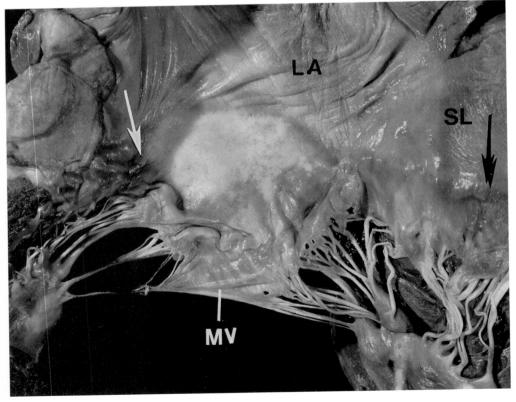

Figure 24: Irregularly thickened mitral valve with thickened elongated chordae and fibrosis of the papillary muscles. LA = left atrium; MV = mitral valve. Arrows point to irregular thickenings.

Anomalies in Three or All Four Valves

There was a total of three cases. All were males and their ages were 75 years, 53 years, and 29 days.

There was one remarkable case of an incidental abnormality of both the mitral and the tricuspid valves in a 53-year-old man. The anterior leaflet of the tricuspid valve was luxuriant and irregularly thickened. Within its midst, there was a small opening whose margins were connected by chordae. The medial part of the anterior leaflet was separated from the anterior part of the medial leaflet by a length of 0.5 cm with no valvular tissue in this area. Guarding this area on both sides were aneurysmal dilatations and thickenings of both anterior and medial leaflets. The medial and inferior leaflets were likewise luxuriant and irregular in thickening. The connections of the valve were somewhat atypical. There was no inferior papillary muscle. Instead, the inferior and medial leaflets were connected to two small nubbins of papillary muscles on the septum in addition to chordae. The tricuspid orifice was enlarged. There was no evidence of insufficiency. The mitral valve was abnormally formed. The anterior leaflet was elongated and was connected to an atypical group of chordae attached to its aortic side.

Double tricuspid orifice in the medial leaflet, agglutination of the aortic valve, and calcification of the mitral valve were present in the 75-year-old asymptomatic male. There were marked hemodynamic changes in all of the valves in a 29-day-old infant.

Double Tricuspid Orifice

There was a total of three cases. One was a 73-year-old man, one a 47-year-old male, the other a 19-year-old sea lion.

In the 73-year-old man, the medial leaflet had an opening in its valve tissue that was connected by chordae to a papillary muscle. This leaflet was larger than the other two and there was increased hemodynamic change in this leaflet (Fig. 25).

There was a huge accessory tricuspid orifice in the 47-year-old male with severe three-vessel disease, old and recent infarctions and aneurysm of the left ventricle and left superior vena cava entering the coronary sinus, aneurysm of the fossa ovalis, and pulmonary hypertension.

The sea lion had marked irregular thickening and nodulations of the tricuspid valve suggestive of infective endocarditis.

Accessory tricuspid orifice was sometimes present with other anomalies or in sudden death in the young and the healthy in an otherwise normal heart.

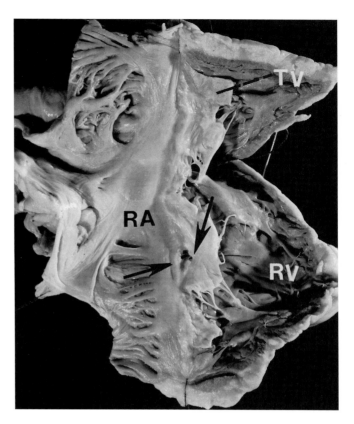

Figure 25: Accessory tricuspid valve in a 73-year-old male. RA = right atrium; TV = tricuspid valve; RV = right ventricle. Arrows point to the accessory opening.

Anomalies in the Right Atrium

There was a total of five cases; four were males and one was female. The ages ranged from 2 days to 60 years.

Aneurysm of the fossa ovalis with acquired heart disease – 1
Bands in the right atrium – 1
Chiari network – 1
Spatio intersepto valvulare with severe coronary artery disease – 1
Displaced coronary sinus to central fibrous body – 1

Anomalous Muscle Band in the Left Atrium

Anomalous muscle band with aneurysm formation was seen in a 49-year-old male. The muscular band extended from the mouth of the atrial appendage to the proximal portion of the atrial septum. This resulted in the production of a pocket or aneurysm in the roof (Fig. 26).

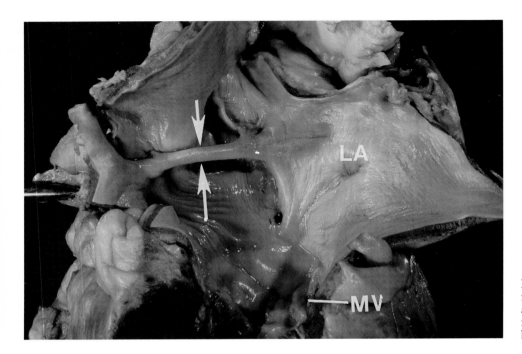

Figure 26: Large muscular band in the left atrium. LA = left atrium; MV = mitral valve. Arrows point to the large muscular band.

Aneurysm of the Sinus of Valsalva of the Pulmonic Valve

This rare anomaly was seen in a 10-day-old infant. It consisted of a pouch that lay in the crista supraventricularis and was continuous with the left posterior sinus of Valsalva (Fig. 27).

Abnormal Origin of the Right Pulmonary Artery

In one case, a huge right pulmonary artery arose almost immediately from the main pulmonary trunk just above the valve in a 6-week-old female (Fig. 28). The left pulmonary artery was distinctly smaller than the right.

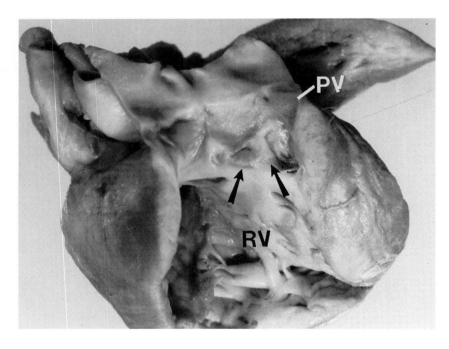

Figure 27: Pouch formation of the sinus of Valsalva of the left pulmonic cusp. RV = right ventricle; PV = pulmonary valve. Arrows point to the pouch formation extending into the endocardium of the outflow tract of the right ventricle.

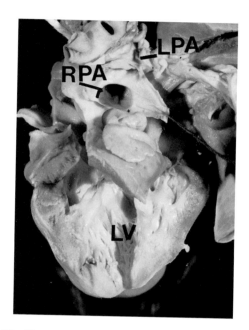

Figure 28: Huge right pulmonary artery emerging immediately distal to the pulmonic valve and small left pulmonary artery. RPA = large right pulmonary artery; LPA = small left pulmonary artery; LV = left ventricle. Note that the main pulmonary trunk has been cut at the level of the valve.

Miscellaneous Anomalies

Other incidental findings were seen in four cases:

Aneurysm of the ascending aorta with a ridge between the ascending aorta and transverse arch in a 30-week gestation fetus – 1

Markedly thickened tricuspid valve in a stillborn male with a papillary muscle going to the base of the valve – 1

Thickened mitral valve, anomalous muscle band in the right atrium, and sclerodema in a 32-year-old female – 1

Pulmonary hypertension, aneurysm of the fossa ovalis, hypoplasia of the aorta, and wide patent ductus arteriosus in a 2-day-old male – 1

91

Undiagnosed Hearts

There was a group of cases in which we could not make a definite diagnosis of the heart, although pathological changes were in evidence grossly.

They fall into five major groups:

		No. of Cases
I.	Stillborns	8
II.	Neonates	41
III.	Infants (5 days to 3 to 5 months)	19
IV.	Younger Age (mostly, except 1)	25
V.	Older Age Group	2
	Total	95

I. Stillborns

In the first group of stillborns (six males, two females), the heart showed a ventricular septal defect or an atrial septal defect and a patent ductus arteriosus (PDA) or hypoplasia of the transverse arch and single ventricle. There was hypertrophy of the right side of the heart, and at times enlargement of the left side. The nature of the hypertrophy could not be explained in our present state of knowledge of fetal hemodynamics. These hearts probably are the end result of abnormal hemodynamics in intrauterine life.

On the other hand, in one the heart was atrophied, in one 24 weeks' gestation fetus there was hemorrhage along the course of the coronaries and in one there were mononuclear cells in the myocardium suggesting intrauterine endocarditis and/or myocarditis.

II. Neonates

The neonatal group (newborn to 72 hours) may be further divided into:

a. Global hypertrophy of heart without cardiac anomaly 10

b. Hypertrophy of the right side of the heart or no hypertrophy (4) 13

c. Hypertrophy of the heart with cardiac anomalies 8

d. Hypertrophy of the heart with thickening of all of the valves and/or blood cyst in the valves 5

e. Hypertrophy of the heart with extracardiac anomalies (and no intracardiac anomalies) 5

a. In the group with global hypertrophy of the heart, there was hypertrophy of both sides of the heart with fibroelastosis in which the presence of myocarditis could not be ruled out at the gross level. There were seven male infants and three female infants.

b. In this group there was right-sided hypertrophy with the ordinary patent foramen ovale and patent ductus arteriosus. In view of the absence of catheterization data, these hypertrophies were not explained. There were 10 male infants and three female infants.

c. There was a group of neonatal hearts that had global hypertrophy of the heart with various types of congenital cardiac anomalies. The anomalies included: small PDA in a 35-weeks' gestation fetus with subaortic stenosis, coarctation, large proximal and fossa ovalis atrial septal defect, straddling inferior vena cava, hypoplasia of the transverse arch with mitral stenosis, stenosis of the pulmonary veins, and multiple VSDs. It is presumed that altered hemodynamics occurred resulting in global hypertrophy of the heart in intrauterine life. However, the reasons for altered hemodynamics are unknown. Four were male infants and four were female.

d. In this group, there were five cases with global hypertrophy of the heart, with associated thickening of all the valves with or without blood cysts. The valvular changes could not be evaluated at this age unless we are dealing with chromosomal anomalies. The presence of blood cysts suggests that there might have been fetal anoxia or distress. In this group there were four male infants and one female infant.

e. In the last group of neonates there was hypertrophy of the heart with no congenital cardiac anomalies but there were associated extracardiac anomalies that included polycystic kidney, one with a small lung, one with partial absence of the pericardium and left diaphragmatic hernia, one with diaphragmatic hernia, and one with hyaline membrane disease. Four were male infants and one was a female infant.

The relationship of extracardiac abnormalities to the hypertrophy of the otherwise normal heart is not known today.

In this group of neonatal hearts there is a distinct male preponderance (29 out of 41, 71%). This deserves further research.

III. Infants (5 days to 3 to 5 months)

This group may be further subdivided into:

a. Infants with otherwise normal hearts
with hypertrophy or no hypertrophy   9
b. Infants with global hypertrophy and
congenital cardiac anomalies   4
c. Infants with cardiac anomalies and
marked thickening of the valves   6

a. This group includes the ages from 5 days to 5 months. In this group, aside from a ordinary patent ductus and patent foramen ovale, there were no other anomalies. There was no hypertrophy in five, there was right-sided hypertrophy in two, and in one there was cardiomegaly, and in one the heart was atrophied. There were five males and four females.

b. In the second group, all had cardiomegaly and congenital heart disease including coarctation, probe patent ductus and mitral stenosis, large left pulmonary artery with a small left pulmonary artery, and sinus venosus atrial septal defect (ASD) with polysplenia and partial visceral heterotaxy. The global hypertrophy could not be explained for the above anomalies. There were three females and one male in this group.

c. In the third group, all had varying degrees of thickening and stenosis of all of the valves, three had VSD (one double), one had PDA and pulmonary stenosis. The valvular thickening was either in the tricuspid, mitral, aortic, or pulmonic valve or in a combination of these. There was one with quadricuspid pulmonic valve, fenestration of the aortic valve, and an ASD. It is not known whether these cases were an exaggerated effect of altered hemodynamics or related to congenital polyvalvular disease. There were three males and three females.

IV. Younger Age

Aside from one 55-year-old female, all were below the age of 41. The hearts belonging to this category can be broadly classified into three groups.

a. Cardiomegaly with diffuse fibroelastosis of all the chambers   17
b. Cardiomegaly with mitral valve anomalies   4
c. Cardiomegaly and thickening of all of
the valves   4

a. In this group there was distinct left atrial and left ventricular hypertrophy and enlargement with diffuse fibroelastosis of the chambers. In some, the histology did not reveal any evidence of myocarditis. In some there were few mononuclear cells in the myocardium. Are these then an end result of a remote myocarditis? It is not known how the hypertrophy occurred in these individuals and therefore an exact diagnosis could not be made. Nevertheless, these are *abnormal hearts* and the nature of cardiomegaly is to be explored. Did hypertrophy and enlargement occur due to some hypersensitivity state in the past? Are these individuals prone or susceptible to developing cardiomegaly due to alterations in the molecular and/or the genetic level, and therefore the hypertrophy occurred due to a previous hypersensitivity state? Can we then detect who will develop hypertrophy and what type of hypertrophy and what type of hypersensitivity mechanism? At any event, these cases have to be explored further in the next century and we should not ignore them. It is of interest that the ages ranged from 5 months to 55 years, and 10 were female subjects, six were male subjects, and one was unknown.

b. In the second group there was tremendous hypertrophy of the heart associated with mitral valve anomalies. In two there was irregular thickening in the mitral valve with insufficiency and diffuse fibroelastosis of the left-sided chambers. In one there was a *partial* cleft in the mitral valve with global hypertrophy. There was one case that appeared to have hemodynamic changes in the mitral valve with rupture of some chordae and mitral insufficiency. Thus, the global hypertrophy could not be explained for the above lesions in the mitral valve unless there is an associated myocardial problem at the genetic and/or at the molecular level. There were three male subjects and one female subject, and the ages were 1 month, 1 year, 2 years, and 16 years.

c. In the third group there were four cases, and all were female subjects. The ages were 6 months, 7 months, 11 years, and 16 years. All had considerable thickening of all of the valves to varying degrees with stenosis and/or insufficiency. All had remarkable hypotrophy and enlargement of all of the chambers.

V. Older Age

In two cases (both male subjects, one 60 and the other 50 years old), there was remarkable thickening of the mitral and aortic valves with hypertrophy and enlargement of all of the chambers. The thickenings are presumed to be due either to aging and/or the effect of aging on abnormally formed valves. These were not due to rheumatic or infective endocarditis.

Comment

The fundamental theme in the majority of the above undiagnosed hearts appears to be inappropriate global hypertrophy of the heart regardless of whether there are intra- or extracardiac associated anomalies. Out of a total of 95 undiagnosed hearts, there were only two in which the heart was actually atrophied. One was a 4½-month-old infant, and another was a stillborn. The valvular thickenings and other anomalies, either intra- or extracardiac, could not explain the global hypertrophy of the heart accompanied with diffuse fibroelastosis.

In the newborn hearts, we are obviously dealing with abnormal hemodynamics in intrauterine life that had resulted in global hypertrophy or hypertrophy of the right-sided chambers. It is conceivable that the abnormal hemodynamics might have originated at the placental level or inferior or superior vena caval level, or at a combination at various levels. The alteration in hemodynamics may be related to an infection in the mother and/or to other immune mechanisms that may, in part, be related to infection. The fundamental problem may possibly lie at the molecular-genetic level. The genes that are responsible for the normal development of the various parts of the heart including the valves may be abnormal (or faulty) to start with, or may be susceptible to the alterations in the environment (such as infection, injury, etc.) to a varying degree. The expression of the altered genes may result in global hypertrophy of the heart with or without other associated cardiac or extracardiac anomalies.

92

Postoperative Congenital Hearts:
Sequelae of Atriotomy, Ventriculotomy on the Myocardium, Endocardium, Conduction System, and General Sequelae After Surgery for Congenital Heart Disease

Today, congenital cardiac anomalies are being operated on with exceedingly good results in the majority of the cases. However, many problems still remain, especially following surgical correction of the complicated congenital anomaly in a growing child. The postoperative congenital hearts, especially those operated several years before death present many pathological changes including (1) cardiomegaly, (2) endocardial fibroelastosis, especially in the operative site, (3) postoperative arrhythmias depending on the site of surgery, (4) insufficiency of the atrioventricular (AV) or semilunar valves (depending on the site of surgery), (5) myocardial fibrosis or fibroelastosis, (6) hypertrophied and enlarged ventricular chambers, and (7) sudden death.

We have now entered a new era in congenital heart disease since operative intervention has produced a new population with a new kind of a heart, the pathological aspects of which are just beginning to be unraveled.

The Normal Endocardium

Normally, the endocardium differs in structure both grossly and histologically from chamber to chamber, and from area to area in the same chamber. The endocardium fundamentally consists of the endocardium proper and the subendocardium. The endocardium proper consists of the epithelium under which there is a small amount of elastic and collagen tissue and an internal elastic lamella. The subendocardium consists of a mixture of thick elastic and collagenous fibers. The endocardium is focally thickened by proliferation of elastic and collagen fibers, and in some areas smooth muscle is also present. In these areas focal endocardial hypertrophy is considered present.

In the normal right atrium, the focal areas of endocardial hypertrophy are present on the limbus and in the fossa ovalis, and also at the entry of the superior vena cava. The right ventricle shows an occasional area of such thickening beneath the pulmonic valve and the crista. The left ventricle presents focal endocardial hypertrophy at the base of the septum, beneath the mitral valve and on the papillary muscles. A *diffuse* endocardial hypertrophy beginning at birth is present only in the left atrium. This consists of a diffuse proliferation of the elastic, collagenous, and ground substance elements of the endocardium and proliferation of the elastic and collagenous elements of the subendocardium. With advancing age, there is a greater involvement of the normal endocardium in focal hypertrophy and of the normal left atrium in diffuse hypertrophy.

Endocardium in Congenital Heart Disease

We studied the endocardium in all types of congenitally malformed hearts. When compared with normal age-matched control hearts, we found that there was an increase in focal hypertrophy in many areas in some hearts *not* operated on as a result of altered hemodynamic status. In some unoperated hearts, there was more than normal diffuse endocardial hypertrophy which we call abnormal fibroelastosis. Thus, distinct fibroelastosis was present (1) on the endocardium of unoperated hearts with hypoplasia of aortic tract complex with aortic atresia and mitral stenosis, and (2) on the endocardium of the right ventricle in pulmonary atresia with tricuspid stenosis (intact ventricular septum). The unoperated hearts were used as controls in evaluating the endocardium in surgically operated hearts.

Endocardium Following Surgery in Congenital Heart Disease

We have studied the endocardium in 99 cases of postoperative congenital cardiac anomalies and compared those with unoperated cases of the same entity with age-matched controls. The surgeries were performed at least 6 weeks before death.

The types of congenital heart disease studied include:

	No. of Cases
Atrial septal defect, secundum type	8
Atrial septal defect, primum type	7
Ventricular septal defect	8
Tetralogy of Fallot	12
Double outlet right ventricle	5
Complete transposition of great arteries	15
Common AV orifice, complete type	3
Corrected transposition of great arteries	4
Ebstein's anomaly of the tricuspid valve	5
Patent ductus arteriosus	6
Isolated pulmonary stenosis	4
Aortic stenosis	10
Paraductal coarctation of the aorta	6
Total anomalous pulmonary venous connections	6
Total	99

There was one distinct common denominator that emerged in all of the hearts examined. There was more endocardial fibroelastosis of the chambers. In general, the hearts with "old" surgical intervention showed more diffuse fibroelastosis in the endocardium of various chambers than those of hearts with the same kind of congenital cardiac anomaly not subjected to surgery (Figs. 1–3). The fibroelastosis was not only present in

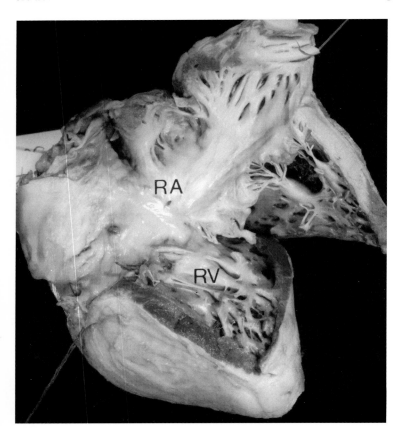

Figure 1: Diffuse fibroelastosis of the right-sided chambers in a case of ostium primum repaired several years before sudden death, with mitral and tricuspid insufficiency. Right atrial, right ventricular view. RA = right atrium; RV = right ventricle. Note the diffuse fibroelastosis of both chambers. (Used with permission from Bharati S, Lev M. See Figure 3.)

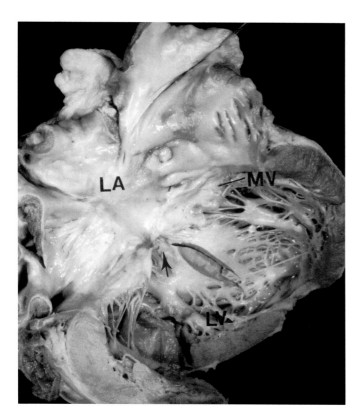

Figure 2: Left atrial, left ventricular view showing mitral insufficiency with enlargement of the left side of the heart with diffuse fibroelastosis. LA = left atrium; MV = mitral valve; LV = left ventricle. Arrow points to the cleft-like malformation in the mitral valve. (Used with permission from Bharati S, Lev M. See Figure 3.)

the chamber in which the surgeon operated, but also was often present in chambers in which the surgeon did not work. This raises the question as to the cause of "surgical fibroelastosis."

Causes for Surgical Fibroelastosis

The possible causes for surgical fibroelastosis are infection, hypoxia, genetics, altered physics, and lymphatic drainage obstruction. It is conceivable that surgical handling of the endocardium itself may be a factor in proliferation of endocardium. This perhaps may account for the fibroelastosis of the chamber that the surgeon opens to excise tissue or suture a defect. Since the entire heart is being manipulated, although not necessarily incised or sutured, this may account for the presence of fibroelastosis in the other chambers. It is also possible that anoxia related to anoxic arrest may

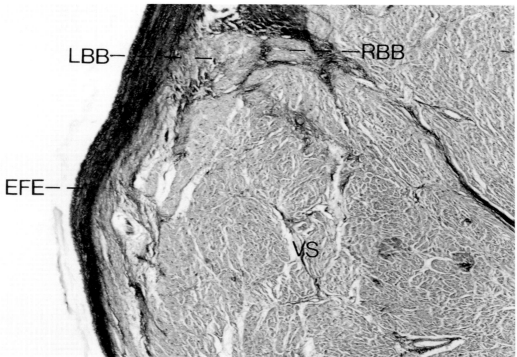

Figure 3: Endocardial fibroelastosis of the left ventricle following old surgical repair of DORV affecting the left and right bundle branches. Photomicrograph, Weigert-van Gieson stain ×45. VS = ventricular septum; EFE = endocardial fibroelastosis; LBB = left bundle branch being compressed and involved in fibroelastosis; RBB = right bundle branch surrounded by fibroelastosis. (Used with permission from Bharati S, Lev M: Sequelae of atriotomy and ventriculotomy of the endocardium, conduction system and coronary arteries. *Am J Cardiol* 1982, 50:580–587.)

play a role as well as cardioplegia by other means. We especially propose the theory of blocked lymphatics as the cause of "surgical fibroelastosis."

Blocked Lymphatic Drainage of the Heart

Normally, the lymph drainage of the heart proceeds from the endocardium to the epicardium. There are right and left currents. The left side of the lymphatic plexus empties into a trunk in the posterior interventricular sulcus and follows the left AV sulcus and unites with two anterior trunks, which emerge from the anterior interventricular sulcus. The left principal lymph-collecting trunk is thus formed and this proceeds along the left and posterior surfaces of the pulmonary trunk and eventually terminates in a node at the tracheal bifurcation or at the right paratracheal chain or, rarely, in the anterior mediastinal nodes. They eventually go to the right jugulosubclavian junction.

The right side of the plexus covers the entire right ventricle, except for a portion close to the anterior longitudinal sulcus. A collecting trunk is formed at the inferior limb of the right AV sulcus that in turn forms the right principal collecting trunk. This ascends on the anterior surface of the aorta, along the aorticopulmonary groove or somewhat to the right of it. It terminates most often in the node in the anterior mediastinal group in front of the origin of the left common carotid artery. These connect with the jugulosubclavian junction. Along these pathways, there are intercalated nodes.

It is possible that surgical manipulation anywhere along the course of the lymphatic pathway may, with time, obstruct the flow of lymph and lead to fibroelastosis of various chambers. It is surprising to find fibroelastosis after surgical repair of coarctation of the aorta, patent ductus arteriosus, and aortic and pulmonary stenosis because these cases did not have atriotomy or ventriculotomy. Fibroelastosis was seen more frequently in these entities when compared with the unoperated specimens of these entities. On the other hand, the amount of fibroelastosis was less than in entities that had atriotomy and ventriculotomy. It is very likely that collateral anastomosis develops in lymphatic channels following obstruction, most likely explaining why certain chambers are especially affected in some cases and others are not. We therefore hypothesize that good collateral anastomosis may occur in some, thereby preventing formation of fibroelastosis.

Coronary Arteries

It is well known that the coronary artery distribution, especially in tetralogy of Fallot, is an important consideration in ventriculotomy. The anterior descending coronary artery, when emerging from the right coronary artery, may proceed in front of the pulmonary trunk very close to the base of the pulmonary trunk or somewhere midway between the base and the apex, or may proceed between the aorta and the pulmonary trunk, or rarely may proceed intramyocardially and course along the superior margin of the defect to enter the anterior interventricular sulcus. Sometimes a single coronary artery may arise from the right sinus and give off the anterior descending coronary artery. In either case, whether the anterior descending coronary artery emerges as a separate ostium from the right sinus or emerges as a part of the single right coronary, it passes beneath the anterior surface of the base of the pulmonary trunk or may take one of the routes already described. In addition, there may be large conal branches.

It is my opinion that during infundibular pulmonary resection, when the ventricular septal myocardium is removed, the septal perforating branches are compromised. This may result in poor contraction of the ventricular septum and may also produce myocardial infarction and, at a later date, aneurysm formation of the ventricular septum.

The Conduction System

Both atriotomy and ventriculotomy can cause damage to the conduction system.

Atriotomy

The sinoatrial (SA) node and its approaches, the AV node, and the atrial preferential pathways may be affected during atriotomy. The SA node is situated in the sulcus terminalis and extends from the hump of the atrial appendage to the Wenckebach bundle. The superior preferential pathway proceeds from the junction of the head of the node with Bachmann's bundle along the superior part of the wall of the atrial septum then swings down to the approaches of the AV node. The middle preferential pathway extends from the proximal middle part of the SA node, swings posteriorly in the atrial septum, and proceeds through the limbus fossae ovalis and joins the superior pathway. The inferior preferential pathway proceeds from the tail end of the node along the crista terminalis, and swings into the lower part of the atrial septum to reach the coronary sinus area.

The approaches to the AV node are thus situated superiorly, inferiorly, and proximal to the AV node. The AV node is situated distal to the upper part of the mouth of the coronary sinus and the medial or septal leaflet of the tricuspid valve.

The atriotomy incision may pass through part of the SA node and/or its approaches. Disruption of the approaches to the SA node may separate the SA node from or diminish its connections to the AV node. As alluded to previously, in the Mustard procedure, the SA and AV nodes may be damaged. In addition, the atrial preferential pathways may be either completely or almost completely cut across and/or removed. Because the middle and inferior preferential pathways are completely or partially severed in this procedure, it would be advisable to keep the superior pathway intact. Today, the Mustard procedure is not being performed.

Ventriculotomy

The basic problem in ventriculotomy is the integrity of the right bundle branch. In addition, the focal fibrotic scars in the right ventricle may become an arrhythmogenic focus.

The right bundle branch is situated in the lower confines of the pars membranacea and proceeds along the lower septal band about 1 mm beneath the muscle of Lancisi, along the lower margin of the septal band into the moderator band. At this region it divides off into three branches. One branch goes to the inferior wall, one to the anterior wall, and one proceeds distally on the ventricular septum for a short distance (upward).

The ventriculotomy incision in closure of ventricular septal defect, tetralogy of Fallot, and double outlet right ventricle may sever most of the secondary branches in the anterior wall of the right ventricle to produce a complete or incomplete right bundle branch block pattern on the electrocardiogram. If the ventriculotomy incision is more on the left portion of the anterior wall, it may cut across the moderator band to give rise to complete right bundle branch block.

In ventricular septal defect, in pure levocardia (concordant chambers), the AV bundle lies on the inferior wall of the defect or slightly to the left of the summit of the septum. The right bundle branch is frequently cut at its junction with the bifurcating bundle or the beginning of the first part of the right bundle branch may be cut, producing right bundle branch block. Likewise, in tetralogy of Fallot, the AV bundle lies more to the left of the summit of the septum. In ventricular septal defect with ventricular inversion (corrected transposition), the AV bundle usually passes over the anterolateral wall of the morphological left ventricle and beneath the pulmonic valve and swings downward over the superior and distal wall of the ventricular septal defect. Thus, the superior distal wall of the defect is in a vulnerable position during the surgical closure of the ventricular septal defect. Ventriculotomy incision near the base of the pulmonary trunk may sever the bundle in repair of pulmonary or subpulmonary stenosis in corrected transposition.

The Myocardium

Sequelae in the postoperative myocardium at the gross level is in the form of focal fibrotic scars or fibrotic scars somewhat diffuse in nature. These are quite prominent, especially after surgery for double outlet right ventricle and Mustard procedures. These scars are also seen in postoperative tetralogy of Fallot (Figs. 4–7), ventricular septal defect closure, and in atrial septal defect closure. There are distinct scars, especially at the site of infundibular pulmonary resection and where the outflow tract of the right ventricle had been enlarged by means of a prosthetic (Figs. 4–7) or homograft material. There may be associated aneurysm formation in and around the scar areas. It is well known that the junctional areas between the healthy myocardium and the scar tissue may provide a milieu for slowing of an impulse and promote a reentry phenomenon or an abnormal automaticity or fractionalization of an impulse that may generate a premature ventricular contraction. The premature ventricular contractions may remain innocuous and silent for a long period of time and eventually, during an altered physiological state, may degenerate into ventricular tachycardia fibrillation and sudden death.

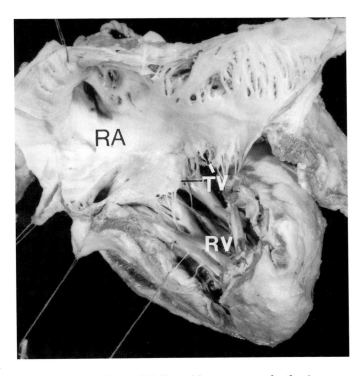

Figure 4: Tetralogy of Fallot, old surgery, arrhythmias, cardiomegaly, and sudden death. Right atrial, right ventricular view. RA = right atrium; RV = right ventricle; TV = tricuspid valve. Note the diffuse fibroelastosis.

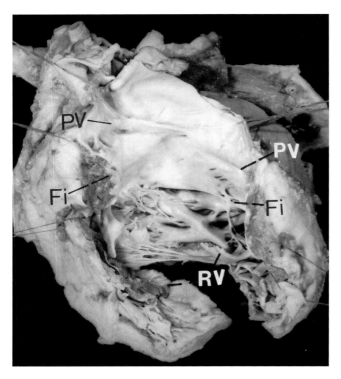

Figure 5: Outflow tract of the right ventricle showing the fibroelastosis, pulmonary insufficiency, and right ventricular hypertrophy and enlargement. PV = surgically altered bicuspid pulmonic valve; RV = right ventricle; Fi = fibroelastosis.

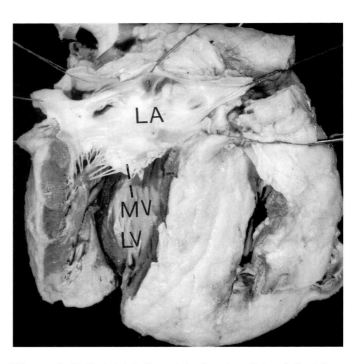

Figure 6: Left atrial, left ventricular view. LA = left atrium; LV = left ventricle; MV = mitral valve.

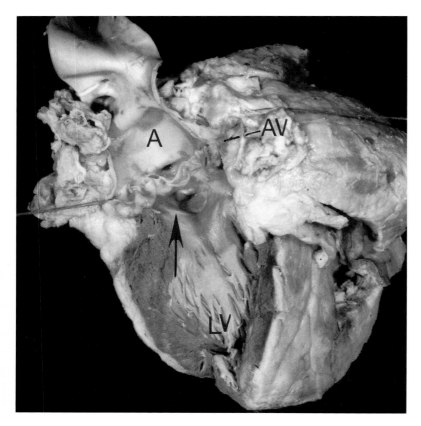

Figure 7: Outflow tract of the left ventricle showing the development of subaortic stenosis and fenestrated aortic valve. A = ascending aorta; AV = aortic valve with fenestration; LV = left ventricle with fibroelastosis. Arrow points to the area beneath the surgical closure of the defect with developing subaortic stenosis.

The Conduction System and Arrhythmias

Surgery following Atrial Septal Defect, Fossa Ovalis Type

Varying types of arrhythmias do occur following surgical closure of a secundum atrial septal defect. These arrhythmias may occur anywhere from a few weeks to several years following surgery. The arrhythmias include atrial fibrillation and flutter, atrial tachycardia, junctional rhythm, junctional nodal rhythm, sinoatrial dysfunction, first- and second-degree as well as complete AV block. If these arrhythmias were present preoperatively, the arrhythmias indeed got worse, especially in older patients. When the defect is quite large, extending close to the coronary sinus or the entry of the inferior vena cava, the approaches to the AV node may be compromised during surgery.

Pathologically, these areas show marked fatty infiltration, fibroelastosis, mononuclear cell infiltration (Fig. 8), and sometimes calcification. These pathological findings obviously interrupt the approaches to the SA and AV nodes and may produce varying types of atrial arrhythmias and/or block. Likewise, direct surgical injury to the approaches to the AV node itself may interrupt the approaches to the AV node and produce varying degrees of block proximal to the His bundle. If a defect is close to the superior vena cava, closure of the defect may result in partial injury to the SA node and its approaches and may produce sick sinus syndrome at a later date. There is a tendency for fatty infiltration to occur more so in postoperative cases, especially in the approaches to the AV node and the atrial septum than the normal population. It is known that fatty infiltration of the atrial septum as such may produce varying types of atrial arrhythmias both in the young as well as in the elderly. Surgical injury to the SA node is also seen in cases of sudden death following surgical closure of atrial septal defect.

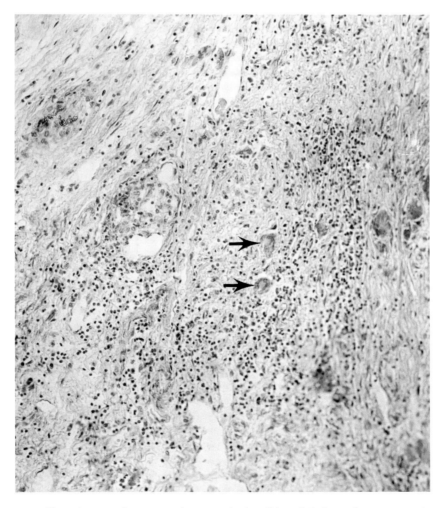

Figure 8: Chronic granulomatous tissue replacing SA nodal tissue in an asymptomatic 38-year-old male with familial ASD and first degree AV block, who died suddenly 8 years after closure of ASD. Hematoxylin-eosin stain ×180. Arrows point to giant cells.

Ventricular Septal Defect, Tetralogy of Fallot, and Double Outlet Right Ventricle

Varying types of arrhythmias have been reported following total surgical correction of these entities. The long-term postoperative arrhythmias include peripheral and central right bundle branch block, and left anterior hemiblock, AV nodal dysfunction, supraventricular and ventricular tachycardia, premature ventricular contractions, abnormal sinus impulse generation, prolonged A-H and H-V time, prolonged intra-atrial time, and complete AV block.

We believe that some cases of right bundle branch block may indeed be due to disruption of the right bundle branch proximally during closure of the ventricular septal defect (Figs. 9–14) or the right bundle branch may be disrupted peripherally during ventriculotomy incision. The bifurcating bundle and the beginning of the bundle branches may be disrupted in the fibrotic process (Fig. 15). AV block probably occurs in some cases from injury to the branching part of the AV bundle (Fig. 16). Further, the fibrosis and fibroelastosis of the various chambers may involve the conduction system.

Common Atrioventricular Orifice

Complete AV block may occur following surgical correction of common AV orifice of a complete type. Junctional rhythm and sinus node dysfunction have been reported. The AV block probably results from injury to the AV bundle during closure of the defect in the AV region.

Complete Transposition, Mustard Procedure, and Senning Procedure

The SA node and its approaches, the AV node and its approaches, and the anterior preferential pathways are frequently injured. The SA node may be interrupted directly while the intra-atrial baffle is placed in the Mustard procedure. Most of the atrial preferential pathways are necessarily removed during the Mustard procedure, thereby setting the stage for various types of supraventricular arrhythmias postoperatively in the long run. Similarly, the fibrotic scars surrounding the AV node and its approaches may result in block proximal to the His bundle in some cases many years after surgery. In the Senning procedure, the atrial septum is interrupted in many ways making it feasible for ar-

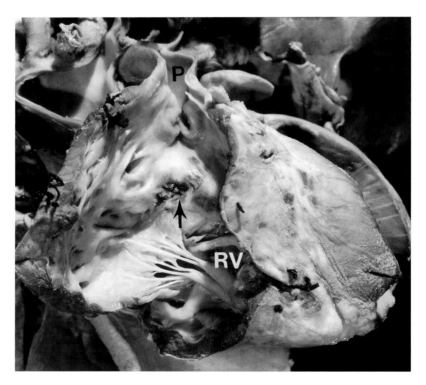

Figure 9: Surgical closure of the ventricular septal defect as seen from the right ventricle with involvement of the proximal part of the right bundle branch. RV = right ventricle; P = pulmonary trunk. Arrow points to the region of the proximal part of the right bundle branch with hemorrhage and sutures.

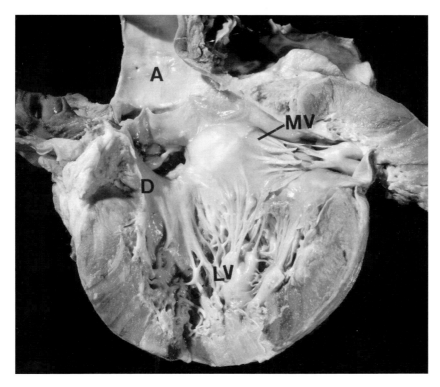

Figure 10: Ventricular septal defect closure as seen from the left ventricle. A = aorta; LV = left ventricle; MV = mitral valve; D = defect.

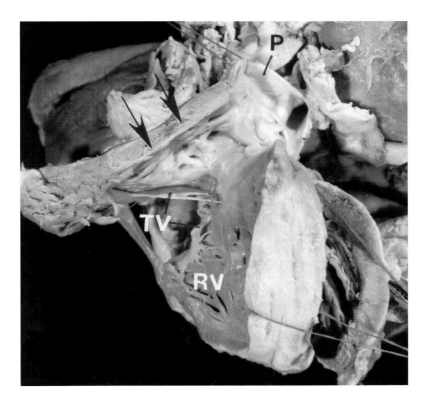

Figure 11: Old surgical closure of ventricular septal defect followed by right bundle branch block, left axis deviation and sudden death in a 16-year-old boy. RV = right ventricle; TV = tricuspid valve; P = pulmonary trunk. Arrows point to the fibroelastosis in the anterior wall of the right ventricle.

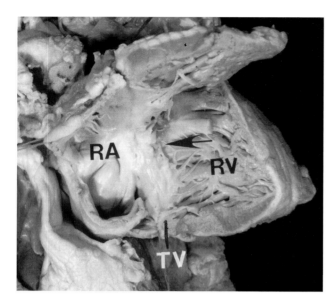

Figure 12: Right atrial, right ventricular view showing fibroelastosis of the right atrium. RA = right atrium; RV = right ventricle; TV = tricuspid valve. Arrow points to the area of closure of the VSD.

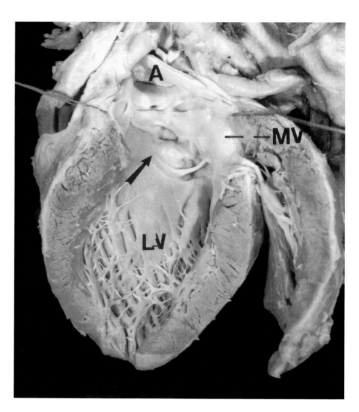

Figure 14: Outflow tract of the left ventricle showing the old surgical closure of the VSD with distinct thickening and fibroelastosis at the region of the closure of the defect with anomalous chordal extension. A = aorta; MV = mitral valve; LV = left ventricle. Arrow points to surgical closure of the defect.

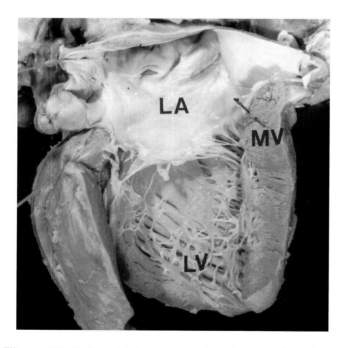

Figure 13: Left atrial, left ventricular view showing fibroelastosis of the left atrium and fine diffuse fibroelastosis of the left ventricle. LA = left atrium; LV = left ventricle; MV = mitral valve.

rhythmias to occur at a later date. Sudden death occurs frequently in longstanding cases of Mustard as well as Senning procedures.

The Central Fibrous Body or the Fibrous Skeleton of the Heart

The central fibrous body indeed undergoes premature aging in postoperative congenital heart disease. This includes the summit of the ventricular septum in some longstanding cases. The aging changes may not only affect the left side of the septum but also affect the right side of the septum. Our previous work on sudden death in the young and the healthy indicates that the aging of the summit of the ventricular septum, especially on the right ventricular side, may increase the risk of sudden death by making the area prone to an arrhythmic event due to reentry phenomena. On the other hand, the aging on the left side of the fibrous skeleton has a tendency to produce AV block. We therefore believe that the aging changes in the form of patchy fibrotic scars seem to have a more lethal out-

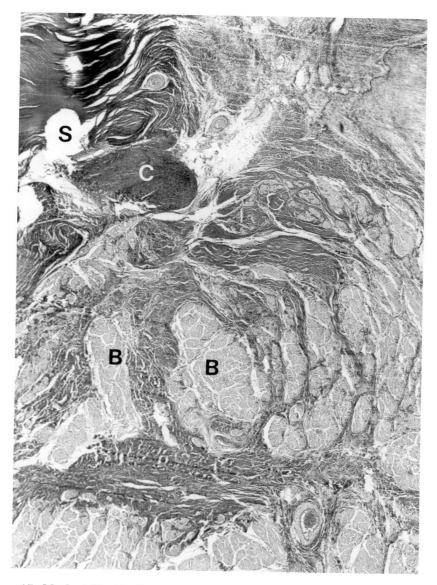

Figure 15: Marked fibrotic disruption of the bifurcating bundle with sutures close to the bundle in a 16-year-old asymptomatic male, with surgical closure of ASD and VSD 9 years before he died suddenly. ECG was normal before surgery; he developed right bundle branch block pattern after surgery, and much later developed atrial fibrillation with a ventricular rate of 70 to 80 beats per minute. Weigert-van Gieson stain ×45. B = bifurcating bundle; S = sutures; C = thickened central fibrous body.

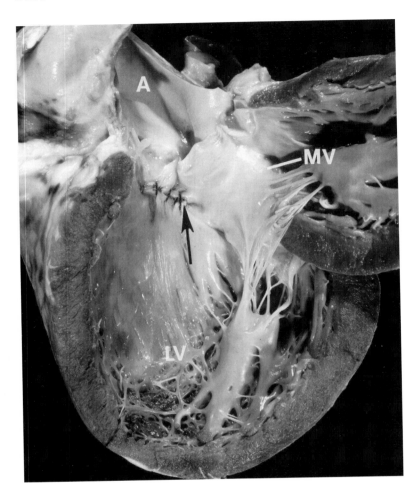

Figure 16: Direct suturing of ventricular septal defect, closure with postoperative heart block. A = aorta; MV = mitral valve; LV = left ventricle. Arrow points to the sutures involving the His bundle and closure of the defect. (Used with permission from Lev M, Fell EH, Arcilla R, Weinberg MH: Surgical injury to the conduction system in ventricular septal defect. Am J Cardiol 1964, 14:464–476.)

come when present on the right ventricular side of the septum than on the left.

Sudden Death after Cardiac Surgery

Sudden death occurs long after repair in literally all types of congenital cardiac anomalies, including atrial septal defect (secundum type) (Fig. 8), ventricular septal defect (Figs. 8–15), ostium primum defect (Figs. 1, 2, 17–25), tetralogy of Fallot (Figs. 4–7, 26–30), common AV orifice, double outlet right ventricle (Figs. 31–34), Mustard procedure (Figs. 35–44), Senning procedure, corrected transposition with ventricular or atrial inversion (Figs. 45–49), and other anomalies. Studies of the conduction system in these cases show varying degrees of interruption of parts of the conduction system with fibrosis, fat, mononuclear cell infiltra-

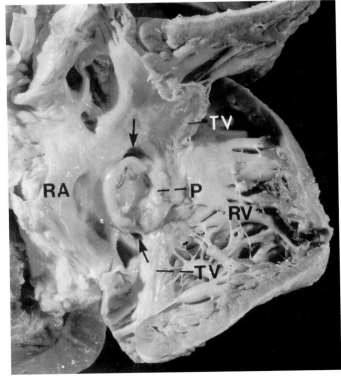

Figure 17: Ostium primum repaired with residual atrial septal defects on either side of the patch, tricuspid insufficiency, and sudden death. Right atrial, right ventricular view. RA = right atrium; RV = right ventricle; TV = tricuspid valve; P = old patch closure of the primum defect. Arrows point to the residual atrial septal defect.

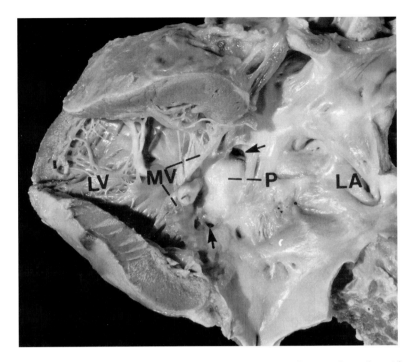

Figure 18: Left atrial, left ventricular view showing mitral stenosis and residual atrial septal defect. LV = left ventricle; LA = hypertrophied and enlarged left atrium with fibroelastosis; P = patch closure of the defect; MV = mitral valve with stenosis. Arrows point to the residual defect in the atrial septum.

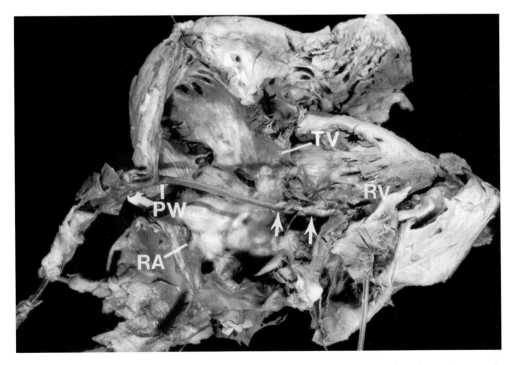

Figure 19: Old ASD primum repaired, with heart block, pacemaker insertion, and sudden death. Right atrial, right ventricular view with tricuspid insufficiency and well-endothelialized pacemaker in the right ventricle. RA = right atrium; RV = right ventricle; TV = tricuspid valve; PW = pacemaker. Arrows point to the well-endothelialized pacemaker as it proceeds towards the apex of the right ventricle. Note that the pacemaker also involves the tricuspid valve with a gap between the patch closure of the primum and the anterior leaflet of the tricuspid valve.

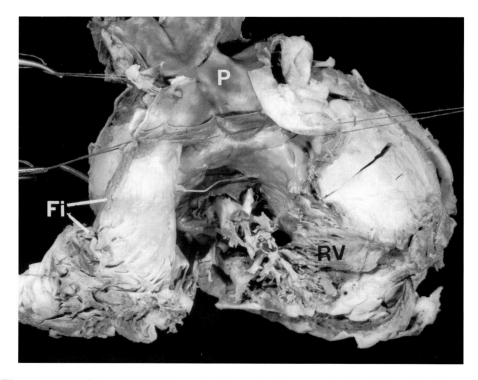

Figure 20: Right ventricular hypertrophy and enlargement with diffuse fibroelastosis of the right ventricle. RV = right ventricle; Fi = fibroelastosis; P = pulmonary trunk.

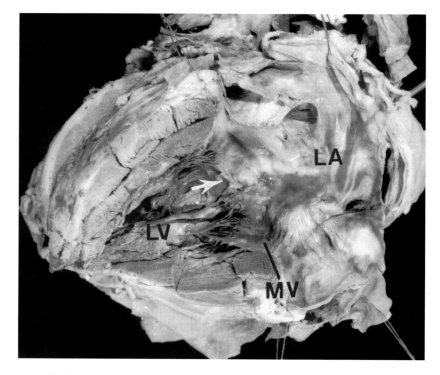

Figure 21: Left atrial, left ventricular view with mitral stenosis. LA = tremendously hypertrophied and enlarged left atrium; LV = left ventricle; MV = mitral valve. Arrow points to the repaired area of cleft with small mitral valve and mitral stenosis.

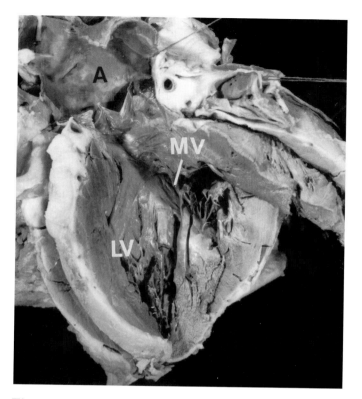

Figure 22: Left ventricular outflow with ventricular septal bulge. A = aorta; LV = left ventricle; MV = mitral valve.

tion, and calcification in some (Figs. 3, 7, 15). The chronic inflammatory cells seen in the operated site, and in some cases the surrounding myocardial tissue, may not be myocarditis in a true sense, and these may represent a form of minor rejection phenomenon occurring as a result of prosthetic material introduced into these hearts.

We therefore hypothesize that a low-grade autoimmune mechanism may play a role when prosthetic materials are introduced into the heart in some cases and may cause a picture similar to myocarditis. In some, the nerves reveal inflammatory phenomena or fibrotic changes. The changes are not only seen at the area of surgery, but the distal part of the conduction system also presents distinct pathological changes in the form of disruption of the His bundle and the bundle branches with varying degrees of scar formation.

The exact cause of sudden death is not clear; however, it is frequently ascribed to ventricular fibrillation produced by a circus movement with reentry or abnormal automaticity.

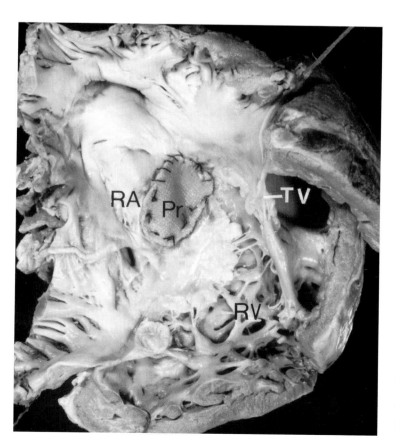

Figure 23: Ostium primum, repaired, with tricuspid insufficiency, large right side of heart with small left side, and sudden death. RA = right atrium; RV = right ventricle; TV = tricuspid valve; Pr = prosthetic closure of ostium primum defect. Note the huge right side of heart.

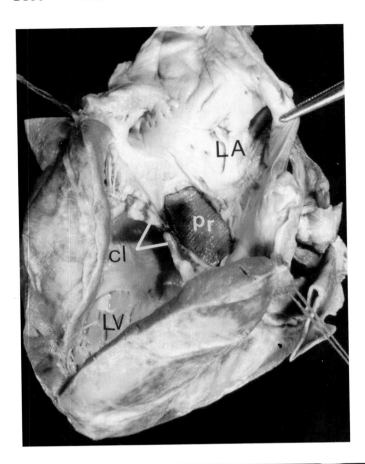

Figure 24: Left atrial, left ventricular view showing lack of mitral valvular tissue with mitral stenosis and possible insufficiency. LA = huge left atrium; LV = small left ventricle; Pr = prosthetic closure of ostium primum defect; Cl = wide cleft with thickened edges and mitral stenosis.

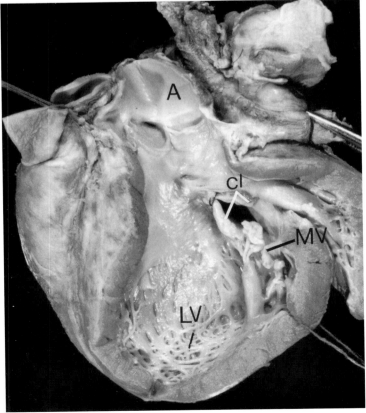

Figure 25: Outflow tract of the left ventricle demonstrating the cleft-like malformation with thickened edges of the mitral valve and fibroelastosis of the left ventricle. A = aorta; LV = left ventricle; MV = mitral valve; Cl = thickened cleft.

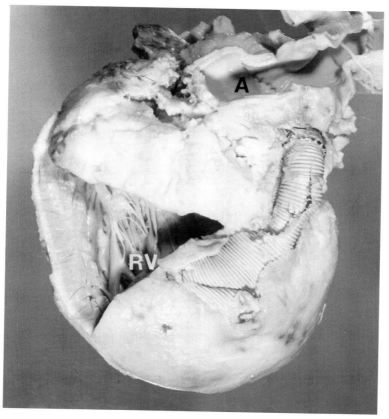

Figure 26: Old tetralogy of Fallot with surgical correction and Hancock prosthesis with cardiomegaly and sudden death. External view of the heart. RV = right ventricle; A = aorta.

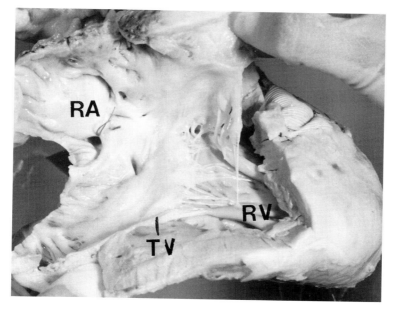

Figure 27: Right atrial, right ventricular view with diffuse fibroelastosis. RA = right atrium; TV = tricuspid valve; RV = right ventricle.

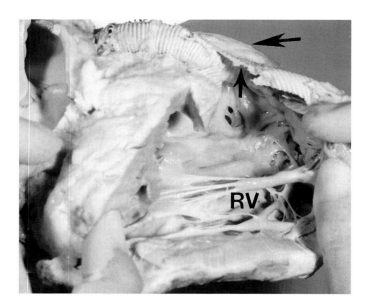

Figure 28: Outflow tract of the right ventricle with diffuse fibroelastosis. Arrows point to the calcification in the prosthesis.

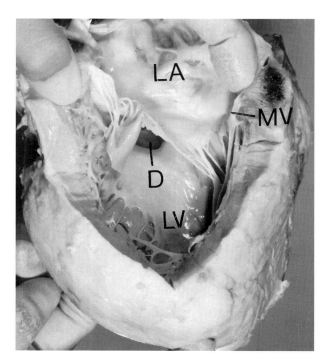

Figure 30: Left atrial, left ventricular view demonstrating closed ventricular septal defect and fibroelastosis. LA = left atrium; D = defect closed surgically; LV = left ventricle; MV = mitral valve.

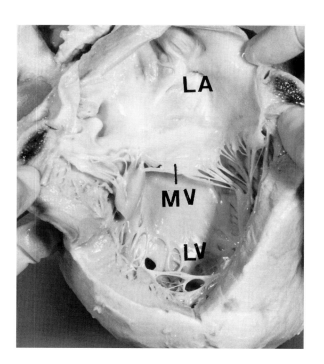

Figure 29: Left atrial, left ventricular view, fibroelastosis. LA = left atrium; LV = left ventricle; MV = mitral valve.

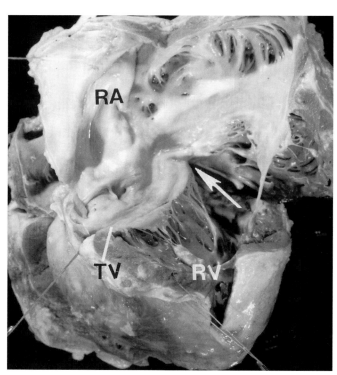

Figure 31: Double outlet right ventricle subaortic ventricular septal defect and subpulmonary and valvular stenosis with old repair and sudden death. Right atrial, right ventricular view. RA = diffuse fibroelastosis of right atrium; TV = thickened tricuspid valve; RV = right ventricle. Arrow points to the area of patch closure of defect.

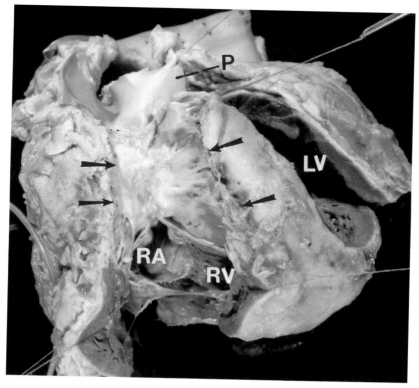

Figure 32: Outflow tract of the right ventricle showing diffuse fibroelastosis in the infundibular area and surgically altered bicuspid pulmonic valve with insufficiency. LV = left ventricle; RA = right atrium; RV = right ventricle; P = pulmonary trunk. Arrows point to diffuse fibroelastosis in the infundibulum.

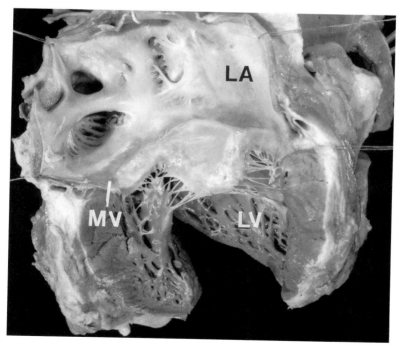

Figure 33: Left atrial, left ventricular view. LA = left atrium; LV = left ventricle; MV = mitral valve.

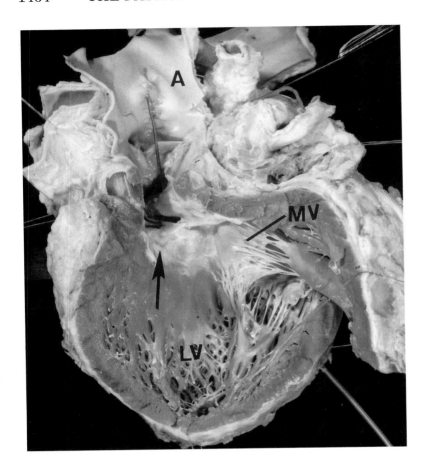

Figure 34: Outflow tract of the left ventricle showing fibroelastosis in the surgically closed area with subaortic obstruction. A = aorta; MV = mitral valve; LV = left ventricle. Arrow points to patch closure with developing subaortic stenosis.

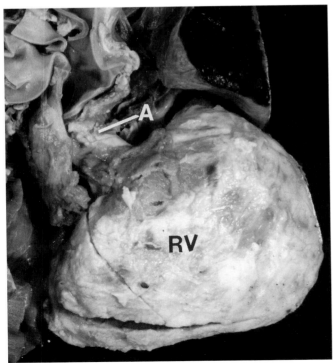

Figure 35: Five-year-old child, old Mustard procedure and sudden death; external view of the heart. RV = right ventricle; A = aorta. Note the cardiomegaly.

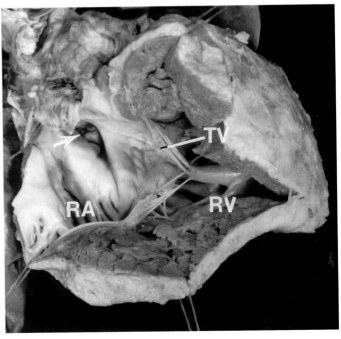

Figure 36: Five-year-old child with old Mustard procedure (2½ years ago) with atrial arrhythmias and sudden death, right-sided view. RA = right atrium; RV = right ventricle; TV = tricuspid valve. Arrow points to the entry of the pulmonary veins. Note the fibroelastosis of the right atrium.

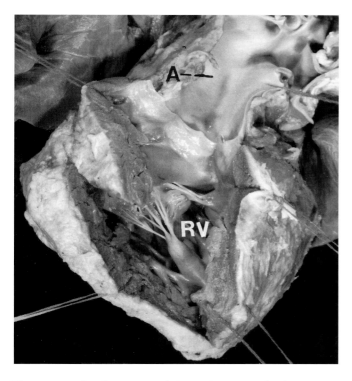

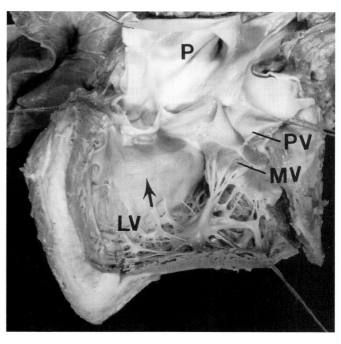

Figure 37: Outflow tract of the right ventricle showing the marked right ventricular hypertrophy. RV = right ventricle; A = aorta.

Figure 39: Outflow tract of the left ventricle demonstrating development of subpulmonary obstruction following long-standing Mustard procedure with intact ventricular septum in complete transposition. MV = mitral valve; PV = pulmonary valve; P = pulmonary trunk; LV = left ventricle. Arrow points to development of subpulmonary obstruction.

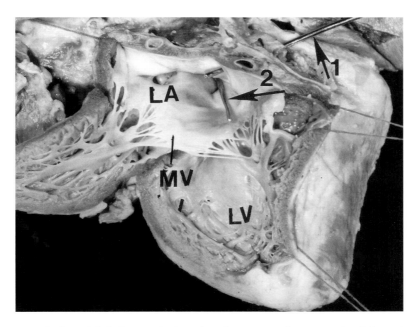

Figure 38: Left atrial, left ventricular view demonstrating stenosis of the entry of the superior vena cava. LA = left atrium; LV = left ventricle; MV = mitral valve. Arrow #1 proceeds through the inferior vena cava; arrow #2 proceeds through the superior vena cava with obstruction.

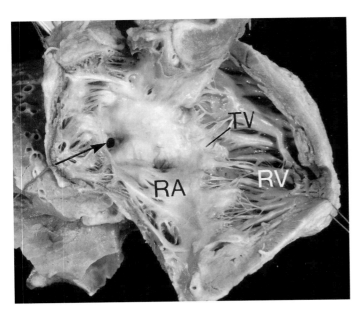

Figure 40: Sudden death following Mustard procedure and closure of ventricular septal defect in a 5-year-old child. Right atrial, right ventricular view, showing stenosis of the entry of the pulmonary veins and tricuspid insufficiency. RA = hypertrophied and enlarged right atrium with diffuse fibroelastosis; RV = right ventricle; TV = enlarged tricuspid with thickened valve and insufficiency. Arrow points to the entry of the pulmonary veins. (Used with permission from Bharati S, et al. See Figure 44.)

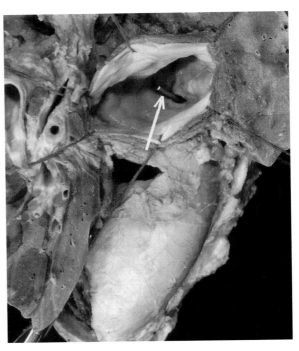

Figure 41: Posterior view of the heart showing the entry of the pulmonary veins resulting in a cor triatriatum type of phenomenon with stenosis of the veins as they enter the right atrium. Arrow points to the probe passing through the stenotic orifice into the right atrium.

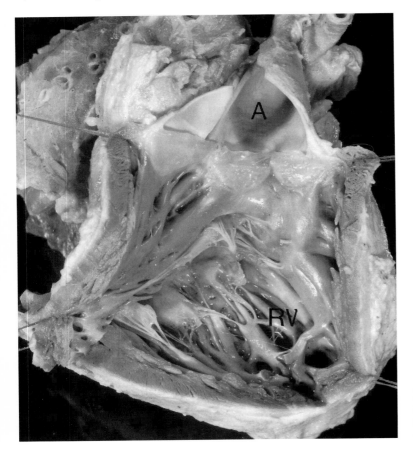

Figure 42: Right ventricular outflow tract demonstrating marked hypertrophy and enlargement with increased trabeculations. RV = right ventricle; A = aorta.

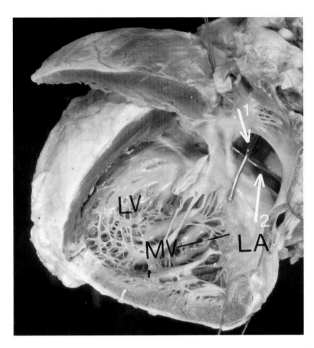

Figure 43: Left atrial, left ventricular view. LA = left atrium; LV = left ventricle; MV = mitral valve. Arrow #1 proceeding into the superior vena cava, arrow #2 proceeding into the inferior vena cava.

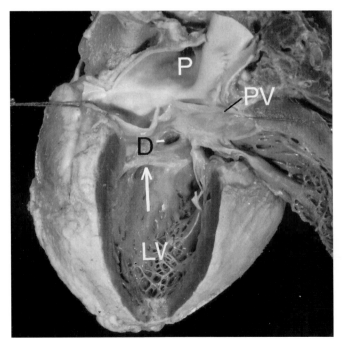

Figure 44: Outflow tract of the left ventricle demonstrating the surgical closure of ventricular septal defect, development of a fibroelastic ridge beneath the pulmonary trunk, and developing subpulmonary stenosis. PV = pulmonary valve; P = pulmonary trunk; LV = left ventricle; D = surgical closure of the defect. Arrow points to the fibroelastic ridge beneath the defect. (Used with permission from Bharati S, Molthan ME, Veasy LG, Lev M: Conduction system in two cases of sudden death two years after the Mustard procedure. *J Thorac Cardiovasc Surg* 1979, 77:101–108.)

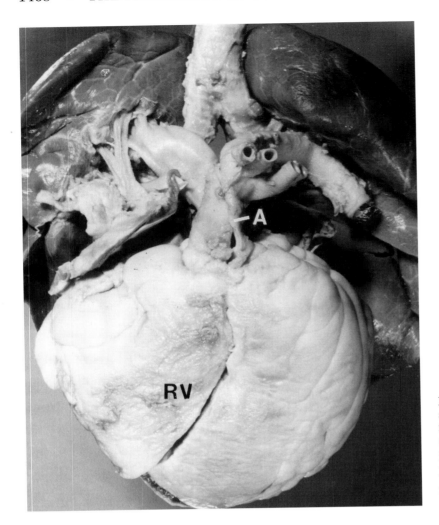

Figure 45: Isolated levocardia with atrial inversion, atrial septal defect and ventricular septal defect, pulmonary stenosis with mild Ebstein's anomaly of the tricuspid valve and old surgery, and sudden death. External view of the heart. Note the hypertrophied and enlarged heart with the aorta situated to the right and anterior, pulmonary left and posterior. RV = right ventricle; A = aorta.

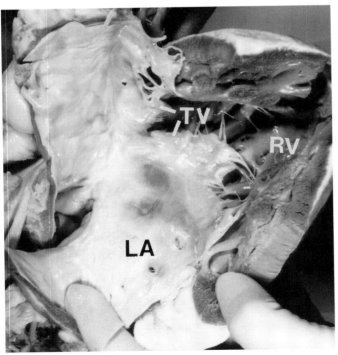

Figure 46: Left atrial, right ventricular view. Note the diffuse fibroelastosis of the left atrium and mild Ebstein's malformation of the tricuspid valve. TV = mild Ebstein's of the tricuspid valve; RV = right ventricle; LA = left atrium.

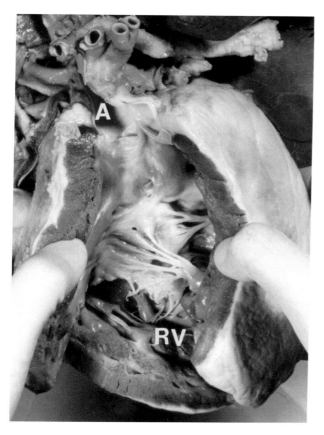

Figure 47: Outflow tract of the right ventricle. Although the aorta is emerging from this chamber, the circulation is physiologically corrected. A = aorta; RV = right ventricle.

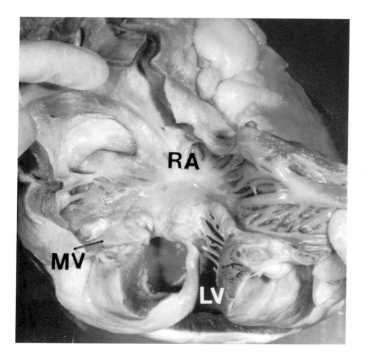

Figure 48: Right atrium situated to the left side connecting with the morphological left ventricle. RA = right atrium; LV = left ventricle; MV = mitral valve.

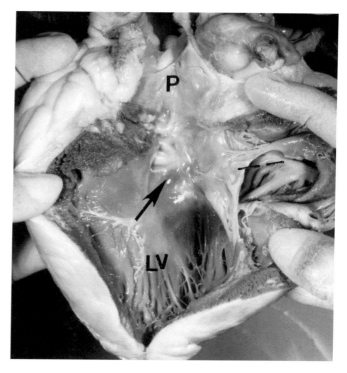

Figure 49: Outflow tract of the morphological left ventricle, pulmonary stenosis, and old surgical closure of ventricular septal defect. P = pulmonary trunk; LV = left ventricle. Note the fibroelastosis in the region of the old surgical closure of the ventricular septal defect and subpulmonary stenosis. Arrow points to the subpulmonary stenosis and the fibroelastosis in the region of the His bundle and the beginning of the left bundle branch fibers.

Sequelae following Repair of the Anomaly Itself

Patent Ductus Arteriosus

Rarely, the persistence of pulmonary hypertension following surgical closure of patent ductus arteriosus resulted in sudden death years after surgery (Fig. 50).

Coarctation of the Aorta

There is a distinct increase in connective tissue proliferation in the anastomotic site in cases of coarctation of the aorta. It is not known why this occurs. This may be due to the development of auto antibodies, which may facilitate the proliferation of connective tissue or the normal increase in the amount of connective tissue that is seen near the coarted area in the adventitia (an increase of connective tissue at the region of coarctation), which may facilitate proliferation postop-

eratively. It is well known that systemic hypertension persists in some or may indeed get worse in some.

The left ventricle in some may retain its hypertrophy and may not come back to its normal level. In some, the hypertrophy may get worse. The reason for the persistence of left ventricular hypertrophy with fibroelastosis is not known today. A bicuspid aortic valve, which is frequently seen with coarctation, may be a nidus for infective endocarditis at a later date, calcification, and aortic insufficiency may occur following infective endocarditis of the valve and/or as a result of the "normal aging phenomena."

It is important to emphasize that there may be an associated mitral valve anomaly in the form of a parachute mitral valve or an arcade mitral valve or a supravalvular mitral ridge that may remain silent for a long period of time and eventually may produce hemodynamically significant stenosis and/or insufficiency at a later date. It is emphasized that these associated abnormalities, especially in the aortic and mitral valves, may not be hemodynamically significant during

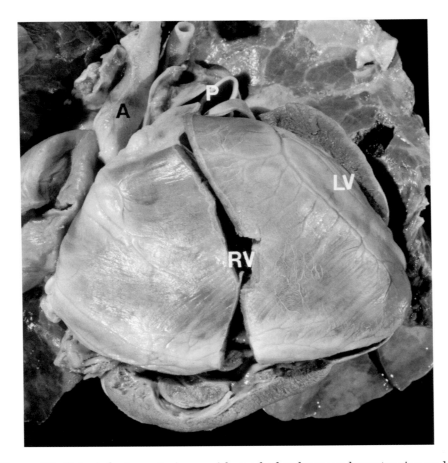

Figure 50: Patent ductus arteriosus with marked pulmonary hypertension and ligation and division of the ductus followed by residual pulmonary hypertension and sudden death many years later. External view of the heart. Note that the apex is formed by the right ventricle. RV = right ventricle; LV = small left ventricle; P = pulmonary trunk; A = aorta.

the time of surgery but may become so postoperatively as the child grows older.

Atrial Septal Defect

Rarely, infective endocarditis may occur at the site of the patch in the secundum area, especially in older people. Rarely, a floppy or abnormally formed mitral valve has resulted in insufficiency following longstanding repair of an atrial septal defect. If a defect is large and is situated close to the superior vena cava, rarely obstruction to the superior vena cava or to the inferior vena cava and still more rarely complete transfer of vena cava into the left atrium may occur.

Ostium Primum Atrial Septal Defect

The majority of cases of ostium primum have hypertrophied and enlarged hearts (Figs. 1, 2, 17–24) with tricuspid and/or mitral insufficiency (Figs. 1, 2, 17–19). Occasionally, they have had mitral stenosis (Fig. 21). The mitral insufficiency that occurs postoperatively may remain silent or may be in the mild form, but as the child starts growing older, the insufficiency becomes significant. The insufficiency may become aggravated by the presence of an accessory mitral orifice, or a floppy leaflet of the mitral valve, or sometimes a parachute mitral valve. The undetected subaortic stenosis preoperatively may progress gradually, resulting in significant subaortic obstruction at a later date.

Ventricular Septal Defect

A bicuspid aortic valve or a dysplastic aortic valve postoperatively after the closure of the ventricular septal defect had produced aortic insufficiency (Fig. 51). Although large anterior defects with or without prolapse of the right aortic cusp may or may not have minimal aortic insufficiency preoperatively, postoperatively, in some, there has been aortic insufficiency. This, we believe, is due to the involvement of the base of the valve during surgical closure of the defect (Figs. 52, 53). Postoperative small ventricular septal defects, when present, serve as nidus for infective endocarditis.

Subaortic stenosis developed rarely several years following surgical closure of the defect (Figs. 54, 55).

Rarely, myocardial abscess formation with rupture was observed (Fig. 56). Acquired diseases of the heart and lung may also complicate the outcome (Fig. 57). Unfortunately, the outflow tract of the right ventricle was closed in one (Figs. 58, 59); and an associated cardiac anomaly that was not detected before surgery had resulted in a fatal outcome (Figs. 60, 61).

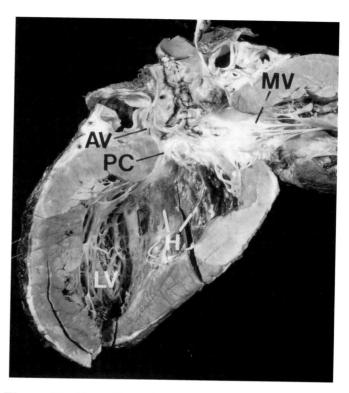

Figure 51: Bicuspid aortic valve with aortic insufficiency and surgical closure of ventricular septal defect. LV = hypertrophied left ventricle; PC = patch closure of defect; AV = surgically altered aortic valve; MV = mitral valve; H = hemorrhage in the region of His bundle and left bundle branch.

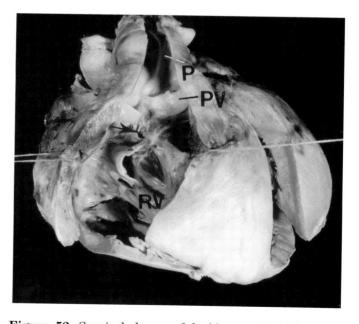

Figure 52: Surgical closure of doubly committed (subarterial or anterior) type of VSD with aortic insufficiency and repair of aortic valve with residual aortic insufficiency. Right ventricular view. RV = right ventricle; P = pulmonary trunk; PV = pulmonary valve. Arrow points to the surgical closure of the defect confluent with the pulmonic valve, in part.

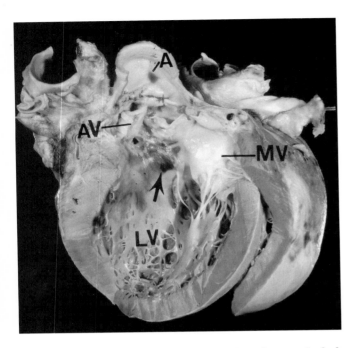

Figure 53: Left ventricular view showing the surgical closure as well as hemorrhage in the region of the His bundle and left bundle branch. LV = left ventricle; MV = mitral valve; A = aorta; AV = thickened aortic valve. Arrows point to the hemorrhage in the AV bundle and left bundle branch.

Tetralogy of Fallot

Postoperatively, there may be residual pulmonary valvular, infundibular, or supravalvular or peripheral pulmonary stenosis, and sometimes pulmonary insufficiency occurs (Fig. 5). Residual ventricular septal defect and subaortic stenosis are rarely seen (Fig. 7). Calcification of the patch area or porcine valved conduit is also seen (Fig. 28). An aneurysmal dilatation of the anterior wall of the right ventricle may occur, especially in cases operated on many years ago. Tricuspid insufficiency and/or stenosis is uncommonly seen following surgery.

Pulmonary insufficiency with or without tricuspid insufficiency may compromise the right ventricle. Aortic insufficiency, rarely seen preoperatively in tetralogy of Fallot, may get worse after surgery. Likewise, an abnormally formed aortic valve (before surgery) may become a site for infective endocarditis at a later date. Rarely, a simple atrial septal defect that was not closed during surgical correction of tetralogy of Fallot may require a second surgery.

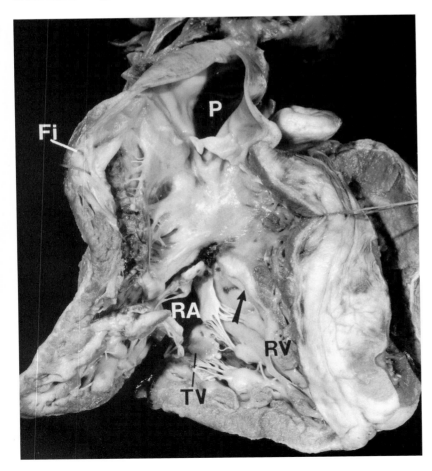

Figure 54: Surgical closure of ventricular septal defect and fibroelastosis of the right ventricle and sudden death. P = pulmonary trunk; RV = right ventricle; TV = tricuspid valve; RA = right atrium; Fi = fibroelastosis. Arrow points to fibroelastosis along the course of the right bundle branch.

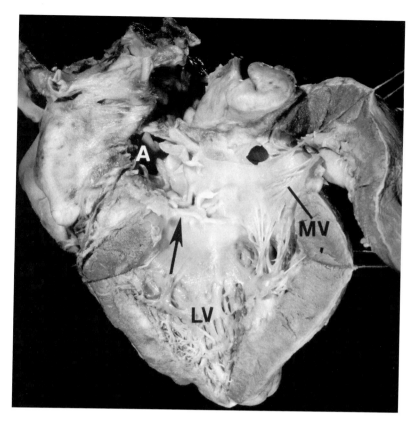

Figure 55: Old surgical closure of ventricular septal defect with sudden death and fibroelastosis and development of subaortic ridges at the region of the defect. A = aorta; LV = left ventricle; MV = mitral valve. Arrow points to the subaortic ridges and the fibroelastosis.

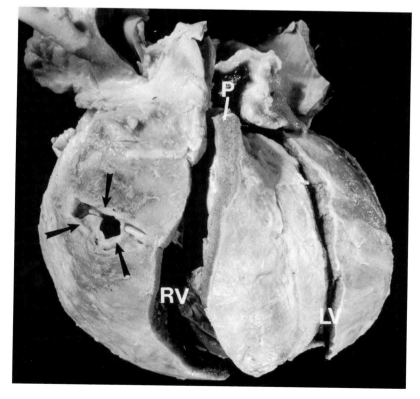

Figure 56: Old ventricular septal defect closure with myocardial abscess and rupture. External view of the heart. RV = right ventricle; LV = left ventricle; P = pulmonary trunk. Arrows point to myocardial abscess with rupture.

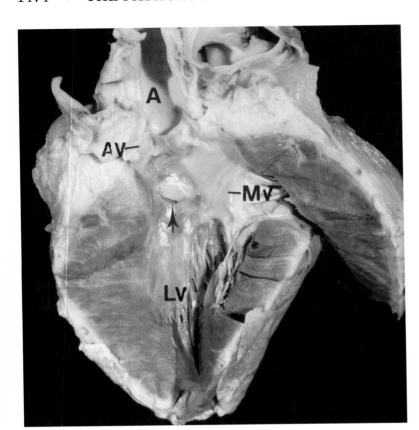

Figure 57: Old surgical closure of ASD, VSD, and repair of infundibular pulmonary stenosis in a case of miliary tuberculosis, tuberculous myocarditis, and epicarditis. Left ventricular view. LV = left ventricle; MV = mitral valve; A = aorta, AV = aortic valve. Arrow points to the surgical closure of the VSD.

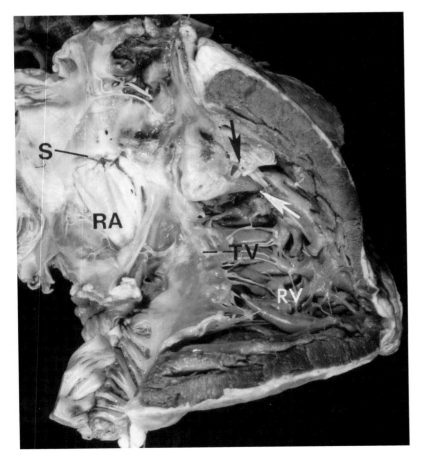

Figure 58: Surgical closure of the outflow tract of the right ventricle into the pulmonary trunk. RA = right atrium; RV = right ventricle; S = surgical sutures in the atrial septum; TV = tricuspid valve. Arrows point to closure of outflow tract to pulmonary trunk.

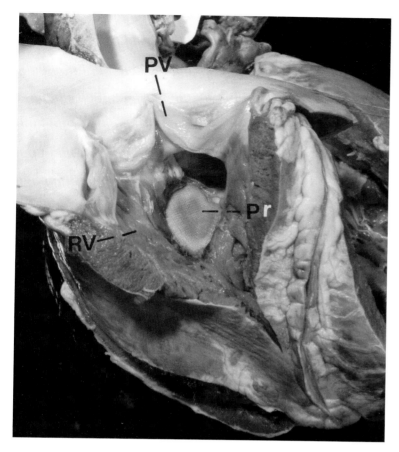

Figure 59: Outflow tract of the right ventricle showing the patch closure. PV = pulmonary valve; Pr = patch closure of the outflow tract; RV = right ventricle.

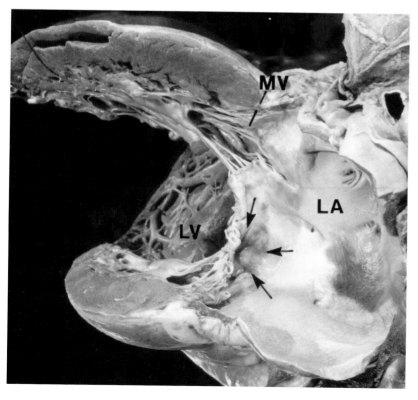

Figure 60: Accessory mitral orifice with mitral insufficiency not diagnosed preoperatively in surgical correction of VSD and patent ductus arteriosus complex. LA = hypertrophied and enlarged left atrium; MV = mitral valve; LV = left ventricle. Arrows point to the accessory mitral orifice with insufficiency.

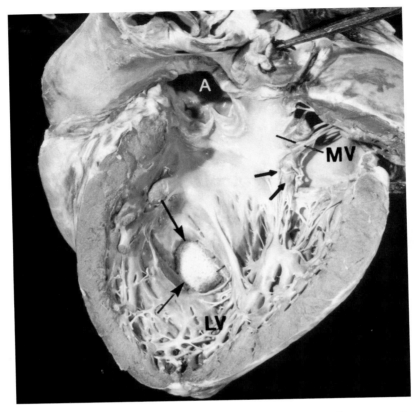

Figure 61: Left ventricular view showing the muscular VSD with surgery. A = aorta; MV = mitral valve; LV = left ventricle. Arrows point to the closure of the defect. Small arrows point to the region of the accessory mitral orifice.

Common AV Orifice (Canal)

Residual atrial and/or ventricular defects are seen after complete correction (Figs. 62, 63). The newly created tricuspid valve in some may be smaller than normal. This may be due to the fact that the valvular tissue on the right side of the common AV leaflet was deficient and the right ventricle was smaller than normal and had resulted in tricuspid stenosis postoperatively. Rarely, the newly created tricuspid valve is quite large, resulting in tricuspid insufficiency (Fig. 62).

In general, in regard to the newly created mitral valve, mitral insufficiency ensues sooner or later. There are multiple factors that produce mitral insufficiency. The mitral component to the AV valve leaflet may have been quite redundant or there might have been an accessory orifice in the mitral component, either in the posterior or the anterior part. In still others, an accessory muscle band may proceed directly to the base of the mitral valve with a poorly developed posterior group of papillary muscles. In others, mitral stenosis had occurred after surgery because of obvious deficiency of valvular tissue (Fig. 63) associated in some with a smaller than normal left ventricle; in addition,

one papillary muscle may be absent or one or both papillary muscles may be hypoplastic.

Subaortic stenosis developed in a few patients postoperatively where there had been no subaortic stenosis preoperatively in cases of ostium primum as well as in common AV canal of the complete or intermediate forms. Postoperatively, the subaortic stenosis develops gradually and becomes hemodynamically significant at a later date. Here again, there are several factors involved in the production of subaortic stenosis in endocardial cushion defects. Fundamentally, the subaortic area in all types of endocardial cushion defect is smaller than a normal outflow tract of the left ventricle. The smallness of the left ventricular outflow tract as such may not produce subaortic stenosis unless it is markedly narrowed. However, insignificant membranous ridges or endocardial tissue not related to the anterior briding leaflet, or excessive endocardial tissue related to the anterior bridging leaflet with or without fibroelastic ridges that are present before surgery proliferates and has a tendency to narrow the outflow tract (Fig. 64). Occasionally, anomalous chordae beneath the aortic valve produced subaortic obstruction. This, we believe, may occur due to the altered mechanism in movement of the anterior leaflet of the mitral valve.

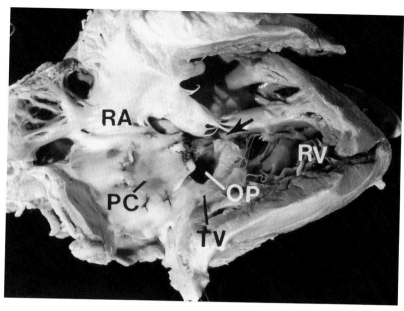

Figure 62: Surgical correction of intermediate type of common AV orifice. Right atrial, right ventricular view. RA = right atrium; RV = right ventricle; TV = tricuspid valve; PC = patch closure of ostium primum defect; OP = residual ostium primum defect.

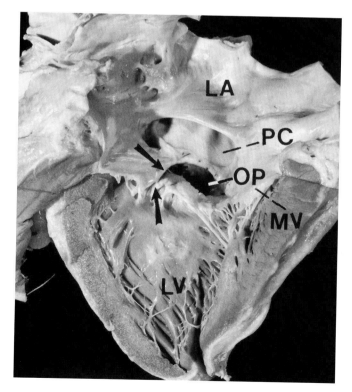

Figure 63: Left atrial, left ventricular view. LA = left atrium; LV = left ventricle; MV = mitral valve; PC = patch closure of ostium primum defect; OP = residual ostium primum defect. Arrows point to the deficiency of the valvular tissue in creating a new mitral valve with mitral stenosis.

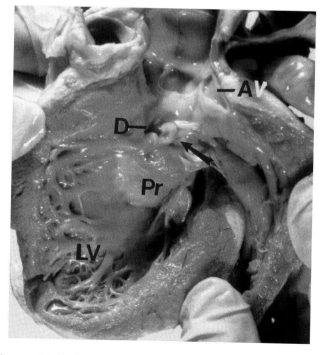

Figure 64: Left ventricular outflow obstruction produced by excess of endocardial tissue beneath the anterior bridging leaflet and residual VSD, in common AV orifice, complete, surgically corrected, old. LV = left ventricle; Pr = patch closure of ventricular component of the defect; AV = aortic valve; D = residual defect. Arrow points to excess of endocardial tissue in the subaortic area.

We hypothesize that the altered movement of the anterior leaflet of the newly created mitral valve produces friction in the subaortic area. This in turn aids in the proliferation of connective tissue in the anatomically narrowed outflow tract of the left ventricle, producing hemodynamically significant obstruction. In other cases, suture material had been present at the base of the anulus of the newly created mitral valve. In still others, anomalous muscle bundles stretched across the left ventricular cavity or the muscle bundles proceeded to the base of the anterior leaflet of the mitral valve, or there may be accessory chordal extensions beneath the aortic valve, producing subaortic stenosis.

Double Outlet Right Ventricle

In subaortic ventricular septal defect, postoperative subaortic obstruction does occur (Fig. 34). This may be due to the fact that the defect in double outlet right ventricle is not as large as that seen in tetralogy of Fallot in many cases. Therefore, this produces a problem for the surgeon in creating the right kind of curve for the patch that will enable the aorta to emerge from the left ventricle without producing subaortic stenosis. In addition, there is usually proliferation of the endocardium at the lower margin of the defect. This may aid in the subaortic obstruction. Likewise, mitral valve anomalies are frequently seen in double outlet right ventricle. The anterior leaflet of the mitral valve may function abnormally with or without anatomic abnormalities, and may compromise the heart postoperatively.

The anatomic abnormalities include a parachute mitral valve, supravalvular ridge formation, or a straddling mitral valve that may have functioned normally prior to surgery but usually functions abnormally following surgery sooner or later. The anterior leaflet of the mitral valve especially may produce subpulmonic obstruction in cases of double outlet right ventricle with subpulmonary ventricular septal defect. Uncommonly, residual pulmonary stenosis and/or insufficiency results following surgery (Figs. 32, 65).

Arterial Switch Operation

In the beginning there was compromise to the coronary arteries that resulted in myocardial infarction. Likewise, in the beginning there were cases with supravalvular pulmonary stenosis or supravalvular aortic stenosis following arterial switch operation. The frequent occurrence of unequal size of pulmonic valve

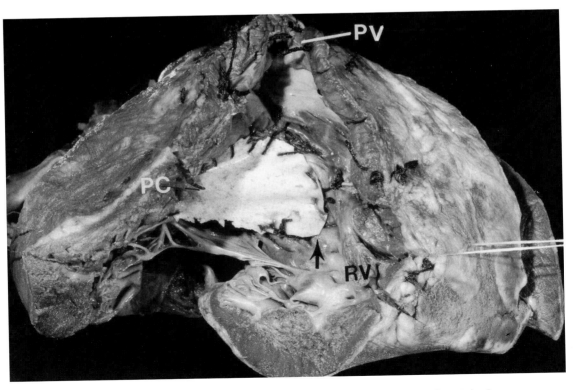

Figure 65: Double outlet right ventricle with doubly committed type of ventricular septal defect with surgical closure of defect with residual pulmonary stenosis. PV = pulmonary valve; RV = right ventricle; PC = patch closure of defect. Arrow points to the patch producing subpulmonary stenosis.

cusps in simple complete transposition may produce aortic valve insufficiency at a later date. Likewise, a straddling parietal band, especially in cases of left-sided Taussig-Bing or subpulmonic ventricular septal defect with marked overriding of the pulmonary trunk may produce subaortic obstruction following arterial switch operation. Likewise, when the arterial switch operation is done for some types of double outlet right ventricle, the straddling mitral valve and/or the cleft-like malformation in the anterior leaflet had produced subaortic obstruction postoperatively.

Corrected Transposition of the Great Arteries

Postoperative AV block occurs frequently in this entity. This is due to the fact that the conduction system is situated anterosuperiorly and along the lateral margins of the ventricular septal defect. The left AV valve abnormality in the form of Ebstein-like malformation is seen frequently in this entity. Although anatomically the valve is abnormally formed, evidently in the presence of a large ventricular septal defect, the

tricuspid stenosis and/or insufficiency were not hemodynamically significant. Following surgical closure of the ventricular septal defect, the insufficiency of the valve became worse in many cases requiring repeat surgery, or occasionally had resulted in sudden death.

The systemic AV valve abnormality has been a cause of death years after surgery. It is our opinion that in practically all cases of corrected transposition, the left AV valve is *anatomically abnormally formed*. However, it is emphasized that most of these valves evidently function normally preoperatively but may fail to function appropriately following surgery. This may indeed also be related to the lack of high technology to detect subtle insufficiency in the presence of a large ventricular septal defect.

Mustard Procedure for Complete Transposition of the Great Arteries

In the early stages we used to find stenosis of the pulmonary veins or stenosis of the superior vena cava and/or the inferior vena cava (Figs. 35–44, 66, 67). In the majority of the cases following longstanding

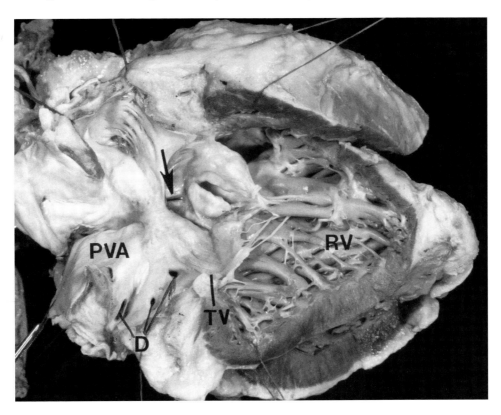

Figure 66: Simple complete transposition, Mustard procedure done a long time ago with residual defect at the entry of the inferior and superior venae cavae and subpulmonary stenosis. Pulmonary venous atrium (right atrium). PVA = pulmonary venous atrium; RV = right ventricle; D = defect; TV = small tricuspid with redundant valve and tricuspid stenosis and tricuspid insufficiency. Arrow points to the defect at entry of the superior vena cava into the left atrium, thus there is straddling of both superior and inferior venae cavae into both atrial chambers.

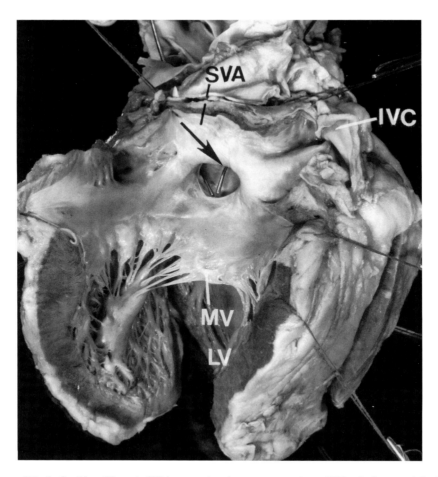

Figure 67: Left side of heart. SVA = systemic venous atrium; LV = left ventricle; MV = mitral valve; IVC = entry of inferior vena cava. Arrow points to entry of probe into the superior vena cava.

surgery, tricuspid insufficiency is present. This is associated with right ventricular dysfunction. In some, as we have already discussed, the tricuspid valve is congenitally abnormally formed.

In others where the valve is normally formed, we believe that the fibroelastosis of the right ventricle which is present in the papillary muscles probably results in functional incompetency of the valve. This may also be due to the effect of the right ventricle due to the altered surgery at the atrial level. The altered geometry of the right ventricle, as such, may cause right ventricular dysfunction in the long run. On the left ventricular side, endocardial ridges beneath the pulmonary valve and/or fibroelastic thickenings usu-

ally progress to form subpulmonary obstruction following Mustard and/or Senning procedures (Fig. 68).

Juxtaposition of the atrial appendages to the left side produced a small systemic venous atrium following the Mustard procedure (Figs. 69–71).

Procedures in the atrium for complete transposition such as atrial septectomy or Blalock-Hanlon done in infancy had resulted in fibroelastosis of the atria, tricuspid insufficiency, atrial arrhythmias, or narrowing of the orifice at the surgical site (Figs. 72–74) and, rarely, had resulted in pericarditis and giant pulmonary arteries (Fig. 75). Likewise, Baffe's procedure had produced diffuse fibroelastosis of the right atrium (Fig. 76) and atrial arrhythmias.

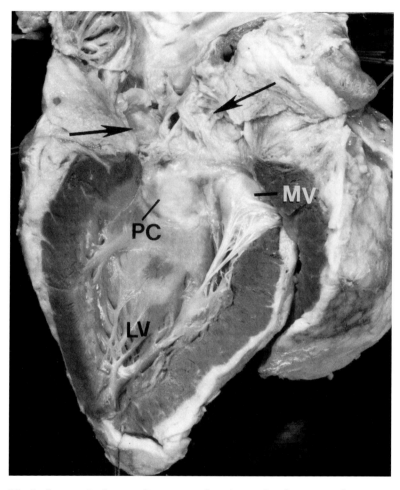

Figure 68: Left ventricular outflow tract showing subpulmonary obstruction (residual) and diffuse fibroelastosis. LV = left ventricle; MV = mitral valve; PC = patch closure of large ventricular septal defect with fibroelastosis. Arrows point to the surgically altered bicuspid valve and subpulmonary stenosis.

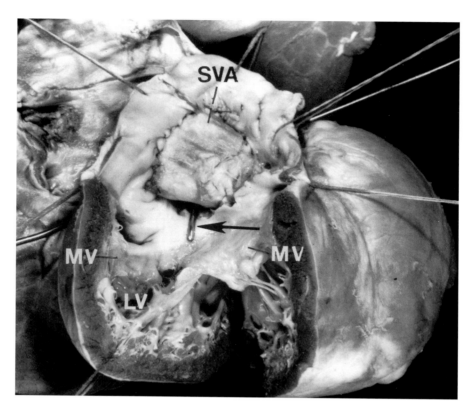

Figure 71: Small left atrium (systemic venous atrium) after Mustard procedure and juxtaposed atrial appendages. SVA = systemic venous atrium; MV = mitral valve; LV = left ventricle with fibroelastosis. Arrow points to the probe passing into the superior vena cava.

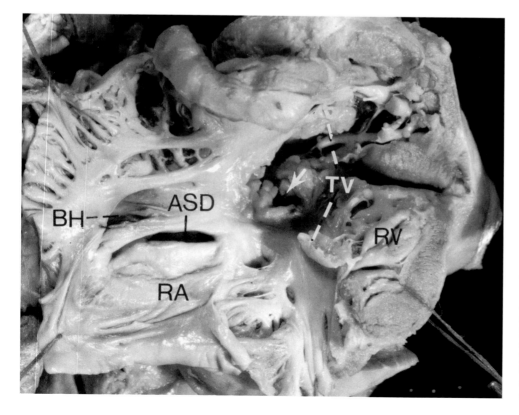

Figure 72: Old Blalock-Hanlon procedure, hypertrophy, and enlargement of the right atrium with diffuse fibroelastosis, dysplastic tricuspid valve, and tricuspid insufficiency. RA = right atrium; ASD = atrial septal defect, fossa ovalis type; BH = Blalock-Hanlon procedure, old; RV = right ventricle; TV = tricuspid valve. Arrow points to the irregular cleft-like malformation with thickened tricuspid valve and tricuspid insufficiency.

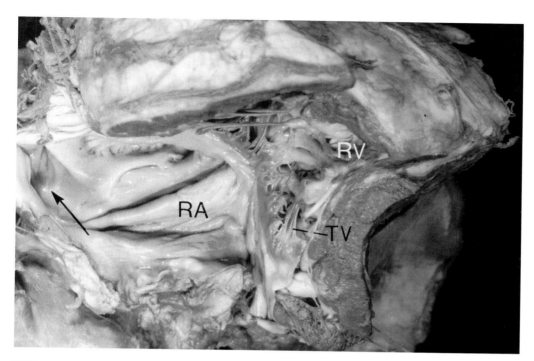

Figure 73: Old Blalock-Hanlon procedure with diffuse fibroelastosis of the right atrium. RA = hypertrophied and enlarged right atrium; RV = right ventricle; TV = tricuspid valve. Arrow points to the area of old Blalock-Hanlon procedure.

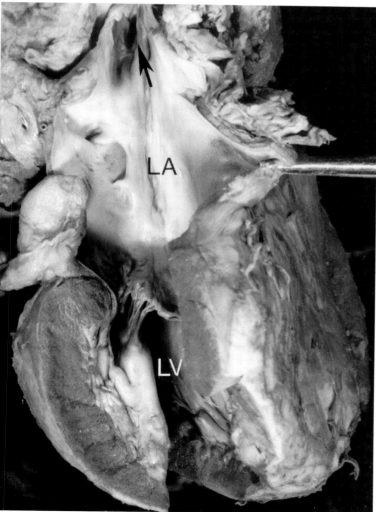

Figure 74: Left atrial, left ventricular view demonstrating the diffuse fibroelastosis of the left atrium. Arrow points to the old Blalock-Hanlon procedure. LA = left atrium; LV = left ventricle.

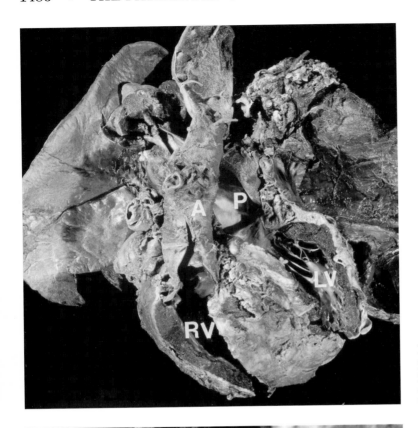

Figure 75: Old atrial septectomy for complete transposition with pericarditis, aneurysmal dilatation of pulmonary trunk, and first-degree AV block. A = aorta; P = giant pulmonary trunk; RV = right ventricle; LV = left ventricle.

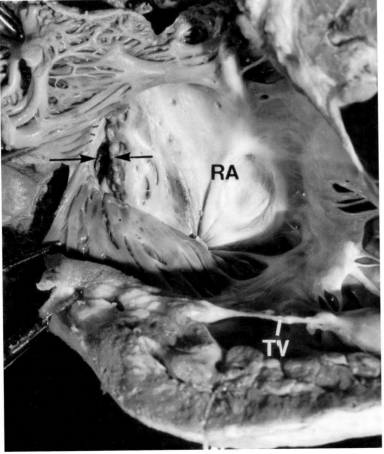

Figure 76: Entry of the pulmonary veins following old Baffe's procedure with diffuse fibroelastosis of the right atrium in complete transposition. RA = hypertrophied and enlarged right atrium with diffuse fibroelastosis; TV = tricuspid valve. Arrows point to entry of the right pulmonary veins into the right atrium.

Fontan Type of Procedures

In general, in longstanding cases following Fontan procedures and/or the modifications thereof, there is cardiomegaly in autopsied hearts. There is immense left atrial and left ventricular hypertrophy and enlargement in cases of tricuspid atresia hearts, and left atrial hypertrophy and enlargement with hypertrophy and enlargement of the main ventricular chamber in single ventricle hearts, thereby giving anatomic evidence of significant mitral valve and/or the left AV valve insufficiency, clinically. There is also significant right atrial hypertrophy and enlargement.

The atrial arrhythmias that frequently occur in longstanding cases are probably related to the hypertrophy and enlargement of both atria that were present before surgery as well as to the presence of chronic inflammatory cells, fibrosis, fat, and disruption of atrial myocardium that occurred following surgery. To this is added the significant insufficiency of the mitral and/or the left AV valve that is usually seen in most cases. The above pathological findings, especially in the atrial preferential pathways, the approaches to the SA and the AV nodes, and injury that sometime occurs to the SA node itself during the Fontan procedure may form a milieu for abnormal automaticity, fractionization of an impulse, or a reentry mechanism that might be responsible for the various types of supraventricular tachycardias or bradyarrhythmias.

It is emphasized that the function of the left AV valve or the mitral valve is probably altered hemodynamically due to the alteration in the geometry of the left ventricle and/or the single ventricular mass following the Fontan procedure.

Efforts should be taken to study the function of an altered AV valve following cardiac surgery and its relationship to the growth of the ventricular myocardium at the molecular-genetic level. Likewise, future research should be directed to study the effects of surgery on the growing altered atrial myocardium and its reaction to altered hemodynamics following cardiac surgery.

Hancock Prosthetic Conduits with Porcine Valves and Homograft Valves

These valves are used for the repair of pulmonary atresia with ventricular septal defect, tetralogy of Fallot, and selected cases of transposition of the great arteries with pulmonary stenosis. There is tremendous calcification in the prosthesis as well as in the porcine valve, and homograft valves resulting in marked stenosis, insufficiency, or both with cardiomegaly (Figs. 26–30).

Likewise, a pericardial patch appears to be susceptible to calcification than other material used for closure of defects or in enlargement of the outflow tract of the right ventricle or both. Calcification does occur following Dacron patch closure or any other type of material used for closure of a defect, either in closure of the defect for tetralogy of Fallot, ventricular septal defect, or double outlet right ventricle.

Any type of a prosthetic valve used at the aortic or mitral valve locations, or both, especially in relatively young children, produces stenosis as a result of calcification (tissue valves), and is prone to infective endocarditis.

Norwood Type of Procedures

Here again, the autopsied hearts are immensely hypertrophied and enlarged with diffuse fibroelastosis of the endocardium following the first stage of the Norwood procedure with sudden death. The tricuspid orifice is enlarged with increased hemodynamic change and hypoplastic anterolateral papillary muscle. The tricuspid valve is unable to function for a systemic chamber. There probably are multiple factors for tricuspid insufficiency and right ventricular dysfunction following this type of a procedure. It is very likely that the genes that are responsible for the development and function of the tricuspid valve and the right ventricle are considerably altered. It is conceivable that the specificity of these genes is predetermined for the appropriate development and function of these structures, and any alteration that may occur at a later date may result in malfunction.

Future work in these areas at the molecular-genetic level will certainly help us in understanding the functional capabilities of the tricuspid valve and the right ventricle during altered hemodynamics.

Homograft conduits likewise result in thickening and calcification over the course of time (Fig. 77).

Hemorrhage in the Operative Site

Although some amount of hemorrhage is expected near the surgical site, a considerable amount of hemorrhage in the vital parts of the conduction system may produce AV block or arrhythmias postoperatively (Figs. 78–82).

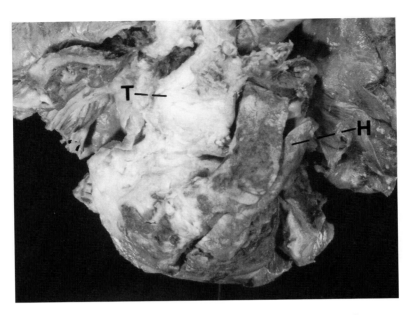

Figure 77: External view of the heart after total surgical correction of truncus arteriosus. T = truncus converted into aorta; H = homograft conduit from the right ventricle to pulmonary arteries with calcification.

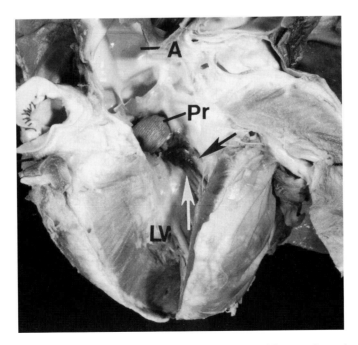

Figure 78: Marked hypertrophy of the left ventricle and hemorrhage in the region of the bundle of His and the left bundle branch with AV block. A = aorta; LV = left ventricle; Pr = patch closure of the defect. Arrows point to the hemorrhage. Note the tremendous left ventricular hypertrophy. Arrow points to area of course of the left bundle branch.

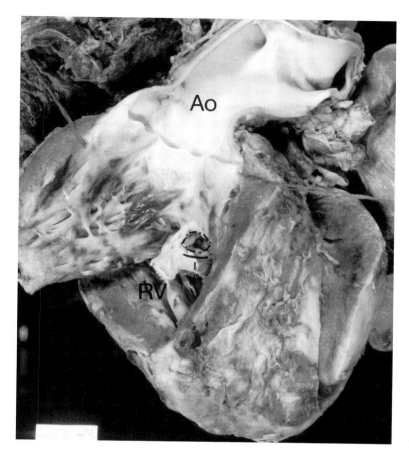

Figure 79: AV block following Mustard procedure and tricuspid stenosis, outflow tract of right ventricle with hemorrhage. RV = right ventricle; Ao = aorta. Dashed and dotted lines depict surgical closure of ventricular septal defect, hemorrhage, and AV block.

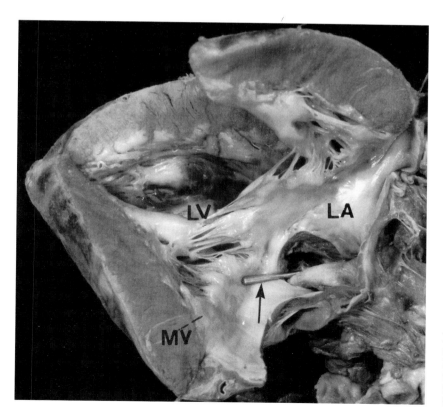

Figure 80: Left atrial, left ventricular view showing hemorrhage in the left ventricle. LA = left atrium; MV = mitral valve; LV = left ventricle. Arrow points to probe passing through the superior vena cava. Note the hemorrhage (dark area) in the left ventricle.

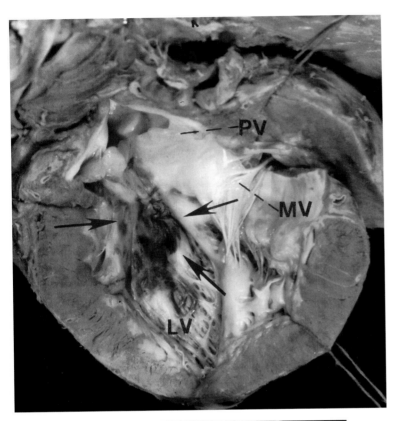

Figure 81: Outflow tract of left ventricle following Mustard procedure with surgical closure of the ventricular septal defect, marked hemorrhage throughout the region of the His bundle and left bundle branch, and complete AV block. PV = pulmonary valve; MV = mitral valve; LV = left ventricle. Arrows point to the hemorrhage.

Interventional Procedures

Interventional procedures of any type may unfortunately tear the valves or, rarely, perforate the myocardium (Fig. 83).

Summary

The long-term effects of cardiac surgery in congenital heart disease are yet to be defined. Today we know that the size of the heart may not return to normal size for months or years after surgery in some. Indeed, cardiomegaly is present in practically all *autopsied postoperative* congenital hearts. Whether this is due to changes related to surgery in the endocardium, myocardium, conduction system, or coronary arteries or due to residual valvular abnormalities, singly or in combination, remains to be determined. On the other hand, the cardiomegaly may indeed be the end result of a previously hypertrophied heart due to altered hemodynamics (Figs. 84–91), or a combination of any of the above.

It is conceivable that a markedly hypertrophied myocardium may react differently to cardiac surgery than a mild to moderately hypertrophied myocardium. The altered geometry of a ventricular mass following cardiac surgery may respond differently to altered hemodynamics.

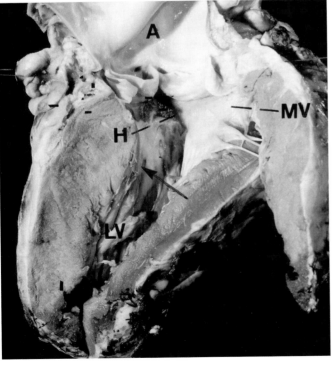

Figure 82: Hypertrophic cardiomyopathy with surgical intervention followed by hemorrhage in the region of the His bundle and left bundle branch with AV block. MV = mitral valve; A = aorta; LV = left ventricle; H = hemorrhage in His bundle and beginning of main left bundle branch. Arrow points to hypertrophied ventricular septum.

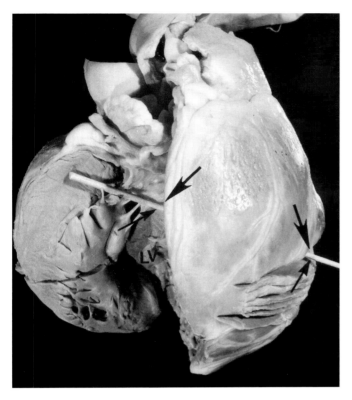

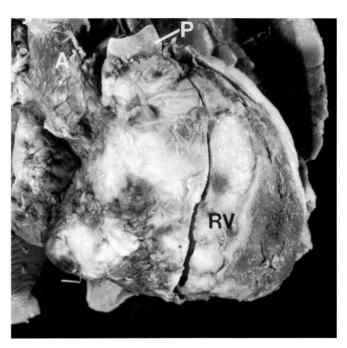

Figure 84: Closure of atrial and ventricular septal defects in a child with immense cardiomegaly. External view of the heart. RV = right ventricle; P = pulmonary trunk; A = aorta.

Figure 83: Catheter perforation of the left ventricle. LV = left ventricle. Arrows point to the probe passing through the perforation created by the catheter.

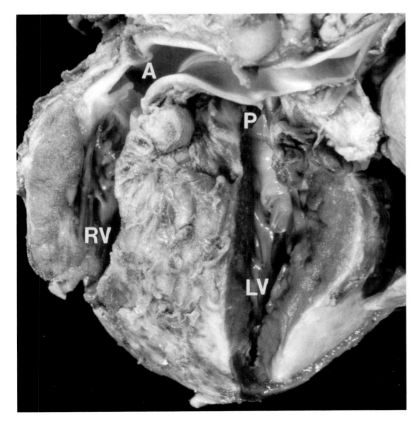

Figure 85: Complete transposition with Mustard procedure and postoperative heart block in a child. External view of the heart showing cardiomegaly. RV = right ventricle; LV = left ventricle; A = aorta; P = pulmonary trunk.

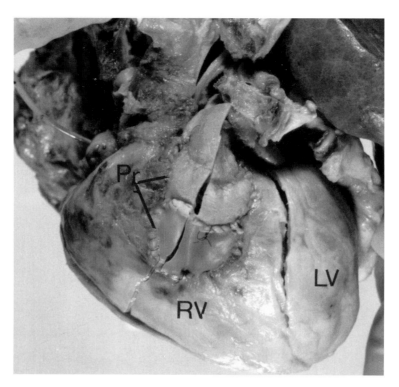

Figure 86: External view of the heart after total surgical correction in double outlet right ventricle, doubly committed type of defect, common AV orifice, and cardiomegaly in an infant. RV = right ventricle; LV = left ventricle; Pr = prosthesis extension from outflow tract of the right ventricle into the pulmonary trunk with pulmonary stenosis.

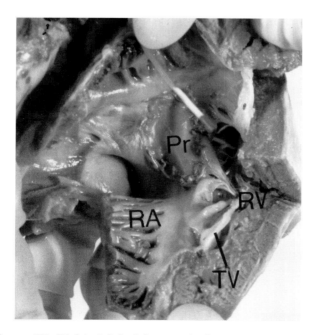

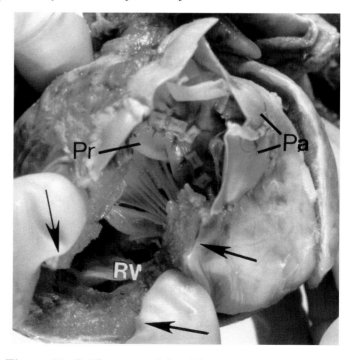

Figure 87: Right atrial, right ventricular view. TV = newly created tricuspid valve with stenosis; Pr = prosthetic closure of common AV orifice; RV = right ventricle, hypertrophied; RA = right atrium.

Figure 88: Outflow tract of the right ventricle showing prosthetic patch extending close to the base of the pulmonary trunk, and tremendous right ventricular hypertrophy. RV = right ventricle, markedly hypertrophied; Pa = patch enlargement of the outflow tract; Pr = prosthetic closure of defect. Arrows point to right ventricular hypertrophy.

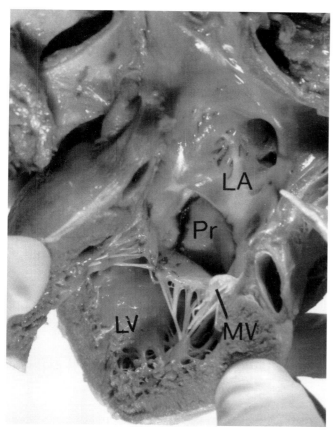

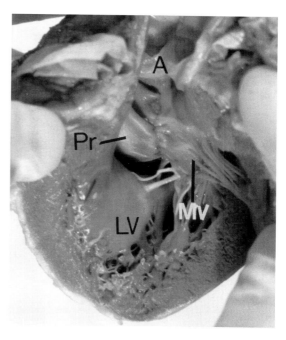

Figure 90: Outflow tract of the left ventricle. Aorta now emerging completely from this chamber with left ventricular hypertrophy and enlargement. MV = newly created mitral valve; LV = left ventricle, hypertrophied and enlarged; Pr = patch closure of common AV orifice defect; A = aorta.

Figure 89: Left atrial, left ventricular view showing the newly created mitral valve. LA = hypertrophied and enlarged left atrium; Pr = patch closure of common AV orifice; LV = left ventricle; MV = newly created mitral valve.

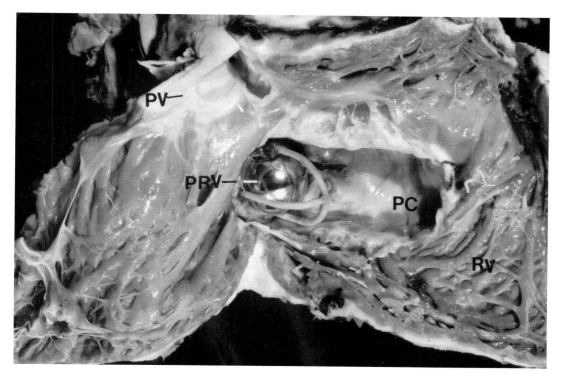

Figure 91: Prosthetic valve replacement in Ebstein's malformation of the tricuspid valve with huge right ventricle and cardiomegaly. PV = pulmonary valve; RV = markedly enlarged right ventricle; PRV = prosthetic valve; PC = proximal atrialized portion of right ventricle.

The Role of Fibroelastosis Due to Blocked Lymph Drainage

The ubiquitous finding of fibroelastosis not only in the chamber that the surgeon operated but also in other chambers in many cases after old surgical intervention raises the question of whether the lymphatics are disturbed and obstructed during cardiac surgery, at least in part. The production of fibroelastosis following surgery may not be an innocuous phenomenon. It may be the reason for cardiomegaly and may be responsible for the delay in the heart's return to normal size following cardiac surgery. In some, the condition may result in sudden death. Every effort should be undertaken to avoid the lymphatic channels during surgical procedures.

The Role of Ventricular Patch

The presence of a patch in the wall of the right ventricle may in some susceptible cases facilitate an aneurysm formation. This may in turn form a nidus for an arrhythmic event.

The Effect on the Conduction System

Damage to the conduction system in ventriculotomy may cause long-lasting results. Right bundle branch block with left axis deviation is an especially vulnerable condition. As aging occurs, over the course of time further fibrosis of the bundle branches, bifurcating bundle, and bundle proximal to it may result in complete heart block years after surgical correction (Figs. 92–94). This may be yet another factor responsible for sudden death in some.

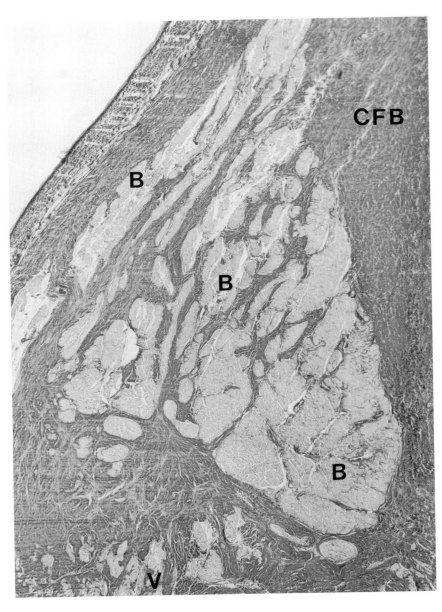

Figure 92: Sudden death in a 16-year-old boy 9 years after closure of ASD and VSD. ECG normal sinus rhythm before surgery, right bundle branch block after surgery, and much later atrial fibrillation with a ventricular rate of 70–80 beats per minute. Photomicrograph fragmented penetrating bundle. Weigert-van Gieson stain ×30. B = penetrating bundle; V = ventricular septum; CFB = thickened central fibrous body.

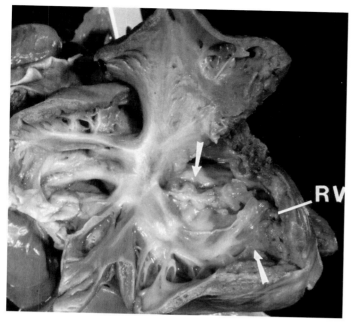

Figure 7: Ebstein's anomaly of the heart in a 3-day-old female infant with preexcitation, cardiomegaly, and sudden death. Right atrial, right ventricular view. RV = right ventricle. Arrows point to the downward displacement and plastering of the septal and inferior leaflets of the tricuspid valve with redundant valvular tissue.

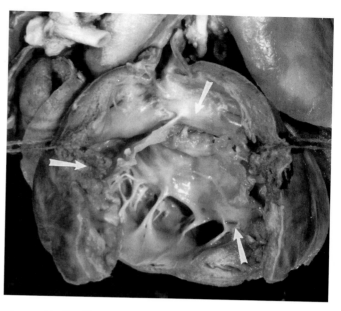

Figure 8: Outflow tract of the right ventricle demonstrating the Ebstein's anomaly of the tricuspid valve extending up to the base of the lower septal band and muscle of Lancisi. Note the immense cardiomegaly. Arrows point to the Ebstein's malformation of the tricuspid valve.

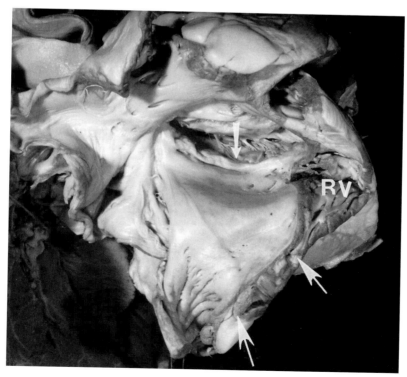

Figure 9: Ebstein's anomaly with pulmonary stenosis and insufficiency in a 35-year-old female with preexcitation and sudden death. Right atrial, right ventricular view. RV = right ventricle. Arrows point to the marked displacement of the combined septal and inferior leaflets with plastering into the inlet or the sinus of the right ventricle.

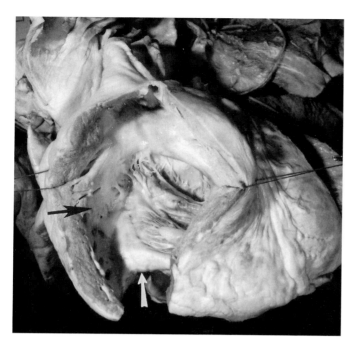

Figure 10: Outflow tract of the right ventricle demonstrating the anomalous connections of the tricuspid valve. Note the marked right ventricular hypertrophy. Arrows point to the tricuspid valve.

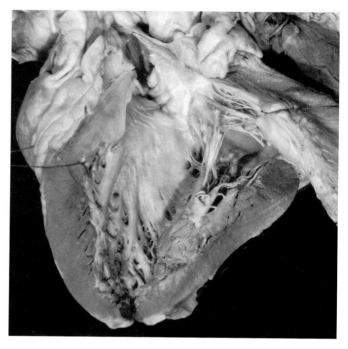

Figure 12: Outflow tract to the left ventricle. Note the diffuse fibroelastosis and anomalous muscle bands from the apex up to the mid-part.

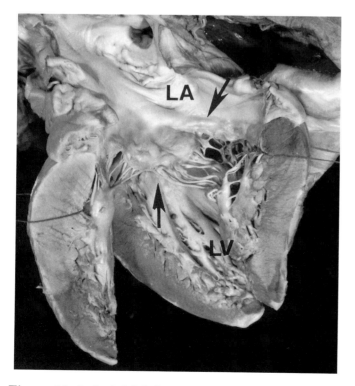

Figure 11: Left atrial, left ventricular view demonstrating redundancy of the mitral valve. LA = left atrium; LV = left ventricle. Arrows point to the redundant anterior leaflet of the mitral valve.

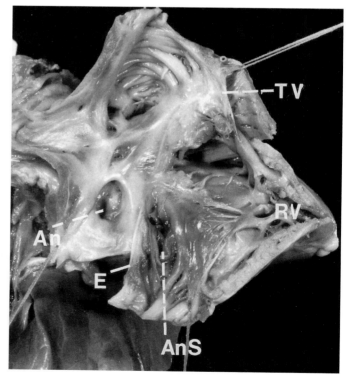

Figure 13: Paroxysmal supraventricular tachycardia in a 5-month-old male child. Cardiomegaly and sudden death. Right-sided view. An = aneurysm of the fossa ovalis; E = enlarged eustachian valve; AnS = aneurysm of space of His; RV = right ventricle; TV = tricuspid valve. Note that the coronary sinus is displaced close to the central fibrous body.

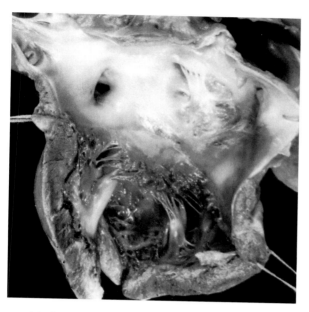

Figure 14: Left side of the heart demonstrating the huge left atrium with fibroelastosis of the left ventricle and the left atrium.

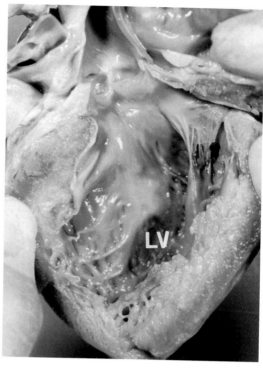

Figure 15: Left ventricular hypertrophy and enlargement with fibroelastosis in a child with paroxysmal supraventricular tachycardia and sudden death. LV = left ventricle.

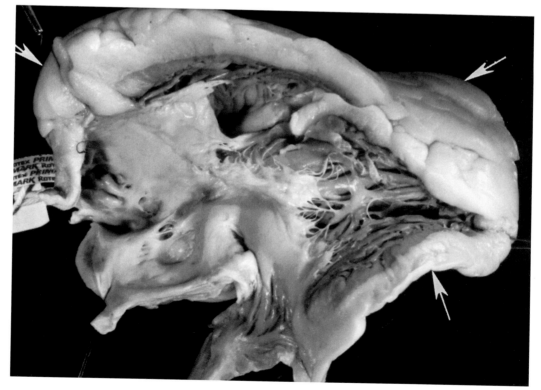

Figure 16: Marked adiposity of the heart in a 41-year-old female, with preexcitation, paroxysmal tachycardia, and sudden death. Right atrial, right ventricular view. Arrows point to marked fatty infiltration throughout the epicardium.

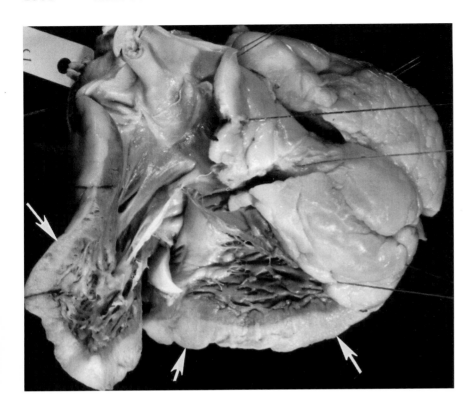

Figure 17: Right ventricular outflow tract view. Arrows point to tremendous fatty infiltration and fat replacing the anterior wall from mid-third to the apex.

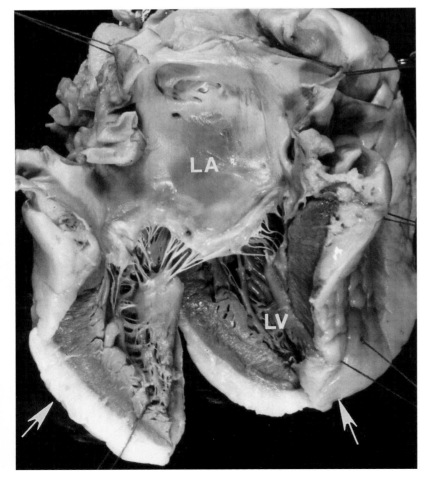

Figure 18: Left atrial, left ventricular view showing the marked fatty infiltration in the epicardium extending to the myocardium. LA = left atrium; LV = left ventricle. Arrows point to fatty infiltration.

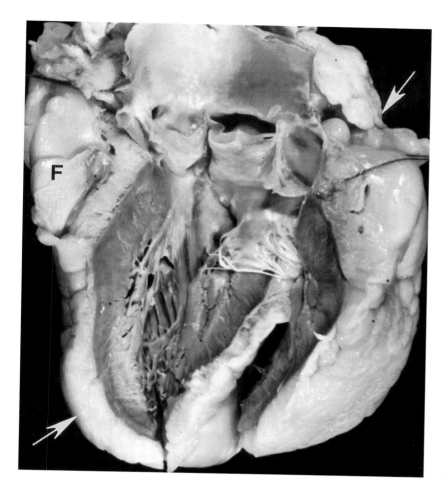

Figure 19: Outflow tract to the left ventricle. F = fat. Arrows point to marked fatty infiltration. Note the fenestrated aortic valve and the high origin of the right coronary ostium.

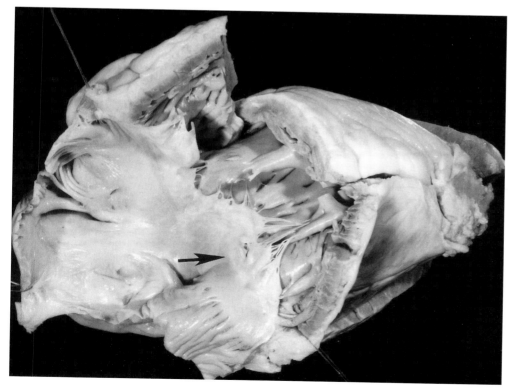

Figure 20: Coronary artery disease (three-vessel disease) in a 72-year-old male with old myocardial infarctions, preexcitation, ventricular tachycardia, and sudden death. Right side of the heart. Arrow points to the accessory tricuspid orifice.

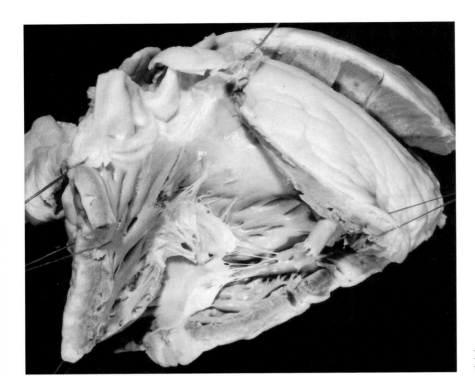

Figure 21: Outflow tract of the right ventricle showing the ventricular septal bulge.

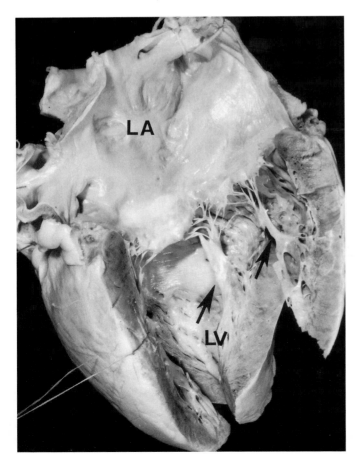

Figure 22: Left atrial, left ventricular view demonstrating fibrotic papillary muscles, old scars in the ventricular myocardium, and mitral insufficiency. LA = left atrium; LV = left ventricle. Arrows point to fibrotic papillary muscles.

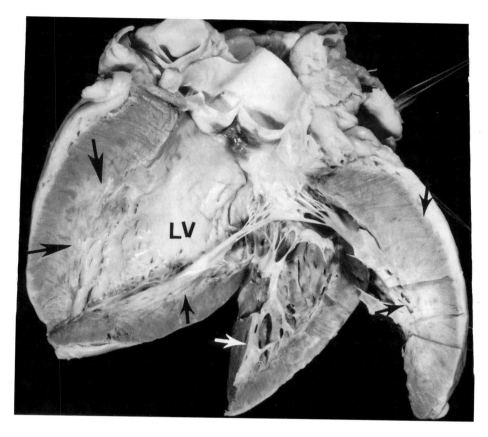

Figure 23: Left ventricle demonstrating old myocardial infarction in the anteroseptal and lateral walls with fibrosis of the papillary muscles. LV = left ventricle. Arrows point to old infarction and fibrosis of the papillary muscles.

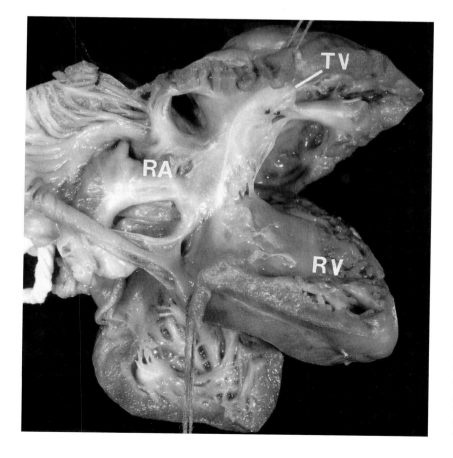

Figure 24: Familial paroxysmal atrial tachycardia with block (first degree, second degree, third degree AV block) in a 6-year-old female who died suddenly. Three other boys died of similar findings. Right side of the heart. Note the immense cardiomegaly. RA = Right atrium; RV = Right ventricle; TV = Tricuspid valve with markedly abbreviated chordae.

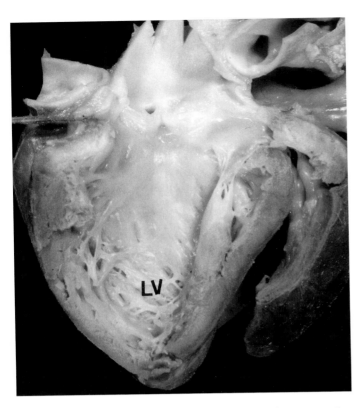

Figure 25: Left ventricular outflow tract demonstrating marked hypertrophy and enlargement of the left ventricle with diffuse fibroelastosis. LV = left ventricle.

5. Redundant tricuspid valve with hypoplastic anterolateral papillary muscle
6. Enlarged eustachian valve (Fig. 13)
7. Aneurysm of space of His (Fig. 13).

These areas are closely associated with the AV node, AV bundle, and the beginning of the bundle branches. Anomalies in these areas may therefore affect the conduction system. For example, a displaced coronary sinus close to the central fibrous body or a huge coronary sinus receiving a large left superior vena cava may alter the approaches to the AV node, and the AV node (Fig. 26). The AV node may then be entrapped within the central fibrous body and may give rise to intractable junctional tachycardia. Purkinje tumors of the heart may also give rise to intractable atrial and ventricular arrhythmias.

The occurrence of arrhythmias in individual congenital cardiac anomalies has already been discussed. Briefly, congenital AV block has a tendency to occur in mixed levocardia with ventricular *inversion* (corrected transposition of the heart). There is a distinct tendency for congenital AV block to occur in mesocardia, dextrocardia, and isolated levocardia, especially with polysplenia. Likewise, there is a tendency for preexci-

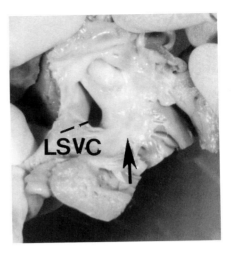

Figure 26: Ten-week-old female child with a huge coronary sinus receiving a large left superior vena cava. LSVC = left superior vena cava. Arrow points to the area of the AV node.

tation to occur with Ebstein's anomaly with or without ventricular inversion (Figs. 7–12). However, it is emphasized that congenital AV block or preexcitation can occur in any type of a congenital cardiac anomaly. There is an association of maternal lupus with AV block in infants. This most likely is related to the maternal immune complexes affecting the fetus. In the majority, however, the AV nodal area is affected and rarely the distal bundle branches. The preferential involvement of the proximal conduction system may at least in part be related to the lymphatic drainage of the heart. This area deserves further research.

The conduction system in various types of congenital cardiac anomalies and its significance in cardiac surgery has been previously published. The interested reader is encouraged to read *Cardiac Surgery and the Conduction System*, revised second edition.

Likewise, the reader can obtain the details of the conduction system findings in sudden death from the book *The Cardiac Conduction System in Unexplained Sudden Death*. The interested reader is also encouraged to read our prior work in the conduction system with various arrhythmias, with or without varying diseases (congenital and acquired).

As observed from our material, the most frequently seen congenital cardiac anomalies with sudden death in the young, especially those who are clinically considered "normal and healthy" are:

1. Coronary artery anomalies (Figs. 27–29)
2. Floppy mitral valve (Figs. 30–38)
3. Hypertrophic cardiomyopathy and its variants (Figs. 39–43)
4. Uhl's anomaly and its variants (Figs. 44–47)

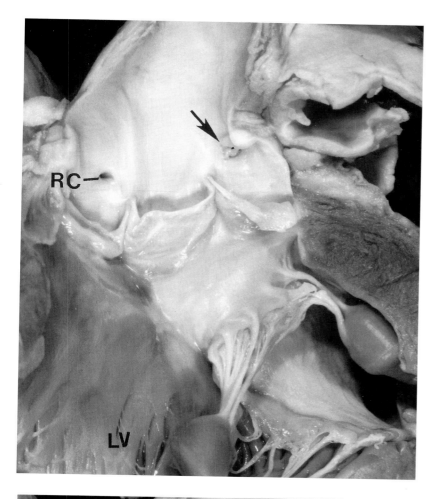

Figure 27: Irregular fold at the mouth of the left coronary artery in a 6-year-old male child who died suddenly. LV = left ventricle; RC = high origin of the right coronary. Arrow points to the fold obstructing the main left coronary ostium.

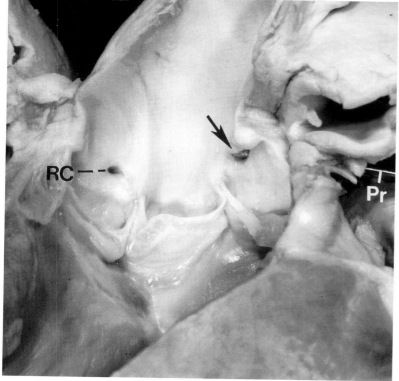

Figure 28: A probe is passing through the left main coronary ostium lifting the fold. RC = right coronary artery; Pr = probe passing through the left coronary artery. Arrow points to the fold lifted by the probe.

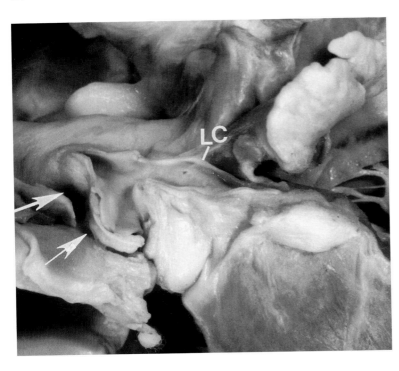

Figure 29: Dilatation of the left main coronary and the left circumflex coronary arteries. LC = left circumflex coronary artery. The two arrows point to the aneurysmal dilatation or poststenotic dilatation of the beginning of the left main and the anterior descending coronary arteries.

On the other hand, tumors of the heart and muscular dystrophy may manifest clinically in the form of varying types of arrhythmias in the young (Fig. 48).

We will therefore discuss those anomalies that are usually or presumably "silent" in nature and sudden death may be the first manifestation of the disease.

Coronary Artery Anomalies Causing Sudden Death

There was a total of 28 cases. Twenty one were male subjects and seven were female subjects.

The heart was normal in size only in four. All others showed varying degrees of hypertrophy of the cardiac chambers and focal scars in the left ventricle. The youngest, a 34 hours, 35 weeks' gestation infant, showed mild hypertrophy and enlargement of the heart.

Left Coronary Artery (L) Emerging from the Right Sinus (R) and Proceeding Between the Aorta and Pulmonary Trunk

There was a total of eight cases. Five were females and three males.

Small left superior vena cava entering coronary sinus, cardiomegaly, pulmonary emboli	female, 47 yr
L from R with small L – heart normal size	female, 15 yr
L from R cardiomegaly Aneurysm at base of ascending aorta	female, 7 yr
L from R sinus, small R coronary artery, cardiomegaly	male, 2 mo
L from R, – heart normal size	female, 7 yr
Cardiomegaly	male, 16 yr
Coronary sinus entering left atrium, heart normal size	female, 23 yr
Cardiomegaly with scars in left ventricle	male, 11 yr

Left Coronary Artery Close to Right Cusp (Junction of Left and Right)

Cardiomegaly	male, 1½ mo
History of bronchial asthma, cardiomegaly	male, 17 yr
Cardiomegaly, spontaneously closed small VSD, history	male, 11 yr

Left Coronary Above Posterior Cusp at Its Junction with the Left Cusp

Cardiomegaly	male, 14 yr

Anomalous Fold above Left Coronary Artery (Figs. 27–29)

Dominant left circulation, heart normal size   male, 6 yr

Single Left Coronary Artery

Hypertrophy and enlarged heart, my-ocarditis   female, 11 yr

Dominant Right and Hypoplasia of Left Coronary Artery and Narrowing of Both Coronary Arteries

Cardiomegaly, ventricular fibrillation   female, 44 yr

Dominant Right and Intramyocardial Left Anterior Descending Artery

Cardiomegaly and fibroelastosis of the left ventricle   male, 20 yr

Intramyocardial Left Anterior Descending Artery

Cardiomegaly   male, 14 yr

Hypoplastic Left Coronary Artery

Cardiomegaly, fibroelastosis   male, 5 mo

Right Coronary Artery (R) from Left (L) and Coursing between Aorta and Pulmonary Trunk

High origin of R from L with dominant L circulation, hypertrophy and en-largement of all chambers   male, 35 yr

Mild cardiomegaly   male, 34 hr, 35 weeks' gestation

Small Right Coronary Artery

Hypertrophy and enlarged right atrium and right ventricle, mild   male, 18 yr

Minute right coronary artery with thickening around coronary artery, left atrial, and ventricular hypertro-phy and enlargement, mild, huge

LSVC entering coronary sinus, re-dundant tricuspid valve and tricus-pid insufficiency, right ventricular hypertrophy and enlargement, large membranous part of atrioventricular septum   male, 35 yr

Single Right Coronary Artery

Single right and left coronary artery proceeding between aorta and pul-monary trunk, history of bronchial asthma, hypertrophic cardiomyopa-thy   male, 16 yr

Right Coronary Ostium Near Posterior Sinus

Cardiomegaly   male, 1 yr

Extra Coronary Artery from Pulmonary

Anomalous coronary artery from the pulmonary trunk forming vascular plexus at base of the pulmonary valve and anastomosis with right and left coronary arteries, in part in-tramyocardial LAD coronary artery, cardiomegaly with fibroelastosis   male, 20 yr

One large (main) coronary artery from the pul-monary trunk and a small coronary artery from the left aortic cusp. The larger one giving rise to the left ante-rior descending and the left circumflex coronary arter-ies. The main left coronary artery and the small left coronary artery joined together. Cardiomegaly.

Both Coronary Ostia near Posterior Cusp

Mild cardiomegaly   male, 25 yr

Right and left ventricular hypertrophy   male, 4 yr

Comment

It is thus clear that there are varieties of anomalies in coronary artery distribution that might produce chronic ischemic episodes that may remain silent, asymptomatic, or may produce arrhythmias, anginal pains, or syncopal episodes.

Sudden death was the common dominator in all, and as mentioned earlier, the heart was hypertrophied and enlarged in 24 out of 28 and in four it was normal,

• *THE PATHOLOGY OF CONGENITAL HEART DISEASE*

with varying amounts of fibrosis, fibroelastosis, or focal scars, especially in the left ventricle indicating previous ischemic episodes.

It is well known that scar tissue as such may slow the propagation of an impulse, especially at the junctional areas between the scar and the healthy myocardium. These areas may therefore form a milieu for an arrhythmic event to occur that may degenerate into ventricular tachycardia, fibrillation, and sudden death, especially during an altered physiological state.

It is of interest that practically all of these youngsters are athletically minded, suggesting an elevated level of catecholamines or some other unknown factors due to chronic and/or intermittent ischemia to the ventricular myocardium.

This particular entity certainly deserves further research in the coming century.

Floppy Mitral Valve

In this entity, the leaflets of the mitral valve are quite large, redundant, and ballooned out (Figs. 30, 31).

In general, the anulus of the mitral orifice is enlarged and although there is a tendency for redundancy of the leaflet to occur or involve the posterior leaflet more so than the anterior, it is not uncommon to find marked redundancy of both leaflets from the anulus to the edge as well as from commissure to commissure. In some, only the posterior leaflet may be involved. In others, part of the posterior and part of the anterior leaflet may be involved. The posterior leaflet may be divided off into several segments and there may be associated calcification on the undersurface of the posterior leaflet in an irregular fashion that may elevate the mitral leaflet closer to the atrial side. The chordae, in general, are elongated with anomalous chordal extensions. The papillary muscles may show fibrosis. In some, there were anomalous papillary muscles proceeding to the base of the valve.

In some, the chordae may not be elongated. It may be relatively abbreviated but thickened with several anomalous papillary muscles to the posterior leaflet. Floppy mitral valve, when associated with an enlarged anulus, usually results in hemodynamically significant

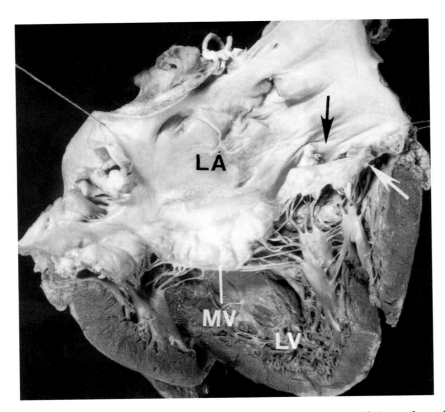

Figure 30: Floppy mitral valve. Left atrial, left ventricular view with irregular calcification of the posterior leaflet. This was a 44-year-old physician who died suddenly. LA = left atrium; LV = left ventricle; MV = mitral valve. Arrows point to the irregular calcification of the posterior leaflet. Note that the floppy mitral valve extends throughout the valve with enlarged anulus, fibrosis of the papillary muscles with tremendous enlargement of the left atrium and left ventricle.

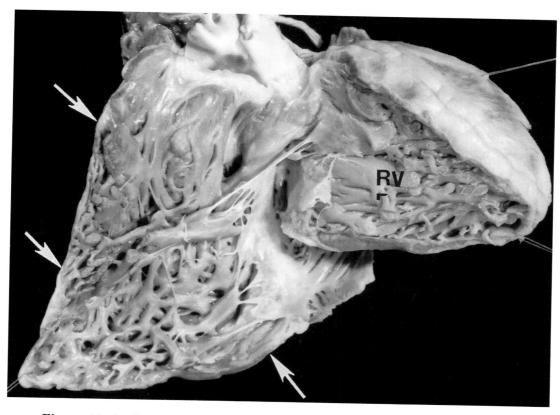

Figure 46: Outflow tract of the right ventricle demonstrating the practical absence of the myocardium in the anterior wall. RV = right ventricle. Arrows point to fatty infiltration. Note also the focal fibrotic scars in the right ventricle.

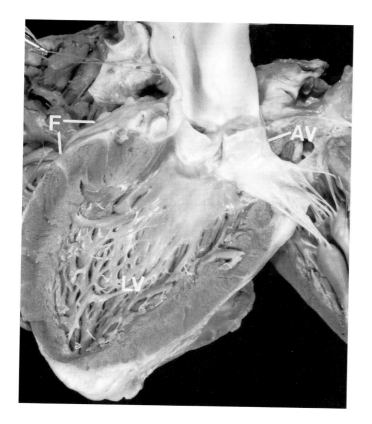

Figure 47: Outflow tract of the left ventricle demonstrating fat in the epicardium as well fatty streaks entering the myocardium. LV = left ventricle; AV = aneurysm of the sinus of Valsalva of the aortic valve; F = fat.

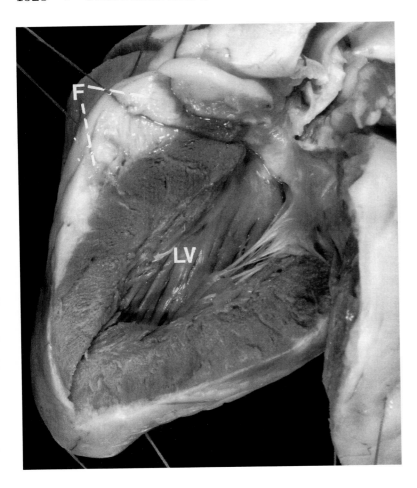

Figure 48: Muscular dystrophy in a teenager with AV dissociation, atypical delta waves, short PR interval, and abnormal intraventricular conduction. Left ventricular view. LV = left ventricle; F = fat. Note the left ventricular hypertrophy with fatty infiltration in the epicardium.

have to be developed to diagnose these anomalies. It is conceivable that patients may have atypical symptoms and these symptoms have obviously been neglected by either the patient and/or the family and/or the physicians. One should therefore be careful in evaluating these atypical symptoms, if any.

It is our opinion that at least in the majority, there *are clues* given by the patient and unfortunately, however, we are not able to appreciate them in our current knowledge. If and when we discover or develop new methodologies to uncover these anomalies and are able to diagnosis them accurately, we may then think in terms of how we could treat the anomalies and/or prevent them, if at all possible. The question of how we are going to prevent sudden death in the young will be a challenge for the coming century.

94

Congenital Cardiac Malformations Related to Cocaine and/or Other Drug Addiction in the Mother

There was a total of 13 infants born to cocaine-addicted mothers; 12 were black and one was Hispanic. In some, there was a history of use of other drugs and/or cigarettes and alcohol. Ten were male infants and three were female infants, with a median age of 3 months, 6 days.

Since this is an important socioeconomic issue, all cases are listed below:

90-minute-old male (44-weeks' gestation)

Common atrium, common atrioventricular orifice (CAVO), paraductal coarctation, patent ductus arteriosus (PDA), and multiple extracardiac anomalies. Small left pulmonary artery. Accessory orifice in mitral component of CAVO with possible insufficiency. Bicuspid AV with possible stenosis. Small pulmonary veins on the right with hypoplastic pulmonary veins on the left.

6-month-old male (36-weeks' gestation)

Dextrocardia, dextroversion, asplenia with partial visceral heterotaxy. Complete transposition, CAVO, pulmonary atresia, large ASD, fossa ovalis defect (FOD), proximal type. Right aortic arch (RAA) right PDA, LSVC, CS and IVC → LA. Both atrial appendages resembling left. Incomplete lobation of both lungs.

1-hour-old male (28-weeks' gestation)

Premature closure of foramen ovale with aneurysm of fossa ovalis, VSD, CAVO type. Overriding aorta and coarctation. Bicuspid pulmonary valve (PV) with PDA, blood cysts in all the valves. High origin of both coronaries. Hypertrophy and enlargement of the heart. Trisomy 13–15 with multiple congenital anomalies.

5-month-old male

Congenital polyvalvular disease, VSD, overriding aorta. Patent ductus arteriosus, pulmonary stenosis (PS), tricuspid stenosis. Bicuspid pulmonary valve, unicuspid aortic valve. Abbreviated chordae for tricuspid valve and mitral valve. Coarctation of the aorta. Massive cardiomegaly.

Newborn male

Marked Ebstein's anomaly with marked tricuspid insufficiency (TI) and pulmonary stenosis (PS). Marked ventricular hypertrophy. Spongy primitive ventricular mass. Almost absent tricuspid valve (TV). Paper-thin right ventricle forming aneurysm.

Stillborn male (38-weeks' gestation)

Abnormal formation and aneurysm of base of ventricular septum with absent aortic valve and aortic insufficiency in intrauterine life. Minute PDA. Primitive left ventricular mass. Ventricular septal hypertrophy and bulge. Bicuspid PV. Diverticulum apex of the left ventricle. Mitral-aortic non-continuity.

4½-month female

Cardiomegaly and sudden death. Distinct ventricular septal bulge. Oblique patent foramen ovale (PFO).

14-month-old male

Asplenia. Complete transposition with marked PS → atresia. CAVO, complete dominant right. Total anomalous pulmonary venous drainage (TAPVD), CS, LSVC → left atrium. Cardiomegaly, RAA, multiple extracardiac anomalies (Figs. 1–4).

3½-month male

Double VSD, ASD, redundant TV, abbreviated chordae. Hypoplastic papillary muscles with TI. Cardiomegaly. Overriding aorta. Extracardiac anomalies.

2-hour-old female

Ebstein's anomaly with TI. ASD, FOD, small pulmonary arteries. Immense cardiomegaly.

10-day-old male (35 weeks' gestation)

Interrupted aortic arch with VSD and subaortic stenosis. Bicuspid aortic valve. Both coronary arteries close to posterior commissure. Straddling parietal band → subaortic stenosis. Distal origin of left subclavian artery. Dysmorphic features.

10-day-old female (30–33-weeks' gestation)

Mesocardia with partial visceral heterotaxy. Congenital AV block and pacemaker. CAVO, complete, dominant left. DORV, subaortic type, TAPVD → RA. Normal spleen, RSVC – atretic. Both atrial appendages resembling left. Anterior leaflet → subaortic stenosis, small pulmonaries. Origin of both coronary ostia close to posterior cusp.

8-month-old male

Immense cardiomegaly with diffuse fibroelastosis and sudden death. Accessory TI with TI, PFO.

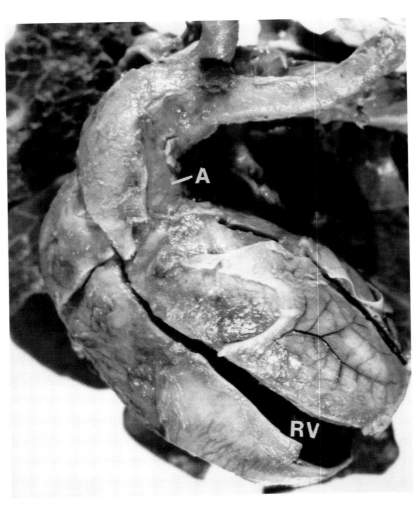

Figure 1: External view of the heart of a 14-month-old born to a cocaine-addicted mother, with complete transposition, marked pulmonary stenosis → pulmonary atresia, and marked cardiomegaly. RV = right ventricle; A = aorta.

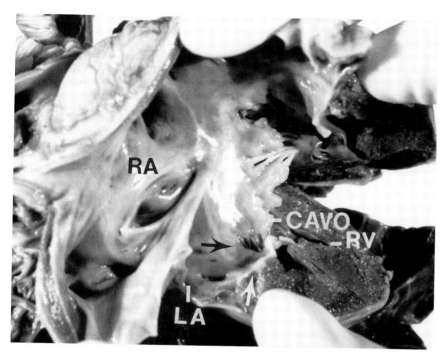

Figure 2: Right-sided view of the heart. RA = right atrium; RV = right ventricle; CAVO = common AV orifice; LA = left atrium. Arrows point to the left side of CAVO.

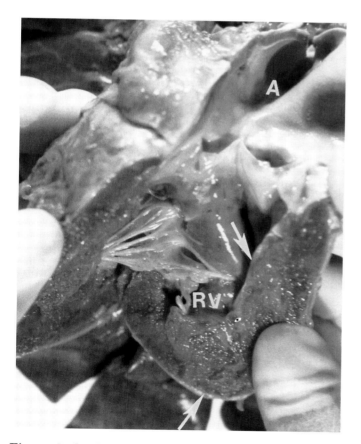

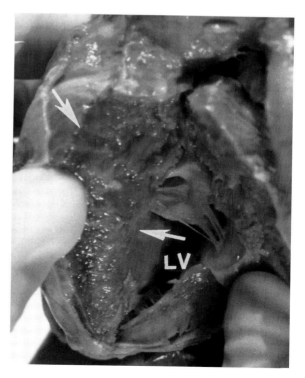

Figure 3: Outflow tract of right ventricle showing marked right ventricular hypertrophy. RV = right ventricle; A = aorta. Arrow points to marked right ventricular hypertrophy.

Figure 4: Left ventricle outflow tract demonstrating marked left ventricular hypertrophy. LV = left ventricle. Arrows point to left ventricular hypertrophy.

Comment

The mechanism or mechanisms of cocaine-induced congenital cardiac anomalies are yet to be elucidated. However, the immense hypertrophy of the heart is most likely related to chronic use of cocaine by the mother. This may perhaps be accentuated by use of other drugs such as amphetamine and alcohol by some of the mothers. Since 12 out of 13 (92%) exhibited major cardiac anomalies, it is conceivable that prolonged use of cocaine might alter the development of myocytes at the molecular and/or genetic level in susceptible individuals. The heart was markedly hypertrophied in 12. In one, it was moderately hypertrophied and enlarged. The hypertrophy was marked, especially in the ventricular septum. Two (15%) with immense cardiomegaly died suddenly.

In summary, our findings suggest: (1) cocaine addiction in the mother may result in congenital cardiac malformation in the fetus in some susceptible individuals, (2) the cardiac malformation may not be a simple anomaly but a major complicated lesion affecting the valves and the ventricular septum predominantly, (3) multiple extracardiac anomalies may be associated with the cardiac malformation, (4) there is marked hypertrophy of the heart in all, (5) sudden death in some infants may be related to chronic cocaine use by the mother, and finally, (6) the high incidence of male infants being affected by cocaine certainly deserves more attention, (7) the effects of cocaine on the growing (developing) myocyte during the embryogenesis of the heart should be futher explored at the molecular-genetic level in the future.

95

Normal or Acquired Heart Diseases

In this group of 35 hearts, some were normal, some had normal aging changes, and others had acquired heart desease. In addition to the above-categorized hearts, we have examined innumerable hearts with varying types of acquired heart diseases that have not been included in this series.

Normal Hearts

17- to 18-weeks' gestation female fetus
  Normal heart

Stillborn male
  Normal heart

11-hours-old male
  Normal heart

Stillborn female
  Normal heart

5-month-old female
  Levocardia, asplenia and partial visceral heterotaxy
  Normal heart

Aging Changes

74-year-old female
  Redundant tricuspid and mitral valves with calcification, tricuspid insufficiency, partial cleft in mitral valve, subaortic stenosis, and Mönckeberg's calcification of the aortic valve

65-year-old male
  Mitral anular calcification with irregular thickening, and questionable floppy valve

77-year-old male
  Aging of mitral valve, huge mitral orifice, redundant posterior leaflet, calcification – floppy valve, and mitral insufficiency

68-year-old female
  Floppy mitral valve with calcification of mitral anulus and mitral and tricuspid insufficiency

69-year-old male
  Floppy mitral valve and calcification of the aortic sinuses of Valsalva

72-year-old male
  Mönckeberg's sclerosis of the aortic valve with aortic stenosis, aging changes of the mitral valve with mitral stenosis, and aneurysm of fossa ovalis

81-year-old female
  Floppy mitral valve, aging of the mitral valve, aneurysm of the fossa ovalis, small tricuspid valve, irregularly thickened, abbreviated chordae, tricuspid insufficiency (clinical), and patent ductus arteriosus

90-year-old female
  Ballooning of the mitral and tricuspid valves with mitral insufficiency–aging changes

Rheumatic Hearts

Female
  Rheumatic mitral stenosis with thrombus of the left atrium

12-year-old male
  Old rheumatic mitral stenosis and previous mitral anuloplasty followed by porcine valve replace-

ment, calcification of porcine valve with stenosis and insufficiency, calcification of papillary muscles and rheumatic tricuspid valve with insufficiency, hypertrophy, and enlargement of heart

65-year-old male
Rheumatic aortic valve with aortic insufficiency and stenosis with marked calcification, hypertrophy, enlargement of all the chambers, mural thrombus in both atrial appendages

31-year-old male
Rheumatic mitral stenosis with mitral valve replacement and infective myocarditis and myocardial infarction, hypertrophy, and enlargement of all the chambers

56-year-old female
Rheumatic mitral stenosis, insufficiency, and mild aortic stenosis, hypertrophy, and enlargement of all the chambers

Myoarditis

3-month-old male
Myocarditis, history, clinical, and cardiomegaly

1-year, 4-month-old male
Acute viral myocarditis

1-year, 11-month-old female
Myocarditis

6-year, 6-month, 21-day-old female
Acute myocarditis

32-year-old
Chronic myocarditis

15-month-old male
Measles, pericardial effusion, fatty infiltration, and cardiomegaly

49-year-old female
Primary amyloidosis with cardiomegaly

19-year-old female
Severe anemia, and cardiomegaly with marked fatty infiltration

38-year-old male
Hemosiderosis and anemia

Left superior vena cava entering coronary sinus, left bundle branch block

14-year, 9-month, 14-day-old male
Thalassemia, hemosiderosis, hypertrophy, and enlargement of all the chambers

Acquired Immune Deficiency Syndrome (AIDS)

2-year, 8-month-old female
Acquired immune deficiency syndrome, fusiform aneurysm of the right coronary artery, calcification and complete thrombus occlusion, infarction of the ventricular septum, aneurysm and dilatation of the ascending aorta, high origin of right coronary ostium, small aneurysm of fossa ovalis, and accessory tricuspid orifice with possible tricuspid insufficiency

7-year-old male
Acquired immune deficiency syndrome, cardiomegaly

2½-year-old male
Acquired immune deficiency syndrome, mild to moderate cardiomegaly

13-month-old female
Acquired immune deficiency syndrome, mild cardiomegaly

4-year-old female
Acquired immune deficiency syndrome, cardiomegaly, fatty infiltration in the AV sulcus, and high origin of both coronary ostia

7-month-old female
Acquired immune deficiency syndrome, cardiomegaly, aneurysmal dilatation of the ascending aorta, tortuous anomalous distribution of the right coronary artery, and possible supravalvular stenosis

33-year-old male
Acquired immune deficiency syndrome, clinical toxoplasmosis of the brain, Kaposi's sarcoma, cytomegalovirus infection, myocarditis histologically, diffuse fibroelastosis of left ventricle, and fibrosis of papillary muscles

96

Hearts Not Examined or Animal Hearts

There were seven hearts—four human and three animal hearts that were not examined. This is due to the fact that the heart specimens were either inadequate for proper evaluation and/or not significantly sufficient to diagnose them in any of the categories.

The reason for including this as a chapter is due to the fact that aside from the above-mentioned seven hearts, there were innumerable instances where our opinion has been requested where the heart has been opened inadequately and/or only part of the heart has been forwarded to us for further evaluation.

In the beginning when the project was initiated, the above seven hearts had been numbered and included in our series. However, in the last 25 years we have tried not to undertake examination of such material unless we are forced to do so.

Today, we are living in a litigious society and therefore urge the pathologists and the medical examiners to be cautious in evaluating the heart specimens and to seek expert opinion when the need arises.

It is our opinion that a true expert in the field of pathology of congenital heart disease and the conduction system of the heart should first evaluate the heart at the gross level and preferably open the heart by herself or himself and take the various measurements as accurately as possible and compare these with the normal hearts of similar age, height, and weight and issue a detailed gross report. If necessary, this should be followed by a histological examination of the myocardium, the valves, the coronary arteries, and the conduction system, depending on the gross diagnosis. Only under these circumstances may the expert opinion be considered complete and therefore legal. Giving opinions based on a few slides prepared elsewhere is in our opinion totally inadequate and improper from the standpoint of the patient, the family, and, above all, the knowledge obtained by such work. We therefore make a special plea to all those interested in this field to obtain an autopsy permit to examine the heart when death occurs following surgery and/or unexpectedly, or under other conditions. This would hopefully eliminate the pressure by the legal system on the few of us who spend our entire lives studying hearts. We foresee no problem in the next century with the emerging information superhighway that the experts can be reached anywhere, any time, and at any place, and thereby a fairly good opinion of the heart may be obtained.

Again, we reiterate, the expert opinion is *not* valid, at least scientifically, when such opinion is obtained based on inadequate tissue samples and improper examination of the heart. The purpose of this chapter is to emphasize this very important issue which is on the rise today. Obtaining a thorough examination of the heart by an expert will hopefully create a better understanding between the family, the physicians, the legal system, the pathologists, and the medical examiners in this country. We hope the coming twenty-first century will provide new ways of dealing with expert opinions concerning the heart.

97

Congenital Hearts Seen According to Complex

	No of Cases		
Tetralogy of Fallot	512 (8.11%)	Complete transposition with mitral atresia	15 (0.23%)
Double outlet right ventricle with subaortic VSD	81 (1.30%)	Complete transposition with common AV orifice	28 (0.44%)
Double outlet right ventricle with doubly committed and noncommitted VSD	38 (0.60%)	Unusual complete transposition complexes – double outlet left ventricle	12 (0.20%)
Double outlet right ventricle, complicated types	98 (1.55%)	Truncus communis	142 (2.25%)
Double outlet right ventricle with subpulmonic VSD – Taussig-Bing right ventricle type and mild overriding of the pulmonary trunk	51 (0.80%)	Pulmonary atresia with ventricular septal defect – pseudotruncus	195 (3.09%)
Taussig-Bing – intermediate and left ventricular types	72 (1.14%)	Tricuspid atresia without transposition	96 (1.52%)
		Tricuspid stenosis with pulmonary atresia	194 (3.07%)
Complete transposition with normal architecture without VSD	223 (3.53%)	Unusual tricuspid stenosis without transposition – with normal or increased pulmonary flow	10 (0.15%)
Complete transposition with normal architecture with VSD	135 (2.14%)	Atrial septal defect, secundum	156 (2.47%)
Complete transposition with pulmonary stenosis	62 (1.00%)	Atrial septal defect, primum	57 (0.90%)
Complete transposition with common ventricle	6 (0.09%)	Atrial septal defect, proximal septum	22 (0.34%)
		Atrial septal defect, coronary sinus type	3 (0.04%)
Complete transposition with tricuspid stenosis	27 (0.42%)	ASD, combined secundum and primum, or common atrium	23 (0.36%)
		Ventricular septal defect	254 (4.02%)
Complete transposition with tricuspid atresia	42 (0.66%)	Common AV orifice	256 (4.05%)
		Common AV orifice intermediate type	79 (1.25%)

Total anomalous pulmonary venous drainage	151 (2.40%)
Partial anomalous pulmonary venous drainage	16 (0.25%)
Patent ductus arteriosus	129 (2.04%)
Aorticopulmonary septal defect	19 (0.30%)
Atrial septal defect and ventricular septal defect	54 (0.90%)
Atrial septal defect and patent ductus arteriosus	112 (1.80%)
Atrial septal defect, ventricular septal defect, and patent ductus arteriosus	109 (1.72%)
Ventricular septal defect and patent ductus arteriosus	54 (0.90%)
Hypoplasia of the aortic tract complex	302 (4.80%)
Fetal coarctation	238 (3.80%)
Transitional coarctation	104 (1.64%)
Adult coarctation	105 (1.66%)
Pure pulmonary stenosis (normal aortic root)	65 (1.03%)
Ventricular septal defect with pulmonary stenosis	6 (0.10%)
Aortic stenosis	165 (2.61%)
Idiopathic hypertrophy with fibroelastosis	81 (1.30%)
Coronary from pulmonary	23 (0.36%)
Ebstein's anomaly	67 (1.06%)
Vascular rings	21 (0.33%)
Mixed Levocardia	79 (1.25%)
Dextroposition	11 (0.17%)
Dextrocardia	137 (2.17%)
Isolated levocardia	79 (1.25%)
Mesocardia	55 (0.90%)
Single ventricle with small outlet chamber	101 (1.60%)
Straddling and displaced tricuspid and mitral orifice (83 included in other entities)	20 (0.31%)
Inverted transposition with left AV valve atresia	26 (0.41%)
Glycogen storage	12 (0.20%)
Gargoylism	6 (0.10%)
Connective tissue dyscrasia – Marfan's syndrome	26 (0.41%)
Congenital polyvalvular disease	101 (1.60%)
Congenital mitral stenosis	8 (0.12%)
Mitral insufficiency	10 (0.15%)
Mitral atresia complex	21 (0.33%)
Aortic atresia with VSD	10 (0.15%)
Pulmonary atresia with tricuspid insufficiency	21 (0.33%)
Aortic and mitral stenosis complex	16 (0.25%)
Cor triatriatum (double left atrium)	17 (0.26%)
Ruptured aneurysm – aortic sinus of Valsalva (or fistula)	6 (0.10%)
Aneurysm of the coronary artery	6 (0.10%)
Abnormal course or narrowing of the pulmonary trunk and its branches	4 (0.06%)
Origin of the right pulmonary artery from the ascending aorta (hemitruncus)	13 (0.20%)
Abnormal blood supply to a lung from the thoracic or abdominal aorta	3 (0.04%)
Double heart	7 (0.11%)
Primary pulmonary hypertension	18 (0.30%)
Premature closure or narrowing of the foramen ovale	86 (1.36%)
Absence of the (interrupted) transverse arch with VSD	67 (1.06%)
Stenosis or atresia of the pulmonary veins	8 (0.12%)
Other complexes	152 (2.41%)
Incidental anomalies	114 (1.80%)
Undiagnosed hearts	95 (1.50%)
Conduction system problems (including sudden death, Uhl's, floppy mitral valve, coronary artery anomalies, and atypical hypertrophic cardiomyopathy)	207 (3.30%)
Cardiac malformations related to cocaine use by the mother	13 (0.20%)

Normal or acquired heart diseases	35 (0.55%)
Not examined or animal hearts	7 (0.11%)
	6,307 (100.00%)

Comment

The above incidence of various types of anomalies represents our experience in this field for the last several years. Regardless of this fact, the material can be analyzed in various ways. If one included all types of transposition complexes, complete, incomplete, including tetralogy of Fallot, double outlet right ventricle, truncus, and pseudotruncus, the incidence of conotruncal anomalies is 27.55%.

Likewise, all shunts (without obstruction) made up 23.74% of our material. Thus, conotruncal anomalies and shunts alone represented 51.29%. On the other hand, left-sided lesions, including origin of coronary from the pulmonary, idiopathic hypertrophy with fibroelastosis of the left ventricle, and congenital anomalies of the mitral valve constituted 20.17%. Positional abnormalities of the heart were found in 5.74%. In autopsied material, one may conclude that conotruncal anomalies, shunts, left-sided lesions, and abnormal position of the heart and its chambers totaled 77.20%. All other anomalies were found in the remainder.

However, it is emphasized that this material represents the *autopsied* hearts during a *given period of time*. Nevertheless, this information may be found useful in the long run.

98

The Future

The enormous amount of material presented in this book has opened our eyes to the wide variations occurring in congenital heart disease. The variations in each entity are mind-boggling. The student of congenital heart disease should develop an open mind and not approach this fascinating field with an idea of a "classic" type of an anomaly. Congenital heart disease may be classified as the most "unclassic," and it represents a gray area, and the anatomy is not as clear-cut as one would like it to be, especially in the autopsied material.

The wide variation probably is the most intriguing aspect of congenital heart disease and raises the possibility of multifactorial etiogenesis and embryogenesis for the same malformation. Is congenital heart disease preventable? Perhaps a few malformations can be prevented. In order to take further steps in preventing congenital heart disease, it is important that we try to understand the following:

1. The exact number of genes that are responsible for the normal development of the heart, including the entire heart, such as the atrial myocardium, the ventricular myocardium, the conduction system, and their associated components, such as the elastic tissue, the collagen connective tissue, the nerves, the blood vessels, and the ubiquitous fat in some areas (normal ?) are to be elucidated at the molecular-genetic level in the next century.

2. Hemodynamics of the normal embryogenesis of the heart.

3. Altered hemodynamics and its relationship to the normal and/or abnormal embryogenesis of the heart.

4. Attempts should be made to study the changes that may occur at the molecular-genetic level during the very early stages of development of the heart.

5. The relationship of normal versus abnormal hemodynamics at the molecular and genetic levels should be explored.

6. Alterations in environment (including food, infective agents, drugs, and other factors) and their effects on the developing heart at the molecular-genetic level need to be explored.

7. The above may shed some light as to the etiology of congenital cardiac malformations.

In regard to treating the disease itself, the most important factors that require further research are:

1. Hypertrophy of a muscle mass to varying types of altered hemodynamics.

2. What is reversible hypertrophy?

3. What is irreversible hypertrophy?

4. The function of a geometrically altered hypertrophied muscle mass in various types of congenital cardiac malformations before and after total surgical correction.

5. The normal variations in all age groups, especially in regard to sizes and wall thickness of the chambers and valves.

6. The aging changes in congenital heart disease.

7. The growth factors in postoperative congenital hearts.

8. The relationship of lymphatic drainage in postoperative congenital hearts.

9. The relationship of the immune system to congenital heart disease and the conduction system.

10. The aging changes in the conduction system in congenital heart disease.

If and when we understand the above, in my opinion, we have only reached the stage of appreciating the variations in congenital heart disease and are only treating the symptoms and not the disease itself.

Approach to Congenital Heart Disease

As gleaned from our material, congenital heart disease may be considered or dealt with broadly in two groups: (1) symptomatic, and seen in infants and younger age groups, (2) asymptomatic or mildly symptomatic, and seen in older age groups. Or, congenital cardiac malformations may be grouped into simple and complicated categories. This approach may help in better understanding congenital heart disease and thereby in providing the best care possible.

This is fundamental because when the entity is seen in infants, the anatomy is quite complicated, with obvious differences in clinical manifestation, diagnosis, and in providing the appropriate corrective procedure. Further, such an approach also indicates the possibility of different etiogenesis of the same malformation, suggesting alteration at the molecular/genetic level.

It is self-evident that the outcome following surgery or any kind of intervention is different in the two groups, although the cardiac anomaly is the same. Newer methodologies should be developed to correct the anomaly at the molecular/genetic level, if possible.

Sudden Death in Congenital Heart Disease

Sudden death does occur in congenital heart disease before or after surgery. The fundamental problem in these hearts is the *cardiomegaly* and *fibroelastosis* of the endocardium, especially in those following surgical procedures.

Arrhythmias Following Surgical Correction

Further research is also needed to explore the possibility of reducing the size of scar formation following corrective procedures. If possible, efforts should be aimed at altering the mechanics of the healing process and thereby preventing scar formation in part or completely. In other words, eliminating the process of scar formation should be the aim.

Methods should be directed to improve the immune system rather than depress it.

The Relationship of Fat in Postoperative Congenital Heart Disease and Its Significance

The most important area is the modification and/or reduction of the amount of fat accumulation near the vital areas of the conduction system, such as the sinoatrial node and its approaches, the atrial preferential pathways, the atrioventricular (AV) node and its approaches, the AV bundle, and the bundle branches. There is a *distinct* tendency for fat and degenerative process to set in in the above areas in cases of sudden death several years following total surgical correction, especially in the so-called "asymptomatic or silent or healthy or normal youngsters."

Likewise, the exact mechanism of how fat that is present, especially in the anterior wall of the right ventricle (focal or diffuse), triggers an arrhythmic event needs to be explored. This is an important area since sudden death may occur with or without intractable arrhythmias in the asymptomatic youngster.

The exact mechanism of normal versus abnormal fat accumulation in the various parts of the heart and its functional significance should be explored at the molecular-genetic level.

The Relationship of Valvular Anomalies to Sudden Death

Dysplastic changes in the valves are seen in the adult hearts that were said to be "asymptomatic" and sudden death was the first manifestation. This again raises the question as to whether we are dealing with changes in elastic tissue, collagen connective tissue, and/or some other unknown factors that may or may not be related to Marfan or forme fruste Marfan's syndrome. Newer technologies have to be developed to identify these changes and further research is obviously indicated to explore this area.

Asymptomatic Versus Symptomatic

This brings in the bigger issue of the definition of asymptomatic versus symptomatic. Are the asymptomatic truly asymptomatic? It is our opinion that we have *not* learned to understand the minor or trivial complaints of the patient. Or, the high level of technology that is used today is not yet sophisticated enough to enable us to detect the subtle, minor to moderate changes in the hemodynamics, as well as to evaluate the sizes and wall thickness of chambers and the valvular anomalies.

Correction of "Silent" Congenital Heart Disease

Noninvasive techniques must be developed that would detect the minor to moderate alterations in physiology and anatomy. Likewise, correcting the lesions, preferably by nonsurgical methods, is to be entertained as a method of prophylaxis. Correcting the anomalies during the asymptomatic stage would prevent further complications.

Is the Flora of Congenital Heart Disease Changing Vis-a-Vis a Quarter of a Century Ago?

There appears to be a tendency for unusual and complicated congenital cardiac abnormalities to occur, especially in the last decade. Whether this is due to the influence of the environment per se, food, water, drugs, and/or other factors such as infective agents or other unknown factors or forces is to be determined in the years to come.

Hearts That Cannot Be Categorized

Furthermore, it was difficult to categorize a group of hearts into a specific known entity and/or into a complex. For example, abnormalities in the valves in the form of mild to moderate redundancy of the leaflet, short or elongated chordae, absent or hypoplastic papillary muscles, hypertrophy and enlargement of the chambers with multiple defects and/or obstructive phenomena without obvious evidence of chromosomal anomalies are seen in infants. This raises the issue of whether we are dealing with minor changes in the chromosomes that are yet to be identified.

The Familial Tendency

Today we know that the incidence of congenial cardiac anomalies in the children born to parents who had congenital cardiac anomalies is higher than in the general population. The incidence is said to be between 4% to 14% regardless of whether the cardiac anomaly was present on the maternal or the paternal side, although there is increased incidence of cardiac anomalies in the progeny of affected mothers over that of fathers with VSDs.

It is obvious that more research should be aimed at the molecular genetic, environmental, infective agents, and other unknown factors or forces that are responsible for the familial occurrence of congenital cardiac anomalies.

Philosophic Concepts

Although for the sake of simplification and practical purposes, one may group the various types of cardiac anomalies and classify them into various complexes, it is again emphasized that the variations have to be kept in mind regarding the clinical presentation, the management, the treatment (surgical or nonsurgical), and the prognosis of the patient in the long run.

The one striking feature in congenital heart disease is the variation that occurs within one anomaly itself. The variations are innumerable, even in the so-called simple anomalies. Many of the variations can be explained at the genetic level; however, it is empha-

sized that they may not necessarily be familial or inherent in nature. This may be explained as follows.

If, for whatever reasons (the reasons may be numerous), the genes that are responsible for the development of the heart are altered, this may result in a malformed heart. For example, one particular gene or genes responsible for the future myocyte may be affected at the critical stage of the development of the heart, giving rise to one type of anomaly. On the other hand, several genes may be affected, giving rise to several types of anomalies. The reasons for the abnormalities in the genes may be many in that there may be several types of etiogenesis that may affect a gene or genes that are responsible for the future development of a myocyte, elastic tissue, collagen, connective tissue, nerves, fat, blood vessels, etc. at the critical stage of development of the heart and may produce either the same or a modification or a different type of an anomaly.

The congenital cardiac malformations may be related to the following factors:

1. The inherent ability of that particular gene or genes responsible for one part or a specific area of the myocardium, and this may or may not include other elements that are considered a part of the myocardium, such as elastic tissue, collagen, etc.

2. The injury that may occur in the form of various types of infective agents, hormonal, stress, and other unknown causes of injury at a critical time during the early period of embryogenesis of the embryo and/or the heart, may affect the specific part of the developing myocardium and/or its accompanying constituents.

3. The ability of the inherently altered (or the weak gene) to overcome the obstacle or the normal gene to overcome that particular type of an injury and its outcome.

4. The reaction or the antibodies that may develop at the placental level to overcome the genetically altered (inborn) gene and/or the injury obtained by the normal gene due to various causes.

5. The effects of the above on the hemodynamics.

6. The mechanism of further alteration of the myocardium to the altered hemodynamics.

7. Thus, one may say that in a sense all anomalies are the end result of alteration or the arrest that might have occurred during the critical stage of the developing myocyte and/or its accompanying constituents at the molecular-genetic level, and its response to the alteration (or its ability to overcome the alteration or modify the outcome).

As indicated previously, the etiogenesis for alteration of the specific myocyte at the given period of development during the embryogenesis of the heart may be numerous. Thus, although most of the cardiac malformations may show some type of genetic alterations, only some may be familial. Therefore, numerous or different types of genes will be discovered for the same type of malformation, out of which only a few may be familial. Even among the familial there may be different variations, and the different variations may express themselves clinically as congenital cardiac malformations, and some, although they are genetically altered, may be normally developed hearts and may or may not carry the expression of the anomaly in the future.

Future research should be aimed at discovering at the genetic level what type of myocyte will be vulnerable during what stage of the development of the heart to what type of injurious agent, infectious agent, etc., that may alter its future growth. If we can identify one type of myocyte or one type of injury at the genetic level and the critical period during which the alteration occurs, and the outcome of the altered myocyte and the future growth that may result in a particular type of anomaly, this may shed some light as to the mechanisms involved in congenital malformations of the heart. It is important to remember that not all congenital cardiac anomalies may have an altered gene and that not all altered genes may be familial in nature. There will be innumerable variations in the familial gene itself with varying degrees of expression, including the normal heart.

The Accumulated Knowledge and Its Usefulness to Humanity at Large

Finally, what have we learned from studying more than 7,000 congenitally malformed hearts in this century? The accumulated knowledge, as such, is obviously useful in its practical applicability in enhancing the management of congenital heart disease patients clinically, surgically, or nonsurgically.

The material clearly demonstrates the innumerable variations and the variants that are present within an entity itself. The only way we can hypothesize the variability is that there probably are innumerable genes involved in creating the same anomaly, making the congenital cardiac anomaly a complex one. However, there appears to be a dominance of one genetic mutation over the other. It is, however, emphasized that not all genetically altered anomalies may be familial.

From an evolutionary point of view, one may consider some of the variations as follows. (1) Some anomalies may represent the evolutionary stages in the development of a mammalian heart. (2) On the other hand, one may also entertain the idea that some of the cardiac anomalies may represent an attempt for survival by the altered gene. In other words, the

heart, though malformed, makes every attempt to maintain a function, although faultily (the best possible function). Thus, the inherent genetic tendency to survive is being expressed in the form of a congenital anomaly of the heart, which by itself is a representation of an alteration at the genetic level. In other words, although the genetic alteration may result in an anomaly, the presence of other genetic components may try to overcome the anomaly, thereby becoming a part of the anomaly (or not), both anatomically and functionally.

The question then emerges of whether this is an anomaly or an altered "normal" with an attempt at survival. Thus, in a true sense one may never be able to prevent congenital heart disease. It is also to be noted that as the global population increases with time, so also will the variations which will also grow in direct proportion. As long as mankind survives, there will be variations, and variations are probably one method by which the species may be preserved on earth. Future genetic manipulations of the human may be attempted judiciously *only* after the complete understanding of the normal development of the human embryo at the molecular-genetic level.

Be that as it may, we have to focus our study on one particular malformation to the fullest at the molecular-genetic level. This of course is tedious, but it would be useful in the long run. Understanding of *one* particular entity will shed some light as to the best possibilities that may be offered to an individual with congenital heart disease. In a sense, the intragenetic variability is an impetus and a challenge to those who have an indefatigable quest for knowledge. This also suggests that the master switch or the commander that orchestrates which part of the developing cell proceeds to become heart muscle, brain tissue, etc., may or may not be affected to a varying degree. It is obvious that if the master switch itself is markedly altered, the future growth of the developing cell may not proceed any further (or may not occur at all). Most of the congenital cardiac anomalies that are amenable for surgical correction are those where the alteration of a specific myocyte occurred at a genetic level.

Chromosomal loci and genes will be assigned to various types of familial congenital cardiac malformations. The variations seen at the anatomic level suggest the possibility of involvement of a cascade effect from multiple genes and a multiplicity of genetic alterations (inherently altered or altered due to injury, infection, toxin, etc.), resulting in multiple genetic mutations. More than one gene can be mutated to cause a similar phenotype. Genetic heterogeneity should be recognized because this will provide the opportunity to identify several genes that may participate in (be involved in), or independently, as such, may yield a similar phenotype.

The inherent ability includes the varying types of familial alterations in the specific gene or genes with or without expressing the disease (i.e., clinically manifest, or silent, or manifest at a later date, etc.). To this is added the susceptibility of these genes to other effects, such as infection, injury, etc., which may still further alter the gene or genes.

Finally, this material may serve as a reference book to compare the changes in flora of congenital heart disease that may occur, for centuries to come.

99

References

1. Lev M, Saphir O: Transposition of the large vessels. *J Tech Methods* 1937, 17:126–162.
2. Lev M, Saphir O: Congenital aneurysm of the membranous septum. *Arch Pathol* 1938, 25:819–837.
3. Lev M, Neuwelt F, Necheles H: Congenital defect of the interventricular septum, aortic regurgitation and probable heart block in a dog. *Am J Vet Res* 1941, 2:91–94.
4. Saphir O, Lev M: Tetralogy of Eisenmenger. *Am Heart J* 1941, 21:31–46.
5. Lev M, Strauss S: Stenosis of the infundibulum. *Arch Int Med* 1942, 70:53–60.
6. Lev M, Killian ST: Hypoplasia of the aorta without transposition with electrocardiographic and histopathologic studies of the conduction system. *Am Heart J* 1942, 24:794–806.
7. Weinstein W, Lev M: Apical diastolic murmurs without mitral stenosis. *Am Heart J* 1942, 23:809–816.
8. Lev M, Saphir O: Truncus arteriosus communis persistens. *J Pediatr* 1943, 20:74–88.
9. Lev M, Saphir O: A theory of transposition of the arterial trunks based on the phylogenetic and ontogenetic development of the heart. *Arch Pathol* 1945, 39:172–183.
10. Simkins CC, Lev M: The architecture of the human ventricular myocardium. Trans. III. Interamerican Cardiol Congress, 1948. *Acta Cardiologica* 1948, Suppl III, p. 114.
11. Lev M, Volk BW: The pathologic anatomy of the Taussig-Bing heart: Riding pulmonary artery. Report of a case. *Bull Internat Am Med Museums* 1950, 31:54–64.
12. Lev M, Vass A: *Spitzer's Architecture of the Normal and Malformed Hearts*. (Translation of Spitzer A: Uber den Bauplan des normalen und missbildeten Herzens. Versuch einer phylogenetischen Theorie. Vir. Arch. Path. Anat. 243:81–201, 1923). Charles C. Thomas & Co., Springfield, Illinois, 1951.
13. Lev M: The pathologic anatomy and interrelationship of cardiac transposition complexes. *Proc Inst Med of Chicago* 1951, 8:326–28.
14. Lev M: Pathologic anatomy and interrelationship of hypoplasia of the aortic tract complexes. *Lab Invest* 1952, 1:61–70.
15. Lev M: *Autopsy Diagnosis of Congenitally Malformed Hearts*. Charles C. Thomas, Springfield, Illinois, 1953.
16. Lev M: The pathologic anatomy of cardiac complexes associated with transposition of arterial trunks. *Lab Invest* 1953, 2:296–311.
17. Lev M: The pathologic diagnosis of positional variations in cardiac chambers in congenital heart disease. *Lab Invest* 1954, 3:71–82.
18. Lev M, Gibson S, Miller RA: Ebstein's disease with Wolff-Parkinson-White syndrome. *Am Heart J* 1955, 49:724–741.
19. Lev M, Simkins CS: Architecture of the human ventricular myocardium. Technic for study using a modification of the Mall-MacCallum Method. *Lab Invest* 1956, 5:396–409.
20. Lev M: Congenital heart disease. In *Saphir's Systemic Pathology*. Vol 1, Grune and Stratton, New York, 1958, pp. 127–180.
21. Lev M: The architecture of the conduction system in congenital heart disease: I. Common atrioventricular orifice. *AMA Arch Pathol* 1958, 65:174–191.
22. Novell HA, Asher LA Jr, Lev M: Marfan's syndrome associated with pregnancy. *Am J Obstet Gynecol* 1958, 75:802–812.
23. Lev M: The architecture of the conduction system in congenital heart disease: II. Tetralogy of Fallot. *AMA Arch Pathol* 1959, 67:572–587.
24. Lev M: Pathology of congenital heart disease. Chap 2, part 6, Congenital heart disease. In *Cardiology*, Vol 3. *Clinical Cardiology*, edited by AA Luisada. McGraw-Hill Book Co., Inc. NY, Blakiston Div, pp. 15–35, 1959.
25. Lev M: The pathologic anatomy of ventricular septal defect. *Dis Chest* 1959, 35:533–545.
26. Lev M, Kaveggia E: Etiology and pathogenesis of congenital heart disease. Chap 1, part 6, Congenital heart disease. In *Cardiology* Vol 3, *Clinical Cardiology* edited by AA Luisada. McGraw-Hill Book Co., Inc., NY, Blakiston Div., 1959, pp. 3–14.
27. Lev M: Pathologic anatomy of congenital intra and extra-cardiac shunts unassociated with intracardiac obstruction to flow. In *Congenital Heart Disease*, edited by AD Bass and GK Moe. Am Assoc for the Adv of Science, Washington, DC, 1960, pp. 105–140.
28. Paul MH, Lev M: Tricuspid stenosis with pulmonary atresia, a cineangiographic-pathologic correlation. *Circulation* 1960, 22:198–203.

29. Wilkinson AH, Potts WJ, Lev M: The postmortem external appearance of congenitally malformed hearts as an aid to surgical diagnosis. *J Thoracic Cardiovasc Surg* 1960, 39:363–379.

30. Lev M: The architecture of the conduction system in congenital heart disease. III. Ventricular septal defect. *AMA Arch Pathol* 1960, 70:529–549.

31. Baffes TG, Lev M, Paul MH, Miller RA, Riker WL, DeBoer A, Potts WJ: Surgical correction of transposition of great vessels: A five year survey. *J Thoracic Cardiovasc Surg* 1960, 40:298–309.

32. Lev M, Rowlatt UF, Rimoldi HJA: Pathologic methods for study of congenitally malformed hearts: Methods for electrocardiographic and physiologic correlation. *AMA Arch Pathol* 1961, 72:493–511.

33. Lev M, Alcalde VM, Baffes TG: Pathologic anatomy of complete transposition of the arterial trunks. *Pediatrics* 1961, 28:293–306.

34. Lev M, Rowlatt UF: The pathologic anatomy of mixed levocardia: A review of thirteen cases of atrial or ventricular inversion with or without corrected transposition. *Am J Cardiol* 1961, 8:216–263.

35. DeBoer A, Grana L, Potts WJ, Lev M: Coarctation of the aorta: A clinico-pathologic study. *AMA Arch Surg* 1961, 82:801–812.

36. Lev M, Agustssen MH, Arcilla R: The pathologic anatomy of a common atrioventricular orifice associated with tetralogy of Fallot. *Am J Clin Pathol* 1961, 36:408–416.

37. Lev M, Rowlatt UF: Pathologic observations on congenital heart disease before and after surgery. *Chicago Med* 1961, 63:13–25.

38. Molthan ME, Paul MH, Lev M: Common AV orifice with pulmonary valvular and hypertrophic subaortic stenosis: A case report. *Am J Cardiol* 1962, 10:291–297.

39. Lev M: Pathologic anatomy of septal defects. In *Congenital Heart Disease Pathogenetic Factors, Natural History, Diagnosis and Surgical Treatment*, edited by DP Morse. Sponsored by Deborah Hospital. FA Davis Co., Philadelphia, PA, 1962, pp. 98–111.

40. Miller RA, Lev M, Paul MH: Congenital absence of pulmonary valve: The clinical Syndrome of tetralogy of Fallot with pulmonary regurgitation. *Circulation* 1962, 26:266–278.

41. Lev M, Riker WL, DeBoer A, Baffes TG, Licata RH, Potts WJ: (Exhibit published). (Conduction System as Related to Cardiac Surgery) *Congenital Heart Disease* in Abbott's *What's New* 1962, 227:10–12.

42. Lev M, Paul MH, Miller RA: A classification of congenital heart disease based on the pathologic complex. *Am J Cardiol* 1962, 10:733–737.

43. Licata RH, Lev M, Brown ER: Cardiac malformations produced by specific heart antibodies. *Quarterly Bull, Northwestern Univ. Med. School*, Chicago, 36(2):107–108, Summer Quarter, 1962.

44. Licata RH, Lev M, Brown ER: The production of congenital malformations utilizing specific anti-heart tissue antibodies: Preliminary report. (Abstract) *Anat Rec* 1962, 142:252–253.

45. Lev M, Licata RH, May RC: Conduction system in mixed levocardia with ventricular inversion: Corrected transposition. (Abstract) *Circulation* 1962, 26:749–50.

46. Rowlatt UF, Rimoldi HJA, Lev M: The quantitative anatomy of the normal child's heart. Edited by LI Gardner. *Pediatr Clin North Am* 1963, 10(2):499–588.

47. Riker WL, Potts WJ, Grana L, Miller RA, Lev M: Tricuspid stenosis or atresia complexes: A surgical-pathologic analysis. *J Thoracic Cardiovas Surg* 1963, 45:423–433.

48. Lev M, Arcilla R, Rimoldi HJA, Licata RH, Gasul BM: Premature narrowing or closure of the foramen ovale. *Am Heart J* 1963, 65:638–647.

49. Rimoldi HHA, Lev M: A note on the concept of normality and abnormality in quantitation of pathologic findings in congenital heart disease. Edited by LI Gardner. *Pediatr Clin North Am* 1963, 10(2):589–591.

50. Lev M, Licata RH, May RC: The conduction system in mixed levocardia with ventricular inversion (corrected transposition). *Circulation* 1963, 28:232–237.

51. Glagov S, Eckner FAO, Lev M: Controlled pressure distention and perfusion: Fixation of human hearts for improved quantitative study. (Abstract-read by title- Am Assoc of Pathol & Bacteriol, April 26–28, 1963). Published in *Programs and Abstracts of the 60th Annual Meeting Scientific Proceedings*, p. 33a, Number 10.

52. Lev M, Fielding RT, Zaeske D: Mixed levocardia with ventricular inversion (corrected transposition) with complete atrioventricular block: A histopathologic study of the conduction system. *Am J Cardiol* 1963, 12:875–883.

53. Hastreiter AR, Oshima M, Miller RA, Lev M, Paul MH: Congenital aortic stenosis syndrome in infancy. *Circulation* 1963, 28:1084–95.

54. Glagov S, Eckner FAO, Lev M: A controlled pressure fixation apparatus for human hearts. *AMA Arch Pathol* 1963, 76:640–646.

55. Lev M: The pathology of congenital heart disease. In *Advances in Cardiopulmonary Disease*. Vol II. Edited by Al Banyai and BL Gordon. Year Book Medical Publishers, Inc., Chicago, Illinois, pp. 146–174, 1964.

56. Lev M, Rimoldi HJA, Rowlatt UF: Examination of the congenitally malformed Heart. In *Recent Advances in Clinical Pathology*, edited by SC Dyke. J & A Churchill Ltd., London, England, 1964, pp. 226–275.

57. Lev M, Eckner FOA: The pathologic anatomy of tetralogy of Fallot and its variations. *Dis Chest* 1964, 45:251–261.

58. Hanlon CR, Diehl AM, Lev M, Neville WE: Surgery for cardiovascular diseases in the newborn. *Dis Chest* 1964, 45:383–395.

59. Lev M, Rimoldi HJA, Rowlatt UF: The quantitative anatomy of cyanotic tetralogy of Fallot. *Circulation* 1964, 30:531–538.

60. Lev M, Cassels DE: Atrial septal defect (fossa ovalis type) with congenital complete atrioventricular dissociation: A conduction system study. (Abstract) *Circulation* 1964, 30:(Suppl #III) p. III-111.

61. Lev M, Rimoldi HJA, Eckner FAO, Paul MH: Taussig-Bing heart: Qualitative and quantitative anatomy. (Abstract) *Circulation* 1964, 30:Suppl #III, p. III-111–2.

62. Straus F, Lev M, Cassels D: Clinical pathologic conference. *Am Heart J* 1964, 68:804–816.

63. Lev M, Fell EH, Arcilla R, Weinberg MH: Surgical injury to the conduction system in ventricular septal defect. *Am J Cardiol* 1964, 14:464–476.

64. Meng CCL, Eckner FAO, Lev M: The coronary artery distribution in tetralogy of Fallot. *AMA Arch Surg* 1965, 90:363–366.

65. Lev M, Eckner FAO, Meng CCL, Rimoldi HJA: Partial transposition complexes (Abstract) *Am J Cardiol* 1965, 15:136–7.

66. Gasul BM, Arcilla RA, Lev M: *Heart Disease in Children: Diagnosis and Treatment.* JB Lippincott Co, Philadelphia, PA, 1966.

67. Lev M, Eckner FAO: Anatomic considerations. In *Heart Disease in Children: Diagnosis and Treatment.* By BM Gasul, RA Arcilla, M Lev, JB Lippincott Co., Philadelphia, PA, pp. 3–10, 1966.

68. Lev M, Eckner FAO: Embryologic, pathogenetic and pathologic considerations. In *Heart Disease in Children: Diagnosis and Treatment.* By BM Gasul, RA Arcilla, M. Lev, JB Lippincott Co., Philadelphia, PA, 1966, pp. 11–25.

69. Lev M: Congenital heart disease. In *Pathology*, Vol 1, Chap 19, edited by WAD Anderson, 5th edition. The CV Mosby Co., St. Louis, MO, 1966, pp. 547–569.

70. Lev M: Some newer concepts of the pathology of congenital heart disease. *Med Clin North Am* 1966, 50:3–14.

71. Lev M, Rimoldi HJA, Eckner FAO, Melhuish BP, Meng CCL, Paul MH: The Taussig-Bing heart: Qualitative and quantitative anatomy. *AMA Arch Pathol* 1966, 81:24–35.

72. Navarro Lopez F, Dobben GG, Rabinowitz M, Ferguson LA, Reisler H, Casels DE, Lev M: Taussig-Bing complex with pulmonary stenosis. *Dis Chest* 1966, 50:1–12.

73. Lev M, Paul MH, Casels DE: Complete atrioventricular block associated with atrial septal defect of the fossa ovalis secundum) type: A histopathologic study of the conduction system. *Am J Cardiol* 1967, 19:266–274.

74. Lev M, Craenen J, Lambert EC: Infantile coronary sclerosis with atrioventricular block. *J Pediatr* 1967, 70:87–94.

75. Lev M: Transposition of the arterial trunks in levocardia. In *Pathology Annual*, Vol 2, edited by SC Sommers NY, Appleton-Century Crofts, 1967, p. 111.

76. Lev M, Okada R, Kerstein MD, Paiva R, Rimoldi HJA: Blood groups and congenital heart disease. *Dis Chest* 1967, 52:616–620.

77. Okada R, Rosenthal IM, Scaravelli G, Lev M: A histopathologic study of the heart in Gargoylism. *AMA Arch Pathol* 1967, 84:20–30.

78. Shaffer AB, JF, Kline IK, Lev M: Truncal inversion with biventricular pulmonary trunk and aorta from right ventricle (variant of Taussig-Bing complex). *Circulation* 1967, 36:783–788.

79. Hait G, Lev M, Rudolph AM: Size of interatrial communication in mitral atresia and stenosis: Anatomical, physiological, and surgical consideration. (Abstract) *Circulation* 1967, 36:Suppl II, p. II-130.

80. Blackstone EH, Moulder PV, Eckner FAO, Daily PO, LEV M: Pressure-derivative loop as a visual aid in ventricular functional assessment. (Abstract) *Circulation* 1967, 36:Suppl II, p. II-71.

81. Lev M: The conduction system in congenital heart disease. *Am J Cardiol* 1968, 21:619–627.

82. Okada R, Glagov S, Lev M: Different effects of increased volume and increased pressure on endocardial structure in hearts with atrial septal defect. *Am Heart J* 1968, 75:474–486.

83. Moulder PV, Blackston EH, Eckner FAO, Lev M: Pressure-derivative loop for left ventricular resuscitation. *Arch Surg* 1968, 96:323–327.

84. Cole RB, Muster AJ, Lev M, Paul MH: Pulmonary atresia with intact ventricular septum. *Am J Cardiol* 1968, 21:23–31.

85. Okada R, Johnson D, Lev M: Extracardiac malformations associated with congenital heart disease. *Arch Pathol* 1968, 85:649–657.

86. Lev M, Liberthson RR, Eckner FAO, Arcilla RA: Pathologic anatomy of dextrocardia and its clinical implications. *Circulation* 1968, 37:979–999.

87. Lev M, Rimoldi HJA, Paiva R, Arcilla RA: The quantitative anatomy of simple complete transposition. *Am J Cardiol* 1969, 23:409–416.

88. Lev M: Certain anatomic cardiac data and their functional import. In *Clinical Cardiopulmonary Physiology*, edited by BL Gordon, RA Carleton, and LP Faber, 3rd edition, NY, NY, Grune & Stratton, 1969, pp. 3–12.

89. Lev M, Liberthson RR, Kirkpatrick JR, Eckner FAO, Arcilla RA: Single (primitive) ventricle. *Circulation* 1969, 39:577–591.

90. Okada R, Glagov S, Lev M: Relation of shunt flow and right ventricular pressure to heart valve structure in atrial septal defect. *Am Heart J* 1969, 78:781–795.

91. Liberthson RR, Arcilla RA, Eckner FAO, Lev M: Straddling and displaced atrioventricular orifices. (Abstract) *Circulation* 1969, 40:III-133 (Suppl III).

92. Fixler DE, Cole R, Paul MH, Lev M, Girod D: Familial occurrence of contracted endocardial fibroelastosis. *Am J Cardiol* 1970, 26:208–213.

93. Lev M, Liberthson RR, Joseph RH, Seten CE, Kunske RD, Eckner FAO, Miller RA: The pathologic anatomy of Ebstein's disease. *AMA Arch Pathol* 1970, 90:334–343.

94. Fisher EHR, Muster AJ, Lev M, Paul MH: Angiocardiographic and anatomic findings in transposition of the great arteries with left ventricular outflow tract gradients. (Abstract) *Am J Cardiol* 1970, 25:95–96.

95. Lev M: Relationship of the development of the ventricular septum to the position of ventricular septal defects (editorial). *Chest* 1970, 58:451.

96. Lev M, Liberthson RR, Golden JG, Eckner FAO, Arcilla RA, Miller RA: Pathologic anatomy of mesocardia. (Abstract) *Circulation* 1970, 41:(Suppl III):III-178.

97. Liberthson RR, Eckner FAO, Lev M: Pathologic anatomy of isolated levocardia. (Abstract) *Circulation* 1970, 41:(Suppl III):III-179.

98. Lev M, Joseph RH, Rimoldi HJA, Paiva R, Arcilla RA: The quantitative anatomy of isolated ventricular septal defect. *Am Heart J* 1971, 81:315–320.

99. Liberthson RR, Paul MH, Muster AJ, Arcilla RA, Eckner FAO, Lev M: Straddling and displaced atrioventricular orifices and valves with primitive ventricles. *Circulation* 1971, 43:213–226.

100. Lev M, Liberthson RR, Golden JG, Eckner FAO, Arcilla RA: The pathologic anatomy of mesocardia. *Am J Cardiol* 1971, 28:428–435.

101. Rimoldi HJHA, Paiva REA, McAuley PC, Lev M: Mass indices of the ventricles at autopsy in children. *Am Heart J* 1971, 81:770–780.

102. Lev M, Eckner FAO, Meng CCL, Liberthson RR, Bharati S: A concept of double outlet right ventricle, (Abstract) *Circulation* 1971, 44:(Suppl II):II:115.

103. Lev M: Congenital heart disease. In *Pathology*, edited by WAD Anderson, 6th edition (2 Vol), Vol I, The C.V. Mosby Co., St. Louis, Missouri, 1971, pp. 706–727.

104. Bharati S, Lev M: Congenital polyvalvular disease. (Abstract) *Am J Cardiol* 1972, 29:253–254.

105. Lev M, Bharati S, Meng CCL, Liberthson RR, Paul MH, Idriss F: A concept of double-outlet right ventricle. *J Thoracic Cardiovas Surg* 1972, 64:271–281.

106. Bharati S, Lev M: Congenital anomalies of the pulmonary veins. *Cardiovasc Clin* 1973, 5:23–41.

107. Liberthson RR, Hastreiter AR, Sinha SN, Bharati S,

Novak GM, Lev M: Levocardia with visceral heterotaxy–isolated levocardia: Pathologic anatomy and its clinical implications. *Am Heart J* 1973, 85:40–54.

108. Bharati S, Lev M, Cassels DE: Aortico-right ventricular tunnel. *Chest* 1973, 63:198–202.

109. Lev M, Bharati S: Double outlet right ventricle associated with other cardiovascular anomalies. *AMA Arch Pathol* 1973, 95:117–122.

110. Bharati S, Lev M: Congenital polyvalvular disease. *Circulation* 1973, 47:575–586.

111. Bharati S, Lev M: The spectrum of common atrioventricular orifice (canal). *Am Heart J* 1973, 86:553–561.

112. Edwards JE, Lev M, Abella MR: *The Heart*, Editors (International Academy of Pathology Monograph-course) *Pathophysiology and Anatomy of the Heart*, Washington D.C. 2/28–3/1/73). Baltimore, Maryland, The Williams & Wilkins Co., 1974.

113. Ingham R, Paiva REA, Engle MA, Hagstrom JWC, Bharati S, Lev M: Outflow tract of the left ventricle in children, a method for measuring. *AMA Arch Pathol* 1974, 97:239–241.

114. Bharati S, McAllister HA Jr., Rosenquist GC, Miller RA, Tatooles CJ, Lev M: The surgical anatomy of truncus arteriosus communis. *J Thoracic Cardiovas Surg* 1974, 67:501–510.

115. Idriss FS, Lev M, Bharati S, Nikaidoh H, Muster AJ, Paul MH: Surgical anatomy of obstructing muscle bands of the right ventricle in tetralogy of fallot. (Abstract) *Am J Cardiol* 1974, 33:450.

116. Idriss FS, Aubert J, Paul M, Nikaidoh H, Lev M, Newfeld EA: Transposition of the great vessels with ventricular septal defect: Surgical and anatomic considerations. *J Thoracic Cardiovas Surg* 1974, 68:732–741.

117. Lev M, Bharati S: Abnormal position of the heart and its chambers. In *The Heart*, edited by JE Edwards, M Lev, MR Abella, Baltimore, Maryland, The Williams and Wilkins Co, Chap 16, 1974, pp. 327–331.

118. Liberthson RR, Dinsmore RE, Bharati S, Rubenstein JJ, Caulfield J, Wheeler EO, Harthorne JW, Lev M: Aberrant coronary artery origin from the aorta: Diagnosis and clinical significance. *Circulation* 1974, 50:774–779.

119. Bharati S, Lev M: Conduction system in single ventricle with inverted (L-) transposition. (Abstract) *Circulation* 1974, 50:Suppl III to Vol 49 & 50:III-39.

120. Lev M, Bharati S: Lesions of the conduction system and their functional significance. In Pathology Annual 1974, edited by SC Sommers. Appleton-Century Crofts, NY, 9:157–208.

121. Bharati S, Rowen M, Camarata SJ, Ostermiller Jr WE, Singer M, Lev M: Diverticulum of the right ventricle. *Arch Pathol* 1975, 99:383–386.

122. Bharati S, Fisher EA, Yaniz RA, Hastreiter AR, Lev M: Infarct of the myocardium with aneurysm in a 13-year-old girl. *Chest* 1975, 67:369–373.

123. Lev M, Bharati S: Transposition of arterial trunks in levocardia. In *Cardiovascular Pathology Decennial 1966–1975*, edited by SC Sommers, Appleton-Century Crofts, NY, 1975, pp. 1–46.

124. Bharati S, Paul MH, Idriss FS, Potkin RET, Lev M: The surgical anatomy of pulmonary atresia with ventricular septal defect-pseudotruncus. *J Thoracic Cardiovas Surg* 1975, 69:713–721.

125. Cassels DE, Bharati S, Lev M: The natural history of the ductus arteriosus in association with other congenital heart defects. *Perspectives in Biol Med* 1975, 18(4):541–572.

126. Bharati S, Lev M: The course of the conduction system in single ventricle with inverted (L-) loop and inverted (L-) transposition. *Circulation* 1975, 51:723–730.

127. Falicov RE, Resnekov L, Bharati S, Lev M: A variant of hypertrophic obstructive cardiomyopathy: Midventricular obstruction. (Abstract) *Am J Cardiol* 1975, 35:136.

128. Liberthson RR, Szidon JP, Bharati S, Lev M, Fishman AP: Hemodynamic consequences of delayed ventriculoconal conduction in the frog *Rana catesbeiana*. *Am J Physiol* 1975, 229:1085–1093.

129. Lev M, Bharati S: Conduction system in simple complete regular (D) transposition with ventricular septal defect. (Abstract) *Circulation* 1975, 52:Suppl II, II-208.

130. Bharati S: Letter to Editor. *Ann Thoracic Surg* 1975, 22(5):596.

131. Ruschhaupt DG, Bharati S, Lev M: Mitral valve malformation of the Ebstein type in absence of corrected transposition. *Am J Cardiol* 1976, 38:109–112.

132. Falicov RE, Resnekov L, Bharati S, Lev M: Mid-ventricular obstruction: A variant of obstructive cardiomyopathy. *Am J Cardiol* 1976, 37:432–437.

133. Rosenquist GC, Bharati S, McAllister HA, Lev M: Truncus arteriosus communis: truncal valve anomalies associated with small conal or truncal septal defects. *Am J Cardiol* 1976, 37:410–412.

134. Bharati S, Lev M: The conduction system in double outlet right ventricle with subpulmonic ventricular septal defect. (Abstract) *Am J Cardiol* 1976, 37:121.

135. Bharati S, Lev M: The conduction system in simple regular (d-) complete transposition with ventricular septal defect. *J Thoracic Cardiovasc Surg* 1976, 72:194–201.

136. Bharati S, Lev M: The conduction system in double outlet right ventricle with subpulmonic ventricular septal defect and related hearts (the Taussig-Bing group). *Circulation* 1976, 54:174–190.

137. Bharati S, McAllister Jr HA, Tatooles CJ, Miller RA, Weinberg Jr M, Bucheleres HG, Lev M: Anatomic variations in underdeveloped right ventricle related to tricuspid atresia and stenosis. *Thoracic Cardiovasc Surg* 1976, 72:383–400.

138. Lev M, Bharati S: Replies to letters to the editor. *Am J Cardiol* 1976, 38:670.

139. Bharati S, Lev M: The conduction system in tricuspid atresia with regular D-transposition. (Abstract) *Circulation* Suppl 1976, 54(II):170.

140. Bharati S: Letter to the Editor. *Am Heart J* 1976, 92(3):410.

141. Thilenius O, Bharati S, Lev M: Subdivided left atrium: An expanded concept of cor triatriatum sisistrum. *Am J Cardiol* 1976, 37:743–752.

142. Lev M, Bharati S: Congenital heart disease. In *Pathology*, edited by WAD Anderson and John M. Kissane, 7th Edition, The CV Mosby Co., St. Louis, Missouri, Vol 1, Chapter 20, 1977, pp. 856–878.

143. Lev M, Bharati S: The course of the conduction system in surgically important types of congenital heart disease (presented at 2nd Henry Ford Hospital International Symposium on Cardiac Surgery, October 6–9, 1975), NY, edited by J.C. Davila, Appleton-Century Crofts NY, Chapter 38, 1977, pp. 233–238.

144. Lev M, Bharati S: The anatomy of the conduction system in normal and congenitally abnormal hearts. In *Cardiac Arrhythmias in the Neonate Infant and Child*,

edited by N. Roberts and H. Gelband. Appleton-Century Crofts, Chapter 2, 1977, pp. 29–54.

145. Cole RB, Lawson E, Newfeld EA, Paul MH, Bharati S, Lev M: The atrial septal defect–patent ductus arteriosus complex. *Am J Dis Child* 1977, 131:281–285.

146. Bharati S, Lev M: Letter to the Editor. *J Thoracic Cardiovasc Surg* 1977, 73:321.

147. Bharati S, McAllister HA Jr, Chiemmongkoltip P, Lev M: Congenital pulmonary atresia with tricuspid insufficiency: A morphologic study. *Am J Cardiol* 1977, 40:70–75.

148. Bharati S, Lev M: The conduction system in dextrocardia. (Abstract) *Am J Cardiol* 1977, 39:304.

149. Lev M, Ciraulo DA, Bilitch M, Rosen KM, Bharati S: Inexcitable right ventricle and bilateral bundle branch block in Uhl's disease. (Abstract) *Am J Cardiol* 1977, 39:325.

150. Bharati S, Lev M: Letter to the Editor: *J Thoracic Cardiovasc Surg* 1977, 74:328–329.

151. Bharati S, Lev M: The conduction system in tricuspid atresia with and without regular (d-) transposition. *Circulation* 1977, 56:423–429.

152. Bharati S, Lev M, McAllister Jr HA, Kirklin JW: The morphologic spectrum of double outlet left ventricle and its surgical significance. (Abstract) *Circulation* 1977, Part II, 56(4):III-43.

153. Bharati S, Lev M: Letter to the Editor. *Am Heart J* 1977, 94:669–670.

154. Bharati S, Lev M: Anatomic variations in underdeveloped right ventricle related to tricuspid atresia and stenosis. (Abstract) A reprint from *Teratology* 1977, 16:102–103.

155. Agarwala B, Agarwala R, Thomas W Jr, Bharati S: Anomalous origin of the left coronary artery from the main pulmonary artery. *Ill Med J* 1977, 151(6):437–42.

156. Bharati S: Letter to the Editor. *Circulation* 1977, 56(3):499.

157. Rosen KM, Bharati S, Dhingra R, Lev M: Letter to the Editor: *Am J Cardiol* 1978, 41:621.

158. Bharati S, Lev M: The course of the conduction system in dextrocardia. *Circulation* 1978, 57:163–171.

159. Bharati S, Ciraulo DA, Bilitch M, Rosen KM, Lev M: Inexcitable right ventricle and bilateral bundle branch block in Uhl's disease. *Circulation* 1978, 57:636–644.

160. Brenner JI, Bharati S, Winn WC, Lev M: Absent tricuspid valve with aortic atresia in mixed levocardia (atria situs solitus, L-loop): A hiterto undescribed entity. *Circulation* 1978, 57:836–840.

161. Bharati S, McCue CM, Tingelstad JB, Mantakas M, Shiel F, Lev M: Lack of connection between the atria and the peripheral conduction system in a case of corrected transposition with congenital atrioventricular block. *Am J Cardiol* 1978, 42:147–153.

162. Aziz K, Paul MH, Bharati S, Lev M, Shannon K: Echocardiographic features of total anomalous pulmonary venous drainage into the coronary sinus. *Am J Cardiol* 1978, 42:108–113.

163. Bharati S, Lev M, Stewart R, McAllister HA Jr, Kirklin JW: The morphologic spectrum of double outlet left ventricle and its surgical significance. *Circulation* 1978, 58:558–565.

164. Lev M: Letter to the Editor. *Am Heart J* 1978, 96:134.

165. Cheitlin M, Robinowitz M, McAllister HA Jr, Hoffman J, Bharati S, Lev M: The distribution of fibrosis in left ventricle in congenital aortic stenosis and coarctation of

the aorta. (Abstract) *Circulation* 1978, Part II, 58:II 243.

166. Muster AJ, Bharati S, Aziz KU, Paul MH, Idriss FA, Lev M: Taussig-Bing heart with straddling mitral valve: Diagnosis and surgical correction. (Abstract) *Circulation* 1978, Part II, 58:II-69.

167. Lev M, Bharati S: Embryology of the Heart and Pathogenesis of Congenital Malformations of the Heart. In *Pediatric Surgery*, Third Edition, Vol 1, edited by MM Ravitch, KJ Welch, CD Benson, E Aberdeen, JG Randolph, Year Book Medical Publishers, Inc., Chicago and London, Chapter 49, 1979, pp. 582–590.

168. Bharati S, Lev M: The relationship between single ventricle and small outlet chamber and straddling and displaced tricuspid orifice and valve. *J Herz* 1979, 4:176–183.

169. Bharati S, Molthan ME, Veasy LG, Lev M: Conduction system in two cases of sudden death two years after the Mustard procedure. *J Thoracic Cardiovasc Surg* 1979, 77:101–108.

170. Muster AJ, Bharati S, Paul MH, Aziz KU, Idriss FS, Lev M, Carr I, DeBoer A, Anagnostopoulos C: Taussig-Bing anomaly with straddling mitral valve. *J Thoracic Cardiovasc Surg* 1979, 77:832–842.

171. Bharati S, Lev M: Positional variations of the heart and its component chambers. Editorial. *Circulation* 1979, 59:886–887.

172. Bharati S, Lev M: The conduction system in hypoplasia of aortic tract complex. *Circulation* 1979, 59:1324–1332.

173. Carr I, Bharati S, Kusnoor VS, Lev M: Truncus arteriosus communis with intact ventricular septum. *Br Heart J* 1979, 42:97–102.

174. Lev M, Bharati S, McAllister HA Jr, Kirklin JW: The surgical anatomy of the atrioventricular valve in the intermediate type of common atrioventricular orifice. (Abstract) *Am J Cardiol* 1979, 43:364.

175. Bharati S, McAllister HA Jr, Lev M: Straddling and displaced atrioventricular orifices and valves. (Abstract) *Am J Cardiol* 1979, 43:364.

176. Bharati S, McAllister HA Jr, Lev M: Straddling and displaced atrioventricular orifices and valves. *Circulation* 1979, 60:673–684.

177. Bharati S, Lev M: The concept of tricuspid atresia complex as distinct from that of the single ventricle complex. *Pediatr Cardiol* 1979, 1:57–62.

178. Thilenius OG, Vitullo D, Bharati S, Luken J, Lamberti JJ, Tatooles C, Lev M, Carr I, Arcilla RA: Endocardial cushion defect associated with cor triatriatum sinistrum or supravalvular mitral ring. *Am J Cardiol* 1979, 44:1339–1343.

179. Bharati S, Kirklin JW, McAllister HA Jr, Lev M: The surgical anatomy of common AV orifice associated with tetralogy of Fallot, double outlet right ventricle and complete transposition. (Abstract). *Circulation* 1979, Pt II, 60:II 169.

180. Bharati S, Rosen K, Steinfeld L, Miller RA, Lev M: Anatomic substrate for preexcitation in corrected transposition. (Abstract) *Circulation* 1979, Pt II, 60:II 113.

181. Rosenquist GC, Clark EB, McAllister HA Jr, Bharati S, Edwards JE: Increased mitral-aortic separation in discrete subaortic stenosis. *Circulation* 1979, 60(1):70–74.

182. Bharati S, Lev M: Reply to letter to the Editor. *Pediatr Cardiol* 1979–80, 1:165–166.

183. Yu LC, Bharati S, Thilenius O, Lamberti J, Lev M, Ar-

cilla RA: Congenital aortico-left atrial tunnel. *Pediatr Cardiol* 1979–80, 1:153–158.

184. Thilenius OG, Bharati S, Arcilla RA, Lev M: Cardiac pathology of Marfan's syndrome: Can dissection and rupture of aortic aneurysms be prevented? *Cardiology* 1980, 65:193–204.

185. Bharati S, Lev M, McAllister HA Jr, Kirklin JW: The surgical anatomy of atrioventricular valve in the intermediate type of common atrioventricular orifice. *J Thoracic Cardiovas Surg* 1980, 79:884–889.

186. Bharati S, Kirklin JW, McAllister HA Jr, Lev M: The surgical anatomy of common atrioventricular orifice associated with tetralogy of Fallot, double outlet right ventricle and complete regular transposition. *Circulation* 1980, 61:1142–9.

187. Ruschhaupt DG, Moshiree M, Lev M, Bharati S: Echocardiogram in mitral-aortic atresia: False positive identification of the ventricular septum and left ventricle. *Pediatr Cardiol* 1980, 1:281–285.

188. Bharati S, McAllister HA Jr, Lev M: Left ventricular outflow obstruction in complete transposition. (Abstract) *Circulation* 1980, Part II, 62:III-71.

189. Bharati S, Rosen K, Steinfield L, Miller RA, Lev M: The anatomic substrate for preexcitation in corrected transposition. *Circulation* 1980, 62:831–842.

190. Bharati S, McAnulty JH, Lev M, Rahimtoola SH: Idiopathic hypertrophic subaortic stenosis with split His bundle potentials: Electrophysiologic and pathologic correlation. *Circulation* 1980, 62:1373–1380.

191. Cheitlin M, Robinowitz M, McAllister HA Jr, Hoffman J, Bharati S, Lev M: The distribution of fibrosis in left ventricle in congenital aortic stenosis and coarctation of the aorta. *Circulation* 1980, 62:823–830.

192. Bharati S, Rosen K, Bilitch M, Salibi H, Mandel W, Lev M: Anatomic substrate for preexcitation in idiopathic hypertrophy with fibroelastosis. (Abstract) *Circulation* Part II, 1980, 62:III-270.

193. Carr I, Bharati S, Lev M: Reply to letter to the Editor. *Br Heart J* 1980, 43:605–606.

194. Berry TA, Bharati S, Muster AJ, Idriss FS, Santucci BA, Lev M, Paul MH: Aorticopulmonary septal defect and aortic origin of the right pulmonary artery. (Abstract) *Circulation* 1980, Part II, 62:III-164.

195. Khoury L, Bharati S, Lev M, Replogle R, Ruschhaupt D: Two-dimensional echo identification of common AV orifice. (Abstract) *Circulation* 1980, Part II, 62:III-73.

196. Lacina S, Thilenius O, Hamilton W, Bharati S, Arcilla RA: Congenital absence of ductus arteriosus (ADA). (Abstract) *Circulation* 1980, Pt II 62(4):III-71.

197. Lev M, Bharati S: The Fibrous Skeleton of the Heart. In Update IV: *The Heart*, edited by J. Willis Hurst, published by McGraw Hill, New York, 1981, Chapter 2, pp. 7–17.

198. Sharma D, Mehta AB, Bharati S, Lev M: Tricuspid atresia with persistent truncus arteriosus. *Chest* 1981, 79:363–365.

199. Cole RB, Abman S, Aziz KU, Bharati S, Lev M, Paul MH: Prolonged PGE infusion: Histologic effects on the patent ductus arteriosus. *Pediatrics* 1981, 67:816–819.

200. Aziz KU, Paul MH, Bharati S, Cole RB, Muster AJ, Lev M, Idriss FS: Two-dimensional echocardiographic evaluation of Mustard operation for D-transposition of the great arteries. *Am J Cardiol* 1981, 47:654–664.

201. Bharati S, Granston AS, Liebson PR, Loeb HS, Rosen KM, Lev M: The conduction system in mitral valve pro-

lapse syndrome with sudden death. *Am Heart J* 1981, 101:667–670.

202. Sanyal SK, Johnson WW, Bharati S, Lev M: Morphologic basis for electrocardiographic evidence of conduction system involvement in Duchenne's muscular dystrophy (DMD). (Abstract) *Am J Cardiol* 1981, Part 2, 47:402.

203. Bharati S, Strasberg B, Bilitch M, Salibi H, Mandel W, Rosen KM, Lev M: Anatomic substrate for preexcitation in idiopathic myocardial hypertrophy with fibroelastosis of the left ventricle. *Am J Cardiol* 1981, 48:47–58.

204. Ow EP, Replogle RL, Thilenius OG, Bharati S, Lev M, Arcilla RA: Angiographic recognition of dominant right or left common AV canal. (Abstract) *Circulation* 1981, Part II, 64:IV-236.

205. Bharati S, Serratto M, DuBrow I, Paul MH, Swiryn S, Miller RA, Rosen KM, Lev M: The conduction system in Pompe's disease. *Pediatr Cardiol* 1982, 2:25–32.

206. Bharati S, Lev M: The conduction system in tricuspid atresia. In *Tricuspid Atresia*, edited by PS Rao, Futura Publishing Co., Mt. Kisco, NY, Chapter 7, pp. 69–80, 1982.

207. Lev M, Bharati S: The surgical anatomy of the sinoatrial and atrioventricular nodes and their approaches and the atrial preferential pathways. In *Second Clinical Conference on Congenital Heart Disease*, edited by BL Tucker, GG Lindesmith, M Takahashi, Grune and Stratton, Inc., New York, 1982, pp. 49–70.

208. Lev M, Bharati S: The surgical anatomy and the conduction pathways in endocardial cushion defects and their surgical implications. In *Second Clinical Conference on Congenital Heart Disease*, edited by BL Tucker, GG Lindesmith, M Takahashi, Grune and Stratton, Inc., New York, 1982, pp. 367–384.

209. Berry TE, Bharati S, Muster AJ, Idriss FS, Santucci B, Lev M, Paul MH: Distal aortopulmonary septal defect, aortic origin of the right pulmonary artery, intact ventricular septum, patent ductus arteriosus and hypoplasia of the aortic isthmus: A newly recognized syndrome. *Am J Cardiol* 1982, 49:108–116.

210. Hamilton WT, Lacina SJ, Bharati S, Lev M, Arcilla RA: Failure of clinical response to prostaglandin E in a cyanotic infant with congenital absence of the ductus arteriosus. *Cathet Cardiovasc Diagn* 1982, 8:273–276.

211. Bharati S, Lev M: Sequelae of atriotomy and ventriculotomy of the endocardium, conduction system and coronary arteries. *Am J Cardiol* 1982, 50:580–587.

212. Parr GVS, Bharati S, Lev M, Waldhausen JA: Fetal coarctation in complete transposition with ventricular septal defect vs. Taussig-Bing group of hearts: Surgical significance. (Abstract) *Circulation* 1982, Part II, 66:II-195.

213. Lappen RS, Muster AJ, Riggs TW, Bharati S, Idriss FS, Paul MH: Masked subaortic stenosis in patients with ostium primum atrial septal defect: Preoperative angiographic recognition. (Abstract) *Pediatr Cardiol* 1982, 3(4):344.

214. Bharati S, Lev M, Kirklin JW: *Cardiac Surgery and the Conduction System*. John Wiley & Sons, Inc., New York, NY, 1983, pp. 1–107.

215. Bharati S, Feld A, Bauernfeind R, Kattus A Jr, Lev M: A case of hypoplasia of the right ventricular myocardium with ventricular tachycardia. *Arch Pathol Lab Med* 1983, 107:249–253.

216. Parr GVS, Fripp RR, Whitman V, Bharati S, Lev M:

Anomalous mitral arcade: Echocardiographic and angiographic recognition. *Pediatr Cardiol* 1983, 4:163–165.

217. Parr GVS, Waldhausen JA, Bharati S, Lev M, Fripp R, Whitman V: Coarctation in Taussig-Bing malformation of the heart: Surgical significance. *J Thorac Cardiovasc Surg* 1983, 86:280–287.

218. Lappen RS, Muster AJ, Idriss FS, Riggs TW, Ilbawi M, Paul MH, Bharati S, Lev M: Masked subaortic stenosis in ostium primum atrial septal defect: Recognition and treatment. *Am J Cardiol* 1983, 52:336–340.

219. Lacina SJ, Hamilton WT, Thilenius OG, Bharati S, Lev M, Arcilla RA: Angiographic evidence of absent ductus arteriosus in severe right ventricular outflow obstruction. *Pediatr Cardiol* 1983, 4:5–11.

220. Bharati S, Lev M: Sequela of atriotomy on the endocardium, conduction system and coronary arteries, 12:229–246, The myocardium, the conduction System, and general sequelae after surgery for congenital heart disease, 13:247–260. In *Congenital Heart Disease after Surgery, Benefits, Residua, Sequelae*, edited by Engle and Perloff. Published by Yorke Medical Books, Technical Publishing, a Division of Dun-Donnelly Publishing Corp., New York, 1983.

221. Brenner JI, Bharati S, Berman MA, Lev M: A rare type of intrapulmonary drainage of one lung by the other with total anomalous pulmonary venous return. *J Am Coll Cardiol* 1983, 2:1174–1177.

222. Muster AJ, Bharati S, Herman JJ, Easterly NB, Crussi FG, Holbrook KA: Fatal cardiovascular disease and cutis laxa following acute febrile neutrophilic dermatosis. *J Pediatr* 1983, 102(2):243–248.

223. Bharati S: Reply to Letter to Editor. *Am J Cardiol* 1983, 51(7):1242.

224. Thilenius OG, Ruschhaupt DG, Replogle RL, Bharati S, Herman T, Arcilla RA: Spectrum of pulmonary sequestration: Association with anomalous pulmonary venous drainage in infants. *Pediatr Cardiol* 1983, 4:97–103.

225. Bharati S, Lev M: Pathology of Complete Atrioventricular Orifice. In *Recent Progress in Mitral Valve Disease*, Butterworths & Co. Ltd., edited by C Duran, WW Angell, AD Johnson, JH Oury. Section 9, Chapter 29, London, England, 1984, pp. 358–367.

226. Lev M, Bharati S: Pathology of Congenital Mitral Valve Disease. In *Recent Progress in Mitral Valve Disease*, Butterworths & Co., Ltd., edited by C Duran, WW Angell, AD Johnson , JH Oury. Section 9, Chapter 28, London, England, 1984, pp. 349–357.

227. Bharati S, Szarnicki RJ, Popper R, Fryer A, Lev M: Origin of both coronaries from the pulmonary trunk, associated with hypoplasia of the aortic tract complex: A new entity. *J Am Coll Cardiol* 1984, 3:437–441.

228. Bharati S, Lev M: The surgical anatomy of hypoplasia of aortic tract complex. *J Thoracic Cardiovasc Surg* 1984, 88:97–101.

229. Bharati S, Lev M: Direct entry of the right superior vena cava into the left atrium with aneurysmal dilatation and stenosis at its entry into the right atrium with stenosis of the pulmonary veins: A rare case. *Pediatr Cardiol* 1984, 5:123–126.

230. Bharati S, Chandra N, Stephenson L, Wagner HR, Weinberg PM, Lev M: Origin of left coronary artery from the right pulmonary artery. *J Am Coll Cardiol* 1984, 3:1565–1569.

231. Bharati S, Nordenberg A, Ponct RR, Lev M: Hypoplas-

tic left heart syndrome with dysplastic pulmonary valve with stenosis. *Pediatr Cardiol* 1984, 5:127–130.

232. Lev M, Bharati S: Congenital Heart Disease. In *Anderson's Pathology*, edited by John M. Kissane, 8th edition, CV Mosby Co., St. Louis, Missouri, Vol I, Chapter 17, pp. 663–683, 1985.

233. Lev M, Bharati S: Embryology of the heart and great vessels, In *Pediatric Cardiac Surgery*, edited by E. Arciniegas, Year Book Medical Publishers, Inc., Chicago, Illinois, Chapter 1:1–12, 1985.

234. Davis JT, Ehrlich R, Blakemore WS, Lev M, Bharati S: Truncus arteriosus with interrupted aortic arch: Report of successful total surgical correction. *Ann Thorac Surg* 1985, 39:82–85.

235. Muster AJ, Idriss FS, Bharati S, Riggs TW, Lev M, Culpepper WS III: Functional aortic valvular atresia in transpostion of the great arteries. *J Am Coll Cardiol* 1985, 6:630–634.

236. Weinreich DJ, Burke JF, Bharati S, Lev M: Isolated prolapse of the tricuspid valve: Report of three cases and a review of the literature. *J Am Coll Cardiol* 1985, 6:475–481.

237. Campbell DJ, Bharati S, Thilenius OG, Lev M, Arcilla RA: The aortic valve in congenital subaortic stenosis. (Abstract) *Circulation* 1985, Part II 72:III-256.

238. Bharati S: Reply to Letter to Editor. *J Thorac Cardiovasc Surg* 1985, 89:149–150.

239. Bharati S, Lev M: The surgical anatomy of the heart in tubular hypoplasia of the transverse aorta (preductal coarctation). *J Thoracic Cardiovasc Surg* 1986, 91:79–85.

240. Bharati S, Lev M: Conduction system in cases of sudden death in congenital heart disease many years after surgical correction. (Abstract) *J Am Coll Cardiol* 1986, 7:48A.

241. Davis JT, Ehrlich R, Hennessey JR, Levine M, Morgan RJ, Bharati S, Lev M: Long term follow-up of cardiac rhythm in repaired total anomalous pulmonary drainage. *J Thoracic Cardiovasc Surg* 1986, 34:172–175.

242. Bharati S, Lev M: Conduction system in cases of sudden death in congenital heart disease many years after surgical correction. *Chest* 1986, 90:861–868.

243. Eldredge WJ, Bharati S, Flicker S, Clark DL, Lev M: Cine CT Scanning in the diagnosis of congenital heart disease: Analysis of the first 42 cases. In *Pediatric Cardiology, Proceedings of the Second World Congress*. Edited by EF Doyle, MA Engle, WM Gersony, WJ Rashkind, NS Talner. Springer-Verlag, New York, Berlin, Heidelberg, Tokyo, 1986, pp. 404–405.

244. Bharati S, Lev M: Sudden death long after repair of atrial septal defect: A study of four cases. (Abstract) *Circulation* 1986, Part II, 74:II-121.

245. El-Habbal MH, Bharati S, Rubin IS, Arcilla RA: Cardiac positional abnormalities after transient hyperthermia. (Abstract) *Circulation* 1986, Part 2, Vol 74(4) p. II-294.

246. Rubin I, El-Habbal N, Bharati S, Arcilla R: Effect of transient hyperthermia upon cardiac development. *Pediat Res* 1986, 20:175A.

247. Thilenius OG, Bharati S, Lev M, Karp RB, Arcilla RA: Horizontal ventricular septum with dextroversion: Hearts with and without aortic atresia. *Pediatr Cardiol* 1987, 8:187–193.

248. Issenberg HJ, Mathew R, Kim ES, Bharati S: Congenital absence of the noncoronary aortic cusp. *Am Heart J* 1987, 113(2):1;400–402.

249. Sen D, Muster AJ, Duffy CE, Bharati S, Ilbawi MN, Deleon SY, Idriss FS: Perimembranous ventricular septal defect and aortic valve prolapse: An unexpectedly frequent association. (Abstract) *Pediatr Cardiol* 1987, 8:75.

250. Bharati S, Lev M: Cardiac tumors. In Moss' *Heart Disease in Infants, Children and Adolescents*, Fourth edition, edited by Forrest H. Adams, George C. Emmanouilides and Thomas A. Reimanschneider, Williams and Wilkins, Baltimore, MD, Chapter 43:886–890, 1989.

251. Lev M, Bharati S: Pathologic basis of Dysrhythmias in Children. In Moss' *Heart Disease In Infants, Children and Adolescents*, Fourth edition, edited by George C. Emmanouilides and Thomas A. Remeinschneider, Williams and Wilkins, Baltimore, MD, Chapter 54:1008–1016, 1989.

252. Thilenius OG, Campbell D, Bharati S, Lev M, Arcilla RA: Small aortic valve annulus in children with fixed subvalvar aortic stenosis. *Pediatr Cardiol* 1989, 10:195–198.

253. Lev M, Bharati S: Congenital heart disease. In Andersons Pathology, edited by John M. Kissane, 9th edition, C.V. Mosby Co, St. Louis, MO, Vol. I, Chap 16, pp. 730–751, 1990.

254. Bharati S, Engle MA, Fatica NS, Bussell JB, Sulayman RF, Lev M, Lynfield J: The heart and conduction system in acute Kawasaki disease: Report of fraternal cases: One lethal, one relapsing. *Am Heart J* 1990, 120:359–365.

255. de Oliveira e Silva, Snyder MS, O'Loughlin JE, Klein AA, Magid MS, Engle MA, Lev M, Bharati S: Unique variant of Taussig-Bing heart – double outlet right ventricle with double ventricular septal defects and double overriding of great arteries. *Pediatr Cardiol* 1991, 12:123–125.

256. Bharati S, Patel AG, Varga P, Husain AN, Lev M: In utero echocardiographic diagnosis of a unique case of premature closure of foramen ovale with mitral insufficiency and large left atrium. *Am Heart J* 1991, 122:597–600.

257. DeLeon SY, Ilbawi MN, Wilson WR Jr, Arcilla RA, Thilenius OG, Bharati S, Lev M, Idriss FS: Surgical options in subaortic stenosis associated with endocardial cushion defects. *Ann Thoracic Surg* 1991, 52:1076–1083.

258. Kovalchin JP, Allen HD, Cassidy C, Bharati S: Pulmonary valve eccentricity in d-transposition: Implica-

tion for arterial switch operation. (Abstract) *Circulation* 1991, Suppl II, Vol 84: No. 4, II-512.

259. Bharati S, Lev M, Kirklin JW: *Cardiac Surgery and the Conduction System*. Second Revised Edition. Futura Publishing Co., Inc., Mount Kisco, New York, pp. 1–176, 1992.

260. Bharati S, Karp R, Lev M: The conduction system in truncus arteriosus and its surgical significance: A study of five cases. *J Thoracic Cardiovasc Surg* 1992, 104:954–960.

261. Bharati S, Lev M: The conduction system in tricuspid atresia. In *Tricuspid Atresia*, Second Edition, edited by PS Rao. Futura Publishing Co., Mt. Kisco, New York, Chapter 7, pp. 101–113, 1992.

262. Gould NS, Bharati S, Fronda G, Jones C: Anomalous origin of left coronary artery from the pulmonary artery leading to demise in a neonate. *Human Pathol* 1991, 22:1044–1045.

263. Bharati S, Lev M: Embryology of the heart and great vessels. In *Pediatric Cardiac Surgery*, Second Edition, edited by C Mavroudis, and CL Backer. Mosby Year Book Inc., St. Louis, MO, Chapter 1, pp. 1–13, 1994.

264. Kovalchin JP, Allen HD, Cassidy SC, Lev M, Bharati S: Pulmonary valve eccentricity in d-transposition of the great arteries and implications for arterial switch operation. *Am J Cardiol* 1994, 73:186–190.

265. Husain AN, Kowal-Vern A, Bharati S: Congenital polyvalvular disease without chromosomal abnormalities. (Abstract) *Pediatr Pathol* 1994, 14(No. 3):541.

266. Young S, Bharati S: Hypertrophic cardiomyopathy as a cause of fetal demise in three stillborn macrosomic infants of diabetic mothers. (Abstract) *Pediatr Pathol* 1994, 14, No. 3:542.

267. Kowal-Vern A, Bharati S, Melnyk A, Husain AN: Congenital polyvalvular cardiac disease without chromosomal abnormalities. *Pediatr Pathol Lab Med* 1995, 15:299–308.

268. DeLeon SY, Ow EP, Chiemmongkoltip P, Vitullo DA, Quinones JA, Fisher EA, Bharati S, Ilbawi M, Pifarre R: Alternatives in biventricular repair of double outlet left ventricle. *Annals Thoracic Surg* 1995, 60:213–216.

269. Remmell-Dow DR, Bharati S, Davis JT, Lev M, Allen HD: Hypoplasia of the eustachian valve and abnormal orientation of the limbus of the foramen ovale in hypoplastic left heart syndrome. *Am Heart J* 1995, 130:148–152.

Index

Fibroelastic ridge subaortic stenosis,
780–788
Fibroelastosis
due to blocked lymph drainage, 1494
idiopathic hypertrophy with, 801–807
of left ventricle, 794–796
surgical, 1447–1448
Fistula
in aneurysm of coronary artery,
1309–1317
coronary arterio-cardiac, 60
between noncoronary aortic cusp and
right atrium and ventricle, 1304
Floppy mitral valve, 1388
conduction disturbances and, 1514–1521
polyvalvular disease and, 1244–1245
Fontan procedure, 418, 1487
Foramen ovale, 32, 48
premature closure of, 55, 1345–1360
classification of, 60
valves in, 1346–1351
Fossa ovalis, 700–701, 702
Fossa ovalis defect, 451–466
associated cardiac anomalies, 463–464
endocardium and, 457
septal morphology in, 458–461
valves and, 456–457
Friedreich's ataxia, 1396

Gargoylism, 1181–1187, 1538
Glycogen storage disease, 1177–1179, 1538
Great vessels
in complete transposition
with common atrioventricular orifice,
335–339
with common ventricle, 295
with double outlet left ventricle, 352
with Ebstein's anomaly, 351
with mitral atresia or stenosis,
331–334
with pulmonary stenosis, 269–274
with tricuspid atresia, 321–323
with ventricular septal defect, 247,
249–251
without ventricular septal defect,
229–231
in double outlet right ventricle, 135,
187–190
in inverted transposition with left
atrioventricular valve atresia,
1163–1176
in mesocardia, 1047
in mixed levocardia with relatively
normally placed chambers with criss-
cross connection of AV valves, 852
in pseudotruncus, 381–384
in single ventricle, 1059

Hancock prosthetic conduits with porcine
valves and homograft valves, 1487
Heart
anatomy of, 29–36
dissection of, 15–20
double, 1335–1337, 1538
embryogenesis of, 45–50
incidental anomalies of, 1423–1439
aberrant origin of right subclavian
artery, 1432, 1433
abnormal origin of right pulmonary
artery, 1438–1439
aneurysm of membranous septum,
1431–1432
aneurysm of membranous septum

associated with ventricular septal
defect, 1430–1431
aneurysm of pars membranacea, 1430
aneurysm of sinus of Valsalva of
pulmonic valve, 1438
bicuspid aortic valve, 1426, 1427–1428
chordae and bands in left ventricle,
1434
coronary artery, 1423–1427
diverticulum of left ventricle,
1432–1434
double mitral orifice, 1434–1435
double tricuspid orifice, 1437
left superior vena cava entering
coronary sinus, 1428–1429
mitral valve, 1435–1436
muscle band in left atrium, 1437–1438
quadricuspid aortic valve, 1428
quadricuspid pulmonic valve,
1429–1430
right atrial, 1437
valvular, 1437
methods of examination, 7–14
anterior descending coronary artery,
10–12
arterial trunk orifices at base, 12–13
atrial appendages, 13
composition of apex, 10–12
direction of longitudinal axis, 8–10
dissection in, 15–20
external, 7, 8
internal, 21–28
normal or acquired diseases of,
1533–1534
origin of valves, vessels, and arches,
51–55
positional variations of, 909–911
postoperative; *see* Postoperative
congenital heart
undiagnosed, 1441–1443
univentricular, 1161
Hemitruncus, 1323–1332, 1538
Hemorrhage in operative site, 1487–1490
Hepatic vein, 15
High origin of coronary ostium, 1424, 1425
Hypertrophic cardiomyopathy
atypical forms or variants, 1521–1524
polyvalvular disease and, 1245
Hypertrophy, 5
classification of, 60
diagrammatic sketches of, 27
idiopathic with fibroelastosis, 801–807
Hypoplasia of aortic tract complex,
687–695
atrial septal morphology in, 691–693
classification of, 58
single ventricle and, 1111
truncus arteriosus communis and, 359,
365–367
Hypoplasia of transverse arch with
coarctation
anterior descending coronary artery and
composition of apex in, 11
aorticopulmonary septal defect with,
1329–1330
embryogenesis of, 54
mixed levocardia, 868–872
preductal or fetal, 699
transitional, 719–721
Hypoplastic left ventricle syndrome, 58

Idiopathic hypertrophy
classification of, 60
with fibroelastosis, 801–807, 1538

Incidental anomalies of heart, 1423–1439
aberrant origin of right subclavian
artery, 1432, 1433
abnormal origin of right pulmonary
artery, 1438–1439
aneurysm of membranous septum,
1431–1432
aneurysm of membranous septum
associated with ventricular septal
defect, 1430–1431
aneurysm of pars membranacea, 1430
aneurysm of sinus of Valsalva of
pulmonic valve, 1438
bicuspid aortic valve, 1426, 1427–1428
chordae and bands in left ventricle, 1434
coronary artery, 1423–1427
diverticulum of left ventricle, 1432–1434
double mitral orifice, 1434–1435
double tricuspid orifice, 1437
left superior vena cava entering coronary
sinus, 1428–1429
mitral valve, 1435–1436
muscle band in left atrium, 1437–1438
quadricuspid aortic valve, 1428
quadricuspid pulmonic valve, 1429–1430
right atrial, 1437
valvular, 1437
Incision
to open heart, 16–17
for quantitative analysis, 24
Infective endocarditis
aneurysm of right aortic sinus of
Valsalva and, 1303–1304
in tetralogy of Fallot, 108–111
Inferior vena cava
dissection of heart and, 15
embryology of, 51
right atrium and, 29
Infundibular pulmonary stenosis
aneurysm of right aortic sinus of
Valsalva and, 1302, 1303, 1304–1306
embryogenesis of, 54
in tetralogy of Fallot, 73, 74, 96–100
tricuspid atresia with, 407–411
Infundibular septum, 380
Internal examination, 21–28
measurement of left ventricle outflow
tract, 26–27
qualitative analysis, 21, 22
quantitative analysis, 21–26
in tetralogy of Fallot, 67–72
in tricuspid atresia, 403–406
Interrupted aortic arch, 1361–1370, 1538
Interventional procedures, 1490, 1491
Intracristal ventricular septal defect,
529–530
Inversion of atria, 909
Inverted transposition
with left atrioventricular valve atresia,
1163–1176
isolated ventricular inversion and
normally related great arteries,
1172–1176
position of great arteries in, 1163–1171
mesocardia and, 1017
single ventricle and, 1052
with inverted loop in levocardia,
1054–1056
with presumed inverted loop,
1075–1098
Ischemic hypertrophy, 5
Isolated levocardia, 983–1016
definition of terminology, 983–984
identification of chambers, 984

associated cardiac abnormalities, 646–647
atrial and ventricular septal defects with, 673–680
atrial septal defect and, 667–672
atrioventricular valve anomalies with stenosis or insufficiency, 1388–1395
classification of, 59
embryogenesis of, 54
morphology of ductus, 642–646
origin of pulmonary artery from ascending aorta and, 1323
postoperative, 1470
premature closure of foramen ovale and, 1356
pseudotruncus and, 395–396, 401
tetralogy of Fallot with, 81
tricuspid atresia and, 411
tricuspid stenosis with pulmonary atresia and, 436
valves and, 635–641
ventricular septal defect and, 681–685
Paternal conditions, 62
Pectus excavatum, 62
Peripheral type of straddling and displaced valve
mitral, 1129–1130
tricuspid, 1123–1127
Persistence of fetal circulation, 668–671
Persistent left superior vena cava, 55
Persistent ostium primum, 467–478
associated cardiac abnormalities, 476–477
complex of, 467–471
valves and, 471–476
Polyvalvular disease, 1211–1246
brachiocephalic vessel anomalies in, 1242
classification of, 62
coronary artery anomalies in, 1242
with insufficiency of valves, 1241
with intracardiac obstruction with or without extracardiac obstruction, 1232–1233
with major cardiac abnormalities, 1238–1240
mitral valve, 1228–1230
with obstruction and shunts, 1233–1237
semilunar valve, 1225–1227
with shunts with or without extracardiac obstructions, 1230–1231
size of valves, 1217
tricuspid valve, 1219–1225
ventricular abnormalities in, 1242–1244
without shunts or obstructions, 1237–1238
Posterior descending coronary artery, tricuspid atresia *versus* single ventricle and, 1155–1156
Posterobasal ventricular septal defect, 259
Postoperative congenital heart, 1445–1498
arrhythmias and, 1451–1456
arterial switch operation, 1478–1479
atrial septal defect, 1471
blocked lymphatic drainage, 1448
coarctation of aorta, 1470–1471
common atrioventricular orifice, 1476–1478
conduction system and, 1448–1451, 1494–1496
coronary arteries and, 1448
double outlet right ventricle, 1478
endocardium and, 1445–1447
fibroelastosis due to blocked lymph drainage, 1494
Fontan procedure, 1487

Hancock prosthetic conduits with porcine valves and homograft valves, 1487
hemorrhage in operative site, 1487–1490
interventional procedures, 1490, 1491
Mustard procedure, 1479–1486
myocardium and, 1449–1450
Norwood procedure, 1487, 1488
patent ductus arteriosus, 1470
sinoatrial nodal damage, 1497
sudden death and, 1456–1469
surgical fibroelastosis, 1447–1448
tetralogy of Fallot, 1472
ventricular patch, 1494
ventricular septal defect, 1471, 1472–1476
Preductal coarctation of aorta, 697–710
preductal, 699–701
tubular hypoplasia of transverse arch with, 699
with ventricular septal defect, 702–707
Premature closure of foramen ovale, 55, 1345–1360
classification of, 60
valves in, 1346–1351
Pressure atrophy, 27
Pressure hypertrophy, 5, 27
Presumptive dextroversion, 926–927
Presumptive mesoversion with atrial situs solitus and normal ventricles, 1026–1027
Presumptive mirror-image dextrocardia, 957–964
Primary pulmonary hypertension, 1339–1343
Primum atrial septal defect, 467–478
associated cardiac abnormalities, 476–477
complex of, 467–471
secundum defect with, 491–494
valves and, 471–476
Proampulla, 45–47
Prolapse of aortic valve, 530–533
Proximal atrial septal defect, 479–486
Pseudotruncus, 381–402
amount of pulmonary flow in, 400
associated cardiac abnormalities, 398
bronchial circulation and, 392, 393–395, 400–401
complete transposition with, 390–392
coronary artery distribution in, 396–397
embryogenesis of, 402
endocardium and, 387
origin of aorta, 401
patent ductus arteriosus and, 395–396, 401
position of vessels in, 381–384
pulmonary trunk and arteries and, 392, 393
right ventricle morphology in, 387–388
spleen and, 399
valves and, 384–387
Pulmonary artery
abnormal origin of right, 1438–1439
morphology of, 1319–1321
origin from ascending aorta, 1323–1332
tetralogy of Fallot and, 100–103, 133
Pulmonary atresia
classification of, 60
with complete transposition
tricuspid atresia and, 325–327
tricuspid stenosis and, 303–306
Ebstein's anomaly with, 819
tetralogy of Fallot with, 82
tricuspid atresia with, 411–416
with tricuspid insufficiency, 1267–1279
atrial septal morphology in, 1277, 1278

embryogenesis of, 1278
endocardium and, 1277
microscopic examination in, 1271–1275
right ventricle and, 1275–1276
treatment of, 1279
valves in, 1267–1271
tricuspid stenosis with, 421–445
atrial septum morphology in, 431–434
coronary artery anomalies, 436–438
patent ductus arteriosus anomalies, 436
severe stenosis with intact ventricular septum, 421–428
valves and, 428–431
ventricular septum morphology in, 435–436
with ventricular septal defect, 381–402
amount of pulmonary flow in, 400
associated cardiac abnormalities, 398
bronchial circulation and, 392, 393–395, 400–401
complete transposition with, 390–392
coronary artery distribution in, 396–397
embryogenesis of, 402
endocardium and, 387
origin of aorta, 401
patent ductus arteriosus and, 395–396, 401
position of vessels in, 381–384
pulmonary trunk and arteries and, 392, 393
right ventricle morphology in, 387–388
spleen and, 399
valves and, 384–387
Pulmonary hypertension, 1339–1343
classification of, 61
ventricular septal defect and, 522–523
Pulmonary stenosis
classification of, 60
with complete transposition, 269–294
associated cardiac anomalies, 275–277
great vessels position, 269–274
incomplete double outlet left ventricle, 285–294
tricuspid atresia and, 323–325
tricuspid stenosis and, 303–306
valves in, 274–275
with ventricular septal defect, 280–285
without ventricular septal defect, 277–279
with double outlet right ventricle
with mitral atresia or stenosis, 151, 179–180
with subaortic ventricular septal defect, 144
Ebstein's anomaly with, 819
embryogenesis of, 54
isolated pure, 747–756
endocardium and, 754
right ventricle and, 754–756
valves and, 747–753
mixed levocardia with ventricular septal defect and left AV valve stenosis, 860–861, 864
in tetralogy of Fallot, 73, 74
with tricuspid atresia, 407–411
ventricular septal defect with, 757–759
Pulmonary trunk
abnormal course or narrowing of, 1319–1322
complete transposition and, 228
double outlet right ventricle and, 199–203
origin from truncus, 354–356, 361–363, 374–376